AF249008

CPT·PLUS!

MILLENNIUM EDITION

A Comprehensive Guide To Current Procedural Terminology

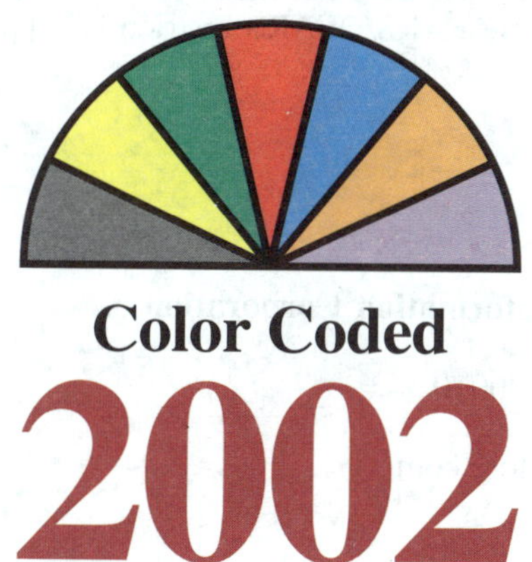

Color Coded

2002

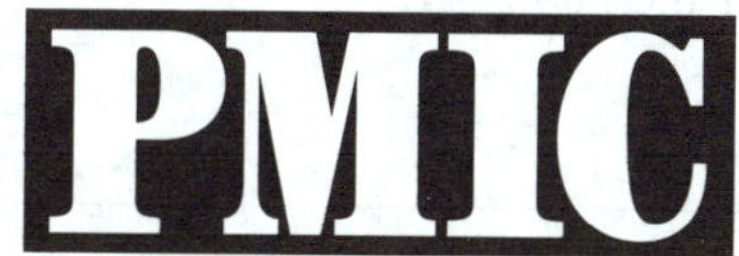

ISBN 1-57066-229-0

Practice Management Information Corporation
4727 Wilshire Boulevard
Los Angeles, California 90010
1-800-MED-SHOP
http://www.medicalbookstore.com/

Printed in China

INTRODUCTION

CPT® PLUS! 2002 is an enhanced CPT® coding resource which includes all official CPT 2002 codes and complete descriptions plus comprehensive CPT coding instructions, full-color anatomical illustrations, a unique color-coding system to help identify CPT codes subject to special coding rules, and a new and improved alphabetic index.

The CPT coding system includes over 7,900 codes and descriptions for reporting medical services, procedures, supplies and materials. Accurate CPT coding provides an efficient method of communicating medical services and procedures among health care providers, health care facilities, and third party payers and enhances the health care provider's control of the reimbursement process.

The CPT coding system is revised annually by the American Medical Association (AMA) and is usually published in late October or November. Each year hundreds of additions, changes and deletions are made the CPT coding system. These changes become effective on January 1st. CPT is required by federal law for all health insurance claim forms filed with Medicare, Medicaid, CHAMPUS and Federal Employee Health Plans and is accepted or required by all other third party payers.

CPT® PLUS! 2002 provides valuable instructions, coding tips, and other information to help providers maximize reimbursement while minimizing audit liability. Our objective is to make CPT coding faster, easier and more accurate for medical office, healthcare facility and third party payer coding and billing staff, while setting a new standard for CPT coding references.

James B. Davis, Publisher

CONTENTS

CPT CODING FUNDAMENTALS

CPT® is an acronym for Current Procedural Terminology. *Physicians' Current Procedural Terminology*, Fourth Edition, known as CPT-4 or more commonly CPT, is a systematic listing of codes and descriptions which classify medical services and procedures. CPT codes are used by physicians, hospitals, and other health care professionals, to report specific medical, surgical and diagnostic services and procedures for statistical and third party payment purposes.

The CPT coding system is maintained by the American Medical Association (AMA) and a revised edition of the CPT book is published each fall. The new CPT codes become effective on January 1st of the following year. The revisions in each new edition are prepared by the CPT Editorial Panel with the assistance of physicians representing all specialties of medicine.

A thorough understanding of the CPT coding system is essential in order to provide accurate reporting of medical services and procedures, maximize payments from third parties, minimize denials, rejections and reductions from third parties, and to protect the medical practice from audit liability.

KEY POINTS REGARDING THE CPT CODING SYSTEM

- CPT codes describe medical procedures, services and supplies.

- All CPT codes are five digit codes.

- CPT codes are mandated by federal law for Medicare, Medicaid, CHAMPUS and Federal Employee Health Plan (FEHP) reporting and are accepted or required by all other third party payers.

- CPT codes are self-definitive, eg. with the exception of CPT codes for unlisted procedures and/or the few CPT codes which include the term *specify* in the description, each CPT *code number* represents the universal definition of the service or procedure.

- CPT codes are revised and updated annually by the AMA and the revisions become effective each January 1st. Hundreds of CPT codes are added, changed or deleted each year. All health care professionals, third party payers, and health care facilities must maintain copies of the current code books.

- Accurate CPT coding provides an efficient method of communicating medical, surgical and diagnostic services and procedures among health care professionals, health care facilities, and third party payers.

- Accurate CPT coding enhances the health care provider's control of the reimbursement process.

STRUCTURE OF THE CPT CODING SYSTEM

The CPT coding system includes over 7,900 codes and definitions for medical services, procedures and diagnostic tests. Each procedure or service is identified by a five digit code, followed by the definition.

The CPT coding system is divided into seven **SECTIONS**. The seven sections of are:

Evaluation and Management	99200-99499
Anesthesiology	00100-01999
Surgery	10000-69999
Radiology	70000-79999
Pathology and Laboratory	80000-89999
Medicine	90000-99199
Category III Emerging Technology	0001T-0026T

Each section of the CPT book includes subsections with anatomic, procedural, condition, or descriptor subheadings. The Evaluation and Management (E/M) section is presented first because 1) these codes are used by virtually all health care providers and 2) are the most frequently used CPT codes.

HOW TO USE THE CPT CODING SYSTEM

A provider or coder using the CPT coding system for coding first chooses the name and associated code of the procedure or service which most accurately identifies and describes the service(s) performed. The provider or coder then chooses names and codes for additional services or procedures. If necessary, modifiers are chosen and added to the selected service and procedure codes. All services or procedures coded must also be documented in the patient's medical record.

According to *CPT 2002*, "The listing of a service or procedure and its CPT code number in a specific section of the CPT coding system does not restrict its use to a specific specialty group. Any procedure or service in any section of the CPT coding system may be used to report the services rendered by any qualified physician or other health care professional."

The codes and descriptions listed in the CPT coding system are those that are generally consistent with contemporary medical practice and being performed by health care professionals in clinical practice. Inclusion in the CPT coding system does not represent endorsement by the American Medical Association of any particular diagnostic or therapeutic procedure. In addition, inclusion or exclusion of a procedure does not imply any health insurance coverage or reimbursement policy.

CPT FORMAT AND CONVENTIONS

The descriptions associated with CPT codes have been developed by the AMA to provide complete descriptions of medical services and procedures.

Many CPT descriptions include the definition of basic procedures followed by supplemental descriptions for variations or modifications of the basic procedure. In the CPT coding book, the basic procedure description ends with a semicolon (;), followed by the additional description.

If a CPT description includes the same basic procedure as the preceding listing, the basic procedure is not listed. Only the supplemental description is listed, preceded by an indentation. For example:

25100 Arthrotomy, wrist joint; with biopsy

25105   with synovectomy

SYMBOLS

- • A filled BLACK CIRCLE preceding a CPT code indicates that the code is new to this revision of the CPT coding system. A symbol key appears on all left-hand pages.

- ▲ A filled BLACK TRIANGLE preceding a CPT code indicates that there is a revision to the description. Wherever possible, the revised text is identified with underlining.

- ( ) CPT codes enclosed within parenthesis have been deleted from the CPT coding system and should no longer be used.

- + A bold plus sign preceding a CPT code indicates that the code is an "add-on" code and must be listed in addition to the main CPT code.

- Ⓢ This symbol preceding a CPT code indicates that the code is exempt from the use of modifier -51.

- * A star symbol preceding a CPT code indicates that the service identifies the surgical procedure only and that pre- or post-operative services are not included in the basic procedure.

Note that a CPT code may be preceded by the add-on, star symbol or modifier-51 exempt symbol, in addition to new or changed code symbols.

COLOR CODING

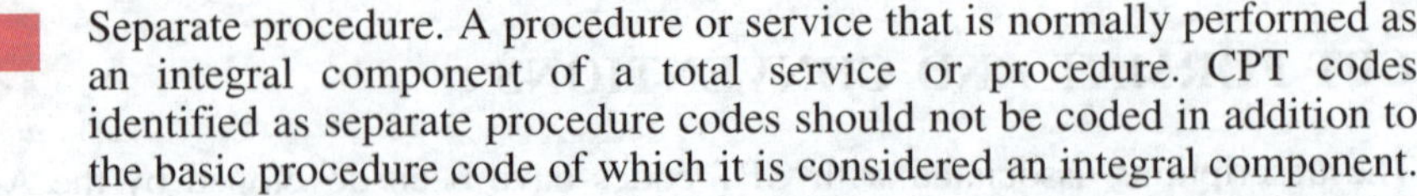

Separate procedure. A procedure or service that is normally performed as an integral component of a total service or procedure. CPT codes identified as separate procedure codes should not be coded in addition to the basic procedure code of which it is considered an integral component.

However, if the procedure or service that is usually designated as a separate procedure is performed independently or is considered to be unrelated or distinct from other procedures or services provided at that time, the separate procedure may be coded by itself. The modifier -59 should be added to the separate procedure code to indicate that the procedure is not considered to be a component of another procedure, but is a distinct, independent procedure.

Unlisted code. Descriptions include the term "unlisted." Use only when a CPT code which specifically describes the service or procedure is unavailable. A report is usually required by third party payers.

Nonspecific code. Descriptions include the term "specify" instructing the coder to include additional information such as the quadrant, the nerve, the muscle, the level of spine, the number of joints, the type of study, the method of dosimetry, the hormone, the receptor, the assay method, the type of kit, the material injected, the type of tests, the number of tests, the doses provided.

CCI comprehensive code. Indicates codes identified as comprehensive codes in the Comprehensive Coding Initiative, Version 7.3 released October 1, 2001. Per CMS (HCFA) rules, all identifiable component procedures are included in the comprehensive code and should not be billed separately to Medicare.

SECTION OVERVIEW

Specific guidelines are presented at the beginning of each of the six sections of the CPT coding system. The guidelines define items that are necessary to interpret and report the procedures and services contained in that section. CPT guidelines also provide explanations regarding terms that apply only to a particular section.

CPT CODING & BILLING ISSUES

Most billing, coding and reporting issues involving the CPT® coding system apply generally to all medical specialties and professions. However, there are some specialty specific issues defined in each section of the CPT coding system that apply only to the specific medical specialty represented.

SUPPORTING DOCUMENTATION

Documentation in the patient's medical report must clearly support the procedures, services and supplies coded on the health insurance claim form. Most medical chart reviewers take the position that if something is not documented in the medical record, then the service or procedure was not performed and therefore is not subject to reimbursement.

If a medical practice is selected for an audit by Medicare or other third party payer, the accuracy and completeness of the documentation of the medical records, or lack thereof, will have a significant impact on the outcome of the audit. The current emphasis on "fraud" and "abuse" by Medicare, Medicaid and private third party payer necessitates a review of documentation by all health care professionals.

SPECIAL MEDICARE CONSIDERATIONS

To satisfy Medicare requirements, there must be sufficient documentation in the medical record to verify the services coded and the level of care required. Section 1833(e) of Title XVIII, Social Security Act requires "available information that documents a claim." If there is no documentation to justify the services or level of care, the claim cannot be considered for Medicare benefits.

If there is insufficient documentation to support claims that have already been paid by Medicare, the reimbursement will be considered an overpayment and a refund will be requested by Medicare. Medicare has the authority to review any information, including medical records, when such information pertains to a Medicare claim.

UNLISTED PROCEDURES OR SERVICES

There are services or procedures performed by health care professionals that are not found in the CPT coding system. These services or procedures may be either new procedures which have not yet been assigned a CPT code or simply a variation of a procedure which precludes using the existing CPT code. Each section of the CPT coding system includes codes for reporting these unlisted procedures.

Unlisted procedure codes should not be coded unless the coder has reviewed the CPT coding system carefully to ensure that a more specific code is not available. If a specific CPT code is not located, check for HCPCS codes that may be reportable.

As a rule, a report needs to be enclosed with the health insurance claim form when reporting unlisted procedure codes. Because unlisted procedure codes are subject to manual medical review, payment is usually slower than for normal processing time.

CPT ADDITIONS, CHANGES, AND DELETIONS

Each year hundreds of codes are added, changed or deleted from the CPT coding system. A summary of these changes is found in Appendix B of the CPT code book which provides a quick reference for coding review. In addition to the appendix, these modifications are identified throughout the CPT code book.

ADDITIONS TO THE CPT CODING SYSTEM

New codes are added to the CPT coding system each year. New CPT codes are identified with a small black circle placed to the left of the code number. Examples of new codes found in CPT 2002 include:

- **44313**   Esophagoplasty for congenital defect, (plastic repair or reconstruction), thoracic approach; without repair of congenital tracheoesophageal fistula

- **64821**   Sympathectomy; radial artery

CHANGES TO CPT CODE DEFINITIONS

Each year the definitions of many CPT codes are revised. CPT codes with changed definitions are identified with a small black triangle placed to the left of the code number. Examples of CPT codes with changed definitions in CPT 2002 include:

- **27132**   Conversion of previous hip surgery to total hip arthroplasty; with or without autograft or allograft

- **48500**   Marsupialization of pancreatic cyst

The only way to determine exactly what part of the definition has been changed is to compare the current changed definition with the definition from the previous edition of the CPT code book.

DELETIONS FROM THE CPT CODING SYSTEM

Each year some CPT codes are deleted. Deleted CPT codes, and references to replacement codes, are enclosed within parenthesis. Examples of CPT codes deleted from CPT 2002 include:

(26585 has been deleted. To report, use 26587)

(93536 has been deleted. To report, use 33967)

NEW SECTIONS AND SUB-SECTIONS

New sections and subsections are frequently added to the CPT coding system to reflect changes in technology or medical practice and to provide additional code sequences for special purposes. Examples of new sub-sections added to CPT 2002 include:

Home Health Procedures/Services	99500-99539
Home Infusion Procedures	99551-99569

In addition, the following new Section was added to CPT 2002:

Category III Emerging Technology Codes	0001T-0026T

CATEGORY II PERFORMANCE MEASUREMENT CODES

Category II, Performance Measurement CPT codes, are designed to facilitate outcomes research. According to the AMA, this new section will not be introduced until the 2003 or 2004 CPT updates. When implemented, Category II codes will include the letter "F" as the fifth digit of the five digit CPT code.

CATEGORY III EMERGING TECHNOLOGY CODES

Emerging Technology Codes are temporary codes for emerging technology, services and procedures. These codes are designed to permit data collection and assessment of new technologies. All Category III codes include the letter "T" as the fifth digit of the five digit CPT code.

CPT 2002 ADDITIONS, CHANGES, AND DELETIONS

Following is a summary listing all additions, deletions, and revisions applicable to CPT 2002 codes. The descriptors of the codes listed as "grammatical change" have not been substantially changed, but involve placement of the semicolon, or other punctuation, or a similar minor change.

MODIFIERS

-22	Modifier revised
-60	Modifier deleted

EVALUATION AND MANAGEMENT SECTION

99289	Patient transport code **added**
99290	Patient transport code **added**
99374	Terminology *revised*
99377	Terminology *revised*
99379	Terminology *revised*
99381	Terminology *revised*
99391	Terminology *revised*

ANESTHESIA

00220	Terminology *revised*
00560	Terminology *revised*
00797	Anesthesia for surgery for morbid obesity code **added**
00850	Code deleted. To report, use 01961
00851	Anesthesia for tubal ligation code **added**
00855	Code deleted. To report, use 01963
00857	Code deleted. To report, see 01968, 01969
00869	Anesthesia for vasectomy code **added**
00884	Code deleted. To report, use 01930
00942	Terminology *revised*
00946	Code deleted. To report, use 01960
00955	Code deleted. To report, use 01967
01214	Terminology *revised*
01402	Terminology *revised*
01904	Code deleted. To report, use 01905
01905	Anesthesia for spinal injection/repair code **added**
01906	Code deleted. To report, use 01905
01908	Code deleted. To report, use 01905
01910	Code deleted. To report, use 01905
01912	Code deleted. To report, use 01905
01914	Code deleted. To report, use 01905
01916	Terminology *revised*
01918	Code deleted. To report, use 01916

01920	Terminology *revised*
01921	Code <u>deleted</u>. To report, see 01924-01926
01924	Anesthesia for therapeutic interventional radiology arterial procedure code **added**
01925	Anesthesia for therapeutic interventional radiology arterial procedure code **added**
01926	Anesthesia for therapeutic interventional radiology arterial procedure code **added**
01930	Anesthesia for therapeutic interventional radiology venous procedure code **added**
01931	Anesthesia for therapeutic interventional radiology venous procedure code **added**
01932	Anesthesia for therapeutic interventional radiology venous procedure code **added**
01933	Anesthesia for therapeutic interventional radiology venous procedure code **added**
01951	Terminology *revised*
01952	Terminology *revised*
01960	Anesthesia for vaginal delivery code **added**
01961	Anesthesia for cesarean delivery code **added**
01962	Anesthesia for urgent hysterectomy following delivery code **added**
01963	Anesthesia for cesarean hysterectomy code **added**
01964	Anesthesia for abortion procedures code **added**
01967	Neuroaxial labor analgesia/anesthesia code **added**
01968	Neuroaxial labor analgesia/anesthesia add-on procedure code **added**
01969	Neuroaxial labor analgesia/anesthesia add-on procedure code **added**
01995	Terminology *revised*

SURGERY-INTEGUMENTARY

10021	Fine needle aspiration code **added**
10022	Fine needle aspiration code **added**
11755	Terminology *revised*
11981	Insertion of drug delivery implant device code **added**
11982	Removal of drug delivery implant device code **added**
11983	Removal and reinsertion of drug delivery implant device code **added**
15732	Terminology *revised*
15860	Terminology *revised*
17000	Terminology *revised*
17004	Terminology *revised*
17110	Terminology *revised*
17260	Terminology *revised*
17270	Terminology *revised*

17280	Terminology *revised*

SURGERY-MUSCULOSKELETAL

20225	Terminology *revised*
20526	Carpal tunnel therapeutic injection code **added**
20550	Terminology *revised*
20551	Injection, tendon origin/insertion code **added**
20552	Trigger point injection code **added**
20553	Trigger point injection code **added**
21182	Terminology *revised*
21183	Terminology *revised*
21184	Terminology *revised*
21750	Terminology *revised*
23000	Terminology *revised*
23350	Terminology *revised*
24075	Terminology *revised*
24076	Grammatical change
24300	Manipulation, elbow, under anesthesia code **added**
24332	Tenolysis of triceps code **added**
24343	Repair of elbow ligament code **added**
24344	Repair of elbow ligament code **added**
24345	Repair of elbow ligament code **added**
24346	Reconstruct elbow ligament code **added**
25001	Incision of flexor tendon sheath, wrist code **added**
25020	Terminology *revised*
25024	Decompression fasciotomy of forearm/wrist code **added**
25025	Decompression fasciotomy of forearm/wrist code **added**
25075	Terminology *revised*
25076	Grammatical change
25259	Manipulation of wrist under anesthesia code **added**
25274	Terminology *revised*
25275	Repair of tendon sheath, forearm/wrist code **added**
25394	Osteoplasty of carpal bone code **added**
25405	Terminology *revised*
25420	Terminology *revised*
25430	Vascular pedicle graft for carpal bone code **added**
25431	Repair of nonunion carpal bone code **added**
25440	Terminology *revised*
25443	Terminology *revised*
25520	Terminology *revised*
25526	Terminology *revised*
25645	Terminology *revised*
25651	Percutaneous skeletal fixation of ulnar styloid fracture code **added**

25652 Open treatment of ulnar styloid fracture code **added**

25671 Percutaneous skeletal fixation of distal radioulnar dislocation code **added**

26115 Terminology *revised*

26116 Terminology *revised*

26160 Terminology *revised*

26340 Manipulation of finger joint under anesthesia code **added**

26350 Terminology *revised*

26356 Terminology *revised*

26390 Terminology *revised*

26392 Terminology *revised*

26415 Terminology *revised*

26416 Terminology *revised*

26426 Terminology *revised*

26428 Terminology *revised*

26445 Terminology *revised*

26510 Terminology *revised*

26585 Code <u>deleted</u>. To report, use 26587

26587 Terminology *revised*

26590 Terminology *revised*

26597 Code <u>deleted</u>. To report, see 11041-11042, 14040-14041, or 15120, 15240)

26607 Terminology *revised*

26670 Terminology *revised*

26676 Terminology *revised*

26685 Terminology *revised*

26843 Terminology *revised*

27110 Terminology *revised*

27130 Terminology *revised*

27132 Terminology *revised*

27140 Terminology *revised*

27185 Terminology *revised*

27447 Terminology *revised*

27475 Grammatical change

28104 Terminology *revised*

28238 Terminology *revised*

28299 Terminology *revised*

28737 Terminology *revised*

29049 Terminology *revised*

29086 Application of finger cast code **added**

29805 Shoulder arthroscopy code **added**

29806 Shoulder arthroscopy code **added**

29807 Shoulder arthroscopy code **added**

29815 Code <u>deleted</u>. To report, use 29805

29819 Grammatical change

29824 Shoulder arthroscopy code **added**

29900 Metacarpophalangeal joint arthroscopy code **added**

29901	Metacarpophalangeal joint arthroscopy code **added**
29902	Metacarpophalangeal joint arthroscopy code **added**
29909	Code <u>deleted</u>. To report, use 29999
29999	Unlisted arthroscopy procedure code **added**

SURGERY-RESPIRATORY

30117	Terminology *revised*
30801	Terminology *revised*
30905	Terminology *revised*
31238	Terminology *revised*
31528	Terminology *revised*
31529	Terminology *revised*
31641	Terminology *revised*
32420	Terminology *revised*
32650	Terminology *revised*

SURGERY-CARDIOVASCULAR

33250	Terminology *revised*
33406	Terminology *revised*
33413	Terminology *revised*
33610	Terminology *revised*
33967	Percutaneous insertion of intra-aortic balloon code **added**
33975	Terminology *revised*
33976	Terminology *revised*
33977	Terminology *revised*
33978	Terminology *revised*
33979	Insertion of intracorporal ventricular assist device code **added**
33980	Removal of intracorporal ventricular assist device code **added**
35001	Terminology *revised*
35005	Terminology *revised*
35021	Terminology *revised*
35045	Terminology *revised*
35081	Terminology *revised*
35091	Terminology *revised*
35102	Terminology *revised*
35111	Terminology *revised*
35121	Terminology *revised*
35131	Terminology *revised*
35141	Terminology *revised*
35151	Terminology *revised*
35161	Terminology *revised*
35646	Terminology *revised*
35647	Aortofemoral bypass graft code **added**
35685	Bypass graft patency/vein patch code **added**
35686	Bypass graft patency/AV fistula code **added**
36002	Pseudoaneurysm injection code **added**
36005	Terminology *revised*
36400	Terminology *revised*
36819	Terminology *revised*

36820	Anastomosis, forearm vein transposition code **added**
36823	Terminology *revised*

SURGERY-HEMIC/LYMPHATIC

38220	Bone marrow aspiration code **added**
38221	Bone marrow biopsy code **added**

SURGERY-DIGESTIVE

42970	Terminology *revised*
43108	Terminology *revised*
43113	Terminology *revised*
43118	Terminology *revised*
43123	Terminology *revised*
43227	Terminology *revised*
43245	Terminology *revised*
43260	Grammatical change
43264	Terminology *revised*
43265	Terminology *revised*
43313	Esophagoplasty for congenital defect code **added**
43314	Esophagoplasty for congenital defect code **added**
43361	Terminology *revised*
43847	Terminology *revised*
43860	Terminology *revised*
44020	Terminology *revised*
44110	Terminology *revised*
44126	Enterectomy of small intestine for congenital atresia code **added**
44127	Enterectomy of small intestine for congenital atresia code **added**
44128	Enterectomy of small intestine for congenital atresia code **added**
44160	Terminology *revised*
44202	Terminology *revised*
44203	Laparoscopic resection of small intestine code **added**
44204	Laparoscopic partial colectomy code **added**
44205	Laparoscopic partial colectomy code **added**
44322	Terminology *revised*
44366	Terminology *revised*
44378	Terminology *revised*
44391	Terminology *revised*
44661	Terminology *revised*
44700	Terminology *revised*
45136	Excision of ileoanal reservoir code **added**
45190	Terminology *revised*
45303	Terminology *revised*
45317	Terminology *revised*
45334	Terminology *revised*
45382	Terminology *revised*
46020	Placement of anal seton code **added**

46604	Terminology *revised*	
46614	Terminology *revised*	
46924	Terminology *revised*	
46940	Terminology *revised*	
47370	Laparoscopic radiofrequency ablation of liver tumor code **added**	
47371	Laparoscopic cryosurgical ablation of liver tumor code **added**	
47380	Open radiofrequency ablation of liver tumor code **added**	
47381	Open cryosurgical ablation of liver tumor code **added**	
47382	Percutaneous radiofrequency ablation of liver tumor code **added**	
47554	Terminology *revised*	
48100	Terminology *revised*	
48160	Terminology *revised*	
48500	Terminology *revised*	
48545	Terminology *revised*	
48547	Terminology *revised*	
49220	Terminology *revised*	
49424	Terminology *revised*	
49491	Inguinal hernia repair on preterm infant code **added**	
49492	Inguinal hernia repair on preterm infant code **added**	
49495	Terminology *revised*	

SURGERY-URINARY

50220	Terminology *revised*
50810	Terminology *revised*
50815	Terminology *revised*
50820	Terminology *revised*
50825	Terminology *revised*
50840	Terminology *revised*
51065	Terminology *revised*
51590	Terminology *revised*
51596	Terminology *revised*
51940	Terminology *revised*
51960	Terminology *revised*
52001	Cystourethroscopy with removal of clots code **added**
52347	Cystourethroscopy with transurethral resection of ejaculatory ducts code **added**
52510	Terminology *revised*
53431	Urethroplasty code **added**
53443	Code <u>deleted</u>. To report, use 53431
53444	Insertion of tandem cuff code **added**
53445	Terminology *revised*
53446	Removal of urethral/bladder neck sphincter code **added**
53447	Terminology *revised*
53448	Removal/replacement of urethral/bladder neck sphincter code **added**

53449 Terminology *revised*

53853 Prostatic water-induced thermotherapy code **added**

SURGERY-MALE GENITAL

54065 Terminology *revised*

54162 Lysis of penile circumcision adhesions code **added**

54163 Repair of incomplete circumcision code **added**

54164 Frenulotomy of the penis code **added**

54402 Code deleted. To report, see 54415, 54416

54405 Terminology *revised*

54406 Removal of penile prosthesis code **added**

54407 Code deleted. To report, see 54406, 54408, 54410

54408 Repair of penile prosthesis code **added**

54409 Code deleted. To report, use 54408

54410 Removal/replacement of penile prosthesis code **added**

54411 Removal/replacement of penile prosthesis code **added**

54415 Removal of penile prosthesis code **added**

54416 Removal/replacement of penile prosthesis code **added**

54417 Removal/replacement of penile prosthesis code **added**

54510 Code deleted. To report, use 54512

SURGERY-FEMALE GENITAL

56501 Terminology *revised*

56515 Terminology *revised*

57022 Terminology *revised*

57061 Terminology *revised*

57065 Terminology *revised*

57155 Insertion of uterine tandems/vaginal ovoids for clinical brachytherapy code **added**

57510 Terminology *revised*

58140 Terminology *revised*

58275 Terminology *revised*

58346 Insertion of Heyman capsules for clinical brachytherapy code **added**

58563 Terminology *revised*

58611 Terminology *revised*

58953 Hysterectomy/removal of tubes/ovaries w/radical dissection code **added**

58954 Hysterectomy/removal of tubes/ovaries w/radical dissection/lymphadenectomy code **added**

59000 Terminology *revised*

59001 Therapeutic amniotic fluid reduction code **added**

SURGERY-NERVOUS SYSTEM

60000	Terminology *revised*
60270	Terminology *revised*
61026	Terminology *revised*
61055	Terminology *revised*
61618	Terminology *revised*
62100	Terminology *revised*
62230	Terminology *revised*
62252	Terminology *revised*
62256	Terminology *revised*
62272	Terminology *revised*
63707	Terminology *revised*
63709	Terminology *revised*
64555	Terminology *revised*
64561	Percutaneous implantation of neurostimulator electrodes code **added**
64575	Terminology *revised*
64581	Incision for neurostimulator electrode implant code **added**
64755	Terminology *revised*
64820	Terminology *revised*
64821	Sympathectomy code **added**
64822	Sympathectomy code **added**
64823	Sympathectomy code **added**

SURGERY-EYE/ADNEXA

65235	Terminology *revised*
65900	Terminology *revised*
65920	Terminology *revised*
65930	Terminology *revised*
66020	Terminology *revised*
66982	Terminology *revised*
67225	Ocular photodynamic therapy code **added**
67515	Terminology *revised*
69310	Terminology *revised*
69990	Terminology *revised*

RADIOLOGY SECTION

74230	Terminology *revised*
74245	Terminology *revised*
74249	Terminology *revised*
74250	Terminology *revised*
74305	Terminology *revised*
74327	Terminology *revised*
74363	Terminology *revised*
75898	Terminology *revised*
75989	Terminology *revised*
76066	Terminology *revised*
76070	Terminology *revised*
76078	Terminology *revised*
76085	Computerized screening mammography code **added**
76120	Terminology *revised*

76125	Terminology *revised*
76355	Terminology *revised*
76360	Terminology *revised*
76362	CAT guidance for tissue ablation code **added**
76370	Terminology *revised*
76375	Terminology *revised*
76380	Terminology *revised*
76394	MRI guidance for tissue ablation code **added**
76490	US guidance for tissue ablation code **added**
76536	Terminology *revised*
76604	Terminology *revised*
76645	Terminology *revised*
76700	Terminology *revised*
76770	Terminology *revised*
76778	Terminology *revised*
76800	Terminology *revised*
76805	Terminology *revised*
76819	Terminology *revised*
76830	Terminology *revised*
76856	Terminology *revised*
76870	Terminology *revised*
76880	Terminology *revised*
76885	Terminology *revised*
76886	Terminology *revised*
76936	Grammatical change
77300	Terminology *revised*
77301	Intensity modulated radiotherapy plan code **added**
77418	Intensity modulated treatment delivery code **added**
78195	Terminology *revised*
78290	Terminology *revised*
78615	Terminology *revised*
78650	Terminology *revised*

PATHOLOGY & LABORATORY

80072	Code <u>deleted</u>. To report, see 84550, 85651, 86255, 86430
82270	Terminology *revised*
82273	Terminology *revised*
82274	Fecal hemoglobin immunoassay test code **added**
82355	Terminology *revised*
83013	Terminology *revised*
83873	Terminology *revised*
83916	Terminology *revised*
83950	Oncoprotein, HER-2/neu code **added**
84445	Terminology *revised*
85095	Code <u>deleted</u>. To report, use 38220
85097	Terminology *revised*
85102	Code <u>deleted</u>. To report, use 38221

85535	Code <u>deleted</u>. To report, use 85536
86140	Grammatical change
86141	High sensitivity C-reactive protein code **added**
86325	Terminology *revised*
86336	Inhibin A code **added**
87045	Terminology *revised*
87198	Cytomegalovirus antibody (DFA) code **added**
87199	Enterovirus antibody (DFA) code **added**
87802	Strep B detection immunoassay detection with optic code **added**
87803	Clostridium difficile toxin A immunoassay detection with optic code **added**
87804	Influenza immunoassay detection with optic code **added**
87902	Hepatitis C genotype analysis code **added**
87903	Terminology *revised*
87904	Terminology *revised*
88170	Code <u>deleted</u>. To report, use 10021
88171	Code <u>deleted</u>. To report, use 10022
88304	Terminology *revised*
88305	Terminology *revised*
88380	Microdissection code **added**
89050	Terminology *revised*

MEDICINE

90471	Terminology *revised*
90473	Immunization administration code **added**
90474	Immunization administration code **added**
90732	Terminology *revised*
90780	Terminology *revised*
90939	Hemodialysis access flow study code **added**
90940	Grammatical change
91123	Pulsed irrigation of fecal impaction code **added**
92136	Ophthalmic biometry code **added**
92532	Terminology *revised*
92534	Terminology *revised*
92973	Percutaneous coronary thrombectomy code **added**
92974	Placement of radiation delivery device for coronary brachytherapy code **added**
93025	Microvolt T-wave assessment code **added**
93536	Code <u>deleted</u>. To report, use 33967
93607	Code <u>deleted</u>. To report, use 93622
93609	Terminology *revised*
93613	3-D intracardiac mapping code **added**
93619	Terminology *revised*

Code	Description
93620	Terminology *revised*
93621	Terminology *revised*
93622	Terminology *revised*
93701	Thoracic bioimpedance code **added**
93737	Code <u>deleted</u>. To report, use 93741 or 93743
93738	Code <u>deleted</u>. To report, use 93742 or 93744
94720	Terminology *revised*
94750	Terminology *revised*
95144	Terminology *revised*
95145	Terminology *revised*
95165	Terminology *revised*
95180	Terminology *revised*
95250	Glucose continuous monitoring code **added**
95875	Terminology *revised*
95904	Terminology *revised*
95965	Magnetoencephalography code **added**
95966	Magnetoencephalography code **added**
95967	Magnetoencephalography code **added**
96000	Motion analysis code **added**
96001	Motion analysis code **added**
96002	Motion analysis code **added**
96003	Motion analysis code **added**
96004	Motion analysis code **added**
96150	Health/behavior assessment code **added**
96151	Health/behavior reassessment code **added**
96152	Health/behavior intervention code **added**
96153	Health/behavior intervention code **added**
96154	Health/behavior intervention code **added**
96155	Health/behavior intervention code **added**
96450	Terminology *revised*
96567	Photodynamic therapy of skin code **added**
97005	Athletic training evaluation code **added**
97006	Athletic training re-evaluation code **added**
97112	Terminology *revised*
97504	Terminology *revised*
97535	Terminology *revised*
97601	Terminology *revised*
99090	Terminology *revised*
99091	Collection and interpretation of patient transmitted data code **added**
99500	Home visit for prenatal assessment code **added**

99501 Home visit for postnatal assessment code **added**

99502 Home visit for newborn care assessment code **added**

99503 Home visit for respiratory therapy care code **added**

99504 Home visit for patients receiving mechanical ventilation code **added**

99505 Home visit for stoma care code **added**

99506 Home visit for intramuscular injections code **added**

99507 Home visit for catheter maintenance code **added**

99508 Home visit for sleep studies code **added**

99509 Home visit for assistance with activities of daily living code **added**

99510 Home visit for individual, family or marriage counseling code **added**

99511 Home visit for fecal impaction code **added**

99512 Home visit for hemodialysis code **added**

99539 Home visit, NOS code **added**

99551 Home infusion for pain management code **added**

99552 Home infusion for pain management code **added**

99553 Home infusion for tocolytic therapy code **added**

99554 Home infusion for hematopoietic hormones code **added**

99555 Home infusion for chemotherapy code **added**

99556 Home infusion for antibiotics, antifungal, antiviral code **added**

99557 Home infusion for continuous anticoagulant therapy code **added**

99558 Home infusion of immunotherapy code **added**

99559 Home infusion of peritoneal dialysis code **added**

99560 Home infusion of enteral nutrition code **added**

99561 Home infusion of hydration therapy code **added**

99562 Home infusion of total parenteral nutrition code **added**

99563 Home infusion of aerosolized pentamidine code **added**

99564 Home infusion for anti-hemophilic agents code **added**

99565 Home infusion of alpha-1 proteinase inhibitor code **added**

99566 Home infusion for long-term intravenous treatment code **added**

99567 Home infusion of sympathomimetic agents code **added**

99568	Home infusion of miscellaneous drugs code **added**
99569	Home infusion, each additional therapy code **added**

CATEGORY III EMERGING TECHNOLOGY CODES

0001T	Endovascular repair of abdominal aortic aneurysm code **added**
0002T	Endovascular repair of abdominal aortic aneurysm code **added**
0003T	Cervicography code **added**
0004T	Code deleted. To report, use 88380
0005T	Percutaneous extracranial cerebrovascular artery stent code **added**
0006T	Percutaneous extracranial cerebrovascular artery stent code **added**
0007T	Percutaneous extracranial cerebrovascular artery stent code **added**
0008T	Upper GI endoscopy with suture of esophagogastric junction code **added**
0009T	Endometrial cryoablation code **added**
0010T	Tuberculosis test, cell mediated immunity code **added**
0012T	Osteochondral knee autograft code **added**
0013T	Osteochondral knee allograft code **added**
0014T	Meniscal transplant of knee code **added**
0016T	Thermotherapy of choroidal eye lesion code **added**
0017T	Photocoagulation of macular drusen code **added**
0018T	Transcranial magnetic stimulation code **added**
0019T	Extracorporeal shock wave therapy code **added**
0020T	Extracorporeal shock wave therapy code **added**
0021T	Fetal oximetry code **added**
0023T	Phenotype drug test for HIV 1 code **added**
0024T	Transcatheter cardiac reduction code **added**
0025T	Ultrasonic pachymetry code **added**
0026T	Remnant lipoproteins code **added**

STARRED PROCEDURES

There are some CPT codes which define minor surgical procedures; for example incision and drainage of an abscess, injection of a tendon sheath, or dilation of the urethra, etc., which do not have well-defined pre-operative and/or post-operative components. These procedures are exempt from the surgical package concept. These procedures are identified in the CPT code book by a star (*) following the procedure code number. These procedures are identified in *CPT® PLUS! 2002* by a star (*) preceding the procedure code number.

Examples of CPT codes identified as starred procedures in CPT 2002 include:

* **20000**   Incision of soft tissue abscess (eg, secondary to osteomyelitis); superficial

* **57150**   Irrigation of vagina and/or application of medicament for treatment of bacterial, parasitic or fungoid disease

INSTRUCTIONAL NOTES

Notes found in the CPT coding system give instructions for using codes. When selecting a code, look for instructions in the section guidelines for any additional information necessary to code accurately. Also, instructional notes take the form of parenthetical statements and paragraphs, which may appear at the beginning of subsections, headings and subheadings, or above and below the code itself.

DEFINITION OF NEW AND ESTABLISHED PATIENT

Solely for the purposes of distinguishing between new and established patients, professional services are those face-to-face services rendered by a physician and coded by a specific cpt code(s). A **new patient** is one who has not received any professional services from the physician or another physician of the same specialty who belongs to the same group practice, within the past three years.

An **established patient** is one who has received professional services from the physician or another physician of the same specialty who belongs to the same group practice, within the past three years.

In the instance where a physician is on call for or covering for another physician, the patient's encounter will be classified as it would have been by the physician who is not available.

No distinction is made between new and established patients in the emergency department. Evaluation and Management services in the emergency department category may be coded for any new or established patient who presents for treatment in the emergency department.

PLACE (LOCATION) OF SERVICE

The CPT coding system makes specific distinctions for place (location) of service for CPT codes defined in the evaluation and management section. The place of service may have considerable impact on reimbursement. The following list defines CPT code ranges for specific places of service:

Office [And Other Outpatient] Services	99201-99215
Home Services	99341-99353
Hospital [Inpatient] Services	99221-99238
Consultations	99241-99245
	99251-99255
	99261-99263
SNF, ICF, Long-Term Care Services	99301-99315
Nursing Home, Custodial Care Services	99321-99333
Emergency Room Services [Assigned Physician]	99281-99288

HOSPITAL CARE

Reporting hospital visits frequently causes reimbursement problems for health care professionals. The three most common coding errors are:

- More than one physician submits an initial hospital care code for the same patient.

- Follow-up hospital visits are coded incorrectly.

- Concurrent care visits by multiple specialists are coded improperly.

If more than one physician is involved in the process of hospitalizing a patient, for example, surgeon and internist, the physicians must decide which is going to actually admit the patient and report the admission services on the health insurance claim form. If both do, the first health insurance claim form to arrive will be processed and paid, and the second will be rejected.

There are valid reasons for visiting a patient more than once daily while hospitalized, however, many physicians and even some insurance billers do not know that subsequent hospital visit codes are for "daily" services. When a physician visits the patient twice in one day, providing a brief level of service each time, the physician or insurance biller may incorrectly report two hospital visit services for the same day, instead of a higher level code incorporating both visits.

Reporting multiple hospital visits provided on the same day separately on the health insurance claim form usually results in either the entire claim being returned for clarification, or the second visit being denied as an apparent duplication.

Unfortunately, insurance billers who are unclear on the proper coding of same day hospital visits may simply accept the rejection without question and write-off the unpaid visit as uncollectible.

The CPT coding system clearly defines subsequent hospital care as "per day", meaning daily services. If the physician visits the patient twice in one day, providing the equivalent of "brief" services each time, report the service using the appropriate evaluation and management code that defines the cumulative level of service provided.

HOSPITAL DISCHARGE

The CPT code for hospital discharge services is evaluation and management code 99238, defined as Hospital discharge day management. Hospital discharge services include final examination of the patient, discussion of the hospital stay, instructions for continuing care, and preparation of discharge records. Many health insurance companies do not recognize and/or do not reimburse this CPT code.

Options for the use of code 99238 include the use of one of the other hospital daily services codes from the evaluation and management series 99231-99233 and perhaps using a code that has a higher value than the routine hospital Visit.

REFERRAL

A referral is the transfer of the total care or specific portion of care of a patient from one physician to another. A referral is not a request for consultation. If a patient is referred to the physician for total care or a portion of their care, use evaluation and management visit codes, and other CPT codes if appropriate, to report the services provided. If a patient is sent to the physician for a consultation, use evaluation and management consultation codes to report the services provided.

SEPARATE OR MULTIPLE PROCEDURES

It is appropriate to designate multiple procedures that are rendered on the same date by separate entries. For example: if a proctosigmoidoscopy was performed in addition to a hospital visit, the proctosigmoidoscopy would be considered a SEPARATE procedure and listed in addition to the hospital visit on the health insurance claim form. Another example would be individual medical psychotherapy rendered in addition to a brief subsequent hospital service. In this instance, both services would be coded.

SUPPLIES AND MATERIALS SUPPLIED BY THE PHYSICIAN

The CPT coding system includes specific codes for identifying certain supplies and materials provided by the physician. HCPCS includes over 3,000 specific codes for identifying supplies, materials and equipment on Medicare claims. CPT or HCPCS supply codes are used to report supplies and materials that are not included in the definition of the basic service.

These codes, along with notes regarding use, may be found in the MEDICINE and RADIOLOGY sections of the CPT book.

CPT CODES FOR SUPPLIES AND MATERIALS

92390-92396	Supply of spectacles, contact lenses, low vision aids and ocular prosthesis.
95144-95170	Provision of antigens for allergen immunotherapy.
96545	Provision of chemotherapy agent.
99070	Supplies and materials (except spectacles) provided by the physician.
99071	Educational supplies, such as books, tapes, and pamphlets, provided by the physician for the patient's education at cost to physician.
78990 & 79900	Diagnostic and therapeutic radiopharmaceuticals.

PURCHASED DIAGNOSTIC SERVICES

It is common for physicians to bill patients and health insurance companies for diagnostic services that were procured or ordered on behalf of the patient but not actually provided by the ordering physician. It is also common for the ordering physician to "mark-up" the fee for the purchased service prior to billing. This is referred to as global billing.

Medical equipment companies, particularly those offering electrocardiography, pulmonary diagnostic equipment, and other diagnostic equipment, have used this global billing concept in the past as a method of selling physicians a new "profit center" for their practice. Some even provided technicians, who were not employees of the practice, to perform the diagnostic tests in the physicians office. OBRA 1987 placed severe restrictions on global billing of certain diagnostic tests as of March 1, 1988.

The Medicare regulations apply to diagnostic tests other than clinical laboratory tests including, but not limited to: EKGs, EEGs, cardiac monitoring, X-rays and ultrasound. Global billing is allowed only when the billing physician personally performs or supervises the diagnostic procedure. To qualify under the supervision definition, the person performing the test must be an employee or the physician or group. Ownership interest in an outside supplier does not meet the supervision requirement.

Billing for purchased services under the new requirement is complicated. The provider must provide the supplier's name, address, provider number and net charge on the health insurance claim form. In addition, a HCPCS Level III modifier must be coded to indicate that the service was purchased. Billing for global services usually will also require a HCPCS Level III modifier to indicate that the service was not purchased. This requirement does not apply to the professional component of these services if provided separately. Continue to bill for this service using modifier -26.

Providers should discontinue billing for the technical component of diagnostic services that were not provided or supervised by the provider as defined in this regulation for the following reasons:

1)   The provider is no longer making any profit on these procedures;

2)   Operating costs are higher due to the increased reporting requirements; and

3)   Risk of audit liability is increased if these services are not coded properly.

UNBUNDLING

Unbundling is defined as reporting multiple CPT codes when one CPT code is sufficient. For example, it is considered unbundling if incidental surgical procedures are coded separately, or office visits for uncomplicated follow-up care are separately coded. This practice often happens unintentionally. However, most third-party payers currently have software in place to catch unbundling when it occurs. When physicians continually break out or itemize services in this manner, they often find themselves under close scrutiny and even the focus of an audit by the insurance company. It is most important to know the guidelines to prevent unbundling when coding and billing for services and/or procedures.

CPT & HCPCS MODIFIERS

The CPT® coding system includes two-digit modifier codes which are used to report that a service or procedure has been "altered or modified by some specific circumstance" without altering or modifying the basic definition or CPT code.

The proper use of CPT modifiers can speed up claim processing and increase reimbursement, while the improper use of CPT modifiers may result in claim delays or claim denials. In addition, using certain CPT modifiers, for example -22, too frequently may trigger a claims audit.

CPT MODIFIERS

-21 Prolonged evaluation and management services

When the face-to-face or floor/unit service(s) provided is prolonged or otherwise greater than that usually required for the highest level of evaluation and management service within a given category, it may be identified by adding modifier -21 to the evaluation and management code number. A report may also be appropriate.

-22 Unusual procedural services

When the service(s) provided is/are greater than that usually required <u>for the listed procedure, it</u> may be identified by adding modifier -22 to the procedure number.

This modifier is not to be used to report procedure(s) complicated by adhesion formation, scarring, and/or alteration of normal landmarks due to late effects of prior surgery, irradiation, infection, very low weight (ie, neonates and infants less than 10kg) or trauma.

Modifier -22 is frequently abused and misused. Some physicians routinely add modifier -22 to CPT procedure codes with the expectation that higher reimbursement will be forthcoming. Many third party payers routinely ignore an undocumented modifier -22 on health insurance claim forms for the same reason.

In most cases, it is more appropriate to choose a CPT code of a higher value than to use modifier -22. If the provider reports modifier -22, documentation in the form of a cover letter or report must be provided with the health insurance claim form to explain the situation or circumstances that make the procedure(s) unusual.

-23   Unusual anesthesia

Modifier -23 is used to report a procedure was performed under general anesthesia that is normally performed without anesthesia.

-24   Unrelated evaluation and management service by the same physician during a postoperative period

The physician may need to indicate that an evaluation and management service was performed during a postoperative period for a reason(s) unrelated to the original procedure. This circumstance may be reported by adding the modifier -24 to the appropriate level of evaluation and management service.

-25   Significant, separately identifiable evaluation and service by the same physician on the same day of a procedure

The physician may need to indicate that on the day a procedure or service identified by a CPT code was performed, the patient's condition required a significant, separately identifiable evaluation and management service above and beyond the usual preoperative and postoperative care associated with the procedure that was performed. This circumstance may be reported by adding the modifier -25 to the appropriate level of evaluation and management service.

This modifier is not used to report an evaluation and management service resulting in a decision to perform surgery (see modifier -57).

-26   Professional component

Used to report the physician component of a procedure that consists of a technical and a professional component. These are typically diagnostic procedures.

-27   Multiple outpatient hospital evaluation and management encounters on the same date

For hospital outpatient reporting purposes, use of hospital resources related to separate and distinct evaluation and management encounters performed in multiple outpatient hospital settings on the same date may be reported by adding modifier -27 to each appropriate outpatient and/or emergency department evaluation and management code(s).

This modifier provides a method of reporting circumstances involving evaluation and management services provided by physician(s) in more than one (multiple) outpatient hospital setting(s) (eg, hospital emergency department, clinic).

This modifier is not to be used for physician reporting of multiple evaluation and management services performed by the same physician on the same date.

-32 Mandated services

Occasionally a consultation and/or related service may be mandated by a third party (eg, peer review organization, third party payer, governmental, legislative or regulatory requirement). Mandated services are identified by adding the modifier -32 to the basic procedure code.

HCPCS modifier -SF is reported instead of CPT modifier -32 if the patient is a Medicare patient.

-47 Anesthesia by surgeon

Regional or general anesthesia may be provided by the surgeon performing the procedure. Report by adding modifier -47 to the basic procedure code.

Modifier -47 is not used for reporting local anesthesia and is also not used with codes from the ANESTHESIA section of CPT.

-50 Bilateral procedure

This modifier is reported when bilateral procedures requiring a separate incision are performed during the SAME operative session.

Proper reporting of this modifier on the HCFA1500 health insurance claim form requires the CPT procedure code to be listed two times: first with no modifier, and the second time with modifier -50.

This modifier may not be used if the definition of the basic procedure code includes the term "bilateral."

-51 Multiple procedures

When multiple procedures, other than evaluation and management services, are performed during the same operative session by the same provider, all secondary, additional, or lessor procedures are listed after the primary procedure with the addition of the modifier -51.

This modifier should not be used with codes designated as "add-on" codes.

-52   Reduced services

Under certain circumstances a service or procedure may be partially reduced or eliminated at the physician's discretion. Under these circumstances the service or procedure provided is identified by reporting the usual procedure code with the addition of modifier -52 to indicate the service was reduced.

The intended use of this modifier is to report the reduction of a service without affecting provider profiles maintained by health insurance companies.

Modifier -52 is another frequently misused modifier. Some medical practices mistakenly use modifier -52 to mean "reduced fee" and use it as a discounting method. Not only is this incorrect, the provider may seriously damage their provider profile with health insurance companies.

The proper use for modifier -52 is to report that a service was not completed, or some part of a multiple-part service was not performed. A fee reduction may be in order as well; however that is not the primary purpose of the modifier.

For hospital outpatient reporting of a previously scheduled procedure or service that is partially reduced or canceled as a result of extenuating circumstances or those that threaten the well-being of the patient prior to or after administration of anesthesia, see modifiers -73 and -74.

-53   Discontinued procedure

Under certain circumstances, the physician may decided to stop a surgical or diagnostic procedure before it is completed due to extenuating circumstances or those that threaten the well being of the patient. This situation is reported by adding modifier -53 to the basic procedure code.

This modifier is not used to report the elective cancellation of a procedure prior to the patient being anesthetized and/or surgical preparation in the operating room.

For hospital outpatient reporting of a previously scheduled procedure or service that is partially reduced or canceled as a result of extenuating circumstances or those that threaten the well-being of the patient prior to or after administration of anesthesia, see modifiers -73 and -74.

-54   Surgical care only

This modifier is reported when one physician performs a surgical procedure and another provides preoperative and/or post-operative care.

-55   Postoperative management only

This modifier is reported when one physician performs the postoperative care after another physician has performed the surgical procedure.

-56   Preoperative management only

This modifier is reported when one physician performs preoperative care and evaluation prior to another physician performing the surgical procedure.

-57   Decision for surgery

This modifier is reported to identify an evaluation and management service that resulted in the initial decision to perform surgery.

-58   Staged or related procedure or service by the same physician during the postoperative period

Modifier -58 is reported when a physician needs to indicate that a procedure or service performed during the postoperative period was: a) planned prospectively at the time of the original procedure (staged); b) more extensive than the original procedure; or c) was for therapy following a diagnostic surgical procedure.

Modifier -58 is not used to report the treatment of a problem that requires a return to the operating room.

-59   Distinct Procedural Service

Under certain circumstances the physician may need to indicate that a procedure or service was distinct or independent from other services performed on the same day. Modifier -59 is used to identify procedures or services that are not normally reported together, but are appropriate under the circumstances. This may represent a different session or patient encounter, different procedure or surgery, different site or organ system, separate incision/excision, separate lesion, or separate injury (or area of injury) not usually encountered on the same day by the same physician.

Modifier -59 should be used only when no more descriptive modifier is available and the use of modifier -59 best explains the circumstances.

(-60   Altered surgical field deleted)

-62   Two surgeons

Modifier -62 is reported when the skills of two surgeons, usually with different skills, are required in the management of a specific surgical procedure.

-66   Surgical team

Modifier -66 is reported when highly complex procedures require the services of several physicians at the same time.

-73   Discontinued outpatient hospital or Ambulatory Surgery Center (ASC) procedure prior to the administration of anesthesia

-74   Discontinued outpatient hospital or Ambulatory Surgery Center (ASC) procedure after administration of anesthesia

-76   Repeat procedure by same physician

This modifier is reported when a procedure or service is repeated by the same physician.

-77   Repeat procedure by another physician

This modifier is reported when a procedure is performed that was previously performed by another physician.

-78   Return to the operating room for a related procedure during the postoperative period

The physician may need to indicate that another procedure was performed during the postoperative period of the initial procedure. When this subsequent procedure is related to the first, and requires the use of the operating room, it is reported by adding modifier -78 to the related procedure. (For repeat procedures on the same day, see -76).

-79   Unrelated procedure or service by the same physician during the postoperative period

The physician may need to indicate that the performance of a procedure or service during the postoperative period was unrelated to the original procedure. This circumstance may be reported by adding the modifier -79 to the procedure or service. (For repeat procedures on the same day, see -76).

-80 Assistant surgeon

This modifier is used to report surgical assistant services provided by the first assistant surgeon.

-81 Minimum assistant surgeon

This modifier is reported to report minimal services provided by a second assistant surgeon.

-82 Assistant surgeon (qualified resident not available)

This modifier is used to report assistant surgeon services provided at teaching hospitals when a qualified resident surgeon was not available to assist.

-90 Reference (outside) laboratory

When laboratory procedures reported on the health insurance claim form are performed by an outside laboratory, add modifier -90 to the basic service.

-91 Repeat clinical diagnostic laboratory test

Occasionally in the course of treatment it may be necessary to repeat laboratory tests on the same day to obtain subsequent (multiple) test results. This situation is reported by added modifier -91 to the basic procedure code.

This modifier may not be used when tests are repeated to confirm initial results, due to testing problems with specimens or equipment, or for any other reason when a normal, one-time, reportable result is all that is required.

This modifier may not be used when other procedure code(s) describe a series of tests results (eg, glucose tolerance tests, evocative/suppression testing).

This modifier may be used only for laboratory test(s) performed more than once on the same day on the same patient.

-99 Multiple modifiers

Occasionally, two or more modifiers may be necessary to completely describe a service. In this situations modifier -99 should be added to the basic procedure, and other applicable modifiers may be listed as part of the description of the service.

HCPCS MODIFIERS

HCPCS modifiers, defined and managed by The Centers for Medicare and Medicaid (CMS), formerly known as HCFA, are two digit modifier codes which may be either alpha (all letters) or alphanumeric (letters plus numbers). HCPCS modifiers are used to modify procedures and services on health insurance claim forms filed for Medicare patients.

HCPCS modifiers may be added, deleted or changed in each new edition of HCPCS, therefore, providers should acquire and review the most current edition of HCPCS each year. HCPCS modifiers may be LEVEL II, which are used nationally, or LEVEL III, which are used only by a local Medicare intermediary.

HCPCS LEVEL II MODIFIERS

Following is the complete list of HCPCS Level II modifiers and descriptions:

-AA   Anesthesia services by anesthesiologist

When anesthesia services are performed personally by the anesthesiologist, add modifier -AA to the basic service.

-AB   Four or less concurrent services by CRNA or AA employed by anesthesiologist

-AC   Four or less concurrent services by CRNA not employed by anesthesiologist

-AD   Supervision of more than four concurrent anesthesia services by anesthesiologist

-AE   Direction of residents in furnishing not more than two concurrent anesthesia services

This modifier is coded to report supervision of residents in a teaching facility.

-AF   Anesthesia complicated by total body hypothermia.

-AG   Anesthesia for emergency surgery on a patient who is moribund or who has an incapacitating systemic disease that is a constant threat to life.

-AH   Clinical psychologist

-AJ   Clinical social worker

-AK   Nurse practitioner (team member service)

-AL   Nurse practitioner, non-rural, team member

-AM   Physician (team member service)

-AN   Physician assistant for other assistant-at-surgery

-AP   Determination of refractive state was not performed

-AR   Ambulance - return trip

-AS   Physician assistant (assisting at surgery)(non-team member).

-AT   Acute treatment

When chiropractic manipulation codes 98940-98943 are coded for acute treatment, add modifier -AT.

-AU   Physician assistant (other than assistant at surgery)(team member)

-AV   Nurse practitioner, non-team member

-AW   Clinical nurse specialist, non-team member

-AY   Clinical nurse specialist, team member

-BP   The beneficiary has been informed of the purchase and rental options and has elected to purchase the item

-BR   The beneficiary has been informed of the purchase and rental options and has elected to rent the item

-BU   The beneficiary has been informed of the purchase and rental options and after 30 days has not informed the supplier of his/her decision

-CC   Portable x-ray (system set)

-DD   Powdered enteral formula

Add modifier -DD to HCPCS codes B4100-B5999 when powdered enteral products are supplied.

-E1   Upper left, eyelid

-E2   Lower left, eyelid

-E3   Upper right, eyelid

-E4   Lower right, eyelid

-EJ   Subsequent EPO injection

-EM   Emergency reserve supply (ESRD)

-EP   Service provided as part of Medicaid early periodic screening, diagnosis and treatment (EPSDT) program

-ET   Emergency treatment

        Modifier -ET is coded with codes D0000-D9999 for dental procedures performed in emergency situations.

-FA   Left hand, thumb

-F1   Left hand, second digit

-F2   Left hand, third digit

-F3   Left hand, fourth digit

-F4   Left hand, fifth digit

-F5   Right hand, thumb

-F6   Right hand, second digit

-F7   Right hand, third digit

-F8   Right hand, fourth digit

-F9   Right hand, fifth digit

-FP   Service provided as part of Medicaid family planning program

-KA   Add on option/accessory for wheelchair

-KH   DMEPOS item, initial claim, purchase or first month rental

-KI   DMEPOS item, second or third month rental

-KJ   DMEPOS item, parenteral enteral nutrition (PEN) pump or capped rental, months four to fifteen

-KK   Inhalation solution compounded from an FDA approved formulation

-KL   Product characteristics defined in medical policy are met

-K0   Lower extremity prosthesis Functional Level 0: Does not have the ability or potential to ambulate or transfer safely with or without assistance and a prosthesis does not enhance their quality of life or mobility

-K1   Lower extremity prosthesis Functional Level 1: Has the ability or potential to use a prosthesis for transfers or ambulation on level surfaces at fixed cadence. Typical of the limited and unlimited household ambulator.

-K2   Lower extremity prosthesis Functional Level 2: Has the ability or potential for ambulation with the ability to traverse low-level environmental barriers such as curbs, stairs or uneven surfaces. Typical of the limited community ambulator.

-K3   Lower extremity prosthesis Functional Level 3: Has the ability or potential for ambulation with variable cadence. Typical of the community ambulator who has the ability to traverse most environmental barriers and may have vocational, therapeutic or exercise activity that demands prosthetic utilization beyond simple locomotion.

-K4   Lower extremity prosthesis Functional Level 4: Has the ability or potential for prosthetic ambulation that exceeds the basic ambulation skills, exhibiting high impact, stress or energy levels, typical of the prosthetic demands of the child, active adult, or athlete.

-LL   Lease/rental

When DME equipment rental is to be applied against the purchase price, add modifier -LL to the basic HCPCS code.

-LR   Laboratory round trip

-LS   FDA-monitored intraocular lens implant

-LT   Left side

This modifier is coded to identify procedures performed on the left side of the body.

-MP   Multiple patients seen

This modifier is coded with evaluation and management codes 99321-99333 to indicate that more than one patient was seen during the visit.

-MS   Six month maintenance and servicing fee for reasonable and necessary parts and labor that are not covered under any manufacturer or supplier warranty

-NR   New when rented

When DME equipment that was new at the time of rental is subsequently purchased, add modifier -NR to the basic HCPCS code.

-NU New equipment

-Q3 Live kidney donor: services associated with postoperative medical complications directly related to the donation

-QB Physician providing services in a rural HMSA

-QC Single channel monitoring

-QD Recording and storage in solid state memory by a digital recorder

-QE Prescribed amount of oxygen is less than one liter per minute

-QF Prescribed amount of oxygen is greater than four liters per minute and portable oxygen also prescribed

-QG Prescribed amount of oxygen is greater than four liters per minute

-QH Oxygen conserving device is being used with an oxygen delivery system

-QI Decision for surgery

-QK Medical direction of two, three or four concurrent anesthesia procedures involving qualified individuals

-QL Ambulatory surgical center (ASC) service

-QM Physician, team member service

-QN Nurse practitioner, team member service

-QS Monitored anesthesia care service

-QT Recording and storage on tape by an analog tape recorder

-QU Physician providing services in an urban HMSA

-QV Nurse practitioner, non-team member

-QW Clinical nurse specialist, non-team member

-QX CRNA service: with medical direction by a physician

-QY Clinical nurse specialist, team member

-QZ CRNA service: without medical direction by a physician

-Q2 HCFA/ORD demonstration project procedure/service

-Q4 Service for ordering/referring physician qualifies as a service exemption

-Q5 Service furnished by a substitute physician under a reciprocal billing arrangement

-Q6 Service furnished by a locum tenens physician

-RP Replacement and repair

Add modifier -RP when reporting HCPCS codes E0000-E9999 and L0000-L9999 to indicate replacement of DME, orthotic and prosthetic devices that have been in use for some time.

-RR Rental

Add modifier -RR when reporting HCPCS codes E0000-E9999 to indicate that DME is rented.

-RT Right side

Modifier -RT is coded to identify procedures performed on the right side of the body.

-SF Second opinion ordered by a professional review organization

Modifier -SF is coded to record a second opinion ordered by a Peer Review Organization (PRO). Reimbursement is 100 percent and there is no deductible or coinsurance.

-SG Ambulatory surgical center (ASC) facility service

-SP Nursing home or SNF visit, single patient seen

-TA Left foot, great toe

-T1 Left foot, second digit

-T2 Left foot, third digit

-T3 Left foot, fourth digit

-T4 Left foot, fifth digit

-T5   Right foot, great toe

-T6   Right foot, second digit

-T7   Right foot, third digit

-T8   Right foot, fourth digit

-T9   Right foot, fifth digit

-TC   Technical component

Under certain circumstances, a charge may be made for the technical component alone. Under those circumstances the technical component charge is identified by adding modifier -TC to the usual procedure number. Technical component charges are institutional charges and are not coded separately by physicians. However, portable x-ray suppliers only bill for technical components and should use modifier -TC. The charge date from portable x-ray suppliers will then be used to build customary and prevailing profiles.

-UE   Used durable medical equipment

-VP   Aphakic patient

-YY   Second surgical opinion

-ZZ   Third surgical opinion

ANATOMICAL ILLUSTRATIONS

A fundamental knowledge and understanding of basic human anatomy and physiology is a prerequisite for accurate CPT® procedure coding. While a comprehensive treatment of anatomy and physiology is beyond the scope of this text, the large scale, full color anatomical illustrations on the following pages are designed to facilitate the procedure coding process for both beginning and experienced coders.

The illustrations provide an anatomical perspective of procedure coding by providing a side-by-side view of the major systems of the human body and a corresponding list of the most common CPT procedural categories used to report medical, surgical and diagnostic services performed on the illustrated system.

The CPT procedural categories listed on the left facing page of each anatomical illustration are code ranges only and should not be used for coding. These categories are provided as "pointers" to the appropriate section of CPT, where the definitive code may be found.

PLATE 1. SKIN AND SUBCUTANEOUS TISSUE-MALE

Skin, Subcutaneous and Accessory Structures

Incision and Drainage	10040-10180
Excision-Debridement	11000-11044
Paring or Cutting	11055-11057
Biopsy	11100-11101
Removal of Skin Tags	11200-11201
Shaving of Epidermal or Dermal Lesions	11300-11313
Excision-Benign Lesions	11400-11471
Excision-Malignant Lesions	11600-11646

Nails
11719-11772

Repair (Closure)

Repair-Simple	12001-12021
Repair-Intermediate	12031-12057
Repair-Complex	13100-13300
Adjacent Tissue Transfer	14000-14350
Free Skin Grafts	15000-15401
Flaps (Skin and/or Deep Tissues)	15570-15738
Pressure Ulcers (Decubitus Ulcers)	15920-15999
Burns	16000-16035

Destruction

Destruction, Benign or Premalignant Lesions	17000-17250
Destruction, Malignant Lesions	17260-17286
Mohs' Micrographic Surgery	17304-17310
Other Destruction Procedures	17340-17999

Laboratory Services

Skin Tests	86485-86585

E/M Services
99200-99499

Male Figure
(Anterior View)

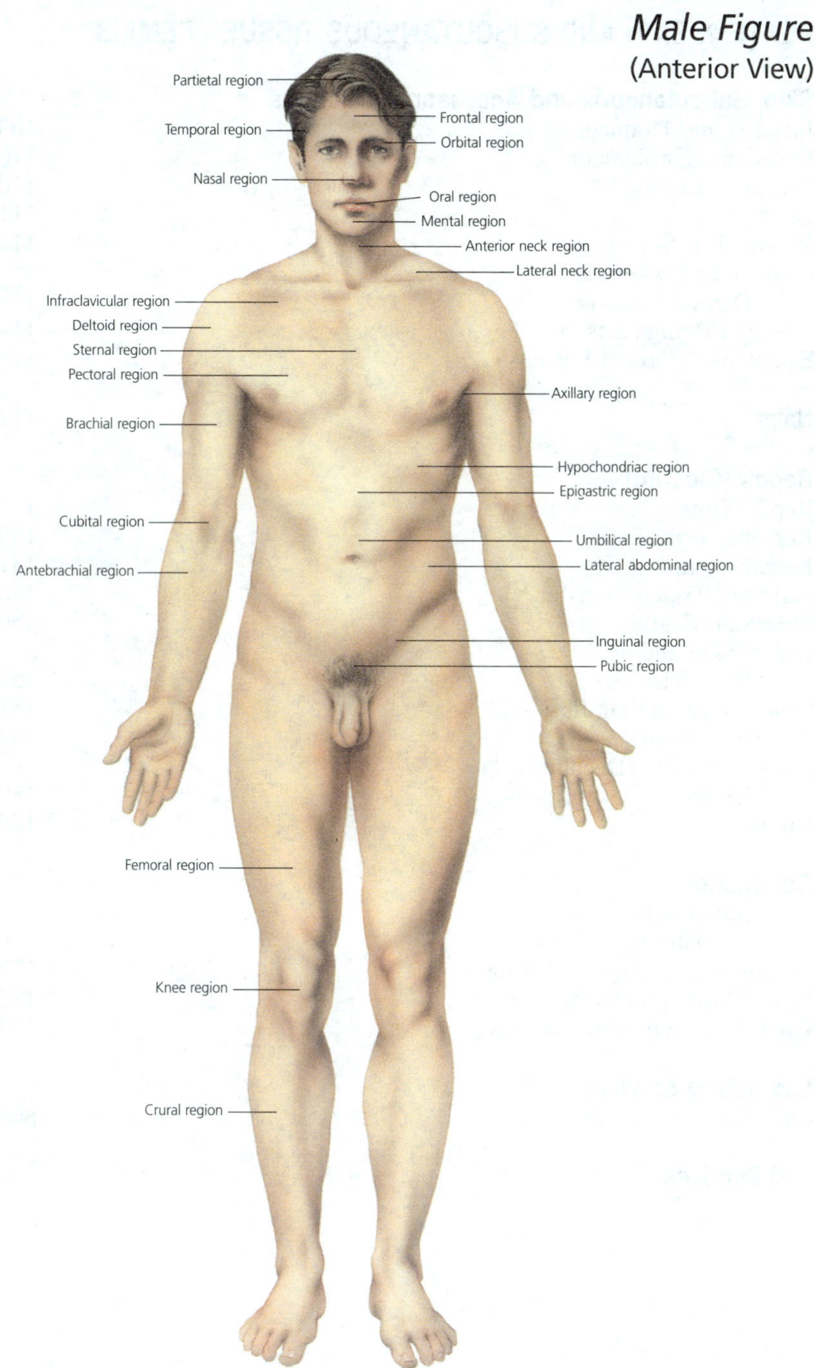

PLATE 2. SKIN AND SUBCUTANEOUS TISSUE - FEMALE

Skin, Subcutaneous and Accessory Structures

Incision and Drainage	10040-10180
Excision-Debridement	11000-11044
Paring or Cutting	11055-11057
Biopsy	11100-11101
Removal of Skin Tags	11200-11201
Shaving of Epidermal or Dermal Lesions	11300-11313
Excision-Benign Lesions	11400-11471
Excision-Malignant Lesions	11600-11646

Nails
11719-11772

Repair (Closure)

Repair-Simple	12001-12021
Repair-Intermediate	12031-12057
Repair-Complex	13100-13300
Adjacent Tissue Transfer	14000-14350
Free Skin Grafts	15000-15401
Flaps (Skin and/or Deep Tissues)	15570-15738
Other Flaps and Grafts	15740-15776
Other Procedures	15780-15879
Pressure Ulcers (Decubitus Ulcers)	15920-15999
Burns	16000-16035

Destruction

Destruction, Benign or Premalignant Lesions	17000-17250
Destruction, Malignant Lesions	17260-17286
Mohs' Micrographic Surgery	17304-17310
Other Destruction Procedures	17340-17999

Laboratory Services

Skin Tests	86485-86585

E/M Services
99200-99499

Female Figure
(Anterior View)

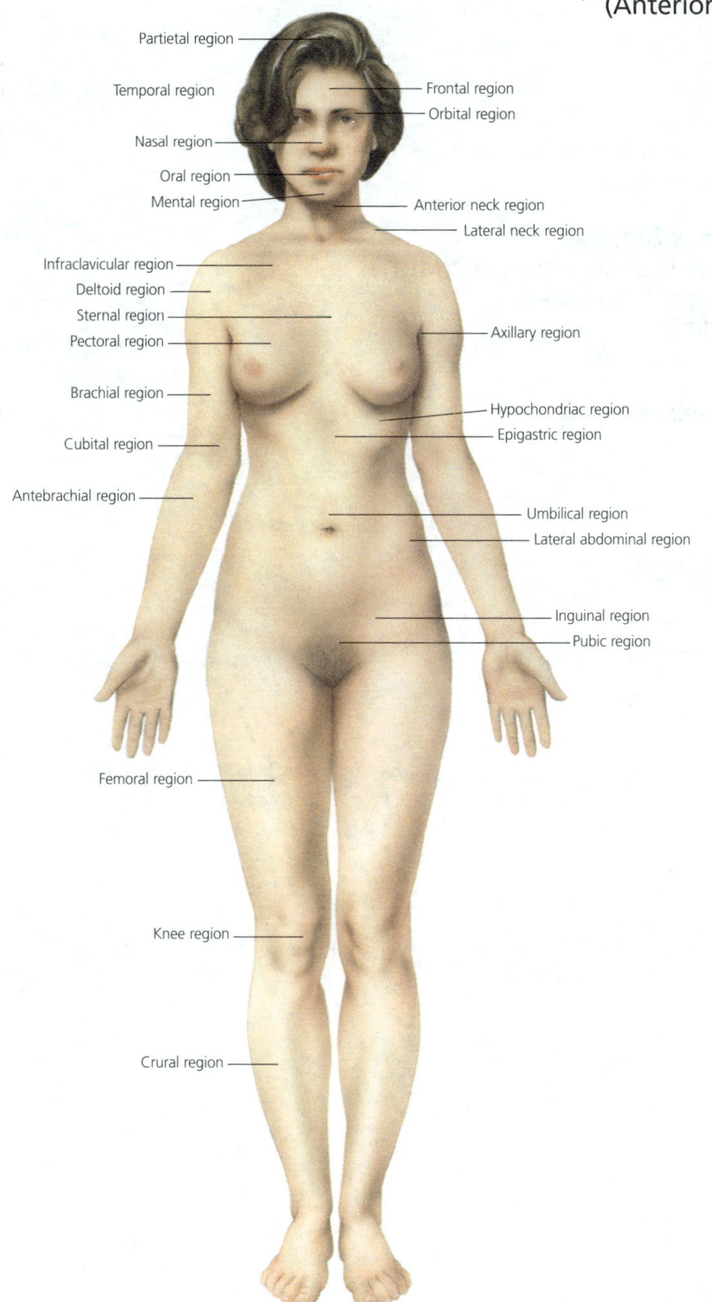

PLATE 3. FEMALE BREAST

Breast

Incision	19000-19030
Excision	19100-19272
Introduction	19260-19291
Repair and/or Reconstruction	19316-19396
Other Procedures	19499

Radiology Services

Magnetic Resonance Imaging (MRI)	76093-76094
Stereotactic Localization	76095
Ultrasound	76645
X-ray	76090-76092

E/M Services

99200-99499

Female Breast

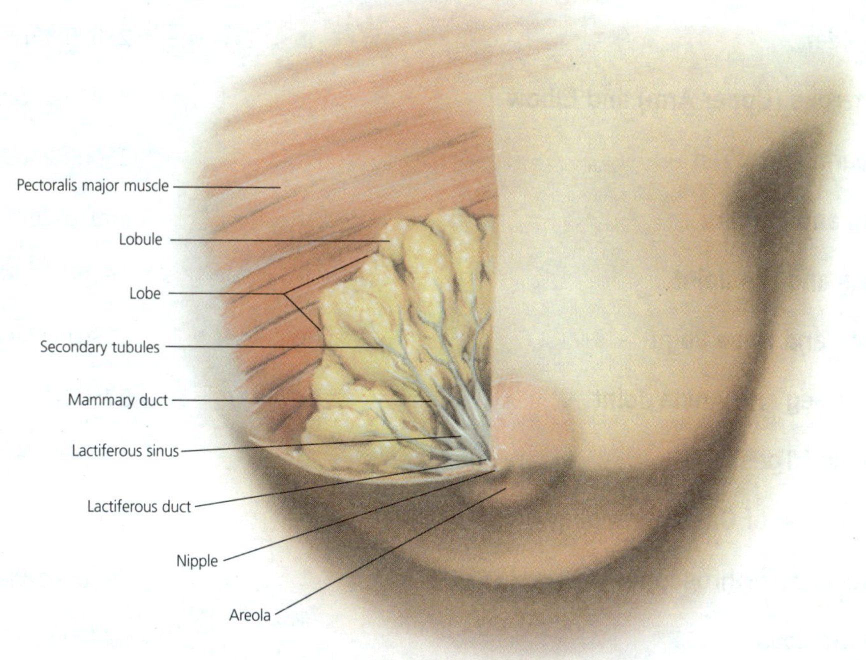

PLATE 4. MUSCULAR SYSTEM AND CONNECTIVE TISSUE - ANTERIOR VIEW

General	20100-20938
Head	21010-21497
Neck (Soft Tissues) and Thorax	21501-21899
Back and Flank	21920-21935
Spine (Vertebral Column)	22100-22855
Shoulder	23000-23680
Humerous (Upper Arm) and Elbow	23930-24685
Forearm and Wrist	25000-25695
Hand and Fingers	26010-26785
Pelvis and Hip Joint	26990-27266
Femur and Knee Joint	27301-27566
Lower Leg and Ankle Joint	27600-27848
Foot and Toes	28001-28675
Application of Casts/Strapping	29000-29799
Endoscopy/Arthroscopy	29800-29909
E/M Services	99200-99499

Muscular System
(Anterior View)

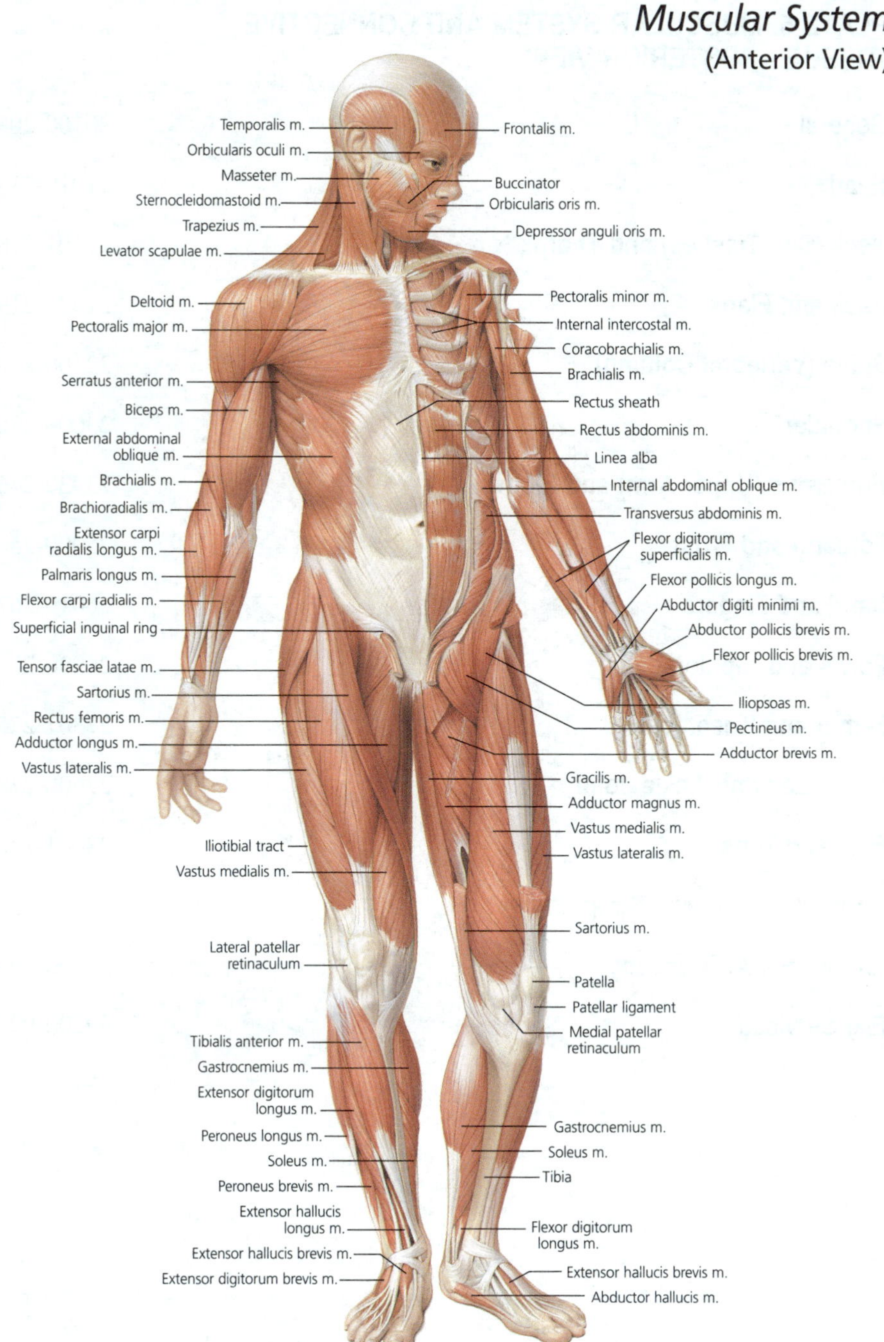

PLATE 5. MUSCULAR SYSTEM AND CONNECTIVE TISSUE - POSTERIOR VIEW

General	20100-20938
Head	21010-21497
Neck (Soft Tissues) and Thorax	21501-21899
Back and Flank	21920-21935
Spine (Vertebral Column)	22100-22855
Shoulder	23000-23680
Humerous (Upper Arm) and Elbow	23930-24685
Forearm and Wrist	25000-25695
Hand and Fingers	26010-26785
Pelvis and Hip Joint	26990-27266
Femur and Knee Joint	27301-27566
Lower Leg and Ankle Joint	27600-27848
Foot and Toes	28001-28675
Application of Casts/Strapping	29000-29799
Endoscopy/Arthroscopy	29800-29909
E/M Services	99200-99499

Muscular System
(Posterior View)

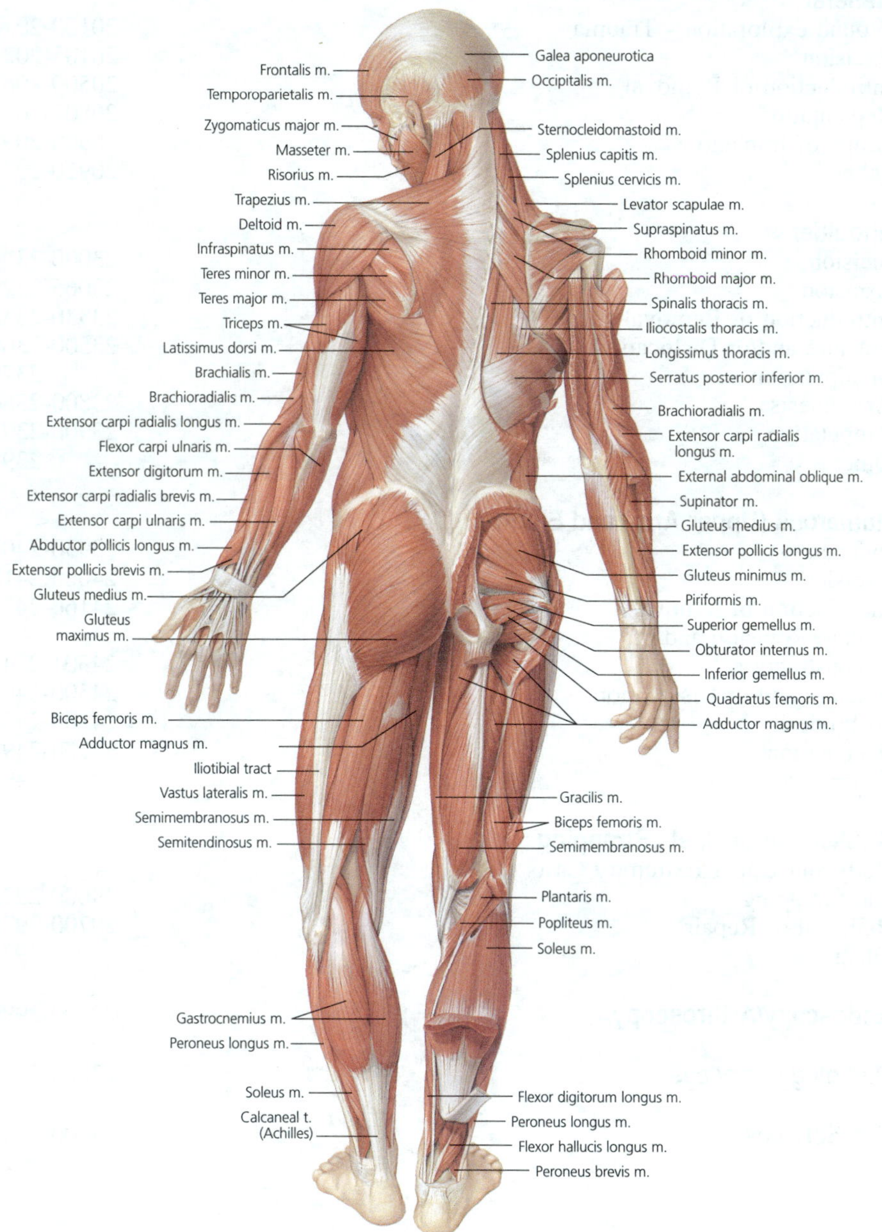

PLATE 6. MUSCULAR SYSTEM - SHOULDER AND ELBOW

General

Wound exploration - Trauma	20100-20103
Excision	20105-20251
Introduction or Removal	20500-20694
Replantation	20802-20838
Grafts of Implants	20900-20938
Other	20950-20999

Shoulder

Incision	23000-23044
Excision	23065-23222
Introduction or Removal	23330-23350
Fracture and/or Dislocation	23500-23680
Manipulation	23700
Arthrodesis	23800-23802
Amputation	23900-23921
Other	23929

Humerous (Upper Arm) and Elbow

Incision	23930-24006
Excision	24065-24155
Introduction or removal	24160-24220
Repair, Revision and/or Reconstruction	24301-24498
Fracture and/or Dislocation	24500-24685
Arthrodesis	24800-24802
Amputation	24900-24940
Other	24999

Application of Casts/Strapping

Body and Upper Extremity Casts and Strapping	29000-29280
Removal or Repair	29700-29750
Other	29799

Endoscopy/Arthroscopy

29800-29909

Radiology Services

73000-73225

E/M Services

99200-99499

Shoulder and Elbow
(Anterior View)

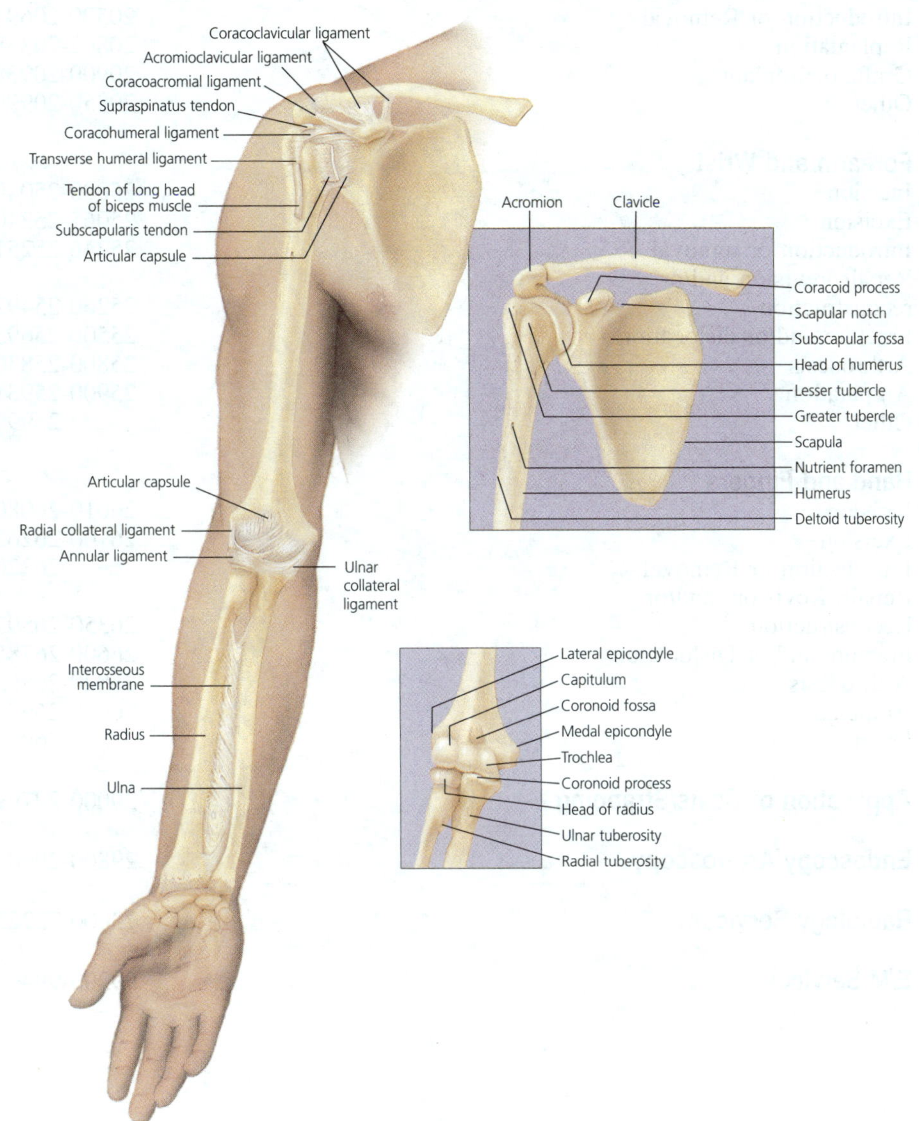

PLATE 7. MUSCULAR SYSTEM - HAND AND WRIST

General

Wound exploration - Trauma	20100-20103
Excision	20105-20251
Introduction or Removal	20500-20694
Replantation	20802-20838
Grafts of Implants	20900-20938
Other	20950-20999

Forearm and Wrist

Incision	25000-25040
Excision	25065-25240
Introduction or removal	25246-25251
Repair, revision and/or reconstruction	25260-25492
Fracture and/or dislocation	25500-25695
Arthrodesis	25800-25830
Amputation	25900-25931
Other	25999

Hand and Fingers

Incision	26010-26080
Excision	26100-26262
Introduction or Removal	26320
Repair, Revision, and/or Reconstruction	26350-26597
Fracture and/or Dislocation	26600-26785
Arthrodesis	26820-26863
Amputation	26910-26952
Other	26989

Application of Casts/Strapping

29000-29799

Endoscopy/Arthroscopy

29800-29909

Radiology Services

73000-73225

E/M Services

99200-99499

Hand and Wrist

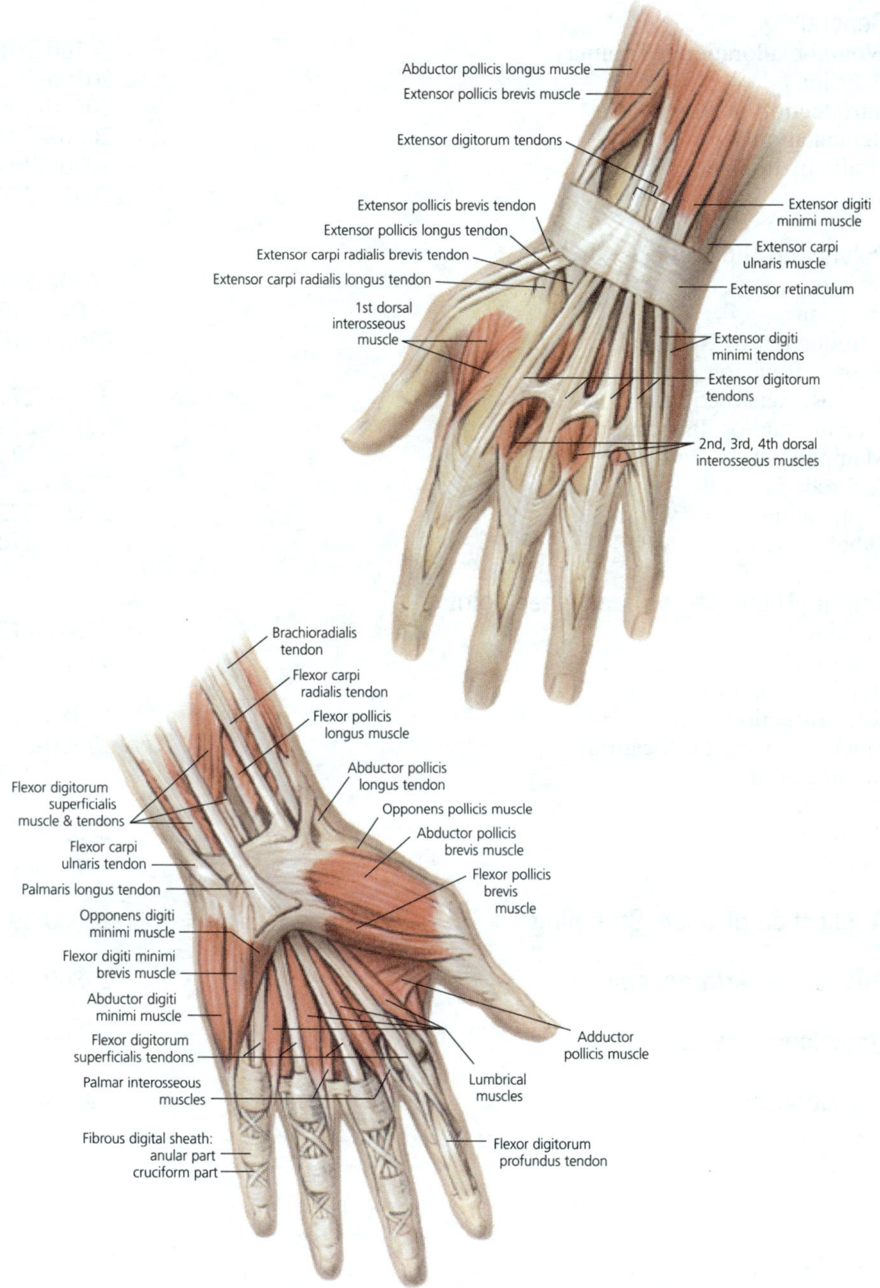

PLATE 8. MUSCULOSKELETAL SYSTEM - HIP AND KNEE

General

Wound exploration - Trauma	20100-20103
Excision	20105-20251
Introduction or Removal	20500-20694
Replantation	20802-20838
Grafts of Implants	20900-20938
Other	20950-20999

Pelvis and Hip Joint

Incision	26990-27036
Excision	27040-27080
Introduction or Removal	27086-27095
Repair, Revision, and/or Reconstruction	27097-27187
Fracture and/or dislocation	27193-27266
Manipulation	27275
Arthrodesis	27280-27286
Amputation	27290-27295
Other	27299

Femur (Thigh Region) and Knee Joint

Incision	27301-27320
Excision	27323-27372
Repair, Revision, and/or Reconstruction	27380-27499
Fracture and/or Dislocation	27500-27566
Manipulation	27570
Arthrodesis	27580
Amputation	27590-27598
Other	27599

Application of Casts/Strapping

29000-29799

Endoscopy/Arthroscopy

29800-29909

Radiology Services

73500-73725

E/M Services

99200-99499

Hip and Knee
(Anterior View)

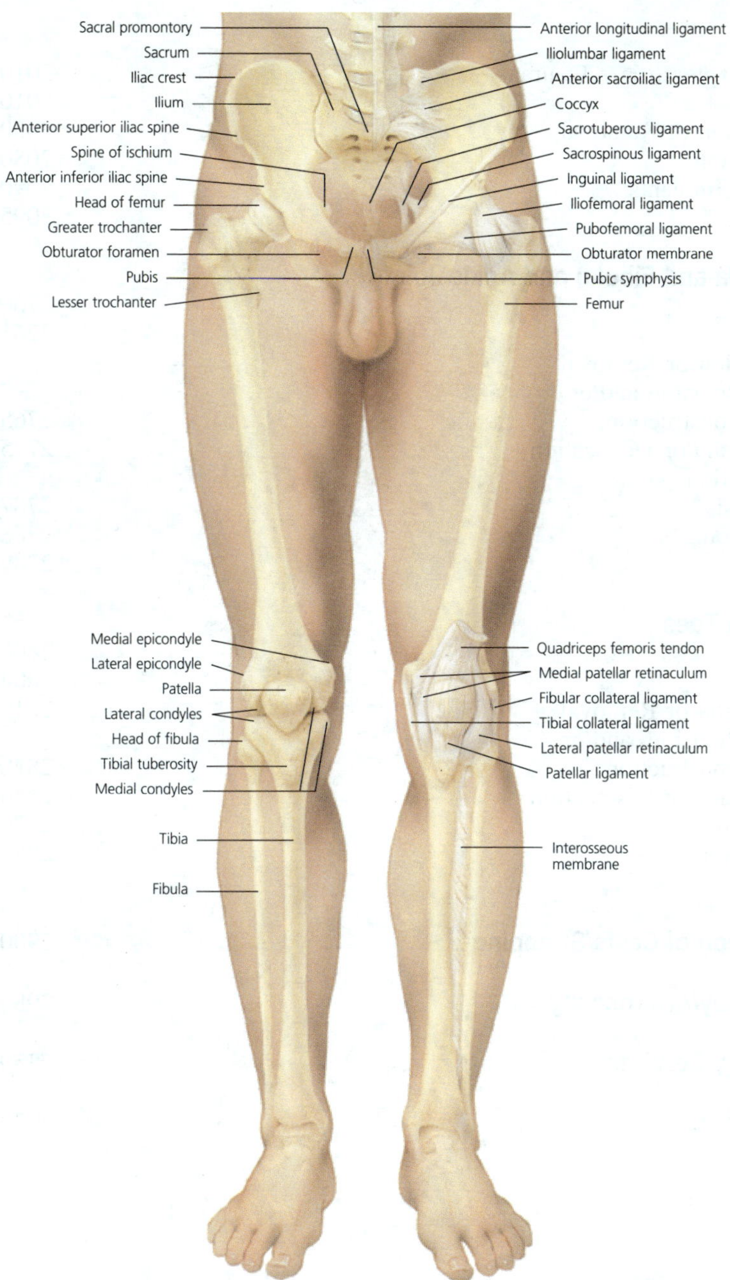

PLATE 9. MUSCULOSKELETAL SYSTEM - FOOT AND ANKLE

General

Wound exploration - Trauma	20100-20103
Excision	20105-20251
Introduction or Removal	20500-20694
Replantation	20802-20838
Grafts of Implants	20900-20938
Other	20950-20999

Leg (Tibia and Fibula) and Ankle Joint

Incision	27600-27612
Excision	27613-27647
Introduction or Removal	27648
Repair, Revision and/or Reconstruction	27650-27745
Fracture and/or Dislocation	27750-27848
Manipulation	27860
Arthrodesis	27870-27871
Amputation	27880-27889
Other	27892-27899

Foot and Toes

Incision	28001-28035
Excision	28043-28175
Introduction or Removal	28190-28193
Repair, Revision, and/or Reconstruction	28200-28360
Fracture and/or Dislocation	28400-28675
Arthrodesis	28705-28760
Amputation	28800-28825
Other	28899

Application of Casts/Strapping 29000-29799

Endoscopy/Arthroscopy 29800-29909

Radiology Services 73500-73725

E/M Services 99200-99499

Foot and Ankle

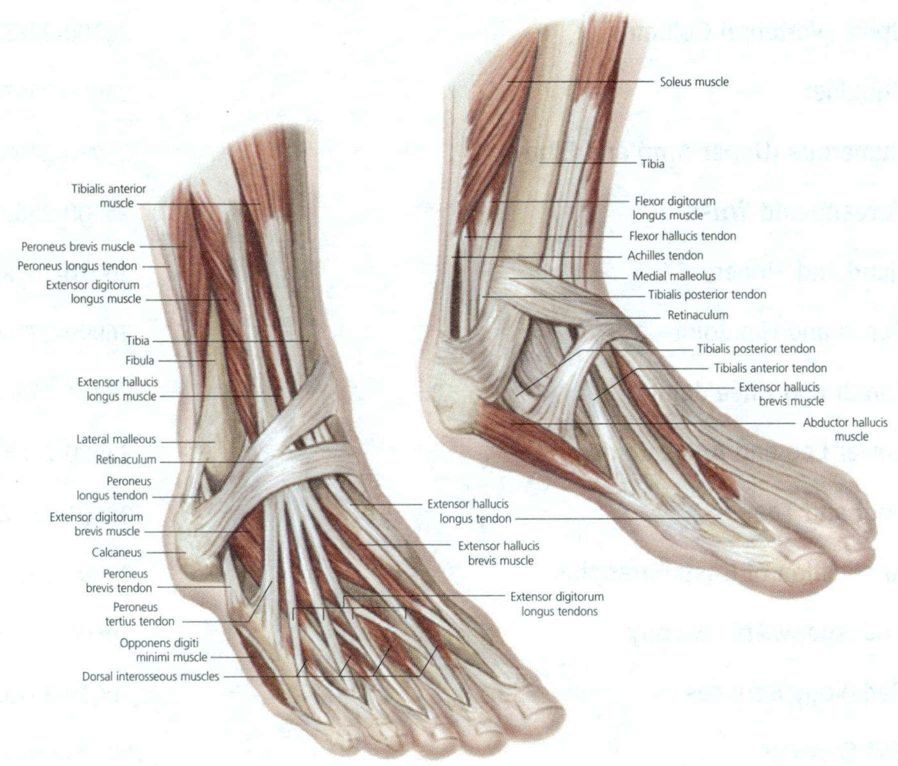

PLATE 10. SKELETAL SYSTEM - ANTERIOR VIEW

General	20100-20938
Head	21010-21497
Neck (Soft Tissues) and Thorax	21501-21899
Back and Flank	21920-21935
Spine (Vertebral Column)	22100-22855
Shoulder	23000-23680
Humerous (Upper Arm) and Elbow	23930-24685
Forearm and Wrist	25000-25695
Hand and Fingers	26010-26785
Pelvis and Hip Joint	26990-27266
Femur and Knee Joint	27301-27566
Lower Leg and Ankle Joint	27600-27848
Foot and Toes	28001-28675
Application of Casts/Strapping	29000-29799
Endoscopy/Arthroscopy	29800-29909
Radiology Services	70010-73725
E/M Services	99200-99499

Skeletal System
(Anterior View)

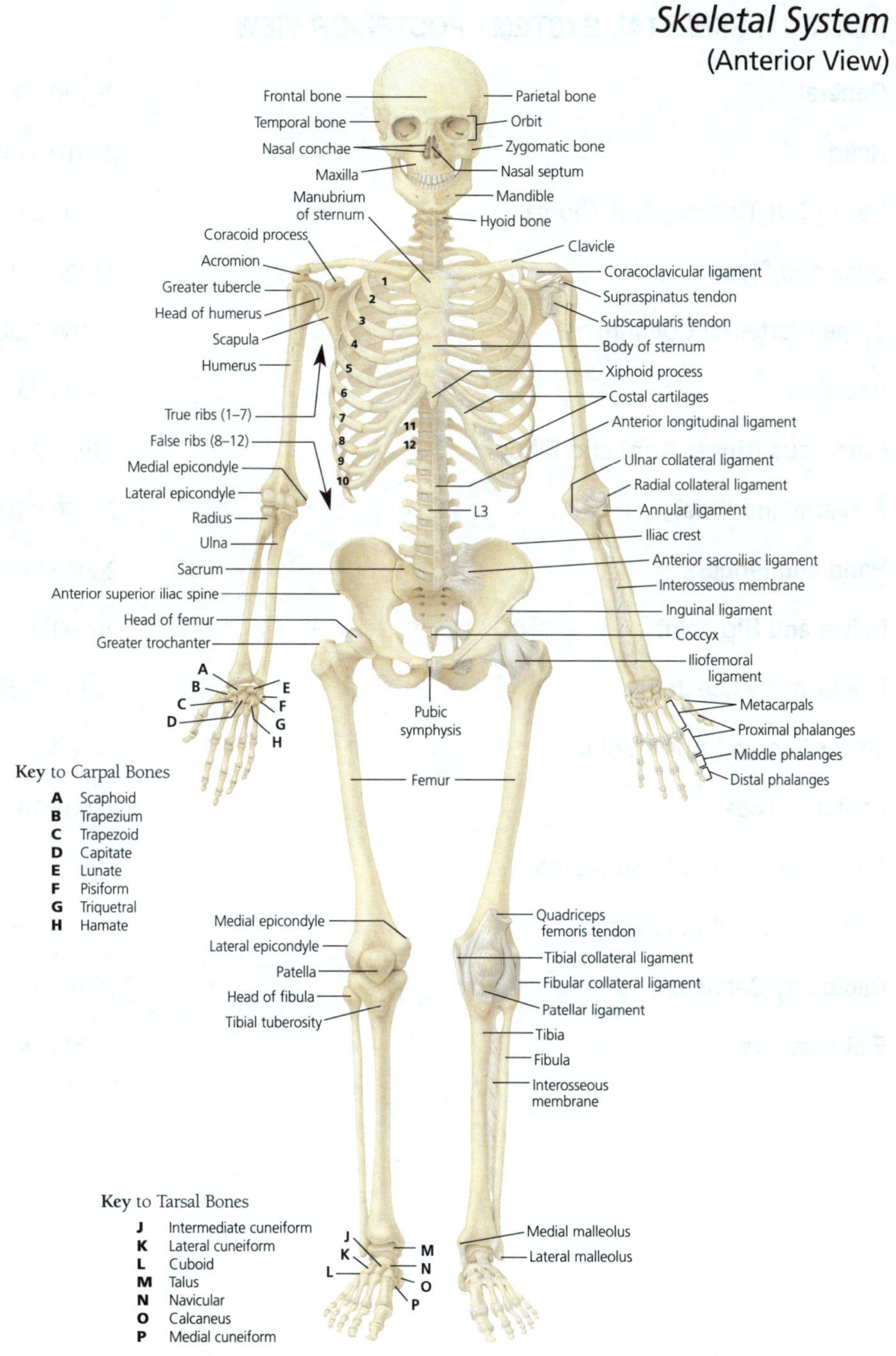

Key to Carpal Bones

A Scaphoid
B Trapezium
C Trapezoid
D Capitate
E Lunate
F Pisiform
G Triquetral
H Hamate

Key to Tarsal Bones

J Intermediate cuneiform
K Lateral cuneiform
L Cuboid
M Talus
N Navicular
O Calcaneus
P Medial cuneiform

PLATE 11. SKELETAL SYSTEM - POSTERIOR VIEW

General	20100-20938
Head	21010-21497
Neck (Soft Tissues) and Thorax	21501-21899
Back and Flank	21920-21935
Spine (Vertebral Column)	22100-22855
Shoulder	23000-23680
Humerous (Upper Arm) and Elbow	23930-24685
Forearm and Wrist	25000-25695
Hand and Fingers	26010-26785
Pelvis and Hip Joint	26990-27266
Femur and Knee Joint	27301-27566
Lower Leg and Ankle Joint	27600-27848
Foot and Toes	28001-28675
Application of Casts/Strapping	29000-29799
Endoscopy/Arthroscopy	29800-29909
Radiology Services	70010-73725
E/M Services	99200-99499

Skeletal System
(Posterior View)

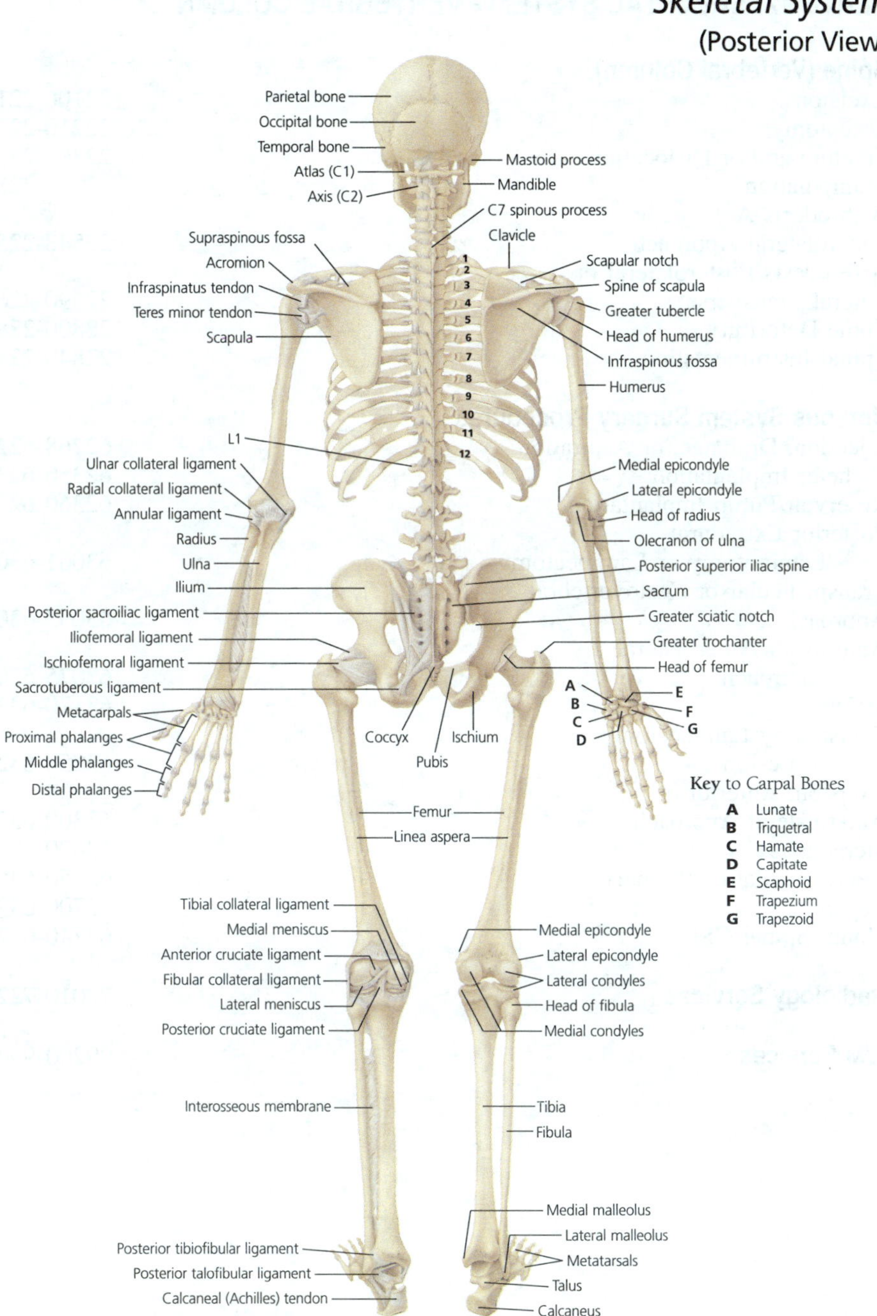

PLATE 12. SKELETAL SYSTEM - VERTEBRAL COLUMN

Spine (Vertebral Column)

Excision	22100-22116
Osteotomy	22210-22226
Fracture and/or Dislocation	22305-22328
Manipulation	22505
Arthrodesis-Anterior or Anterolateral Approach	22548-22585
Arthrodesis-Posterolateral or Lateral Transverse	22590-22632
Spine Deformity	22800-22819
Spinal Instrumentation	22840-22899

Nervous System Surgery Procedures

Injection, Drainage, or Aspiration	62268-62298
Catheter Implantation	62350-62355
Reservoir/Pump Implantation	62360-62368
Posterior Extradural Laminotomy or Laminectomy	63001-63048
Transpedicular or Costovertebral Approach	63055-63066
Anterior or Anterolateral Approach	63075-63091
Incision	63170-63200
Excision by Laminectomy of Lesion	63250-63290
Excision, Anterior or Anterolateral Approach	63300-63308
Stereotaxis	63600-63615
Neurostimulators (Spinal)	63650-63688
Repair	63700-63710
Shunt, Spinal CSF	63740-63746

Radiology Services

22010-72295

Radiology Services   72010-72295

E/M Services   99200-99499

Vertebral Column
(Lateral View)

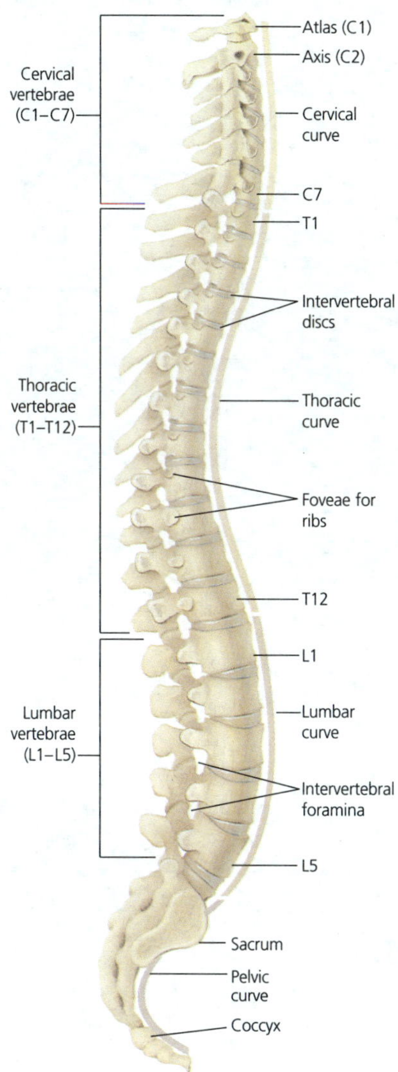

PLATE 13. RESPIRATORY SYSTEM

Nose

Incision	30000-30020
Excision	30100-30160
Introduction	30200-30220
Removal of Foreign Body	30300-30320
Repair	30400-30630
Destruction	30801-30802
Other	30901-30999

Accessory Sinuses

Incision	31000-31090
Excision	31200-31230
Endoscopy	31231-31294
Other	31299

Larynx

Excision	31300-31420
Introduction	31500-31502
Endoscopy	31505-31579
Repair	31580-31590
Destruction	31595
Other	31599

Trachea and Bronchi

Incision	31600-31614
Endoscopy	31615-31656
Introduction	31700-31730
Repair	31750-31830

Lungs and Pleura

Incision	32000-32225
Excision	32310-32540
Endoscopy	32601-32665
Repair	32800-32820
Lung Transplantation	32850-32854
Surgical Collapse Therapy; Thoracoplasty	32900-32960

Radiology Services

	71010-71555

E/M Services

	99200-99499

Respiratory System

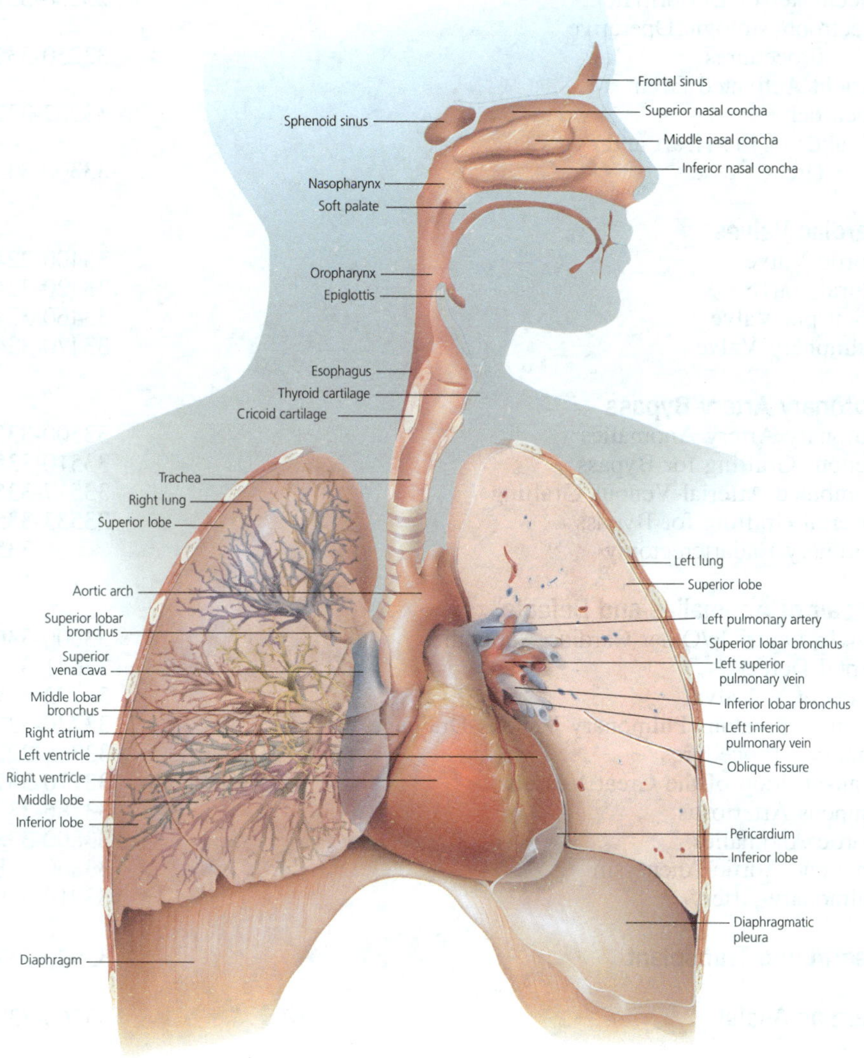

PLATE 14. HEART AND PERICARDIUM

General
Pericardium	33010-33050
Cardiac Tumor	33120-33130
Pacemaker or Defibrillator	33200-33261
Electrophysiologic Operative Procedures	33250-33261
Patient Activated Event Recorder	33282-33284
Wounds of the Heart and Great Vessels	33300-33335

Cardiac Valves
Aortic Valve	33400-22417
Mitral Valve	33420-33430
Tricuspid Valve	33460-33468
Pulmonary Valve	33470-33478

Coronary Artery Bypass
Coronary Artery Anomalies	33500-33506
Venous Grafting for Bypass	33510-33516
Combined Arterial-Venous Grafting	33517-33530
Arterial Grafting for Bypass	33533-33545
Coronary Endarterectomy	33572

Repair of Anomalies and Defects
Single Ventricle/Other Cardiac Anomalies	33600-33619
Septal Defect	33641-33697
Sinus of Valsalva	33702-33722
Total Anomalous Pulmonary Venous Drainage	33730-33732
Shunting Procedures	33735-22767
Transposition of the Great Vessels	33770-33781
Truncus Arteriosus	33786-33788
Aortic Anomalies	33800-33853
Thoracic Aortic Aneurysm	33860-33877
Pulmonary Artery	33910-33924

Heart/Lung Transplant
33930-33945

Cardiac Assist
33960-33978

Radiology Services
75552-75996

E/M Services
99200-99499

Heart
(External View)
Left common carotid artery
Brachiocephalic artery
Left subclavian artery
Aortic arch
Ligamentum arteriosum
Left pulmonary artery
Superior vena cava
Ascending aorta
Pulmonary trunk
Left auricle
Right coronary artery
Circumflex artery
Right atrium
Great cardiac vein
Right ventricle
Anterior descending (interventricular) artery
Anterior cardiac vein
Left ventricle
Right marginal artery
Small cardiac vein
Apex

Heart
(Internal View)
Superior vena cava
Right pulmonary artery branches
Left pulmonary artery
Aorta
Pulmonary trunk
Left pulmonary veins
Right pulmonary veins
Left atrium
Pulmonary semilunar valve
Aortic semilunar valve
Right atrium
Bicuspid (left AV) valve
Left ventricle
Tricuspid (right AV) valve
Papillary muscle
Interventricular septum
Chordae tendineae
Inferior vena cava
Myocardium
Right ventricle
Trabeculae carneae

PLATE 15. CIRCULATORY SYSTEM

Embolectomy/Thrombectomy

Arterial, With or Without Repair   34001-34203
Venous, Direct or w/Catheter   34401-34490

Venous Reconstruction   34501-34530

Repair

Direct Repair of Aneurysm   35001-35162
Repair Arteriovenous Fistula   35180-35190
Repair Blood Vessel Other Than for Fistula   35201-35286

Thromboendarterectomy   35301-35390

Transluminal Angioplasty   35450-35476

Transluminal Atherectomy   35480-35495

Bypass Graft

Vein   35500-35571
In-situ Vein   35582-35587
Composite Grafts   35681-35683

Transposition and Exploration/Revision

Arterial Transposition   35691-35695
Exploration/Revision   35700-35907

Vascular Injection Procedures

Intravenous   36000-36015
Intra-Arterial/Intra-Aortic   36100-36299
Venous   36400-36535
Arterial   36600-36660
Intraosseous   36680

Cannulization or Shunt and Other Procedures

Intervascular Cannulization or Shunt   36800-36861
Portal Decompression Procedures   37140-37181
Transcatheter Procedures   37195-37209
Intravascular Ultrasound Services   37250-37251
Ligation and Other Procedures   37565-37799

Radiology Services   75600-75996

E/M Services   99200-99499

Vascular System

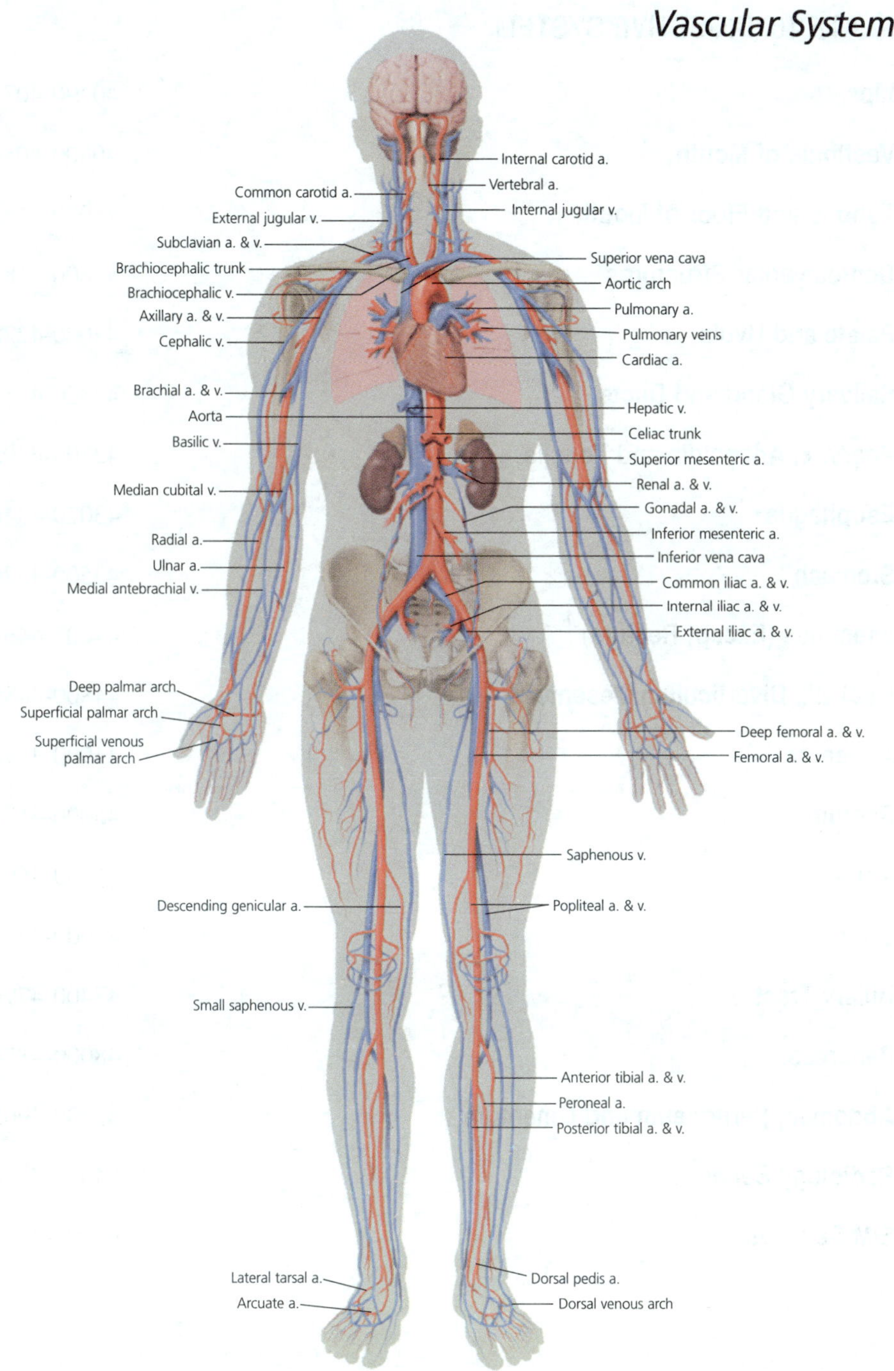

PLATE 16. DIGESTIVE SYSTEM

Lips	40490-40761
Vestibule of Mouth	40800-40845
Tongue and Floor of Mouth	41000-41599
Dentoalveolar Structures	41800-41850
Palate and Uvula	42000-42281
Salivary Gland and Ducts	42300-42510
Pharynx, Adenoids, and Tonsils	42700-42953
Esophagus	43020-43460
Stomach	43500-43761
Intestines (Except Rectum)	44005-44680
Meckel's Diverticulum/Mesentery	44800-44899
Appendix	44900-44979
Rectum	45000-45915
Anus	46030-46942
Liver	47000-47362
Biliary Tract	47400-47900
Pancreas	48000-48547
Abdomen, Peritoneum and Omentum	49000-49659
Radiology Services	74000-74363
E/M Services	99200-99499

Digestive System

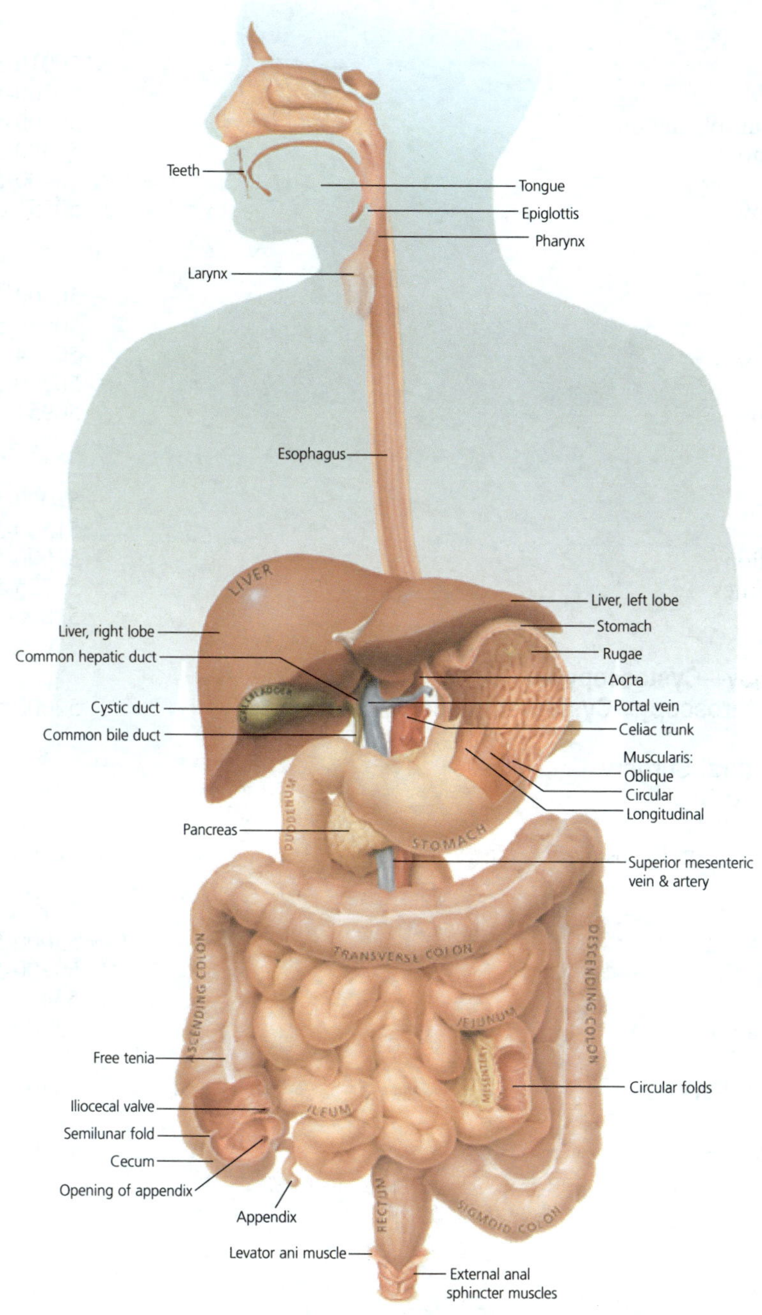

PLATE 17. GENITOURINARY SYSTEM

Kidney

Incision	50010-50135
Excision	50200-50290
Renal Transplantation	50300-50380
Introduction	50390-50398
Repair	50400-50540
Endoscopy	50551-50580

Ureter

Incision	50600-50630
Excision	50650-50660
Introduction	50684-50690
Repair	50700-50940
Endoscopy	50951-50980

Bladder

Incision	51000-51080
Excision	51500-51597
Introduction	51600-51720
Urodynamics	51725-51980
Repair	51800-51980

Endoscopy—Cystoscopy— Urethroscopy—Cystourethroscopy

	52000-52010

Transurethral Surgery

Urethra and Bladder	52204-52318
Ureter and Pelvis	52320-52339
Vesical Neck and Prostate	52340-52700

Urethra

Incision	53000-53085
Excision	53200-53275
Repair	53400-53520
Manipulation	53600-53675

Radiology Services

	74400-74485

E/M Services

	99200-99499

Urinary System

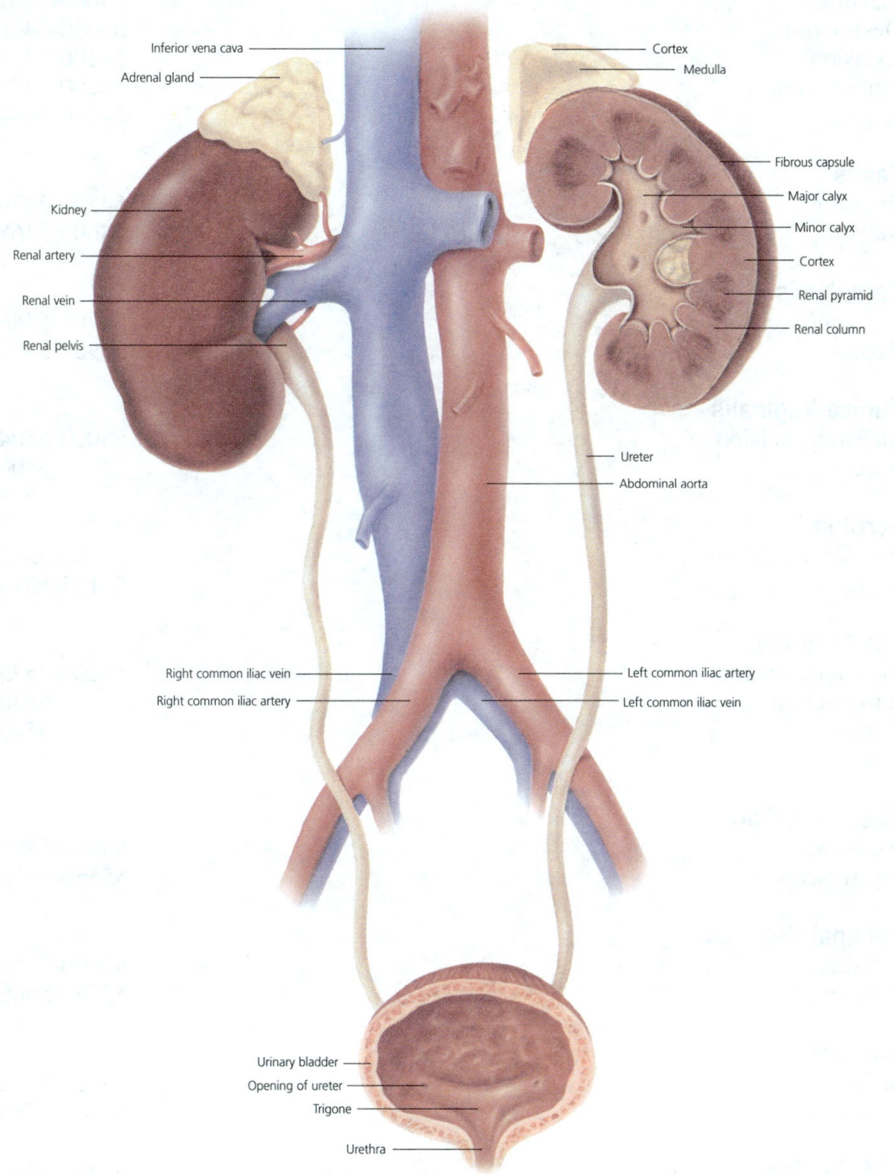

PLATE 18. MALE REPRODUCTIVE SYSTEM

Penis
Incision   54000-54015
Destruction   54050-54065
Excision   54100-54161
Introduction   54200-54250
Repair   54300-54440

Testis
Excision   54500-54560
Repair   54600-54680

Epididymis
Incision/Excision   54700-54861
Repair   54900-54901

Tunica Vaginalis
Incision/Excision   55000-55041
Repair   55060

Scrotum
Incision/Excision   55100-55150
Repair   55175-55180

Vas Deferens
Incision/Excision   55200-55250
Introduction   55300
Repair   55400
Suture   55450

Spermatic Cord
Excision   55500-55540
Laparoscopy   55550-55559

Seminal Vesicles
Incision   55600-55605
Excision   55650-55680

Prostate
Incision   55700-55725
Excision   55801-55865

E/M Services   99200-99499

Male Reproductive System

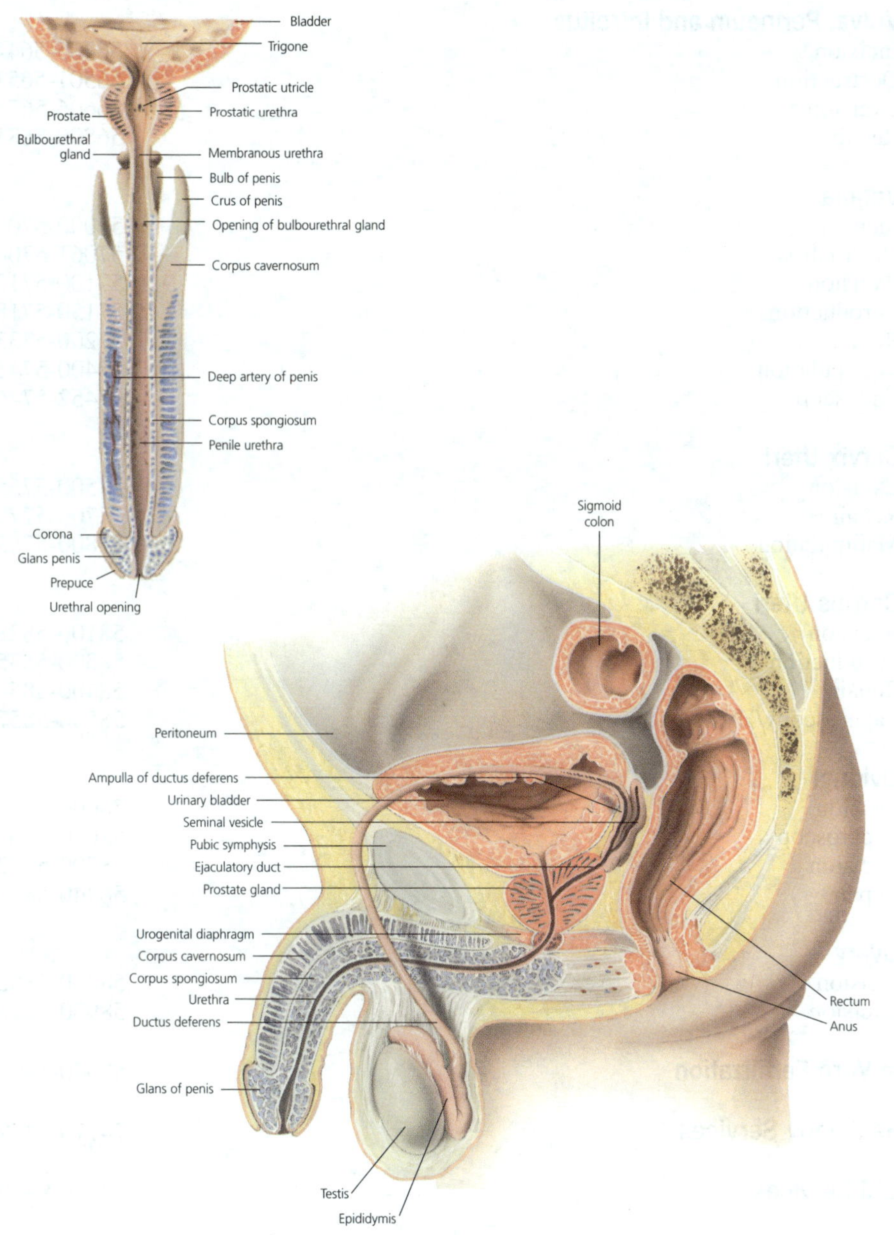

PLATE 19. FEMALE REPRODUCTIVE SYSTEM

Vulva, Perineum and Introitus
Incision	56405-56441
Destruction	56501-56515
Excision	56606-56740
Repair	56800-56810

Vagina
Incision	57000-57020
Destruction	57061-57065
Excision	57100-57135
Introduction	57150-57180
Repair	57200-57335
Manipulation	57400-57415
Endoscopy	57452-57460

Cervix Uteri
Excision	57500-57556
Repair	57700-57720
Manipulation	57800-57820

Corpus Uteri
Excision	58100-58285
Introduction	58300-58350
Repair	58400-58540
Laparoscopy/Hysteroscopy	58550-58579

Oviduct
Incision	58600-58615
Laparoscopy	58660-68679
Excision	58700-58720
Repair	58740-58770

Ovary
Incision	58800-58825
Excision	58900-58960

In Vitro Fertilization
58970-58976

Radiology Services
74710-74775

E/M Services
99200-99499

Female Reproductive System

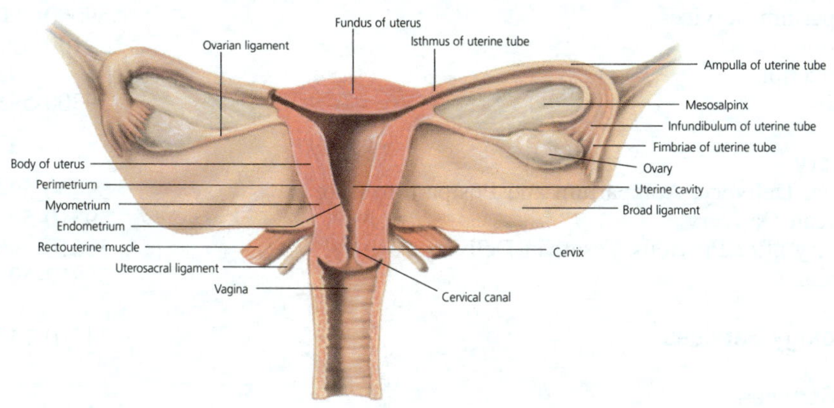

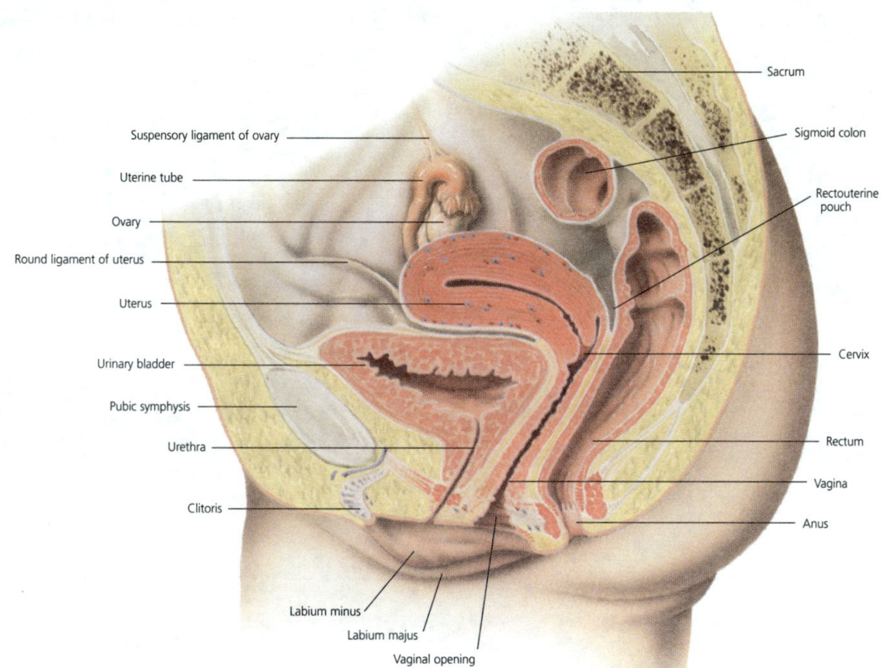

PLATE 20. PREGNANCY, CHILDBIRTH AND THE PUERPERIUM

Antepartum Services
Antepartum Services	59000-59051
Excision	59100-59160
Introduction	59200
Repair	59300-59350

Delivery
Vaginal Delivery, Antepartum and Postpartum Care	59400-59430
Cesarean Delivery	59510-59525
Delivery after Previous Cesarean Delivery	59610-59622
Abortion	59812-59857

Radiology Services
74710-74775

E/M Services
E/M Services	99200-99499
Newborn Care	99431-99440

Female Reproductive System: Pregnancy
(Lateral View)

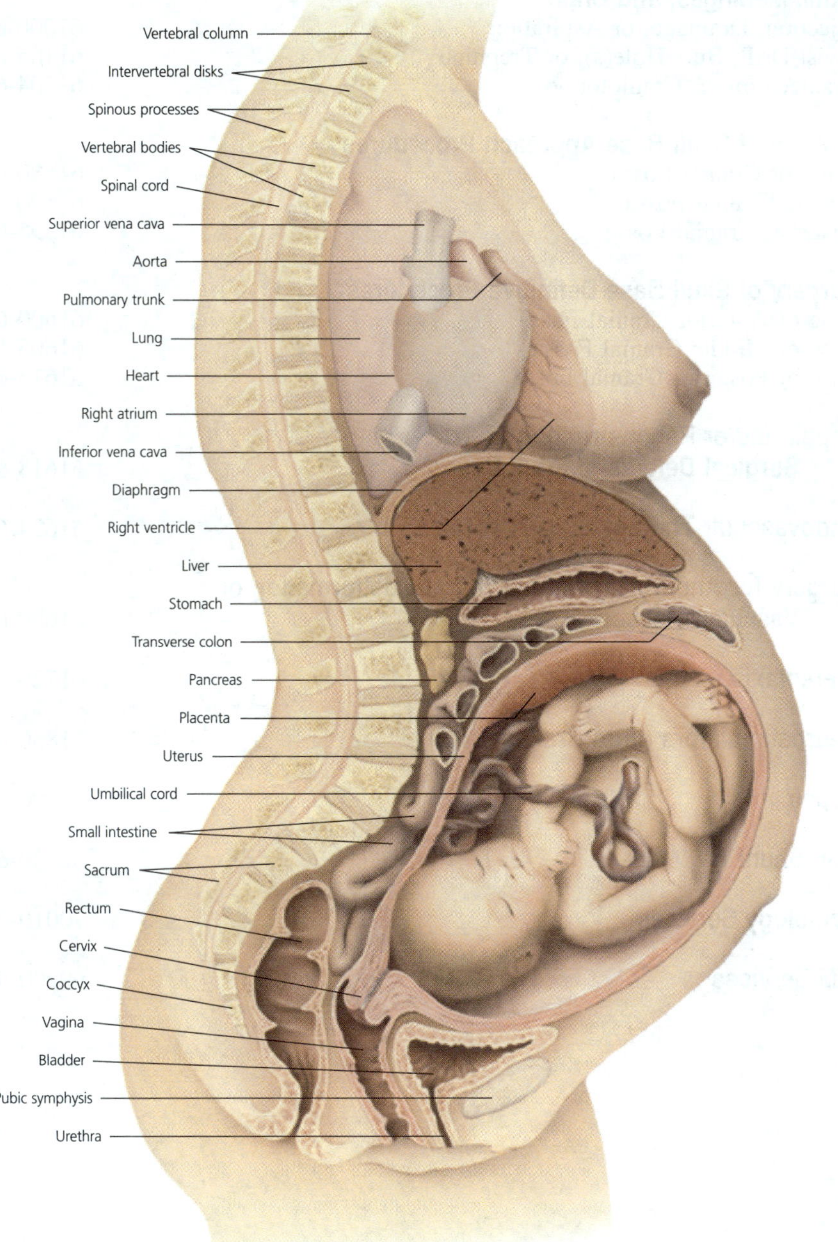

PLATE 21. NERVOUS SYSTEM - BRAIN

Skull, Meninges, and Brain
Injection, Drainage, or Aspiration	61000-61070
Twist Drill, Burr Hole(s), or Trephine	61105-61253
Craniectomy or Craniotomy	61304-61576

Surgery of Skull Base Approach Procedures
Anterior Cranial Fossa	61580-61586
Middle Cranial Fossa	61590-61592
Posterior Cranial Fossa	61595-61598

Surgery of Skull Base Definitive Procedures
Base of Anterior Cranial Fossa	61600-61601
Base of Middle Cranial Fossa	61605-61613
Base of Posterior Cranial Fossa	61615-61616

Repair and/or Reconstruction of Surgical Defects of Skull Base
61618-61619

Endovascular Therapy
61624-61626

Surgery for Aneurysm, Arterio-Venous Malformation or Vascular Disease
61680-61711

Stereotaxis
61720-61795

Neurostimulators (Intra-Cranial)
61850-61888

Repair
62000-62147

CSF Shunt
62180-62258

Radiology Services
70010-70553

E/M Services
99200-99499

Brain
(Base View)

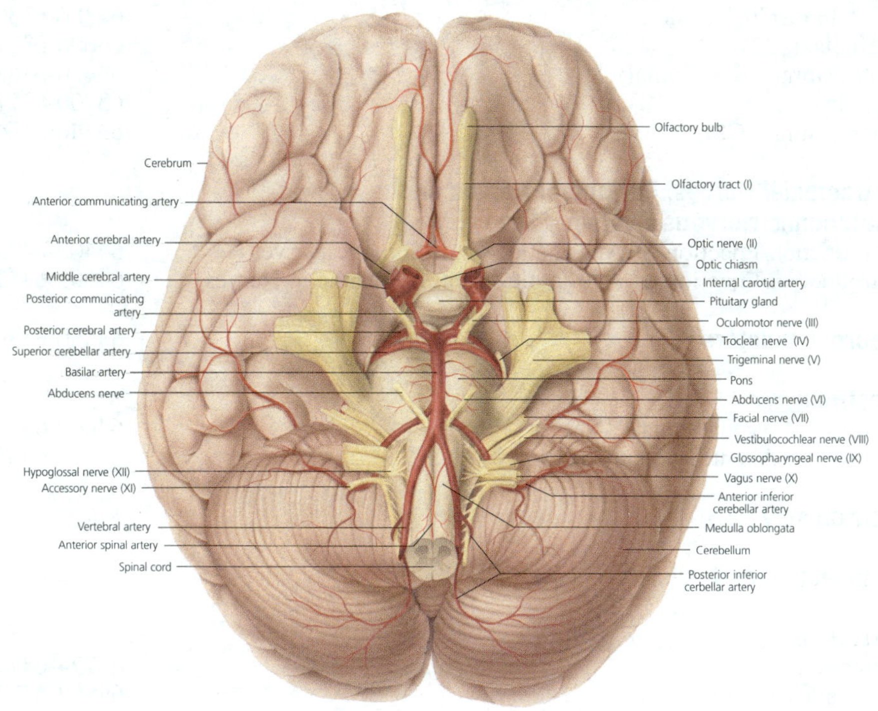

PLATE 22. NERVOUS SYSTEM

Spine and Spinal Cord

Injection, Drainage or Aspiration	62263-62319
Catheter Implantation	62350-62368
Posterior Extradural Laminotomy or Laminectomy	63001-63048
Transpedicular or Costovertebral Approach	63055-63066
Anterior or Anterolateral Approach	63075-63091
Incision	63170-63200
Excision by Laminectomy of Lesion	63250-63290
Excision, Anterior or Anterolateral Approach Intraspinal Lesion	63300-63308
Stereotaxis	63600-63615
Neurostimulators (Spinal)	63650-63688
Repair	63700-63710
Shunt, Spinal CSF	63740-63746

Extracranial Nerves, Peripheral Nerves and Autonomic Nervous System

Introduction/Injection of Anesthetic Agent Somatic Nerves	64400-64450
Introduction/Injection of Anesthetic Agent Sympathetic Nerves	64505-64530

Neurostimulators

64550-64595

Destruction

Neurolytic Agent Somatic Nerves	64600-64640
Neurolytic Agent Sympathetic Nerves	64680

Neuroplasty

64702-64727

Transection or Avulsion

64732-64772

Excision

Somatic Nerves	64774-64795
Sympathetic Nerves	64802-64820

Neurorrhaphy

Without Nerve Graft	64831-64876
With Nerve Graft	64885-64907

E/M Services

99200-99499

Nervous System

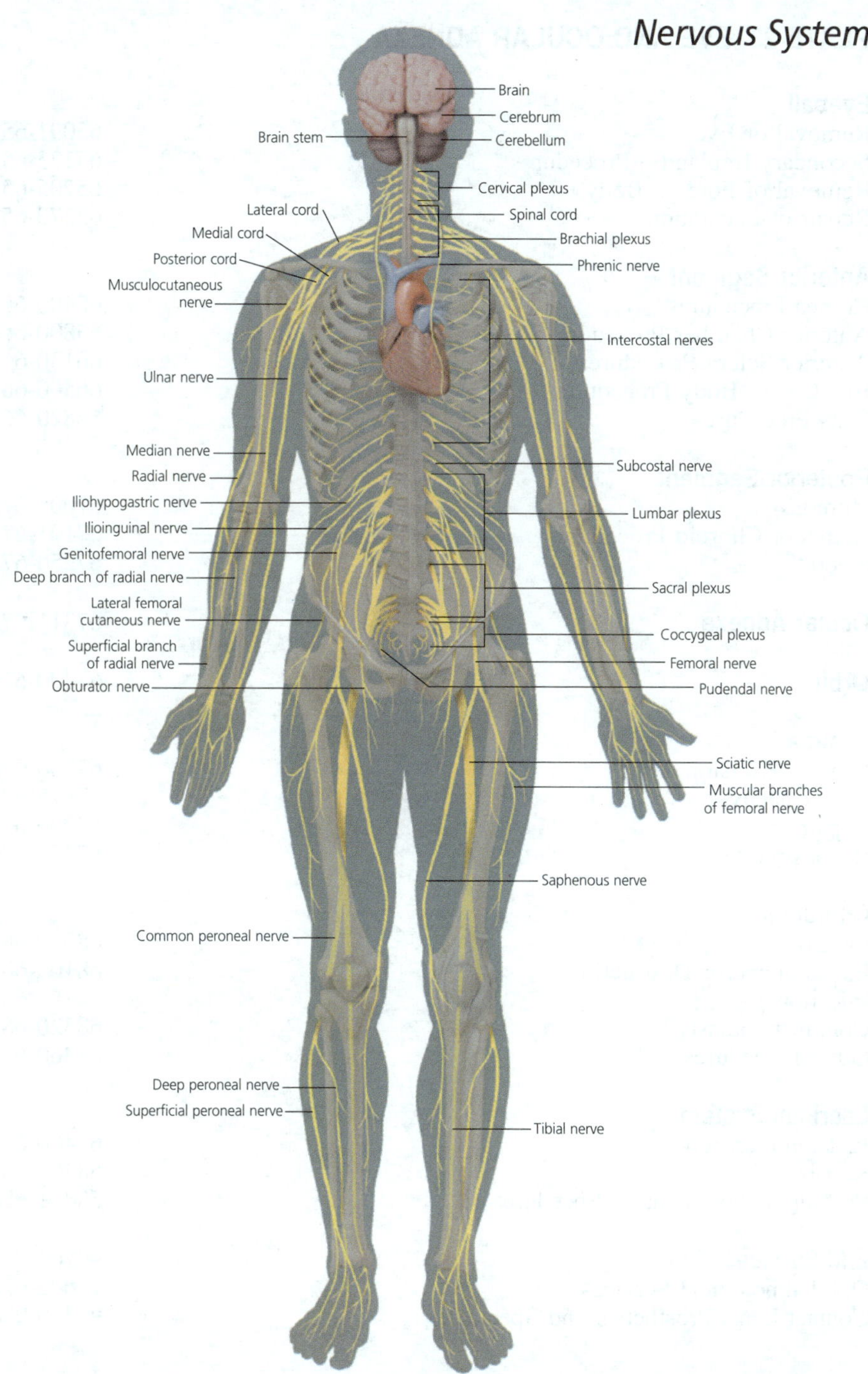

PLATE 23. EYE AND OCULAR ADNEXA

Eyeball
Removal of Eye   65091-65114
Secondary Implant(s) Procedures   65125-65175
Removal of Foreign Body   65205-65265
Repair of Laceration   65270-65290

Anterior Segment
Cornea Procedures   65400-65775
Anterior Chamber Procedures   65800-66030
Anterior Sclera Procedures   66130-66250
Iris, Ciliary Body Procedures   66500-66770
Lens Procedures   66820-66986

Posterior Segment
Vitreous   67005-67040
Retina or Choroid Procedures   67101-67228
Sclera   67250-67255

Ocular Adnexa   67311-67399

Orbit   67400-67599

Eyelids
Incision/Excision   67700-67875
Tarsorrhaphy   67875-67882
Repair   67900-67924
Reconstruction   67930-67975

Conjunctiva
Incision and Drainage   68020-68040
Excision and/or Destruction   68100-68135
Injection   68200
Conjunctivoplasty   68320-68340
Other Procedures   68360-68399

Lacrimal System
Incision/Excision   68400-68550
Repair   68700-68770
Probing and/or Related Procedures   68801-68850

E/M Services   99200-99499
Ophthalmological Services   92002-92887
Contact Lens, Prosthetics and Spectacles   92310-92371

Right Eye
(Horizontal Section)

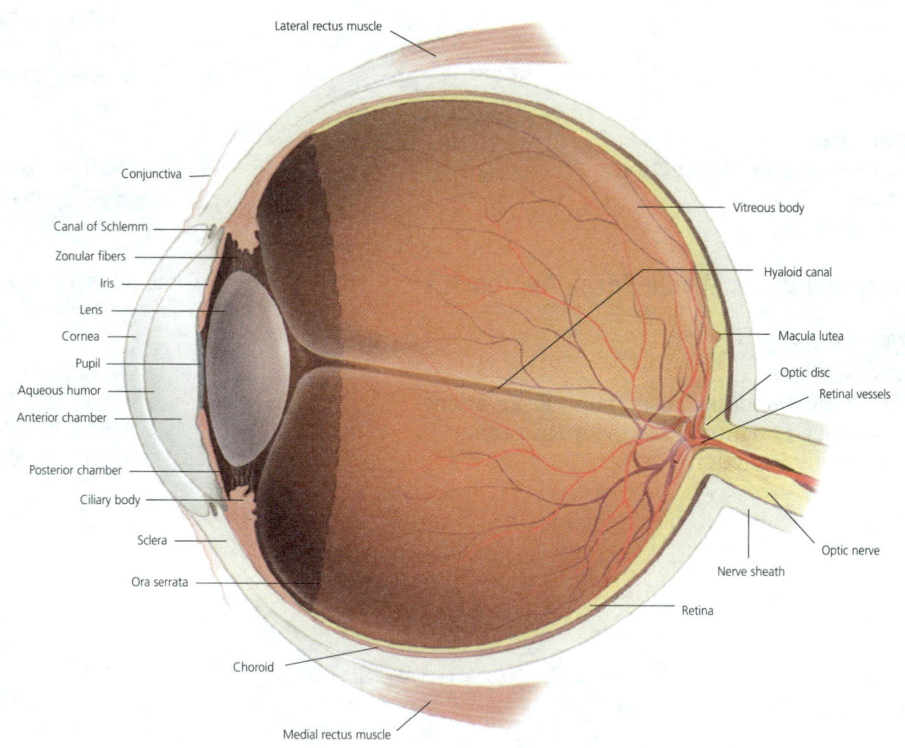

PLATE 24. AUDITORY SYSTEM

External Ear
Incision	69000-69090
Excision	69100-69155
Removal of Foreign Body	69200-69222
Repair	69300-69320

Middle Ear
Introduction	69400-69410
Incision	69420-69554
Repair	69601-69676
Other	69700-69799

Inner Ear
Incision and/or Destruction	69801-69840
Excision	69905-69915
Introduction	69930

Temporal Bone, Middle Fossa Approach
	69950-69970

E/M Services
E/M Services	99200-99499
Vestibular Function Tests with Observation	92531-92534
Vestibular Function Tests with Recording	92541-92548
Audiologic Function Tests	92551-92598

The Ear

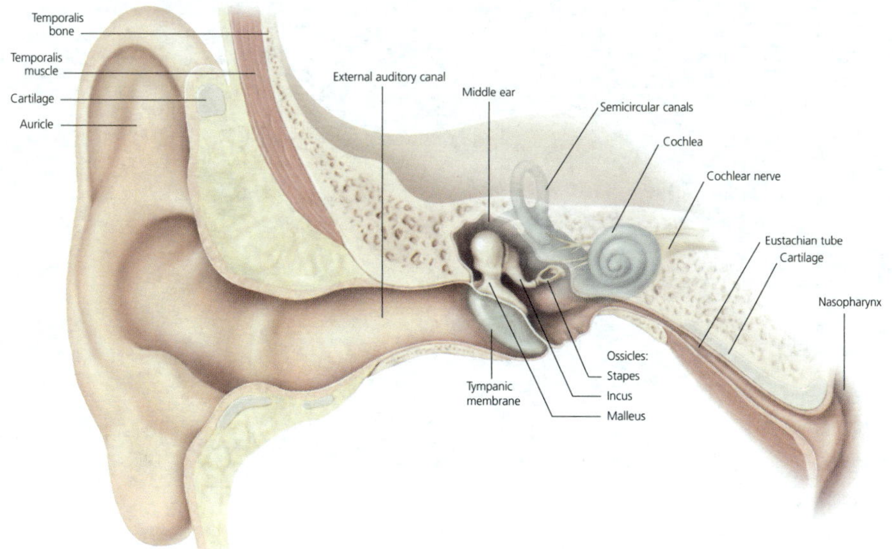

Temporalis bone
Temporalis muscle
Cartilage
Auricle
External auditory canal
Middle ear
Semicircular canals
Cochlea
Cochlear nerve
Eustachian tube
Cartilage
Nasopharynx
Ossicles:
Stapes
Incus
Malleus
Tympanic membrane

EVALUATION & MANAGEMENT SERVICES

EVALUATION AND MANAGEMENT SERVICES OVER-VIEW

The first section of the CPT coding system is the evaluation and management section, which includes procedure codes for visit and special care services. Within each subsection, the CPT codes are arranged by first by patient category, then by level of the service.

The evaluation and management section of the CPT coding system includes codes for reporting visits, consultations, prolonged service, case management services, preventive medicine services, newborn care, and special services. The section is divided into categories such as office visits, hospital visits and consultations. Most of the categories are further divided into two or more subcategories.

The subcategories for evaluation and management services are further classified into levels of service that are identified by specific codes. The level of service classification is important because the physician work required to provide the service varies by the type of service, the place of service, and the patient's clinical status.

The basic format of the evaluation and management service codes and definitions is the same for most categories.

- A unique five-digit CPT code number is listed

- The place and/or type of service is specified, for example "office consultation"

- The content of the service is defined, eg. "comprehensive history and comprehensive examination"

- The nature of the presenting problem(s) usually associated with a given level is described.

- The time typically required to provide the service is specified.

EVALUATION AND MANAGEMENT SERVICES SUBSECTIONS

The Evaluation and Management SECTION of the CPT book is divided into 19 SUBSECTIONS; namely:

Office or Other Outpatient Services	99201-99215
Hospital Observation Discharge Services	99217
Hospital Observation Services	99218-99220
Hospital Inpatient Services	99221-99238
Consultations	99241-99275
Emergency Department Services	99281-99288
Critical Care Services	99291-99292
Neonatal Intensive Care	99295-99297
Nursing Facility Services	99301-99313
Domiciliary, Rest Home or Custodial Care Services	99321-99333
Home Services	99341-99353
Prolonged Services	99354-99359
Standby Services	99360
Case Management Services	99361-99373
Care Plan Oversight Services	99375-99376
Preventive Medicine Services	99381-99249
Newborn Care	99431-99440
Special Evaluation and Management services	99450-99456
Other Evaluation and Management services	99499

All subsections within the Evaluation and Management section have extensive notes that should be reviewed carefully prior to selecting codes for services located within the section.

EVALUATION AND MANAGEMENT (E/M) SERVICES GUIDELINES

In addition to the information presented in the introduction, several other items unique to this section are defined or identified here.

Classification of Evaluation and Management (E/M) Services

The Evaluation and Management section is divided into broad categories such as office visits, hospital visits, and consultations. Most of the categories are further divided into two or more subcategories of evaluation and management services. For example, there are two subcategories of office visits (new patient and established patient) and there are two subcategories of hospital visits (initial and subsequent).

The subcategories of evaluation and management services are further classified into levels of evaluation and management services that are identified by specific codes.

This classification is important because the nature of physician work varies by type of service, place of service, and the patient's status.

The basic format of the levels of evaluation and management services is the same for most categories. First, a unique code number is listed. Second, the place and/or type of service is specified, eg, office consultation. Third, the content of the service is defined, eg, comprehensive history and comprehensive examination. Fourth, the nature of the presenting problem(s) usually associated with a given level is described. Fifth, the time typically required to provide the service is specified.

Definitions of Commonly Used Terms

Certain key words and phrases are used throughout the Evaluation and Management section. The following definitions are intended to reduce the potential for differing interpretations and to increase the consistency of reporting by physicians in differing specialties.

New and Established Patient

Solely for the purposes of distinguishing between new and established patients, professional services are those face-to-face services rendered by a physician and coded by a specific CPT code(s). A **new patient** is one who has not received any professional services from the physician or another physician of the same specialty who belongs to the same group practice, within the past three years.

An **established patient** is one who has received professional services from the physician or another physician of the same specialty who belongs to the same group practice, within the past three years.

In the instance where a physician is on call for or covering for another physician, the patient's encounter will be classified as it would have been by the physician who is not available.

No distinction is made between new and established patients in the emergency department. Evaluation and Management services in the emergency department category may be coded for any new or established patient who presents for treatment in the emergency department.

Chief Complaint

A concise statement describing the symptom, problem, condition, diagnosis or other factor that is the reason for the encounter, usually stated in the patient's words.

Concurrent care

Concurrent care is the provision of similar services, eg, hospital visits, to the same patient by more than one physician on the same day. When concurrent care is provided, no special reporting is required. Modifier '-75' has been deleted.

Counseling

Counseling is a discussion with a patient and/or family concerning one or more of the following areas:

- diagnostic results, impressions, and/or recommended diagnostic studies;
- prognosis;
- risks and benefits of management (treatment) options;
- instructions for management (treatment) and/or follow-up;
- importance of compliance with chosen management (treatment) options;
- risk factor reduction; and
- patient and family education. (For psychotherapy, see 90804-90857)

Family History

A review of medical events in the patient's family that includes significant information about:

- the health status or cause of death of parents, siblings, and children;
- specific diseases related to problems identified in the chief complaint or history of the present illness, and/or system review;
- diseases of family members which may be hereditary or place the patient at risk.

History of Present Illness

A chronological description of the development of the patient's present illness from the first sign and/or symptom to the present. This includes a description of location, quality, severity, timing, context, modifying factors and associated signs and symptoms significantly related to the presenting problem(s).

Levels of Evaluation and Management Services

Within each category or subcategory of evaluation and management service, there are three to five levels of evaluation and management services available for reporting purposes. Levels of evaluation and management services are not interchangeable among the different categories or subcategories of service. For example, the first level of evaluation and management services in the subcategory of office visit, new patient, does not have the same definition as the first level of evaluation and management services in the subcategory of office visit, established patient.

The levels of evaluation and management services include examinations, evaluations, treatments, conferences with or concerning patients, preventive pediatric and adult health supervision, and similar medical services, such as the determination of the need and/or location for appropriate care. Medical screening includes the history, examination, and medical decision making required to determine the need and/or location for appropriate care and treatment of the patient (eg, office and other outpatient setting, emergency department, nursing facility, etc.). The levels of evaluation and management services encompass the wide variations in skill, effort, time, responsibility and medical knowledge required for the prevention or diagnosis and treatment of illness or injury and the promotion of optimal health. Each level of evaluation and management services may be used by all physicians.

The descriptors for the levels of evaluation and management services recognize seven components, six of which are used in defining the levels of evaluation and management services. These components are:

- history;
- examination;
- medical decision making;
- counseling;
- coordination of care;
- nature of presenting problem; and
- time.

The first three of these components (history, examination, and medical decision making) are considered the key components in selecting a level of evaluation and management services. (See "determine the extent of history obtained")

The next three components (counseling, coordination of care, and the nature of the presenting problem) are considered contributory factors in the majority of encounters. Although the first two of these contributory factors are important evaluation and management services, it is not required that these services be provided at every patient encounter.

Coordination of care with other providers or agencies without a patient encounter on that day is coded using the case management codes.

The final component, time, is discussed in detail.

Any specifically identifiable procedure (ie, identified with a specific cpt code) performed on or subsequent to the date of initial or subsequent "Evaluation and management services" should be coded separately. The actual performance and/or interpretation of diagnostic tests/studies ordered during a patient encounter are not included in the levels of evaluation and management services. Physician performance of diagnostic tests/studies for which specific cpt codes are available may be coded separately, in addition to the appropriate evaluation and management code. The physician's interpretation of the results of diagnostic tests/studies (ie, professional component) with preparation of a separate distinctly identifiable signed written report may also be coded separately, using the appropriate cpt code with the modifier '-26' appended.

The physician may need to indicate that on the day a procedure or service identified by a cpt code was performed, the patient's condition required a significant separately identifiable evaluation and management service above and beyond other services provided or beyond the usual preservice and postservice care associated with the procedure that was performed. The evaluation and management service may be caused or prompted by the symptoms or condition for which the procedure and/or service was provided. This circumstance may be coded by adding the modifier '-25' to the appropriate level of evaluation and management service. As such, different diagnoses are not required for reporting of the procedure and the evaluation and management services on the same date.

Nature of Presenting Problem

A presenting problem is a disease, condition, illness, injury, symptom, sign, finding, complaint, or other reason for encounter, with or without a diagnosis being established at the time of the encounter. The evaluation and management codes recognize five types of presenting problems that are defined as follows:

Minimal: a problem that may not require the presence of the physician, but service is provided under the physician's supervision.

Self-limited or minor: a problem that runs a definite and prescribed course, is transient in nature, and is not likely to permanently alter health status or has a good prognosis with management/compliance.

Low severity: a problem where the risk of morbidity without treatment is low; there is little to no risk of mortality without treatment; full recovery without functional impairment is expected.

Moderate severity: a problem where the risk of morbidity without treatment is moderate; there is moderate risk of mortality without treatment; uncertain prognosis or increased probability of prolonged functional impairment.

High severity: a problem where the risk of morbidity without treatment is high to extreme; there is a moderate to high risk of mortality without treatment or high probability of severe, prolonged functional impairment.

Past History

A review of the patient's past experiences with illnesses, injuries, and treatments that includes significant information about:

- prior major illnesses and injuries;
- prior operations;
- prior hospitalizations;
- current medications;
- allergies (eg, drug, food);
- age appropriate immunization status;
- age appropriate feeding/dietary status.

Social History

An age appropriate review of past and current activities that includes significant information about:

- marital status and/or living arrangements;
- current employment;
- occupational history;
- use of drugs, alcohol, and tobacco;
- level of education;
- sexual history;
- other relevant social factors

System Review (Review of Systems)

An inventory of body systems obtained through a series of questions seeking to identify signs and/or symptoms which the patient may be experiencing or has experienced. For the purposes of cpt the following elements of a system review have been identified:

- Constitutional symptoms (fever, weight loss, etc.)
- Eyes
- Ears, nose, mouth, throat
- Cardiovascular
- Respiratory
- Gastrointestinal
- Genitourinary
- Musculoskeletal
- Integumentary (skin and/or breast)
- Neurological
- Psychiatric
- Endocrine
- Hematologic/lymphatic
- Allergic/immunologic

The review of systems helps define the problem, clarify the differential diagnosis, identify needed testing, or serves as baseline data on other systems that might be affected by any possible management options.

Time

The inclusion of time in the definitions of levels of evaluation and management services has been implicit in prior editions of cpt. The inclusion of time as an explicit factor beginning in cpt 1992 is done to assist physicians in selecting the most appropriate level of evaluation and management services. It should be recognized that the specific times expressed in the visit code descriptors are averages, and therefore represent a range of times which may be higher or lower depending on actual clinical circumstances.

Time is not a descriptive component for the emergency department levels of evaluation and management services because emergency department services are typically provided on a variable intensity basis, often involving multiple encounters with several patients over an extended period of time. Therefore, it is often difficult for physicians to provide accurate estimates of the time spent face-to-face with the patient.

Studies to establish levels of evaluation and management services employed surveys of practicing physicians to obtain data on the amount of time and work associated with typical evaluation and management services. Since "work" is not easily quantifiable, the codes must rely on other objective, verifiable measures that correlate with physicians' estimates of their "work". It has been demonstrated that physicians' estimations of intraservice time (as explained on the next page), both within and across specialties, is a variable that is predictive of the "work" of evaluation and management services. This same research has shown there is a strong relationship between intra-service time and total time for evaluation and management services. Intra-service time, rather than total time, was chosen for inclusion with the codes because of its relative ease of measurement and because of its direct correlation with measurements of the total amount of time and work associated with typical evaluation and management services.

Intra-service times are defined as face-to-face time for office and other outpatient visits and as unit/floor time for hospital and other inpatient visits. This distinction is necessary because most of the work of typical office visits takes place during the face-to-face time with the patient, while most of the work of typical hospital visits takes place during the time spent on the patient's floor or unit.

Face-to-face time (office and other outpatient visits and office consultations): for coding purposes, face-to-face time for these services is defined as only that time that the physician spends face-to-face with the patient and/or family. This includes the time in which the physician performs such tasks as obtaining a history, performing an examination, and counseling the patient.

Physicians also spend time doing work before or after the face-to-face time with the patient, performing such tasks as reviewing records and tests, arranging for further services, and communicating further with other professionals and the patient through written reports and telephone contact.

This non-face-to-face time for office services-also called pre- and post-encounter time-is not included in the time component described in the evaluation and management codes. However, the pre- and post-face-to-face work associated with an encounter was included in calculating the total work of typical services in physician surveys.

Thus, the face-to-face time associated with the services described by any evaluation and management code is a valid proxy for the total work done before, during, and after the visit.

Unit/floor time (hospital observation services, inpatient hospital care, initial and follow-up hospital consultations, nursing facility): for reporting purposes, intra-service time for these services is defined as unit/floor time, which includes the time that the physician is present on the patient's hospital unit and at the bedside rendering services for that patient. This includes the time in which the physician establishes and/or reviews the patient's chart, examines the patient, writes notes and communicates with other professionals and the patient's family.

In the hospital, pre- and post-time includes time spent off the patient's floor performing such tasks as reviewing pathology and radiology findings in another part of the hospital.

This pre- and post-visit time is not included in the time component described in these codes. However, the pre- and post-work performed during the time spent off the floor or unit was included in calculating the total work of typical services in physician surveys. Thus, the unit/floor time associated with the services described by any code is a valid proxy for the total work done before, during, and after the visit.

Unlisted Service

An evaluation and management service may be provided that is not listed in this section of cpt. When reporting such a service, the appropriate "unlisted" code may be used to indicate the service, identifying it by "special report", as discussed in the following paragraph. The "unlisted services" and accompanying codes for the evaluation and management section are as follows:

99429	Unlisted preventive medicine service
99499	Unlisted evaluation and management service
99539	Unlisted home visit service or procedure

Special Report

An unlisted service or one that is unusual, variable, or new may require a special report demonstrating the medical appropriateness of the service. Pertinent information should include an adequate definition or description of the nature, extent, and need for the procedure; and the time, effort, and equipment necessary to provide the service. Additional items which may be included are complexity of symptoms, final diagnosis, pertinent physical findings, diagnostic and therapeutic procedures, concurrent problems, and follow-up care.

Clinical Examples

Clinical examples of the codes for evaluation and management services are included in the CPT code book to assist physicians in understanding the meaning of the descriptors and selecting the correct code. The clinical examples are listed in Appendix D of the CPT code book. Each example was developed by physicians in the specialties shown.

The same problem, when seen by physicians in different specialties, may involve different amounts of work. Therefore, the appropriate level of encounter should be coded using the descriptors rather than the examples.

The examples have been tested for validity and approved by the cpt editorial panel. Physicians were given the examples and asked to assign a code or assess the amount of time and work involved. Only those examples that were rated consistently have been included in appendix d.

Instructions for Selecting a Level of Evaluation and Management Service

Identify the Category and Subcategory of Service

The categories and subcategories of codes available for reporting evaluation and management services are shown in Table 1 on the following page.

Review the Reporting Instructions for the Selected Category or Subcategory

Most of the categories and many of the subcategories of service have special guidelines or instructions unique to that category or subcategory. Where these are indicated, eg, "inpatient hospital care," special instructions will be presented preceding the levels of evaluation and management services.

Review the Level of Evaluation and Management Service Descriptors and Examples in the Selected Category or Subcategory

The descriptors for the levels of evaluation and management services recognize seven components, six of which are used in defining the levels of evaluation and management services. These components are:

- history;
- examination;
- medical decision making;
- counseling;
- coordination of care;
- nature of presenting problem; and
- time.

The first three of these components (ie, history, examination, and medical decision making) should be considered the key components in selecting the level of evaluation and management services. An exception to this rule is in the case of visits which consist predominantly of counseling or coordination of care.

The nature of the presenting problem and time are provided in some levels to assist the physician in determining the appropriate level of evaluation and management service.

Determine the Extent of History Obtained

The extent of the history is dependent upon clinical judgment and on the nature of presenting problems(s). The levels of evaluation and management services recognize four types of history that are defined as follows:

Problem focused: chief complaint; brief history of present illness or problem.

Expanded problem focused: chief complaint; brief history of present illness; problem pertinent system review.

Detailed: chief complaint; extended history of present illness; problem pertinent system review extended to include a review of a limited number of additional systems; pertinent past, family, and/or social history directly related to the patient's problems.

Comprehensive: chief complaint; extended history of present illness; review of systems which is directly related to the problem(s) identified in the history of the present illness plus a review of all additional body systems; complete past, family, and social history.

Table 1: Categories and subcategories of service

Category/subcategory	Code Numbers
Office or other outpatient services	
Nursing facility discharge services	99315-99316
New patient	99201-99205
Established patient	99211-99215
Hospital observation discharge services	99217
Hospital observation services	99218-99220
Hospital observation or inpatient care home services	
(including admission and new patient Discharge services)	99234-99236
Hospital inpatient services	
Initial hospital care	99221-99223
Subsequent hospital care	99231-99233
Hospital discharge services	99238-99239
Consultations	
Office consultations	99241-99245
Initial inpatient consultations	99251-99255
Follow-up inpatient consultations	99261-99263
Confirmatory consultations	99271-99275
Emergency department services	99281-99288
Patient transport	99289-99290
Critical care services	99291-99292
Neonatal intensive care	99295-99298
Nursing facility services	
Comprehensive nursing facility Assessments	99301-99303
Subsequent nursing facility care	99311-99313
Nursing facility discharge services	99315-99316
Domiciliary, rest home or custodial Care services new patient	99321-99323
Established patient	99331-99333
Home services	
New patient	99341-99345
Established patient	99347-99350
Prolonged services	
With direct patient contact	99354-99357
Without direct patient contact	99358-99359
Standby services	99360
Case management services	
Team conferences	99361-99362
Telephone calls	99371-99373
Care plan oversight services	99374-99380
Preventive medicine services	
New patient	99381-99387
Established patient	99391-99397
Individual counseling	99401-99404
Group counseling	99411-99412
Other	99420-99429
Newborn care	99431-99440
Special Evaluation and Management services	99450-99456
Other Evaluation and Management services	99499

The comprehensive history obtained as part of the preventive medicine evaluation and management service is not problem-oriented and does not involve a chief complaint or present illness. It does, however, include a comprehensive system review and comprehensive or interval past, family, and social history as well as a comprehensive assessment/history of pertinent risk factors.

Determine the Extent of Examination Performed

The extent of the examination performed is dependent on clinical judgment and on the nature of the presenting problem(s). The levels of evaluation and management services recognize four types of examination that are defined as follows:

Problem focused: a limited examination of the affected body area or organ system.

Expanded problem focused: a limited examination of the affected body area or organ system and other symptomatic or related organ system(s).

Detailed: an extended examination of the affected body area(s) and other symptomatic or related organ system(s).

Comprehensive: a general multi-system examination or a complete examination of a single organ system. Note: the comprehensive examination performed as part of the preventive medicine evaluation and management service is multisystem, but its extent is based on age and risk factors identified.

For the purposes of these cpt definitions, the following body areas are recognized:

- Head, including the face
- Neck
- Chest, including breasts and axilla
- Abdomen
- Genitalia, groin, buttocks
- Back
- Each extremity

For the purposes of these cpt definitions, the following organ systems are recognized:

- Eyes
- Ears, nose, mouth, and throat
- Cardiovascular
- Respiratory
- Gastrointestinal
- Genitourinary
- Musculoskeletal
- Skin
- Neurologic
- Psychiatric

- Hematologic/lymphatic/immunologic

Determine the Complexity of Medical Decision Making

Medical decision making refers to the complexity of establishing a diagnosis and/or selecting a management option as measured by:

- the number of possible diagnoses and/or the number of management options that must be considered;
- the amount and/or complexity of medical records, diagnostic tests, and/or other information that must be obtained, reviewed, and analyzed; and
- the risk of significant complications, morbidity, and/or mortality, as well as comorbidities, associated with the patient's presenting problems(s), the diagnostic procedure(s) and/or the possible management options.

Four types of medical decision making are recognized: straightforward; low complexity; moderate complexity; and high complexity. To qualify for a given type of decision making, two of the three elements in table 2 on the following page must be met or exceeded.

Comorbidities/underlying diseases, in and of themselves, are not considered in selecting a level of evaluation and management services unless their presence significantly increases the complexity of the medical decision making.

Select the appropriate level of Evaluation and Management services based on the following

1. For the following categories/subcategories, **all of the key components**, ie, history, examination, and medical decision making, must meet or exceed the stated requirements to qualify for a particular level of evaluation and management service: office, new patient; hospital observation services; initial hospital care; office consultations; initial inpatient consultations; confirmatory consultations; emergency department services; comprehensive nursing facility assessments; domiciliary care, new patient; and home, new patient.

2. For the following categories/subcategories, **two of the three key components** (ie, history, examination, and medical decision making) must meet or exceed the stated requirements to qualify for a particular level of evaluation and management services: office, established patient; subsequent hospital care; follow-up inpatient consultations; subsequent nursing facility care; domiciliary care, established patient; and home, established patient.

Table 2: Complexity of medical decision making

Number of diagnoses of Management Options	Amount and/or Complexity of Data to be Reviewed	Risk of complications and/or Morbidity or Mortality	Type of Decision Making
minimal	minimal or none	minimal	straightforward
limited	limited	moderate	low complexity
multiple	moderate	moderate	moderate complexity
extensive	extensive	high	high complexity

3.   When counseling and/or coordination of care dominates (more than 50%) the physician/patient and/or family encounter (face-to-face time in the office or other outpatient setting or floor/unit time in the hospital or nursing facility), then **time** may be considered the key or controlling factor to qualify for a particular level of evaluation and management services. This includes time spent with parties who have assumed responsibility for the care of the patient or decision making whether or not they are family members (eg, foster parents, person acting in locum parentis, legal guardian). The extent of counseling and/or coordination of care must be documented in the medical record.

Other Definitions of Nature of the Presenting Problem

In addition to the above five specific definitions found in the CPT coding system, there are other definitions found in the evaluation and management service codes used to report Subsequent Hospital Care and Follow-up Inpatient Consultations. See Table 3 for these additional definitions.

Table 3: Other Definitions of Nature of Presenting Problems

Evaluation and Management Codes	Nature of Presenting Problem(s) Defined	Equivalent To
99231 or 99261	Stable, recovering or improving	Self-limited or minor
99232 or 99262	Inadequate response or minor complication	Low to moderate severity
99233 or 99263	Significant complication or new problem	Moderate to high severity

DIAGNOSTIC TESTS OR STUDIES

The performance of diagnostic tests or studies for which specific CPT codes are available is not included in the levels of evaluation and management services. Any diagnostic tests or studies performed by the physician for which specific CPT codes are available should be coded separately, in addition to the appropriate evaluation and management service code.

EVALUATION AND MANAGEMENT SERVICES MODIFIERS

Evaluation and management services may be modified under certain circumstances. When applicable, the modifying circumstance should be identified by reporting the appropriate modifier code in addition to the basic service. Modifiers which may be used with evaluation and management service codes are:

-21 Prolonged evaluation and management services

-24 Unrelated evaluation and management service by the same physician during a postoperative period

-25 Significant, separately identifiable evaluation and management service by the same physician on the day of a procedure

-32 Mandated services

-52 Reduced services

-57 Decision for surgery

HOW TO CHOOSE EVALUATION AND MANAGEMENT CODE(S)

Choosing the correct evaluation and management service code to report is a nine step process. The most important steps, in terms of both reimbursement and audit liability, are verifying compliance and documentation. The italicized items represent an example of the selection process.

1. **Identify the Category of Service**

    Where was the patient seen and what category of services were provided?

    ☐ Office or Other Outpatient Services
    ☐ Hospital Observation Services
    ☐ Hospital Inpatient Services
    ☐ Consultations
    ☐ Emergency Department Services
    ☐ Critical Care Services

☐ Neonatal Intensive Care
☐ Nursing Facility Services
☐ Domiciliary, Rest Home or Custodial Care Services
☐ Home Services
☐ Prolonged Services
☐ Standby Services
☐ Case Management Services
☐ Preventive Medicine Services
☐ Newborn Care
☐ Special or Other evaluation and management services

2. Identify the Subcategory of Service

Is the patient a new patient or established patient?
Is the service initial care, subsequent care or follow-up?

☐ New Patient
☐ Established Patient
☐ Initial Care
☐ Subsequent Care
☐ Follow-up

3. Determine the Extent of History Obtained

What level of history was taken on this patient?

☐ Problem Focused
☐ Expanded Problem Focused
☐ Detailed
☐ Comprehensive

4. Determine the Extent of Examination Performed

What level of physician examination was performed?

☐ Problem Focused
☐ Expanded Problem Focused
☐ Detailed
☐ Comprehensive

5. Determine the Complexity of Medical Decision Making

What level of medical decision making was required?

☐ Straightforward
☐ Low Complexity
☐ Moderate Complexity

□   High Complexity

6. **Record the Approximate Amount of Time**

How much time was spent either face-to-face with the patient for office visits and consults, or unit or floor time for hospital care, hospital consults, and nursing facilities?

If counseling and/or coordination of care exceeds 50 percent of the total face-to-face physician/patient encounter, then TIME is considered to be the key or controlling factor which qualifies the choice of a particular level of evaluation and management service. The extent of counseling and/or coordination of care must be documented in the medical record.

7. **Verify Compliance with Reporting Requirements**

<u>All Three Key Components Required</u>

To report services to new patients, initial care, office or confirmatory consultations, emergency department services, and comprehensive nursing facility assessments, all three key components must meet or exceed the stated requirements.

□ History component met or exceeded
□ Examination component met or exceeded
□ Medical decision making component met or exceeded

<u>Two of Three Key Components Required</u>

To report services to established patients, subsequent or follow-up care, two of the three key components must meet or exceed the stated requirements.

□ History component met or exceeded; and/or
□ Examination component met or exceeded; and/or
□ Medical decision making component met or exceeded

8. **Verify Documentation**

Make sure that the medical record includes proper documentation of the history, examination, medical decision making, the nature of the problem(s), the approximate amount of time, and when appropriate, the extent of counseling and/or coordination of care.

9. **Assign the Code**

The following is an example of the code selection process.

EXAMPLE OF THE CODE SELECTION PROCESS

1.	Category of Service	*Office*
2.	Subcategory	*New patient*
3.	History	*Problem focused*
4.	Examination	*Problem focused*
5.	Medical Decision Making	*Straightforward*
6.	Intra-service Time	*10 minutes*
7.	Key Components	*Met or exceeded*
8.	Documentation	*Met or exceeded*
9.	Assign the Code	***99201***

EVALUATION AND MANAGEMENT SERVICES DOCUMENTATION GUIDELINES

Documentation in the medical records of all services provided is critical in terms of reimbursement and audit liability. If the provider reported a service or procedure on the health insurance claim form but did not document it, or document it completely, in the patient's medical records, from the point of view of Medicare or private health insurance company auditors, the service was not performed, can't be reported, and therefore will not be paid for.

Millions of dollars are reclaimed from physicians and other medical professionals annually by Medicare and other third party payers because the medical record documentation does not support the services and procedures reported. Providers can protect their medical practices from audit liability by following the most current documentation guidelines published by HCFA.

The following documentation guidelines for evaluation and management services were developed jointly by the American Medical Association (AMA) and HCFA. The stated goal of HCFA in publishing these guidelines is to provide physicians and health insurance claims reviewers with advice about preparing or reviewing documentation for evaluation and management services.

In developing and testing the validity of these guidelines, special emphasis was placed on assuring that they:

- are consistent with the clinical descriptors and definitions contained in CPT,

- would be widely accepted by clinicians and minimize any changes in record-keeping practices, and

- would be interpreted and applied uniformly by users across the country.

WHAT IS DOCUMENTATION AND WHY IS IT IMPORTANT?

Medical record documentation is required to record pertinent facts, findings, and observations about an individual's health history including past and present illnesses, examinations, tests, treatments, and outcomes. The medical record chronologically documents the care of the patient and is an important element contributing to high quality care. The medical record facilitates:

- the ability of the physician and other medical professionals to evaluate and plan the patient's immediate treatment, and to monitor his/her health care over time.

- communication and continuity of care among physicians and other medical professionals involved in the patient's care;

- accurate and timely claims review and payment;

- appropriate utilization review and quality of care evaluations; and

- collection of data that may be useful for research and education.

An appropriately documented medical record can reduce many of the "hassles" associated with claims processing and may serve as a legal document to verify the care provided, if necessary.

WHAT DO THIRD PARTY PAYERS WANT AND WHY?

Because payers have a contractual obligation to enrollees, they may require reasonable documentation that services are consistent with the insurance coverage provided. They may request information to validate:

- the site of service;

- the medical necessity and appropriateness of the diagnostic and/or therapeutic services provided; and/or

- that services provided have been accurately reported.

GENERAL PRINCIPLES OF MEDICAL RECORD DOCUMENTATION

The principles of documentation listed below are applicable to all types of medical and surgical services in all settings. For evaluation and management (E/M) services, the nature and amount of physician work and documentation varies by type of service, place of service and the patient's status. The general principles listed below may be modified to account for these variable circumstances in providing evaluation and management services.

1. The medical record should be complete and legible.

2. The documentation of each patient encounter should include:

   - reason for the encounter and relevant history, physical examination findings and prior diagnostic test results;

   - assessment, clinical impression or diagnosis;

   - plan for care; and

   - date and legible identity of the observer.

3. If not documented, the rationale for ordering diagnostic and other ancillary services should be easily inferred.

4. Past and present diagnoses should be accessible to the treating and/or consulting physician.

5. Appropriate health risk factors should be identified.

6. The patient's progress, response to and changes in treatment, and revision of diagnosis should be documented.

7. CPT and ICD-9-CM codes reported on the health insurance claim form or patient billing statement should be supported by the documentation in the medical record.

DOCUMENTATION OF EVALUATION AND MANAGEMENT SERVICES

This section provides definitions and documentation guidelines for the three key components of evaluation and management services and for visits which consist predominately of counseling or coordination of care. The three key components—history, examination, and medical decision making—appear in the descriptors for office and other outpatient services, hospital observation services, hospital inpatient services, consultations, emergency department services, nursing facility services, domiciliary care services, and home services. Note that documentation guidelines are identified by the symbol ·**DG**.

The descriptors for the levels of evaluation and management services recognize seven components which are used in defining the levels of evaluation and management services. These components are:

- history
- examination
- medical decision making
- counseling
- coordination of care
- nature of presenting problem
- time

The first three of these components (i.e., history, examination and medical decision making) are the key components in selecting the level of evaluation and management services. In the case of visits which consist predominantly of counseling or coordination of care, time is the key or controlling factor to qualify for a particular level of evaluation and management service.

Because the level of evaluation and management service is dependent on two or three key components, performance and documentation of one component (e.g., examination) at the highest level does not necessarily mean that the encounter in its entirety qualifies for the highest level of evaluation and management service.

These documentation guidelines for evaluation and management services reflect the needs of the typical adult population. For certain groups of patients, the recorded information may vary slightly from that described here.

Specifically, the medical records of infants, children, adolescents and pregnant women may have additional or modified information recorded in each history and examination area.

As an example, newborn records may include under history of the present illness, the details of mother's pregnancy and the infant's status at birth; social history will focus on family structure; family history will focus on congenital anomalies and hereditary disorders in the family. In addition, the content of a pediatric examination will vary with the age and development of the child. Although not specifically defined in these documentation guidelines, these patient group variations on history and examination are appropriate.

DOCUMENTATION OF HISTORY

The levels of evaluation and management services are based on four types of history (Problem Focused, Expanded Problem Focused, Detailed, and Comprehensive). Each type of history includes some or all of the following elements:

- Chief complaint
- History of present illness
- Review of systems
- Past, family and/or social history

The extent of history of present illness, review of systems and past, family and/or social history that is obtained and documented is dependent upon clinical judgement and the nature of the presenting problem(s).

The following chart shows the progression of the elements required for each type of history. To qualify for a given type of history all three elements in the table must be met. (A chief complaint is indicated at all levels.)

Present History	Review of Systems	Past, Family or Social History	Type of History
Brief	N/A	N/A	*Problem Focused*
Brief	Problem Pertinent	N/A	*Expanded Problem Focused*
Extended	Extended	Pertinent	*Detailed*
Extended	Complete	Complete	*Comprehensive*

•DG: The chief complaint, review of systems and past, family and/or social history may be listed as separate elements of history, or they may be included in the description of the history of the present illness.

•DG: A review of systems and/or a past, family and/or social history obtained during an earlier encounter does not need to be re-recorded if there is evidence that the physician reviewed and updated the previous information. This may occur when a physician updates his or her own record or in an institutional setting or group practice where many physicians use a common record. The review and update may be documented by:

- describing any new review of systems and/or past, family and/or social history information or noting there has been no change in the information; and

- noting the date and location of the earlier review of systems and/or past, family and/or social history.

•DG: The review of systems and/or past, family and/or social history may be recorded by ancillary staff or on a form completed by the patient. To document that the physician reviewed the information, there must be a notation supplementing or confirming the information recorded by others.

•DG: If the physician is unable to obtain a history from the patient or other source, the record should describe the patient's condition or other circumstance which precludes obtaining a history.

Definitions and specific documentation guidelines for each of the elements of history are listed below.

CHIEF COMPLAINT

The chief complaint is a concise statement describing the symptom, problem, condition, diagnosis, physician recommended return, or other factor that is the reason for the encounter, usually stated in the patient's words.

•DG: The medical record should clearly reflect the chief complaint.

HISTORY OF PRESENT ILLNESS

The history of present illness is a chronological description of the development of the patient's present illness from the first sign and/or symptom or from the previous encounter to the present. It includes the following elements:

- location
- quality
- severity
- duration
- timing

- context
- modifying factors
- associated signs and symptoms

Brief and extended history of present illnesses are distinguished by the amount of detail needed to accurately characterize the clinical problem(s). A brief history of present illness consists of one to three elements of the history of present illness.

•**DG:** The medical record should describe one to three elements of the present illness (history of present illness).

An extended history of present illness consists of at least four elements of the history of present illness or the status of at least three chronic or inactive conditions.

•**DG:** Medical record should describe at least four elements of the present illness (history of present illness), or the status of at least three chronic or inactive conditions.

REVIEW OF SYSTEMS

A review of systems is an inventory of body systems obtained through a series of questions seeking to identify signs and/or symptoms which the patient may be experiencing or has experienced. For purposes of review of systems, the following systems are recognized:

- Constitutional symptoms (e.g., fever, weight loss)
- Eyes
- Ears, Nose, Mouth, Throat
- Cardiovascular
- Respiratory
- Gastrointestinal
- Genitourinary
- Musculoskeletal
- Integumentary (skin and/or breast)
- Neurological
- Psychiatric
- Endocrine
- Hematologic/Lymphatic
- Allergic/Immunologic

A problem pertinent review of systems inquires about the system directly related to the problem(s) identified in the history of present illness.

•**DG:** The patient's positive responses and pertinent negatives for the system related to the problem should be documented.

An extended review of systems inquires about the system directly related to the problem(s) identified in the history of present illness and a limited number of additional systems.

•DG: The patient's positive responses and pertinent negatives for two to nine systems should be documented.

A complete review of systems inquires about the system(s) directly related to the problem(s) identified in the history of present illness *plus* all additional body systems.

•DG: At least ten organ systems must be reviewed. Those systems with positive or pertinent negative responses must be individually documented. For the remaining systems, a notation indicating all other systems are negative is permissible. In the absence of such a notation, at least ten systems must be individually documented.

PAST, FAMILY AND/OR SOCIAL HISTORY

The past, family and/or social history consists of a review of three areas:

- past history (the patient's past experiences with illnesses, operations, injuries and treatments);

- family history (a review of medical events in the patient's family, including diseases which may be hereditary or place the patient at risk); and

- social history (an age appropriate review of past and current activities).

For certain categories of evaluation and management services that include only an interval history, it is not necessary to record information about the past, family and/or social history. Those categories are subsequent hospital care, follow-up inpatient consultations and subsequent nursing facility care.

A pertinent past, family and/or social history is a review of the history area(s) directly related to the problem(s) identified in the history of present illness.

•DG: At least one specific item from any of the three history areas must be documented for a pertinent past, family and/or social history .

A complete past, family and/or social history is of a review of two or all three of the past, family and/or social history areas, depending on the category of the evaluation and management service. A review of all three history areas is required for services that by their nature include a comprehensive assessment or reassessment of the patient. A review of two of the three history areas is sufficient for other services.

•DG: At least one specific item from two of the three history areas must be documented for a complete past, family and/or social history for the following categories of evaluation and management services: office or other outpatient services, established patient; emergency department; domiciliary care, established patient; and home care, established patient.

•DG: At least one specific item from each of the three history areas must be documented for a complete past, family and/or social history for the following categories of evaluation and management services: office or other outpatient services, new patient; hospital observation services; hospital inpatient services, initial care; consultations; comprehensive nursing facility assessments; domiciliary care, new patient; and home care, new patient.

DOCUMENTATION OF EXAMINATION

The levels of evaluation and management services are based on four types of examination:

- Problem Focused — a limited examination of the affected body area or organ system.

- Expanded Problem Focused — a limited examination of the affected body area or organ system and any ther symptomatic or related body area(s) or organ system(s).

- Detailed — an extended examination of the affected body area(s) or organ system(s) and any other symptomatic or related body area(s) or organ system(s).

- Comprehensive — a general multi-system examination, or complete examination of a single organ system and other symptomatic or related body area(s) or organ system(s).

These types of examinations have been defined for general multi-system and the following single organ systems:

- Cardiovascular
- Ears, Nose, Mouth and Throat
- Eyes
- Genitourinary (Female)
- Genitourinary (Male)
- Hematologic/Lymphatic/Immunologic
- Musculoskeletal
- Neurological
- Psychiatric
- Respiratory
- Skin

A general multi-system examination or a single organ system examination may be performed by any physician regardless of specialty. The type (general multi-system or single organ system) and content of examination are selected by the examining physician and are based upon clinical judgement, the patient's history, and the nature of the presenting problem(s).

The content and documentation requirements for each type and level of examination are summarized below and described in detail in tables beginning on page 32. In the tables, organ systems and body areas recognized by CPT for purposes of describing examinations are shown in the left column. The content, or individual elements, of the examination pertaining to that body area or organ system are identified by bullets (■) in the right column.

Parenthetical examples, (e.g., ...), have been used for clarification and to provide guidance regarding documentation. Documentation for each element must satisfy any numeric requirements (such as "Measurement of any three of the following seven...") included in the description of the element. Elements with multiple components but with no specific numeric requirement (such as "Examination of liver and spleen") require documentation of at least one component. It is possible for a given examination to be expanded beyond what is defined here. When that occurs, findings related to the additional systems and/or areas should be documented.

•DG: Specific abnormal and relevant negative findings of the examination of the affected or symptomatic body area(s) or organ system(s) should be documented. A notation of "abnormal" without elaboration is insufficient.

•DG: Abnormal or unexpected findings of the examination of any asymptomatic body area(s) or organ system(s) should be described.

•DG: A brief statement or notation indicating "negative" or "normal" is sufficient to document normal findings related to unaffected area(s) or asymptomatic organ system(s).

General Multi-System Examinations

To qualify for a given level of multi-system examination, the following content and documentation requirements should be met:

■   Problem Focused Examination-should include performance and documentation of one to five elements identified by a bullet (•) in one or more organ system(s) or body area(s).

■   Expanded Problem Focused Examination-should include performance and documentation of at least six elements identified by a bullet (•) in one or more organ system(s) or body area(s).

- Detailed Examination — should include at least six organ systems or body areas. For each system/area selected, performance and documentation of at least two elements identified by a bullet (•) is expected. Alternatively, a detailed examination may include performance and documentation of at least twelve elements identified by a bullet (•) in two or more organ systems or body areas.

- Comprehensive Examination — should include at least nine organ systems or body areas. For each system/area selected, all elements of the examination identified by a bullet (•) should be performed, unless specific directions limit the content of the examination. For each area/system, documentation of at least two elements identified by a bullet is expected.

Single Organ System Examinations

Variations among single organ system examinations in the organ systems and body areas identified in the left columns and in the elements of the examinations described in the right columns reflect differing emphases among specialties. To qualify for a given level of single organ system examination, the following content and documentation requirements should be met:

- Problem Focused Examination — should include performance and documentation of one to five elements identified by a bullet (•), whether in a box with a shaded or unshaded border.

- Expanded Problem Focused Examination — should include performance and documentation of at least six elements identified by a bullet (•), whether in a box with a shaded or unshaded border.

- Detailed Examination — examinations other than the eye and psychiatric examinations should include performance and documentation of at least twelve elements identified by a bullet (•), whether in box with a shaded or unshaded border.

  Eye and psychiatric examinations should include the performance and documentation of at least nine elements identified by a bullet (•), whether in a box with a shaded or unshaded border.

- Comprehensive Examination — should include performance of all elements identified by a bullet (•), whether in a shaded or unshaded box. Documentation of every element in each box with a shaded border and at least one element in each box with an unshaded border is expected.

Documentation of every element in each box with a shaded border and at least one element in each box with an unshaded border is expected.

GENERAL MULTI-SYSTEM EXAMINATION

SYSTEM/BODY AREA	ELEMENTS OF EXAMINATION
Constitutional	• measurement of any three of the following seven vital signs: 1) sitting or standing blood pressure, 2) supine blood pressure, 3) pulse rate and regularity, 4) respiration, 5) temperature, 6) height, 7) weight (May be measured and recorded by ancillary staff) • general appearance of patient (e.g., development, nutrition, body habitus, deformities, attention to grooming)
Eyes	• inspection of conjunctivae and lids • examination of pupils and irises (e.g., reaction to light and accommodation, size and symmetry) • Ophthalmoscopic examination of optic discs (e.g., size, C/D ratio, appearance) and posterior segments (e.g., vessel changes, exudates, hemorrhages)
Ears, Nose, Mouth Throat	• External inspection of ears and nose (e.g., overall **and** appearance, scars, lesions, masses) • Otoscopic examination of external auditory canals and tympanic membranes • Assessment of hearing (e.g., whispered voice, finger rub, tuning fork) • Inspection of nasal mucosa, septum and turbinates • Inspection of lips, teeth and gums • Examination of oropharynx: oral mucosa, salivary glands, hard and soft palates, tongue, tonsils and posterior pharynx
Neck	• Examination of neck (e.g., masses, overall appearance, symmetry, tracheal position, crepitus) • Examination of thyroid (e.g., enlargement, tenderness, mass)

Respiratory	• Assessment of respiratory effort (e.g., intercostal retractions, use of accessory muscles, diaphragmatic movement) • Percussion of chest (e.g., dullness, flatness, hyperresonance) • Palpation of chest (e.g., tactile fremitus) • Auscultation of lungs (e.g., breath sounds, adventitious sounds, rubs)
Cardiovascular	• Palpation of heart (e.g., location, size, thrills) • Auscultation of heart with notation of abnormal sounds and murmurs Examination of: • carotid arteries (e.g., pulse amplitude, bruits) • abdominal aorta (e.g., size, bruits) • femoral arteries (e.g., pulse amplitude, bruits) • pedal pulses (e.g., pulse amplitude) • extremities for edema and/or varicosities
Chest (Breasts)	• Inspection of breasts (e.g., symmetry, nipple discharge) • Palpation of breasts and axillae (e.g., masses or lumps, tenderness)
Gastrointestinal (Abdomen)	• Examination of abdomen with notation of presence of masses or tenderness • Examination of liver and spleen • Examination for presence or absence of hernia • Examination (when indicated) of anus, perineum and rectum, including sphincter tone, presence of hemorrhoids, rectal masses • Obtain stool sample for occult blood test when indicated

Genitourinary Male	• Examination of the scrotal contents (e.g., hydrocele, spermatocele, tenderness of cord, testicular mass) • Examination of the penis • Digital rectal examination of prostate gland (e.g., size, symmetry, nodularity, tenderness)
Genitourinary Female	• Pelvic examination (with or without specimen collection for smears and cultures), including • Examination of external genitalia (e.g., general appearance, hair distribution, lesions) and vagina (e.g., general appearance, estrogen effect, discharge, lesions, pelvic support, cystocele, rectocele) • Examination of urethra (e.g., masses, tenderness, scarring) • Examination of bladder (e.g., fullness, masses, tenderness) • Cervix (e.g., general appearance, lesions, discharge) • Uterus (e.g., size, contour, position, mobility, tenderness, consistency, descent or support) • Adnexa/parametria (e.g., masses, tenderness, organomegaly, nodularity)
Lymphatic	Palpation of lymph nodes in two or more areas: • Neck • Axillae • Groin • Other
Musculoskeletal	• Examination of gait and station • Inspection and/or palpation of digits and nails (e.g., clubbing, cyanosis, inflammatory conditions, petechiae, ischemia, infections, nodes) • Examination of joints, bones and muscles of one or more of the following six areas: 1) head and neck; 2)

spine, ribs and pelvis; 3) right upper extremity; 4) left upper extremity; 5) right lower extremity; and 6) left lower extremity. The examination of a given area includes:

- Inspection and/or palpation with notation of presence of any misalignment, asymmetry, crepitation, defects, tenderness, masses, effusions

- Assessment of range of motion with notation of any pain, crepitation or contracture

- Assessment of stability with notation of any dislocation (luxation), subluxation or laxity

- Assessment of muscle strength and tone (e.g., flaccid, cog wheel, spastic) with notation of any atrophy or abnormal movements

Skin

- Inspection of skin and subcutaneous tissue (e.g., rashes, lesions, ulcers)

- Palpation of skin and subcutaneous tissue (e.g., induration, subcutaneous nodules, tightening)

Neurologic

- Test cranial nerves with notation of any deficits

- Examination of deep tendon reflexes with notation of pathological reflexes (e.g., Babinski)

- Examination of sensation (e.g., by touch, pin, vibration, proprioception)

Psychiatric

- Description of patient's judgment and insight

- Description of patient's judgment and insight. Brief assessment of mental status including:

- orientation to time, place and person

- recent and remote memory

- mood and affect (e.g., depression, anxiety, agitation)

CONTENT AND DOCUMENTATION REQUIREMENTS

Level of Exam	Perform and Document:
Problem Focused	One to five elements identified by a bullet.
Expanded Problem Focused	At least six elements identified by a bullet.
Detailed	At least two elements identified by a bullet from each of six areas/systems OR at least twelve elements identified by a bullet in two or more areas/systems.
Comprehensive	Perform all elements identified by a bullet in at least nine organ systems or body areas and document at least two elements identified by a bullet from each of nine areas/systems.

CARDIOVASCULAR EXAMINATION

SYSTEM/BODY AREA	ELEMENTS OF EXAMINATION
Constitutional	• Measurement of any three of the following seven vital signs: 1) sitting or standing blood pressure, 2) supine blood pressure, 3) pulse rate and regularity, 4) respiration, 5) temperature, 6) height, 7) weight (May be measured and recorded by ancillary staff) • General appearance of patient (e.g., development, nutrition, body habitus, deformities, attention to grooming)
Head and Face	
Eyes	• Inspection of conjunctivae and lids (e.g., xanthelasma)
Ears, Nose, Mouth and Throat	• Inspection of teeth, gums and palate • Inspection of oral mucosa with notation of presence of pallor or cyanosis
Neck	• Examination of jugular veins (e.g., distension; a, v or cannon a waves) • Examination of thyroid (e.g., enlargement, tenderness, mass)
Respiratory	• Assessment of respiratory effort (e.g., intercostal retractions, use of accessory muscles, diaphragmatic movement) • Auscultation of lungs (e.g., breath sounds, adventitious sounds, rubs)
Cardiovascular	• Palpation of heart (e.g., location, size and forcefulness of the point of maximal impact; thrills; lifts; palpable S3 or S4) • Auscultation of heart including sounds, abnormal sounds and murmurs

continued

extremities when indicated (e.g., aortic dissection, coarctation)

Examination of:

- Carotid arteries (e.g., waveform, pulse amplitude, bruits, apical-carotid delay)

- Abdominal aorta (e.g., size, bruits)

- Femoral arteries (e.g., pulse amplitude, bruits)

- Pedal pulses (e.g., pulse amplitude)

- Extremities for peripheral edema and/or varicosities

Chest (Breasts)

Gastrointestinal (Abdomen)

- Examination of abdomen with notation of presence of masses or tenderness

- Examination of liver and spleen

- Obtain stool sample for occult blood from patients who are being considered for thrombolytic or anticoagulant therapy

Genitourinary (Abdomen)

Lymphatic

Musculoskeletal

- Examination of the back with notation of kyphosis or scoliosis

- Examination of gait with notation of ability to undergo exercise testing and/or participation in exercise programs

- Assessment of muscle strength and tone (e.g., flaccid, cog wheel, spastic) with notation of any atrophy and abnormal movements

Extremities	• Inspection and palpation of digits and nails (e.g., clubbing, cyanosis, inflammation, petechiae, ischemia, infections, Osler's nodes)
Skin	• Inspection and/or palpation of skin and subcutaneous tissue (e.g., stasis dermatitis, ulcers, scars, xanthomas)
Neurological/ Psychiatric	Brief assessment of mental status including • Orientation to time, place and person, • Mood and affect (e.g., depression, anxiety, agitation)

CONTENT AND DOCUMENTATION REQUIREMENTS

Level of Exam	Perform and Document:
Problem Focused	One to five elements identified by a bullet.
Expanded Problem Focused	At least six elements identified by a bullet.
Detailed	At least twelve elements identified by a bullet.
Comprehensive	Perform all elements identified by a bullet; document every element in each box with a shaded border and at least one element in each box with an unshaded border.

EAR, NOSE AND THROAT EXAMINATION

SYSTEM/BODY AREA   ELEMENTS OF EXAMINATION

Constitutional

- Measurement of any three of the following seven vital signs: 1) sitting or standing blood pressure, 2) supine blood pressure, 3) pulse rate and regularity, 4) respiration, 5) temperature, 6) height, 7) weight (May be measured and recorded by ancillary staff)

- General appearance of patient (e.g., development, nutrition, body habitus, deformities, attention to grooming)

- Assessment of ability to communicate (e.g., use of sign language or other communication aids) and quality of voice

Head and Face

- Inspection of head and face (e.g., overall appearance, scars, lesions and masses)

- Palpation and/or percussion of face with notation of presence or absence of sinus tenderness

- Examination of salivary glands

- Assessment of facial strength

Eyes

- Test ocular motility including primary gaze alignment

**Ears, Nose,
Mouth and Throat**

- Otoscopic examination of external auditory canals and tympanic membranes including pneumo-otoscopy with notation of mobility of membranes

- Assessment of hearing with tuning forks and clinical speech reception thresholds (e.g., whispered voice, finger rub)

- External inspection of ears and nose (e.g., overall appearance, scars, lesions and masses)

- Inspection of nasal mucosa, septum and turbinates

- Inspection of lips, teeth and gums

continued

	• palates, tongue, tonsils and posterior pharynx (e.g., asymmetry, lesions, hydration of mucosal surfaces) • Inspection of pharyngeal walls and pyriform sinuses (e.g., pooling of saliva, asymmetry, lesions) • Examination by mirror of larynx including the condition of the epiglottis, false vocal cords, true vocal cords and mobility of larynx (Use of mirror not required in children) • Examination by mirror of nasopharynx including appearance of the mucosa, adenoids, posterior choanae and eustachian tubes (Use of mirror not required in children)
Neck	• Examination of neck (e.g., masses, overall appearance, symmetry, tracheal position, crepitus) • Examination of thyroid (e.g., enlargement, tenderness, mass)
Respiratory	• Inspection of chest including symmetry, expansion and/or assessment of respiratory effort (e.g., intercostal retractions, use of accessory muscles, diaphragmatic movement) • Auscultation of lungs (e.g., breath sounds, adventitious sounds, rubs)
Cardiovascular	• Auscultation of heart with notation of abnormal sounds and murmurs • Examination of peripheral vascular system by observation (e.g., swelling, varicosities) and palpation (e.g., pulses, temperature, edema, tenderness)
Chest (Breasts)	
Gastrointestinal (Abdomen)	
Genitourinary	
Lymphatic	• Palpation of lymph nodes in neck, axillae, groin and/or other location

Musculoskeletal

Extremities

Skin

Neurological/ Psychiatric	• Test cranial nerves with notation of any deficits
	Brief assessment of mental status including
	• Orientation to time, place and person,
	• Mood and affect (e.g., depression, anxiety, agitation)

CONTENT AND DOCUMENTATION REQUIREMENTS

Level of Exam	Perform and Document:
Problem Focused	One to five elements identified by a bullet.
Expanded Problem Focused	At least six elements identified by a bullet.
Detailed	At least twelve elements identified by a bullet.
Comprehensive	Perform all elements identified by a bullet; document every element in each box with a shaded border and at least one element in each box with an unshaded border.

EYE EXAMINATION

SYSTEM/BODY AREA	ELEMENTS OF EXAMINATION
Constitutional	
Head and Face	

Eyes

- Test visual acuity (Does not include determination of refractive error)

- Gross visual field testing by confrontation

- Test ocular motility including primary gaze alignment

- Inspection of bulbar and palpebral conjunctivae

- Examination of ocular adnexae including lids (e.g., ptosis or lagophthalmos), lacrimal glands, lacrimal drainage, orbits and preauricular lymph nodes

- Examination of pupils and irises including shape, direct and consensual reaction (afferent pupil), size (e.g., anisocoria) and morphology

- Slit lamp examination of the corneas including epithelium, stroma, endothelium, and tear film

- Slit lamp examination of the anterior chambers including depth, cells, and flare

- Slit lamp examination of the lenses including clarity, anterior and posterior capsule, cortex, and nucleus
- Measurement of intraocular pressures (except in children and patients with trauma or infectious disease)

- Ophthalmoscopic examination through dilated pupils (unless contraindicated) of

- Optic discs including size, C/D ratio, appearance (e.g., atrophy, cupping, tumor elevation) and nerve fiber layer

- Posterior segments including retina and vessels (e.g., exudates and hemorrhages)

Ears, Nose, Mouth and Throat

Neck

Respiratory

Cardiovascular

Chest (Breasts)

Gastrointestinal (Abdomen)

Genitourinary

Lymphatic

Musculoskeletal

Extremities

Skin

Neurological/ Psychiatric	Brief assessment of mental status including • Orientation to time, place and person • Mood and affect (e.g., depression, anxiety, agitation)

CONTENT AND DOCUMENTATION REQUIREMENTS

Level of Exam	Perform and Document:
Problem Focused	One to five elements identified by a bullet.
Expanded Problem Focused	At least six elements identified by a bullet.
Detailed	At least nine elements identified by a bullet.
Comprehensive	Perform all elements identified by a bullet; document every element in each box with a shaded border and at least one element in each box with an unshaded border.

GENITOURINARY EXAMINATION

SYSTEM/BODY AREA   **ELEMENTS OF EXAMINATION**

SYSTEM/BODY AREA	ELEMENTS OF EXAMINATION
Constitutional	• Measurement of any three of the following seven vital signs: 1) sitting or standing blood pressure, 2) supine blood pressure, 3) pulse rate and regularity, 4) respiration, 5) temperature, 6) height, 7) weight (May be measured and recorded by ancillary staff) • General appearance of patient (e.g., development, nutrition, body habitus, deformities, attention to grooming)
Head and Face	
Eyes	
Ears, Nose, Mouth and Throat	
Neck	• Examination of neck (e.g., masses, overall appearance, symmetry, tracheal position, crepitus) • Examination of thyroid (e.g., enlargement, tenderness, mass)
Respiratory	• Assessment of respiratory effort (e.g., intercostal retractions, use of accessory muscles, diaphragmatic movement) • Auscultation of lungs (e.g., breath sounds, adventitious sounds, rubs)
Cardiovascular	• Auscultation of heart with notation of abnormal sounds and murmurs • Examination of peripheral vascular system by observation (e.g., swelling, varicosities) and palpation (e.g., pulses, temperature, edema, tenderness)
Chest (Breasts)	[See genitourinary (female)]
Gastrointestinal (Abdomen)	• Examination of abdomen with notation of presence of masses or tenderness

continued

	• Examination for presence or absence of hernia
	• Examination of liver and spleen
	• Obtain stool sample for occult blood test when indicated
Genitourinary (male)	• Inspection of anus and perineum
	Examination (with or without specimen collection for smears and cultures) of genitalia including:
	• Scrotum (e.g., lesions, cysts, rashes)
	• Epididymides (e.g., size, symmetry, masses)
	• Testes (e.g., size, symmetry, masses)
	• Urethral meatus (e.g., size, location, lesions, discharge)
	• Penis (e.g., lesions, presence or absence of foreskin, foreskin retractability, plaque, masses, scarring, deformities)
	Digital rectal examination including:
	• Prostate gland (e.g., size, symmetry, nodularity, tenderness)
	• Seminal vesicles (e.g., symmetry, tenderness, masses, enlargement)
	• Sphincter tone, presence of hemorrhoids, rectal masses
Genitourinary (female)	Includes at least seven of the following eleven elements identified by bullets:
	• Inspection and palpation of breasts (e.g., masses or lumps, tenderness, symmetry, nipple discharge)
	• Digital rectal examination including sphincter tone, presence of hemorrhoids, rectal masses
	Pelvic examination (with or without specimen collection for smears and cultures) including:

- External genitalia (e.g., general appearance, hair distribution, lesions)

- Urethral meatus (e.g., size, location, lesions, prolapse)

- Urethra (e.g., masses, tenderness, scarring)

- Bladder (e.g., fullness, masses, tenderness)

- Vagina (e.g., general appearance, estrogen effect, discharge, lesions, pelvic support, cystocele, rectocele)

- Cervix (e.g., general appearance, lesions, discharge)

- Uterus (e.g., size, contour, position, mobility, tenderness, consistency, descent or support)

- Adnexa/parametria (e.g., masses, tenderness, organomegaly, nodularity)

- Anus and perineum

Lymphatic
- Palpation of lymph nodes in neck, axillae, groin and/or other location

Musculoskeletal

Extremities

Skin
- Inspection and/or palpation of skin and subcutaneous tissue (e.g., rashes, lesions, ulcers)

Neurological/ Psychiatric

Brief assessment of mental status including:

- Orientation (e.g., time, place and person) and

- Mood and affect (e.g., depression, anxiety, agitation)

CONTENT AND DOCUMENTATION REQUIREMENTS

Level of Exam	Perform and Document:
Problem Focused	One to five elements identified by a bullet.
Expanded Problem Focused	At least six elements identified by a bullet.
Detailed	At least twelve elements identified by a bullet.
Comprehensive	Perform all elements identified by a bullet; document every element in each box with a shaded border and at least one element in each box with an unshaded border.

HEMATOLOGIC, LYMPHATIC, AND/OR IMMUNOLOGIC EXAMINATION

SYSTEM/BODY AREA	ELEMENTS OF EXAMINATION
Constitutional	• Measurement of any three of the following seven vital signs: 1) sitting or standing blood pressure, 2) supine blood pressure, 3) pulse rate and regularity, 4) respiration, 5) temperature, 6) height, 7) weight (May be measured and recorded by ancillary staff) • General appearance of patient (e.g., development, nutrition, body habitus, deformities, attention to grooming)
Head and Face	• Palpation and/or percussion of face with notation of presence or absence of sinus tenderness
Eyes	• Inspection of conjunctivae and lids
Ears, Nose, Mouth and Throat	• Otoscopic examination of external auditory canals and tympanic membranes • Inspection of nasal mucosa, septum and turbinates • Inspection of teeth and gums • Examination of oropharynx (e.g., oral mucosa, hard and soft palates, tongue, tonsils, posterior pharynx)
Neck	• Examination of neck (e.g., masses, overall appearance, symmetry, tracheal position, crepitus) • Examination of thyroid (e.g., enlargement, tenderness, mass)
Respiratory	• Assessment of respiratory effort (e.g., intercostal retractions, use of accessory muscles, diaphragmatic movement) • Auscultation of lungs (e.g., breath sounds, adventitious sounds, rubs)
Cardiovascular	• Auscultation of heart with notation of abnormal sounds and murmurs

continued

	• Examination of peripheral vascular system by observation (e.g., swelling, varicosities) and palpation (e.g., pulses, temperature, edema, tenderness)
Chest (Breasts)	
Gastrointestinal (Abdomen)	• Examination of abdomen with notation of presence of masses or tenderness • Examination of liver and spleen
Genitourinary	
Lymphatic	• Palpation of lymph nodes in neck, axillae, groin, and/or other location
Musculoskeletal	
Extremities	• Inspection and palpation of digits and nails (e.g., clubbing, cyanosis, inflammation, petechiae, ischemia, infections, nodes)
Skin	• Inspection and/or palpation of skin and subcutaneous tissue (e.g., rashes, lesions, ulcers, ecchymoses, bruises)
Neurological/ Psychiatric	Brief assessment of mental status including • Orientation to time, place and person • Mood and affect (e.g., depression, anxiety, agitation)

CONTENT AND DOCUMENTATION REQUIREMENTS

Level of Exam	Perform and Document:
Problem Focused	One to five elements identified by a bullet.
Expanded Problem Focused	At least six elements identified by a bullet.
Detailed	At least twelve elements identified by a bullet.
Comprehensive	Perform all elements identified by a bullet; document every element in each box with a shaded border and at least one element in each box with an unshaded border.

MUSCULOSKELETAL EXAMINATION

SYSTEM/BODY AREA	ELEMENTS OF EXAMINATION
Constitutional	• Measurement of any three of the following seven vital signs: 1) sitting or standing blood pressure, 2) supine blood pressure, 3) pulse rate and regularity, 4) respiration, 5) temperature, 6) height, 7) weight (May be measured and recorded by ancillary staff) • General appearance of patient (e.g., development, nutrition, body habitus, deformities, attention to grooming)
Head and Face	
Eyes	
Ears, Nose, Mouth and Throat	
Neck	
Respiratory	
Cardiovascular	• Examination of peripheral vascular system by observation (e.g., swelling, varicosities) and palpation (e.g., pulses, temperature, edema, tenderness)
Chest (Breasts)	
Gastrointestinal(Abdomen)	
Genitourinary	
Lymphatic	• Palpation of lymph nodes in neck, axillae, groin and/or other location
Musculoskeletal	• Examination of gait and station Examination of joint(s), bone(s) and muscle(s)/ tendon(s) of four of the following six areas: 1) head and neck; 2) spine, ribs and pelvis; 3) right upper extremity; 4) left upper extremity; 5) right lower extremity; and 6) left lower extremity. The examination of a given area includes:

- Inspection, percussion and/or palpation with notation of any misalignment, asymmetry, crepitation, defects, tenderness, masses or effusions

- Assessment of range of motion with notation of any pain (e.g., straight leg raising), crepitation or contracture

- Assessment of stability with notation of any dislocation (luxation), subluxation or laxity

- Assessment of muscle strength and tone (e.g., flaccid, cog wheel, spastic) with notation of any atrophy or abnormal movements

NOTE: For the comprehensive level of examination, all four of the elements identified by a bullet must be performed and documented for each of four anatomic areas. For the three lower levels of examination, each element is counted separately for each body area. For example, assessing range of motion in two extremities constitutes two elements.

Extremities   [See musculoskeletal and skin]

Skin

- Inspection and/or palpation of skin and subcutaneous tissue (e.g., scars, rashes, lesions, cafe-au-lait spots, ulcers) in four of the following six areas: 1) head and neck; 2) trunk; 3) right upper extremity; 4) left upper extremity; 5) right lower extremity; and 6) left lower extremity.

NOTE: For the comprehensive level, all four areas must be examined and documented. For the three lower levels, each body area is counted separately. For example, inspection and/or palpation of the skin and subcutaneous tissue of two extremities constitutes two elements.

Neurological/

- Test coordination (e.g., finger/nose, heel/ **Psychiatric** knee/shin, rapid alternating movements in the upper and lower extremities, evaluation of fine motor coordination in young children)

- Examination of deep tendon reflexes and/or nerve stretch test with notation of pathological reflexes (e.g., Babinski)

- Examination of sensation (e.g., by touch, pin, vibration, proprioception)

Brief assessment of mental status including

- Orientation to time, place and person

- Mood and affect (e.g., depression, anxiety, agitation)

CONTENT AND DOCUMENTATION REQUIREMENTS

Level of Exam	Perform and Document:
Problem Focused	One to five elements identified by a bullet.
Expanded Problem Focused	At least six elements identified by a bullet.
Detailed	At least twelve elements identified by a bullet.
Comprehensive	Perform all elements identified by a bullet; document every element in each box with a shaded border and at least one element in each box with an unshaded border.

NEUROLOGICAL EXAMINATION

SYSTEM/BODY AREA ELEMENTS OF EXAMINATION

SYSTEM/BODY AREA	ELEMENTS OF EXAMINATION
Constitutional	• Measurement of any three of the following seven vital signs: 1) sitting or standing blood pressure, 2) supine blood pressure, 3) pulse rate and regularity, 4) respiration, 5) temperature, 6) height, 7) weight (May be measured and recorded by ancillary staff) • General appearance of patient (e.g., development, nutrition, body habitus, deformities, attention to grooming)
Head and Face	
Eyes	• Ophthalmoscopic examination of optic discs (e.g., size, C/D ratio, appearance) and posterior segments (e.g., vessel changes, exudates, hemorrhages)
Ears, Nose, Mouth and Throat	
Neck	
Respiratory	
Cardiovascular	• Examination of carotid arteries (e.g., pulse amplitude, bruits) • Auscultation of heart with notation of abnormal sounds and murmurs • Examination of peripheral vascular system by observation (e.g., swelling, varicosities) and palpation (e.g., pulses, temperature, edema, tenderness)
Chest (Breasts)	
Gastrointestinal (Abdomen)	
Genitourinary	
Lymphatic	

Musculoskeletal	• Examination of gait and station Assessment of motor function including: • Muscle strength in upper and lower extremities • Muscle tone in upper and lower extremities (e.g., flaccid, cog wheel, spastic) with notation of any atrophy or abnormal movements (e.g., fasciculation, tardive dyskinesia)
Extremities	[See musculoskeletal]
Skin	
Neurological	Evaluation of higher integrative functions including: • Orientation to time, place and person • Recent and remote memory • Attention span and concentration • Language (e.g., naming objects, repeating phrases, spontaneous speech) • Fund of knowledge (e.g., awareness of current events, past history, vocabulary) Test the following cranial nerves: • 2nd cranial nerve (e.g., visual acuity, visual fields, fundi) • 3rd, 4th and 6th cranial nerves (e.g., pupils, eye movements) • 5th cranial nerve (e.g., facial sensation, corneal reflexes) • 7th cranial nerve (e.g., facial symmetry, strength) • 8th cranial nerve (e.g., hearing with tuning fork, whispered voice and/or finger rub)

continued

- 9th cranial nerve (e.g., spontaneous or reflex palate movement)

- 11th cranial nerve (e.g., shoulder shrug strength)

- 12th cranial nerve (e.g., tongue protrusion)

- Examination of sensation (e.g., by touch, pin, vibration, proprioception)

- Examination of deep tendon reflexes in upper and lower extremities with notation of pathological reflexes (e.g., Babinski)

- Test coordination (e.g., finger/nose, heel/knee/shin, rapid alternating movements in the upper and lower extremities, evaluation of fine motor coordination in young children)

Psychiatric

CONTENT AND DOCUMENTATION REQUIREMENTS

Level of Exam	Perform and Document:
Problem Focused	One to five elements identified by a bullet.
Expanded Problem Focused	At least six elements identified by a bullet.
Detailed	At least twelve elements identified by a bullet.
Comprehensive	Perform all elements identified by a bullet; document every element in each box with a shaded border and at least one element in each box with an unshaded border.

PSYCHIATRIC EXAMINATION

SYSTEM/BODY AREA	ELEMENTS OF EXAMINATION
Constitutional	• Measurement of any three of the following seven vital signs: 1) sitting or standing blood pressure, 2) supine blood pressure, 3) pulse rate and regularity, 4) respiration, 5) temperature, 6) height, 7) weight (May be measured and recorded by ancillary staff) • General appearance of patient (e.g., development, nutrition, body habitus, deformities, attention to grooming)
Head and Face	
Eyes	
Ears, Nose, Mouth and Throat	
Neck	
Respiratory	
Cardiovascular	
Chest (Breasts)	
Gastrointestinal (Abdomen)	
Genitourinary	
Lymphatic	
Musculoskeletal	• Assessment of muscle strength and tone (e.g., flaccid, cog wheel, spastic) with notation of any atrophy and abnormal movements • Examination of gait and station
Extremities	
Skin	
Neurological	

Psychiatric

- Description of speech including: rate; volume; articulation; coherence; and spontaneity with notation of abnormalities (e.g., perseveration, paucity of language)

- Description of thought processes including: rate of thoughts; content of thoughts (e.g., logical vs. illogical, tangential); abstract reasoning; and computation

- Description of associations (e.g., loose, tangential, circumstantial, intact)

- Description of abnormal or psychotic thoughts including: hallucinations; delusions; preoccupation with violence; homicidal or suicidal ideation; and obsessions

- Description of the patient's judgment (e.g., concerning everyday activities and social situations) and insight (e.g., concerning psychiatric condition)

Complete mental status examination including:

- Orientation to time, place and person
- Recent and remote memory

- Attention span and concentration

- Language (e.g., naming objects, repeating phrases)

- Fund of knowledge (e.g., awareness of current events, past history, vocabulary)

- Mood and affect (e.g., depression, anxiety, agitation, hypomania, lability)

CONTENT AND DOCUMENTATION REQUIREMENTS

Level of Exam	Perform and Document:
Problem Focused	One to five elements identified by a bullet.
Expanded Problem Focused	At least six elements identified by a bullet.
Detailed	At least nine elements identified by a bullet.
Comprehensive	Perform all elements identified by a bullet; document every element in each box with a shaded border and at least one element in each box with an unshaded border.

RESPIRATORY EXAMINATION

SYSTEM/BODY AREA	ELEMENTS OF EXAMINATION
Constitutional	• Measurement of any three of the following seven vital signs: 1) sitting or standing blood pressure, 2) supine blood pressure, 3) pulse rate and regularity, 4) respiration, 5) temperature, 6) height, 7) weight (May be measured and recorded by ancillary staff) • General appearance of patient (e.g., development, nutrition, body habitus, deformities, attention to grooming)
Head and Face	
Eyes	
Ears, Nose, Mouth and Throat	• Inspection of nasal mucosa, septum and turbinates • Inspection of teeth and gums • Examination of oropharynx (e.g., oral mucosa, hard and soft palates, tongue, tonsils and posterior pharynx)
Neck	• Examination of neck (e.g., masses, overall appearance, symmetry, tracheal position, crepitus) • Examination of thyroid (e.g., enlargement, tenderness, mass) • Examination of jugular veins (e.g., distension; a, v or cannon a waves)
Respiratory	• Inspection of chest with notation of symmetry and expansion • Assessment of respiratory effort (e.g., intercostal retractions, use of accessory muscles, diaphragmatic movement) • Percussion of chest (e.g., dullness, flatness, hyperresonance) • Palpation of chest (e.g., tactile fremitus)

continued

	• Auscultation of lungs (e.g., breath sounds, adventitious sounds, rubs)
Cardiovascular	• Auscultation of heart including sounds, abnormal sounds and murmurs
	• Examination of peripheral vascular system by observation (e.g., swelling, varicosities) and palpation (e.g., pulses, temperature, edema, tenderness)
Chest (Breasts)	
Gastrointestinal (Abdomen)	• Examination of abdomen with notation of presence of masses or tenderness
	• Examination of liver and spleen
Genitourinary	
Lymphatic	• Palpation of lymph nodes in neck, axillae, groin and/or other location
Musculoskeletal	• Assessment of muscle strength and tone (e.g., flaccid, cog wheel, spastic) with notation of any atrophy and abnormal movements
	• Examination of gait and station
Extremities	• Inspection and palpation of digits and nails (e.g., clubbing, cyanosis, inflammation, petechiae, ischemia, infections, nodes)
Skin	• Inspection and/or palpation of skin and subcutaneous tissue (e.g., rashes, lesions, ulcers)
Neurological/ Psychiatric	Brief assessment of mental status including • Orientation to time, place and person • Mood and affect (e.g., depression, anxiety, agitation)

CONTENT AND DOCUMENTATION REQUIREMENTS

Level of Exam	Perform and Document:
Problem Focused	One to five elements identified by a bullet.
Expanded Problem Focused	At least six elements identified by a bullet.
Detailed	At least twelve elements identified by a bullet.
Comprehensive	Perform all elements identified by a bullet; document every element in each box with a shaded border and at least one element in each box with an unshaded border.

SKIN EXAMINATION

SYSTEM/BODY AREA	ELEMENTS OF EXAMINATION
Constitutional	• Measurement of any three of the following seven vital signs: 1) sitting or standing blood pressure, 2) supine blood pressure, 3) pulse rate and regularity, 4) respiration, 5) temperature, 6) height, 7) weight (May be measured and recorded by ancillary staff) • General appearance of patient (e.g., development, nutrition, body habitus, deformities, attention to grooming)
Head and Face	
Eyes	• Inspection of conjunctivae and lids
Ears, Nose, Mouth and Throat	• Inspection of lips, teeth and gums • Examination of oropharynx (e.g., oral mucosa, hard and soft palates, tongue, tonsils, posterior pharynx)
Neck	• Examination of thyroid (e.g., enlargement, tenderness, mass)
Respiratory	
Cardiovascular	• Examination of peripheral vascular system by observation (e.g., swelling, varicosities) and palpation (e.g., pulses, temperature, edema, tenderness)
Chest (Breasts)	
Gastrointestinal (Abdomen)	• Examination of liver and spleen • Examination of anus for condyloma and other lesions
Genitourinary	
Lymphatic	• Palpation of lymph nodes in neck, axillae, groin and/or other location
Musculoskeletal	

Extremities	• Inspection and palpation of digits and nails (e.g., clubbing, cyanosis, inflammation, petechiae, ischemia, infections, nodes)

Skin

• Palpation of scalp and inspection of hair of scalp, eyebrows, face, chest, pubic area (when indicated) and extremities

• Inspection and/or palpation of skin and subcutaneous tissue (e.g., rashes, lesions, ulcers, susceptibility to and presence of photo damage) in eight of the following ten areas:

- Head, including the face and
- Neck
- Chest, including breasts and axillae
- Abdomen
- Genitalia, groin, buttocks
- Back
- Right upper extremity
- Left upper extremity
- Right lower extremity
- Left lower extremity

NOTE: For the comprehensive level, the examination of at least eight anatomic areas must be performed and documented. For the three lower levels of examination, each body area is counted separately. For example, inspection and/or palpation of the skin and subcutaneous tissue of the right upper extremity and the left upper extremity constitutes two elements.

• Inspection of eccrine and apocrine glands of skin and subcutaneous tissue with identification and location of any hyperhidrosis, chromhidroses or bromhidrosis

Neurological/ Psychiatric

Brief assessment of mental status including

• Orientation to time, place and person

• Mood and affect (e.g., depression, anxiety, agitation)

CONTENT AND DOCUMENTATION REQUIREMENTS

Level of Exam	Perform and Document:
Problem Focused	One to five elements identified by a bullet.
Expanded Problem Focused	At least six elements identified by a bullet.
Detailed	At least twelve elements identified by a bullet.
Comprehensive	Perform all elements identified by a bullet; document every element in each box with a shaded border and at least one element in each box with an unshaded border.

DOCUMENTATION OF THE COMPLEXITY OF MEDICAL DECISION MAKING

The levels of evaluation and management services recognize four types of medical decision making (straight-forward, low complexity, moderate complexity and high complexity). Medical decision making refers to the complexity of establishing a diagnosis and/or selecting a management option as measured by:

- the number of possible diagnoses and/or the number of management options that must be considered;

- the amount and/or complexity of medical records, diagnostic tests, and/or other information that must be obtained, reviewed and analyzed; and

- the risk of significant complications, morbidity and/or mortality, as well as comorbidities, associated with the patient's presenting problem(s), the diagnostic procedure(s) and/or the possible management options.

The following chart illustrates the progression of the elements required for each level of medical decision making. To qualify for a given type of decision making, two of the three elements in the table must be either met or exceeded.

Number of Diagnoses	Amount of Data to Review	Risk of Complication	Type of Decision Making
Minimal	Minimal or None	Minimal	*Straightforward*
Limited	Limited	Low	*Low Complexity*
Multiple	Moderate	Moderate	*Moderate Complexity*
Extensive	Extensive	High	*High Complexity*

Each of the elements of medical decision making is described below

NUMBER OF DIAGNOSES OR MANAGEMENT OPTIONS

The number of possible diagnoses and/or the number of management options that must be considered is based on the number and types of problems addressed during the encounter, the complexity of establishing a diagnosis and the management decisions that are made by the physician.

Generally, decision making with respect to a diagnosed problem is easier than that for an identified but undiagnosed problem. The number and type of diagnostic tests employed may be an indicator of the number of possible diagnoses. Problems which are improving or resolving are less complex than those which are worsening or failing to change as expected. The need to seek advice from others is another indicator of complexity of diagnostic or management problems.

•DG: For each encounter, an assessment, clinical impression, or diagnosis should be documented. It may be explicitly stated or implied in documented decisions regarding management plans and/or further evaluation.

- For a presenting problem with an established diagnosis the record should reflect whether the problem is: a) improved, well controlled, resolving or resolved; or, b) inadequately controlled, worsening, or failing to change as expected.

- For a presenting problem without an established diagnosis, the assessment or clinical impression may be stated in the form of differential diagnoses or as a "possible", "probable", or "rule out" (R/O) diagnosis.

•DG: The initiation of, or changes in, treatment should be documented. Treatment includes a wide range of management options including patient instructions, nursing instructions, therapies, and medications.

•DG: If referrals are made, consultations requested or advice sought, the record should indicate to whom or where the referral or consultation is made or from whom the advice is requested.

AMOUNT AND/OR COMPLEXITY OF DATA TO BE REVIEWED

The amount and complexity of data to be reviewed is based on the types of diagnostic testing ordered or reviewed. A decision to obtain and review old medical records and/or obtain history from sources other than the patient increases the amount and complexity of data to be reviewed.

Discussion of contradictory or unexpected test results with the physician who performed or interpreted the test is an indication of the complexity of data being reviewed. On occasion the physician who ordered a test may personally review the image, tracing or specimen to supplement information from the physician who prepared the test report or interpretation; this is another indication of the complexity of data being reviewed.

•**DG:**   If a diagnostic service (test or procedure) is ordered, planned, scheduled, or performed at the time of the evaluation and management encounter, the type of service, e.g., lab or x-ray, should be documented.

•**DG:**   The review of lab, radiology and/or other diagnostic tests should be documented. A simple notation such as "WBC elevated" or "chest x-ray unremarkable" is acceptable. Alternatively, the review may be documented by initialing and dating the report containing the test results.

•**DG:**   A decision to obtain old records or decision to obtain additional history from the family, caretaker or other source to supplement that obtained from the patient should be documented.

•**DG:**   Relevant findings from the review of old records, and/or the receipt of additional history from the family, caretaker or other source to supplement that obtained from the patient should be documented. If there is no relevant information beyond that already obtained, that fact should be documented. A notation of "Old records reviewed" or "additional history obtained from family" without elaboration is insufficient.

•**DG:**   The results of discussion of laboratory, radiology or other diagnostic tests with the physician who performed or interpreted the study should be documented.

•**DG:**   The direct visualization and independent interpretation of an image, tracing or specimen previously or subsequently interpreted by another physician should be documented.

RISK OF SIGNIFICANT COMPLICATIONS, MORBIDITY AND/OR MORTALITY

The risk of significant complications, morbidity, and/or mortality is based on the risks associated with the presenting problem(s), the diagnostic procedure(s), and the possible management options.

•DG: Comorbidities/underlying diseases or other factors that increase the complexity of medical decision making by increasing the risk of complications, morbidity, and/or mortality should be documented.

•DG: If a surgical or invasive diagnostic procedure is ordered, planned or scheduled at the time of the evaluation and management encounter, the type of procedure, e.g., laparoscopy, should be documented.

•DG: If a surgical or invasive diagnostic procedure is performed at the time of the evaluation and management encounter, the specific procedure should be documented.

•DG: The referral for or decision to perform a surgical or invasive diagnostic procedure on an urgent basis should be documented or implied.

The following table may be used to help determine whether the risk of significant complications, morbidity, and/or mortality is *minimal*, *low*, *moderate*, or *high*. Because the determination of risk is complex and not readily quantifiable, the table includes common clinical examples rather than absolute measures of risk. The assessment of risk of the presenting problem(s) is based on the risk related to the disease process anticipated between the present encounter and the next one. The assessment of risk of selecting diagnostic procedures and management options is based on the risk during and immediately following any procedures or treatment. The highest level of risk in any one category (presenting problem(s), diagnostic procedure(s), or management options) determines the overall risk.

DOCUMENTATION OF AN ENCOUNTER DOMINATED BY COUNSELING OR COORDINATION OF CARE

In the case where counseling and/or coordination of care dominates (more than 50%) of the physician/patient and/or family encounter (face-to-face time in the office or other or outpatient setting, floor/unit time in the hospital or nursing facility), time is considered the key or controlling factor to qualify for a particular level of evaluation and management services.

•DG: If the physician elects to report the level of service based on counseling and/or coordination of care, the total length of time of the encounter (face-to-face or floor time, as appropriate) should be documented and the record should describe the counseling and/or activities to coordinate care.

TABLE OF RISK

LEVEL OF RISK	PRESENTING PROBLEM(S)	DIAGNOSTIC PROCEDURES	MANAGEMENT OPTIONS
Minimal	• One self-limited or minor problem, e.g., cold, insect bite, tinea corporis	• Laboratory tests requiring venipuncture • Chest x-rays • EKG/EEG • Urinalysis • Ultrasound, e.g., echocardiography • KOH prep	• Rest • Gargles • Elastic bandages • Superficial dressings
Low	• Two or more self-limited or minor problems • One stable chronic illness, e.g., well controlled hyper-tension, non-insulin dependent diabetes, cataract, BPH • Acute uncomplicated illness or injury, e.g., cystitis, allergic rhinitis, simple sprain	• Physiologic tests not under stress, e.g., pulmonary function tests • Non-cardiovascular imaging studies with contrast, e.g., barium enema • Superficial needle biopsies • Clinical laboratory tests requiring arterial puncture • Skin biopsies	• Over-the-counter drugs • Minor surgery with no identified risk factors • Physical therapy • Occupational therapy • IV fluids without additives
Moderate	• One or more chronic illnesses with mild exacerbation, pro-gression, or side effects of treatment • Two or more stable chronic illnesses • Undiagnsed new problem with un-certain prognosis, e.g., lump in breast • Acute illness with systemic symptoms, e.g., pyelonephritis, pneumonitis, colitis • Acute complicated injury, e.g., head injury with brief loss of consciousness	• Physiologic tests under stress, e.g., cardiac stress test, fetal contraction stress test • Diagnostic endoscopies with no identified risk factors • Deep needle or incisional biopsy • Cardiovascular imaging studies with contrast and no identified risk factors, e.g., arterio-gram, cardiac cath-eterization • Obtain fluid from body cavity, e.g.lumbar puncture, thoracentesis, culdocentesis	• Minor surgery with identified risk factors • Elective major surgery (open, percutaneous or endoscopic) with no identified risk factors • Prescription drug management • Therapeutic nuclear medicine • IV fluids with additives • Closed treatment of fracture or dislocation without manipulation *CONTINUED*

TABLE OF RISK *(continued)*

LEVEL OF RISK	PRESENTING PROBLEM(S)	DIAGNOSTIC PROCEDURES	MANAGEMENT OPTIONS
High	• One or more chronic illnesses with severe exacerbation, progression, or side effects of treatment • Acute or chronic illnesses or injuries that pose a threat to life or bodily function, e.g., multiple trauma, acute MI, pulmonary embolus, severe respiratory distress, progressive severe rheumatoid arthritis, psychiatric illness with potential threat to self or others, peritonitis, acute renal failure • An abrupt change in neuro-logic status, e.g., seizure, TIA, weakness, sensory loss	• Cardiovascular imaging studies with contrast with identified risk factors • Cardiac electrophysiological tests • Diagnostic Endoscopies with identified risk factors • Discography	• Elective major surgery (open, percutaneous or endoscopic) with identified risk factors • Emergency major surgery (open, percutaneous or endoscopic) • Parenteral controlled substances • Drug therapy requiring intensive monitoring for toxicity • Decision not to resuscitate or to de-escalate care because of poor prognosis

EVALUATION AND MANAGEMENT

OFFICE OR OTHER OUTPATIENT SERVICES

Evaluation and management codes 99201-99215 are used to report services provided to new and established patients in the office or other outpatient facility, including the emergency department when the physician is not assigned to the emergency department. The key coding issues are the extent of history obtained, the extent of examination performed, and the complexity of medical decision making. Additional reporting issues include counseling and/or coordination of care, the nature of presenting problem(s), and the duration of face-to-face time spent with the patient and/or family.

CODING RULES

1. A patient is considered an outpatient until admitted as an inpatient to a health care facility.

2. If outpatient evaluation and management services are provided in conjunction with, or result in, an inpatient admission, the service is reported using CPT codes for initial hospital care.

3. CPT codes in this section may also be used to report the services provided by a physician to a patient in an observation area of a hospital.

4. Laboratory tests, radiology services, and diagnostic or therapeutic procedures performed in conjunction with evaluation and management services are reported in addition to the basic evaluation and management service.

5. Supplies and materials provided by the physician over and above those usually included with the evaluation and management or other services rendered may be listed separately. List all drugs, trays, supplies and materials provided.

NEW PATIENT

99201 Office or other outpatient visit for the evaluation and management of a new patient, which requires these three key components:

- a problem focused history;
- a problem focused examination; and

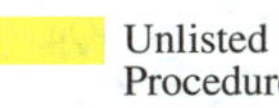

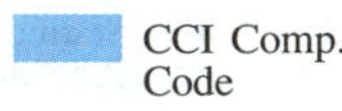

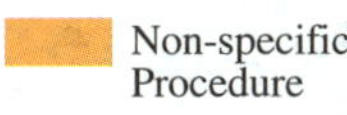

- straightforward medical decision making.

Counseling and/or coordination of care with other providers or agencies are provided consistent with the nature of the problem(s) and the patient's and/or family's needs.

Usually, the presenting problems are self limited or minor. Physicians typically spend 10 minutes face-to-face with the patient and/or family.

99202 Office or other outpatient visit for the evaluation and management of a new patient, which requires these three key components:

- an expanded problem focused history;
- an expanded problem focused examination; and
- straightforward medical decision making.

Counseling and/or coordination of care with other providers or agencies are provided consistent with the nature of the problem(s) and the patient's and/or family's needs.

Usually, the presenting problem(s) are of low to moderate severity. Physicians typically spend 20 minutes face-to-face with the patient and/or family.

99203 Office or other outpatient visit for the evaluation and management of a new patient, which requires these three key components:

- a detailed history;
- a detailed examination; and
- medical decision making of low complexity.

Counseling and/or coordination of care with other providers or agencies are provided consistent with the nature of the problem(s) and the patient's and/or family's needs.

Usually, the presenting problem(s) are of moderate severity. Physicians typically spend 30 minutes face-to-face with the patient and/or family.

99204 Office or other outpatient visit for the evaluation and management of a new patient, which requires these three key components:

- a comprehensive history;
- a comprehensive examination;
- and medical decision making of moderate complexity.

● New Code   ▲ Revised Code   ＊ Starred Procedure   ＋ Add-On Code   ⊘ Modifier -51 Exempt

Counseling and/or coordination of care with other providers or agencies are provided consistent with the nature of the problem(s) and the patient's and/or family's needs.

Usually, the presenting problem(s) are of moderate to high severity. Physicians typically spend 45 minutes face-to-face with the patient and/or family.

99205 Office or other outpatient visit for the evaluation and management of a new patient, which requires these three key components:

- a comprehensive history;
- a comprehensive examination; and
- medical decision making of high complexity.

Counseling and/or coordination of care with other providers or agencies are provided consistent with the nature of the problem(s) and the patient's and/or family's needs.

Usually, the presenting problem(s) are of moderate to high severity. Physicians typically spend 60 minutes face-to-face with the patient and/or family.

ESTABLISHED PATIENT

99211 Office or other outpatient visit for the evaluation and management of an established patient, that may not require the presence of a physician. Usually, the presenting problem(s) are minimal. Typically, 5 minutes are spent performing or supervising these services.

99212 Office or other outpatient visit for the evaluation and management of an established patient, which requires at least two of these three key components:

- a problem focused history;
- a problem focused examination;
- straightforward medical decision making.

Counseling and/or coordination of care with other providers or agencies are provided consistent with the nature of the problem(s) and the patient's and/or family's needs.

Usually, the presenting problem(s) are self limited or minor. Physicians typically 10 minutes face-to-face with the patient and/or family.

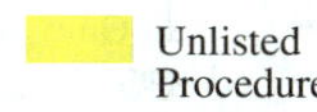
Separate Procedure

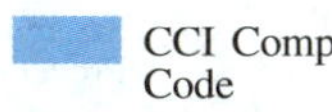
Unlisted Procedure

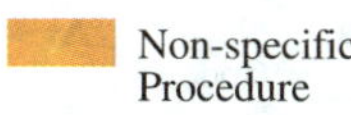
CCI Comp. Code

Non-specific Procedure

163

99213 Office or other outpatient visit for the evaluation and management of an established patient, which requires at least two of these three key components:

- an expanded problem focused history;
- an expanded problem focused examination;
- medical decision making of low complexity.

Counseling and coordination of care with other providers or agencies are provided consistent with the nature of the problem(s) and the patient's and/or family's needs.

Usually, the presenting problem(s) are of low to moderate severity. Physicians typically spend 15 minutes face-to-face with the patient and/or family.

99214 Office or other outpatient visit for the evaluation and management of an established patient, which requires at least two of these three key components:

- a detailed history;
- a detailed examination;
- medical decision making of moderate complexity.

Counseling and/or coordination of care with other providers or agencies are provided consistent with the nature of the problem(s) and the patient's and/or family's needs.

Usually, the presenting problem(s) are of moderate to high severity. Physicians typically spend 25 minutes face-to-face with the patient and/or family.

99215 Office or other outpatient visit for the evaluation and management of an established patient, which requires at least two of these three key components:

- a comprehensive history;
- a comprehensive examination;
- medical decision making of high complexity.

Counseling and/or coordination of care with other providers or agencies are provided consistent with the nature of the problem(s) and the patient's and/or family's needs.

Usually, the presenting problem(s) are of moderate to high severity. Physicians typically spend 40 minutes face-to-face with the patient and/or family.

● New Code   ▲ Revised Code   * Starred Procedure   + Add-On Code   ⊘ Modifier -51 Exempt

HOSPITAL OBSERVATION SERVICES

Occasionally a physician will watch or "observe" a patient in an area of an inpatient hospital designated as an "observation" area. This area is frequently located in or near the emergency room, and the observation typically after any acute care is rendered.

The purpose of the observation is to determine if the patient's condition requires inpatient hospitalization. Patients considered under observation status may be discharge from the observation area or admitted to the hospital as an inpatient.

All observation care services are "per day" and should be coded only once per date of service. CPT code 99217 is used to report all services provided on discharge from "observation status" if the discharge is on other than the initial date of "observation status."

OBSERVATION CARE DISCHARGE SERVICES

99217 Observation care discharge day management (This code is to be utilized by the physician to report all services provided to a patient on discharge from "observation status" if the discharge is on other than the initial date of "observation status." To report services to a patient designated as "observation status" or "inpatient status" and discharged on the same date, use codes for Observation or Inpatient Care Services [including Admission and Discharge Services, 99234-99236 as appropriate]).

INITIAL OBSERVATION CARE

NEW OR ESTABLISHED PATIENT

99218 Initial observation care, per day, for the evaluation and management of a patient which requires these three key components:

- a detailed or comprehensive history;
- a detailed or comprehensive examination; and
- medical decision making that is straightforward or of low complexity.

Counseling and/or coordination of care with other providers or agencies are provided consistent with the nature of the problem(s) and the patient's and/or family's needs.

Usually, the problem(s) requiring admission to "observation status" are of low severity.

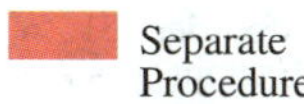

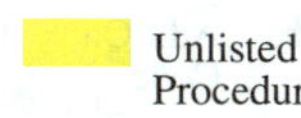

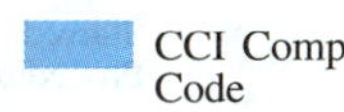

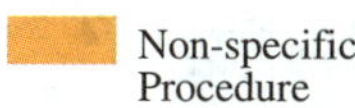

99219 Initial observation care, per day, for the evaluation and management of a patient, which requires these three key components:

- a comprehensive history;
- a comprehensive examination; and
- medical decision making of moderate complexity.

Counseling and/or coordination of care with other providers or agencies are provided consistent with the nature of the problem(s) and the patient's and/or family's needs.

Usually, the problem(s) requiring admission to "observation status" are of moderate severity.

99220 Initial observation care, per day, for the evaluation and management of a patient, which requires these three key components:

- a comprehensive history;
- a comprehensive examination; and
- medical decision making of high complexity.

Counseling and/or coordination of care with other providers or agencies are provided consistent with the nature of the problem(s) and the patient's and/or family's needs.

Usually, the problem(s) requiring admission to "observation status" are of high severity.

HOSPITAL INPATIENT SERVICES

Hospital inpatient services refer to hospital visits during the course of an inpatient hospital stay. The services may be provided by the patient's primary physician and/or other physicians in the event of multiple illnesses or injuries. Evaluation and management codes 99221-99239 are used to report services provided in the hospital. The key coding issues are the extent of history obtained, the extent of examination performed, and the complexity of medical decision making. Additional reporting issues include counseling and/or coordination of care, the nature of presenting problem(s), and the time spent at the bedside and on the patient's facility floor or unit.

CODING RULES

1. CPT codes defined as Initial Hospital Care are used to report the first hospital inpatient encounter with the patient by the admitting physician.

2. The admitting physician should report all service related to the admission provided in all other locations.

| ● New Code | ▲ Revised Code | ✻ Starred Procedure | ✚ Add-On Code | ⊘ Modifier -51 Exempt |

3. For observation care or inpatient hospital care services provided to patients who are admitted and discharged on the same date, report with CPT codes 99234-99236 from the Observation or Inpatient Care services subsections.

INITIAL HOSPITAL CARE

NEW OR ESTABLISHED PATIENT

99221 Initial hospital care, per day, for the evaluation and management of a patient which requires these three key components:

- a detailed or comprehensive history;
- a detailed or comprehensive examination; and
- medical decision making that is straightforward or of low complexity.

Counseling and/or coordination of care with other providers or agencies are provided consistent with the nature of the problem(s) and the patient's and/or family's needs.

Usually, the problem(s) requiring admission are of low severity. Physicians typically spend 30 minutes at the bedside and on the patient's hospital floor or unit.

99222 Initial hospital care, per day, for the evaluation and management of a patient, which requires these three key components:

- a comprehensive history;
- a comprehensive examination; and
- medical decision making of moderate complexity.

Counseling and/or coordination of care with other providers or agencies are provided consistent with the nature of the problem(s) and the patient's and/or family's needs.

Usually, the problem(s) requiring admission are of moderate severity. Physicians typically spend 50 minutes at the bedside and on the patient's hospital floor or unit.

99223 Initial hospital care, per day, for the evaluation and management of a patient, which requires these three key components:

- a comprehensive history;
- a comprehensive examination; and
- medical decision making of high complexity.

 Separate Procedure
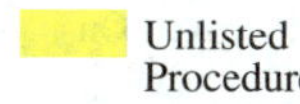 Unlisted Procedure
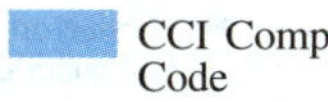 CCI Comp. Code
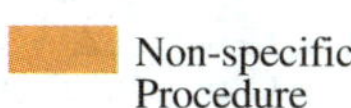 Non-specific Procedure

167

Counseling and/or coordination of care with other providers or agencies are provided consistent with the nature of the problem(s) and the patient's and/or family's needs.

Usually, the problem(s) requiring admission are of high severity. Physicians typically spend 70 minutes at the bedside and on the patient's hospital floor or unit.

SUBSEQUENT HOSPITAL CARE

99231 Subsequent hospital care, per day, for the evaluation and management of a patient, which requires at least two of these three key components:

- a problem focused interval history;
- a problem focused examination;
- medical decision making that is straightforward or of low complexity.

Counseling and/or coordination of care with other providers or agencies are provided consistent with the nature of the problem(s) and the patient's and/or family's needs.

Usually, the patient is stable, recovering or improving. Physicians typically spend 15 minutes at the bedside and on the patient's hospital floor or unit.

99232 Subsequent hospital care, per day, for the evaluation and management of a patient, which requires at least two of these three key components:

- an expanded problem focused interval history;
- an expanded problem focused examination;
- medical decision making of moderate complexity.

Counseling and/or coordination of care with other providers or agencies are provided consistent with the nature of the problem(s) and the patient's and/or family's needs.

Usually, the patient is responding inadequately to therapy or has developed a minor complication. Physicians typically spend 25 minutes at the bedside and on the patient's hospital floor or unit.

99233 Subsequent hospital care, per day, for the evaluation and management of a patient, which requires at least two of these three key components:

- a detailed interval history;
- a detailed examination;

- medical decision making of high complexity.

Counseling and/or coordination of care with other providers or agencies are provided consistent with the nature of the problem(s) and the patient's and/or family's needs.

Usually, the patient is unstable or has developed a significant complication or a significant new problem. Physicians typically spend 35 minutes at the bedside and on the patient's hospital floor or unit.

OBSERVATION OR INPATIENT CARE SERVICES (INCLUDING ADMISSION AND DISCHARGE SERVICES)

99234 Observation or inpatient hospital care, for the evaluation and management of a patient including admission and discharge on the same date which requires these three key components:

- a detailed or comprehensive history;
- a detailed or comprehensive examination; and
- medical decision making that is straightforward or of low complexity.

Counseling and/or coordination of care with other providers or agencies are provided consistent with the nature of the problem(s) and the patient's and/or family's needs.

Usually the presenting problem(s) requiring admission are of low severity.

99235 Observation or inpatient hospital care, for the evaluation and management of a patient including admission and discharge on the same date which requires these three key components:

- a comprehensive history;
- a comprehensive examination; and
- medical decision making of moderate complexity.

Counseling and/or coordination of care with other providers or agencies are provided consistent with the nature of the problem(s) and the patient's and/or family's needs.

Usually the presenting problem(s) requiring admission are of moderate severity.

99236 Observation or inpatient hospital care, for the evaluation and management of a patient including admission and discharge on the same date which requires these three key components:

- a comprehensive history;
- a comprehensive examination; and

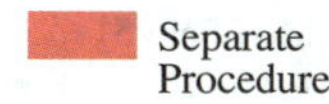
Separate
Procedure

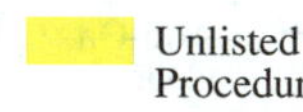
Unlisted
Procedure

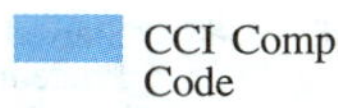
CCI Comp.
Code

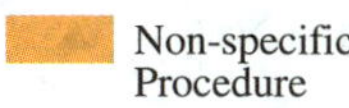
Non-specific
Procedure

169

■ medical decision making of high complexity.

Counseling and/or coordination of care with other providers or agencies are provided consistent with the nature of the problem(s) and the patient's and/or family's needs.

Usually the presenting problem(s) requiring admission are of high severity.

HOSPITAL DISCHARGE SERVICES

99238 Hospital discharge day management; 30 minutes or less

99239 Hospital discharge day management; more than 30 minutes

(These codes are to be utilized by the physician to report all services provided to a patient on the date of discharge, if other than the initial date of inpatient status. To report services to a patient who is admitted as an inpatient, and discharged on the same date, see codes 99234-99236 for observation or inpatient hospital care including the admission and discharge of the patient on the same date. To report concurrent care services provided by a physician(s) other than the attending physician, use subsequent hospital care codes (99231-99233) on the day of discharge.)

(For Observation Care Discharge, use 99217)

(For observation or inpatient hospital care including the admission and discharge of the patient on the same date, see 99234-99236)

(For Nursing Facility Care Discharge, 99315, 99316)

(For discharge services provided to newborns admitted and discharged on the same date, use 99435)

CONSULTATIONS

A consultation is the process of taking a history, performing a physical examination, and ordering and interpreting appropriate diagnostic tests, for the purpose of rendering an expert opinion about a patient's illness and/or injury.

A consultation may be requested by a patient's primary physician, by the patient or by a third party, such as a review organization.

The key coding issues are the location of the service, the extent of history obtained, the extent of examination performed, and the complexity of medical decision making. Additional reporting issues include counseling

● New Code   ▲ Revised Code   ✳ Starred Procedure   ✛ Add-On Code   ⊘ Modifier -51 Exempt

and/or coordination of care, the nature of presenting problem(s), and the time, depending on location, spent either face-to-face with the patient and/or family or at the bedside and on the patient's facility floor or unit.

CODING RULES

1. The request for a consultation from the attending physician or other appropriate source, and the need for a consultation must be documented in the patient's medical record.

2. The consulting physician must document all services provided and the resulting opinion in the patient's medical record.

3. Modifier -32 must be added to the consulting service CPT code if a confirmatory consultation is required by a third party, such as a PRO.

4. If the consulting physician assumes responsibility for the continuing care of the patient, the service is no longer considered a consultation, and any subsequent visit services rendered are coded using evaluation and management codes.

OFFICE OR OTHER OUTPATIENT CONSULTATIONS

NEW OR ESTABLISHED PATIENT

99241 Office consultation for a new or established patient, which requires these three key components:

- a problem focused history;
- a problem focused examination; and
- straightforward medical decision making.

Counseling and/or coordination of care with other providers or agencies are provided consistent with the nature of the problem(s) and the patient's and/or family's needs.

Usually, the presenting problem(s) are self limited or minor. Physicians typically spend 15 minutes face-to-face with the patient and/or family.

99242 Office consultation for a new or established patient, which requires these three key components:

- an expanded problem focused history;
- an expanded problem focused examination;
- and straightforward medical decision making.

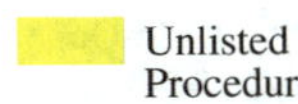
Separate Procedure

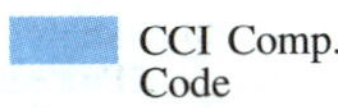
Unlisted Procedure

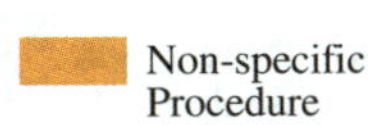
CCI Comp. Code

Non-specific Procedure

171

Counseling and/or coordination of care with other providers or agencies are provided consistent with the nature of the problem(s) and the patient's and/or family's needs.

Usually, the presenting problem(s) are of low severity. Physicians typically spend 30 minutes face-to-face with the patient and/or family.

99243 Office consultation for a new or established patient, which requires these three key components:

- a detailed history;
- a detailed examination; and
- medical decision making of low complexity.

Counseling and/or coordination of care with other providers or agencies are provided consistent with the nature of the problem(s) and the patient's and/or family's needs.

Usually, the presenting problem(s) are of moderate severity. Physicians typically spend 40 minutes face-to-face with the patient and/or family.

99244 Office consultation for a new or established patient, which requires these three key components:

- a comprehensive history;
- a comprehensive examination; and
- medical decision making of moderate complexity.

Counseling and/or coordination of care with other providers or agencies are provided consistent with the nature of the problem(s) and the patient's and/or family's needs.

Usually, the presenting problem(s) are of moderate to high severity. Physicians typically spend 60 minutes face-to-face with the patient and/or family.

99245 Office consultation for a new or established patient, which requires these three key components:

- a comprehensive history;
- a comprehensive examination; and
- medical decision making of high complexity.

Counseling and/or coordination of care with other providers or agencies are provided consistent with the nature of the problem(s) and the patient's and/or family's needs.

● New Code   ▲ Revised Code   ✱ Starred Procedure   ✛ Add-On Code   ⊘ Modifier -51 Exempt

Usually, the presenting problem(s) are of moderate to high severity. Physicians typically spend 80 minutes face-to-face with the patient and/or family.

INITIAL INPATIENT CONSULTATIONS

NEW OR ESTABLISHED PATIENT

The following CPT codes are used to report physician consultations provided to hospital inpatients, residents of nursing facilities, or patients in a partial hospital setting. Only one initial consultation should be reported by the consultant per admission.

99251 Initial inpatient consultation for a new or established patient, which requires these three key components:

- a problem focused history;
- a problem focused examination; and
- straightforward medical decision making.

Counseling and/or coordination of care with other providers or agencies are provided consistent with the nature of the problem(s) and the patient's and/or family's needs.

Usually, the presenting problem(s) are self limited or minor. Physicians typically spend 20 minutes at the bedside and on the patient's hospital floor or unit.

99252 Initial inpatient consultation for a new or established patient, which requires these three key components:

- an expanded problem focused history;
- an expanded problem focused examination; and
- straightforward medical decision making.

Counseling and/or coordination of care with other providers or agencies are provided consistent with the nature of the problem(s) and the patient's and/or family's needs.

Usually, the presenting problem(s) are of low severity. Physicians typically spend 40 minutes at the bedside and on the patient's hospital floor or unit.

99253 Initial inpatient consultation for a new or established patient, which requires these three key components:

- a detailed history;
- a detailed examination; and
- medical decision making of low complexity.

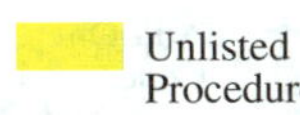 Separate Procedure

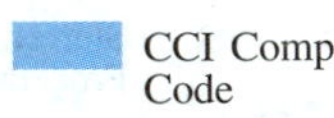 Unlisted Procedure

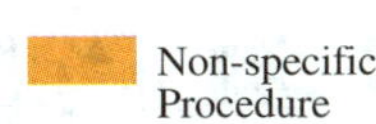 CCI Comp. Code

Non-specific Procedure

Counseling and/or coordination of care with other providers or agencies are provided consistent with the nature of the problem(s) and the patient's and/or family's needs.

Usually, the presenting problem(s) are of moderate severity. Physicians typically spend 55 minutes at the bedside and on the patient's hospital floor or unit.

99254 Initial inpatient consultation for a new or established patient, which requires three key components:

- ■ a comprehensive history;
- ■ a comprehensive examination; and
- ■ medical decision making of moderate complexity.

Counseling and/or coordination of care with other providers or agencies are provided consistent with the nature of the problem(s) and the patient's and/or family's needs.

Usually, the presenting problem(s) are of moderate to high severity. Physicians typically spend 80 minutes at the bedside and on the patient's hospital floor or unit.

99255 Initial inpatient consultation for a new or established patient, which requires these three key components:

- ■ a comprehensive history;
- ■ a comprehensive examination; and
- ■ medical decision making of high complexity.

Counseling and/or coordination of care with other providers or agencies are provided consistent with the nature of the problem(s) and the patient's and/or family's needs.

Usually, the presenting problem(s) are of moderate to high severity. Physicians typically spend 110 minutes at the bedside and on the patient's hospital floor or unit.

FOLLOW-UP INPATIENT CONSULTATIONS

ESTABLISHED PATIENT

Follow-up consultations are visits to complete the initial consultation or subsequent consultative visits requested by the attending physician. A follow-up consultation includes monitoring progress, recommending management modifications or advising on a new plan of care in response to changes in the patient's status.

If the consulting physician initiated treatment following the initial consultation, and participates thereafter in the patient's management,

● New Code   ▲ Revised Code   ＊ Starred Procedure   ✛ Add-On Code   ⊘ Modifier -51 Exempt subsequent hospital care CPT codes should be used instead of follow-up consultation CPT codes.

99261 Follow-up inpatient consultation for an established patient, which requires at least two of these three key components:

- a problem focused interval history;
- a problem focused examination;
- medical decision making that is straightforward or of low complexity.

Counseling and/or coordination of care with other providers or agencies are provided consistent with nature of the problem(s) and the patient's and/or family's needs.

Usually, the patient is stable, recovering or improving. Physicians typically 10 minutes at the bedside and on the patient's hospital floor or unit.

99262 Follow-up inpatient consultation for an established patient which requires at least two of these three key components:

- an expanded problem focused interval history;
- an expanded problem focused examination;
- medical decision making of moderate complexity.

Counseling and/or coordination of care with other providers or agencies are provided consistent with the nature of the problem(s) and the patient's and/or family's needs.

Usually, the patient is responding inadequately to therapy or has developed a minor complication. Physicians typically spend 20 minutes at the bedside and on the patient's hospital floor or unit.

99263 Follow-up inpatient consultation for an established patient which requires at least two of these three key components:

- a detailed interval history;
- a detailed examination;
- medical decision making of high complexity.

Counseling and/or coordination of care with other providers or agencies are provided consistent with the nature of the problem(s) and the patient's and/or family's needs.

Usually, the patient is unstable or has developed a significant complication or a significant new problem. Physicians typically spend 30 minutes at the bedside and on the patient's hospital floor or unit.

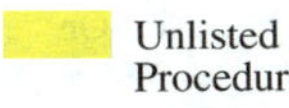 Separate Procedure

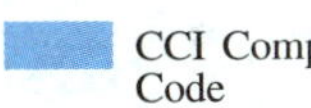 Unlisted Procedure

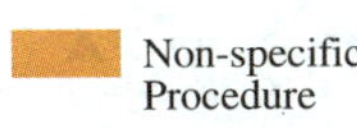 CCI Comp. Code

Non-specific Procedure

CONFIRMATORY CONSULTATIONS

NEW OR ESTABLISHED PATIENT

Confirmatory consultation codes are used when the consultation is requested by the patient, or other agency. Typically the consultation will involve a second or third opinion on the necessity or appropriateness of a medical treatment or surgical procedure recommended by another physician.

Note that there are special modifiers in the CPT coding system which are used to modify these codes. Use the following guidelines when adding modifiers to mandated consultations.

- If the second opinion is mandated by a professional review organization, use CPT modifier -32 if the patient IS NOT a Medicare patient and HCPCS Level II modifier -SF if the patient IS a Medicare patient.

- Many Medicare intermediaries have assigned HCPCS Level III modifiers for second opinions requested by the patient. Check with the local Medicare intermediary before reporting these services.

99271   Confirmatory consultation for a new or established patient, which requires these three key components:

- a problem focused history;
- a problem focused examination; and
- straightforward medical decision making.

Counseling and/or coordination of care with other providers or agencies are provided consistent with the nature of the problem(s) and the patient's and/or family's needs.

Usually, the presenting problem(s) are self limited or minor.

99272   Confirmatory consultation for a new or established patient, which requires these three key components:

- an expanded problem focused history;
- an expanded problem focused examination; and
- straightforward medical decision making.

Counseling and/or coordination of care with other providers or agencies are provided consistent with the nature of the problem(s) and the patient's and/or family's needs.

Usually, the presenting problem(s) are of low severity.

99273   Confirmatory consultation for a new or established patient, which requires these three key components:

- a detailed history;

● New Code   ▲ Revised Code   ✱ Starred Procedure   ✛ Add-On Code   ⊘ Modifier -51 Exempt

- a detailed examination; and
- medical decision making of low complexity.

Counseling and/or coordination of care with other providers or agencies are provided consistent with the nature of the problem(s) and the patient's and/or family's needs.

Usually, the presenting problem(s) are of moderate severity.

99274 Confirmatory consultation for a new or established patient, which requires these three key components:

- a comprehensive history;
- a comprehensive examination; and
- medical decision making of moderate complexity.

Counseling and/or coordination of care with other providers or agencies are provided consistent with the nature of the problem(s) and the patient's and/or family's needs.

Usually, the presenting problem(s) are of moderate to high severity.

99275 Confirmatory consultation for a new or established patient, which requires these three key components:

- a comprehensive history;
- a comprehensive examination; and
- medical decision making of high complexity.

Counseling and/or coordination of care with other providers or agencies are provided consistent with the nature of the problem(s) and the patient's and/or family's needs.

Usually, the presenting problem(s) are of moderate to high severity.

EMERGENCY DEPARTMENT SERVICES

Evaluation and management codes 99281-99288 are used to report services provided to new or established patients in the emergency department. The emergency department is defined as a facility for the treatment of patients with emergent conditions. The emergency department must be attached to a hospital and operate on a 24/7 basis.

The key coding issues for evaluation and management emergency services are the extent of history obtained, the extent of examination performed, and the complexity of medical decision making. Additional reporting issues include counseling and/or coordination of care, and the nature of presenting problem(s).

 Separate Procedure

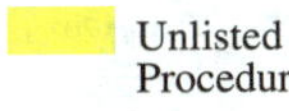 Unlisted Procedure

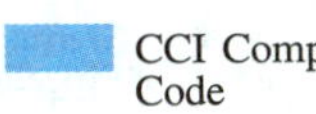 CCI Comp. Code

 Non-specific Procedure

Time is not a descriptive component for evaluation and management services provided in the emergency department. These services are typically provided on a variable intensity basis, often involving multiple encounters with several patients over an extended period of time. Therefore, it is difficult for physicians to provide accurate estimates of the time spent face-to-face with the patient in the emergency department.

CODING RULES

1. No distinction is made between new and established patients in the emergency department.

2. If the emergency department is used for observation or inpatient care services, report using codes from the Observation Care services subsection of the CPT coding system.

3. For critical care services provided in the emergency department, use the appropriate codes from the Critical Care subsection of the CPT coding system.

EMERGENCY DEPARTMENT SERVICES

NEW OR ESTABLISHED PATIENT

99281 Emergency department visit for the evaluation and management of a patient, which requires these three key components:

- a problem focused history;
- a problem focused examination; and
- straightforward medical decision making.

Counseling and/or coordination of care with other providers or agencies are provided consistent with the nature of the problem(s) and the patient's and/or family's needs.

Usually, the presenting problem(s) are self limited or minor.

99282 Emergency department visit for the evaluation and management of a patient, which requires these three key components:

- an expanded problem focused history;
- an expanded problem focused examination; and
- medical decision making of low complexity.

Counseling and/or coordination of care with other providers or agencies are provided consistent with the nature of the problem(s) and the patient's and/or family's needs.

Usually, the presenting problem(s) are of low to moderate severity.

● New Code   ▲ Revised Code   * Starred Procedure   + Add-On Code   ⊘ Modifier -51 Exempt

99283 Emergency department visit for the evaluation and management of a patient, which requires these three key components:

- an expanded problem focused history;
- an expanded problem focused examination; and
- medical decision making of moderate complexity.

Counseling and/or coordination of care with other providers or agencies are provided consistent with the nature of the problem(s) and the patient's and/or family's needs.

Usually, the presenting problem(s) are of moderate severity.

99284 Emergency department visit for the evaluation and management of a patient, which requires these three key components:

- a detailed history;
- a detailed examination; and
- medical decision making of moderate complexity.

Counseling and/or coordination of care with other providers or agencies are provided consistent with the nature of the problem(s) and the patient's and/or family's needs.

Usually, the presenting problem(s) are of high severity, and require urgent evaluation by the physician but do not pose an immediate significant threat to life or physiologic function.

99285 Emergency department visit for the evaluation and management of a patient, which requires these three key components within the constraints imposed by the urgency of the patient's clinical condition and/or mental status:

- a comprehensive history;
- a comprehensive examination; and
- medical decision making of high complexity.

Counseling and/or coordination of care with other providers or agencies are provided consistent with the nature of the problem(s) and the patient's and/or family's needs.

Usually, the presenting problem(s) are of high severity and pose an immediate significant threat to life or physiologic function.

OTHER EMERGENCY SERVICES

99288 Physician direction of emergency medical systems (EMS) emergency care, advanced life support

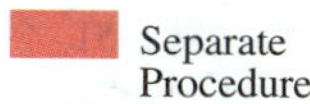 Separate Procedure

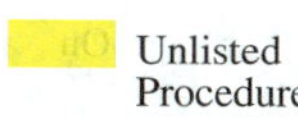 Unlisted Procedure

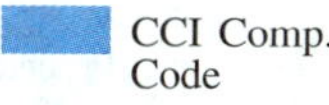 CCI Comp. Code

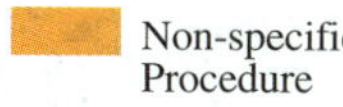 Non-specific Procedure

PATIENT TRANSPORT

Occasionally a seriously ill or injured patient must be transferred from one facility to another under the direct care of a physician. If the total face-to-face time spent in attending to the patient is less than 30 minutes, the patient transport codes should not be coded. Any additional services performed by the physician during the transport period may be coded separately.

- **99289** Physician constant attention of the critically ill or injured patient during an interfacility transport; first 30-74 minutes

- **+99290**   each additional 30 minutes (List separately in addition to code for primary service)

  (Use 99290 in conjunction with 99289)

  (Codes 99289, 99290 may be reported separately from any other procedure/service provided on the date of the transfer. The time spent by the physician performing separately reportable services or procedures should not be included in the face-to-face time reported by codes 99289, 99290)

CRITICAL CARE SERVICES

Critical care includes the care of critically ill patients in a variety of medical emergencies that requires the constant attention of the physician. Cardiac arrest, shock, bleeding, respiratory failure, postoperative complications, or a critically ill neonate are examples of medical emergencies defined in CPT. Critical care is usually, but not always, given in a critical area, such as the coronary care unit, intensive care unit, respiratory care unit, or the emergency care facility.

CPT codes listed in this section are intended to include cardiopulmonary resuscitation (CPR) and the variety of services commonly employed with this procedure as well as other acute emergency situations. Other services, such as catheter placement, cardiac output measurement, dialysis management, control of gastrointestinal hemorrhage, cardioversion, etc. are considered to be included when reporting critical care services under these time-based CPT codes.

Evaluation and management codes 99291-99292 are used to report services for specific conditions (usually) provided in a critical care area. Key coding issues include the condition of the patient (supported by diagnostic coding), the service(s) provided, and the amount of time spent. Follow-up critical care services may be reported using either evaluation and management codes from this section or hospital evaluation and management codes from the series 99231-99233.

● New Code	▲ Revised Code	* Starred Procedure	+ Add-On Code	⊘ Modifier -51 Exempt

CODING RULES

1. The critical care CPT codes are used to report the total duration of time spent by a physician providing constant attention to a critically ill patient.

2. Critical care code 99291 is used to report the first hour of critical care on a given day. It may be reported only once per day even if the time spent is not continuous on that day.

3. Critical care 99292 is used to report each additional 30 minutes beyond the first hour.

4. Other procedures which are not considered included in the critical care services, for example, suturing of lacerations, setting of fractures, reduction of joint dislocations, lumbar puncture, peritoneal lavage and bladder tap, are reported separately.

CORRECT CODING CHART FOR CRITICAL CARE SERVICES

DURATION OF CRITICAL CARE	CODE(S) TO REPORT
less than 30 minutes	appropriate evaluation and management codes
30- 74 minutes	99291 once
75-104 minutes	99291 once and 99292 once
105-134 minutes	99291 once and 99292 twice
135-164 minutes	99291 once and 99292 three times
165-194 minutes	99291 once and 99292 four times

CRITICAL CARE SERVICES

99291   Critical care, evaluation and management of the critically ill or critically injured patient; first 30-74 minutes

+99292   each additional 30 minutes (List separately in addition to code for primary service)

(Use 99292 in conjunction with 99291)

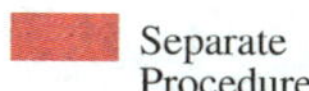

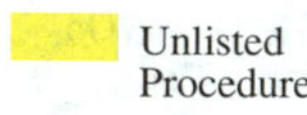

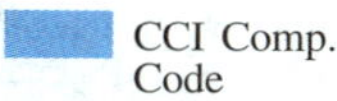

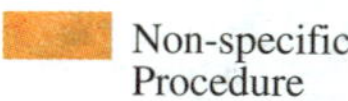

NEONATAL INTENSIVE CARE

Neonatal intensive care refers to services, including management, monitoring and treatment, provided to a critically ill newborn or infant, usually in the neonatal intensive care unit (NICU). Counseling of parents, case management services and personal direct supervision of the NICU team are bundled into these codes.

CODING RULES

1. Neonatal intensive care services start with the date of admission and are coded only once per day, per patient.

2. Once the neonate is no longer considered to be critically ill, report with CPT codes for subsequent hospital care instead of neonatal intensive care.

3. Neonatal intensive care CPT codes are coded in addition to physician stand-by code 99360 or newborn resuscitation code 99440 when the physician is present for the delivery and newborn resuscitation is required.

4. Procedures which are routinely performed as part of NICU care are included in the bundled NICU codes. These routine procedures include: venous/arterial catheterization, bladder catheterization, intubation, lumbar puncture, mechanical ventilation/CPAP, IV and/or blood transfusions, and monitoring.

NEONATAL INTENSIVE CARE SERVICES

99295 Initial neonatal intensive care, per day, for the evaluation and management of a critically ill neonate or infant

This code is reserved for the date of admission for neonates who are critically ill. Critically ill neonates require cardiac and/or respiratory support (including ventilator or nasal CPAP when indicated), continuous or frequent vital sign monitoring, laboratory and blood gas interpretations, follow-up physician reevaluations, and constant observation by the health care team under direct physician supervision. Immediate preoperative evaluation and stabilization of neonates with life threatening surgical or cardiac conditions are included under this code.

| ● New Code | ▲ Revised Code | ✳ Starred Procedure | ✛ Add-On Code | ⊘ Modifier -51 Exempt |

99296 Subsequent neonatal intensive care, per day, for the evaluation and management of a critically ill and unstable neonate or infant.

A critically ill and unstable neonate will require cardiac and/or respiratory support (including ventilator or nasal CPAP when indicated), continuous or frequent vital sign monitoring, laboratory and blood gas interpretations, follow-up physician re-evaluations throughout a 24-hour period, and constant observation by the health care team under direct physician supervision. In addition, most will require frequent ventilator changes, intravenous fluid alterations, and/or early initiation of parenteral nutrition. Neonates in the immediate post-operative period or those who become critically ill and unstable during the hospital stay will commonly qualify for this level of care.

This code encompasses intensive care provided on dates subsequent to the admission date.

99297 Subsequent neonatal intensive care, per day, for the evaluation and management of a critically ill though stable neonate or infant.

Critically ill though stable neonates require cardiac and/or respiratory support (including ventilator and nasal CPAP when indicated), continuous or frequent vital sign monitoring, laboratory and blood gas interpretations, follow-up physician re-evaluations throughout a 24-hour period, and constant observation by the health care team under direct physician supervision. Neonates at this level of care would be expected to require less frequent changes in respiratory, cardiovascular and fluid and electrolyte therapy as those included under code 99296.

This code encompasses intensive care provided on dates subsequent to the admission date.

99298 Subsequent neonatal intensive care, per day, for the evaluation and management of the recovering very low birth weight infant (less than 1500 grams).

Very low birth weight neonates who are no longer critically ill continue to require intensive cardiac and respiratory monitoring, continuous and/or frequent vital sign monitoring, heat maintenance, enteral and/or parenteral nutritional adjustments, laboratory and oxygen monitoring and constant observation by the health care team under direct physician supervision. Neonates of this level of care would be expected to require infrequent changes in respiratory, cardiovascular and/or fluid and electrolyte therapy as those induced under 99296 or 99297.

 Separate Procedure

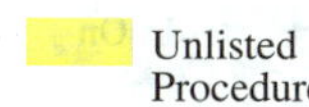 Unlisted Procedure

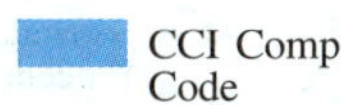 CCI Comp. Code

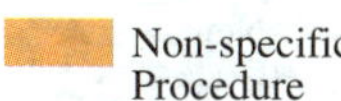 Non-specific Procedure

183

This code encompasses intensive care provided on days subsequent to the admission date.

NURSING FACILITY SERVICE

A patient may be transferred from an inpatient hospital to a nursing facility for supervised care when the patient no longer requires the skill levels of the inpatient hospital. Evaluation and management service codes 99301-99313 are used to report services provided in nursing facilities. The key coding issues are the extent of history obtained, the extent of examination performed, and the complexity of medical decision making. Additional reporting issues include counseling and/or coordination of care, the nature of presenting problem(s), and the time spent at the bedside and on the patient's facility floor or unit.

These CPT codes are also used to report evaluation and management services provided to a patient in a psychiatric residential treatment center. If procedures such as medical psychotherapy are provided in addition to evaluation and management services, these are coded in addition to the evaluation and management services.

CPT codes in this section apply to Comprehensive Nursing Facility Assessments and Subsequent Nursing Facility care. Both subcategories apply to new and established patients. Comprehensive Assessments may be performed at one or more sites during the assessment process; including the hospital, the office, a nursing facility, a domiciliary facility and/or the patient's home.

CODING RULES

1. If a patient is admitted to the nursing facility after receiving services in the physician's office or hospital emergency department, all evaluation and management services are considered inclusive in the initial nursing facility care.

2. With the exception of hospital discharge services, evaluation and management service on the same date provided in locations other than the nursing facility that are related to the admission should not be coded separately.

3. When reporting these CPT codes to Medicare include the HCPCS Level II modifier -SP or -MP, or HCPCS Level III modifier if specified by the local Medicare carrier.

| ● New Code | ▲ Revised Code | ✳ Starred Procedure | ✛ Add-On Code | ⊘ Modifier -51 Exempt |

COMPREHENSIVE NURSING FACILITY ASSESSMENTS

NEW OR ESTABLISHED PATIENT

99301 Evaluation and management of a new or established patient involving an annual nursing facility assessment which requires these three key components:

- a detailed interval history;
- a comprehensive examination; and
- medical decision making that is straightforward or of low complexity.

Counseling and/or coordination of care with other providers or agencies are provided consistent with the nature of the problem(s) and the patient's and/or family's needs.

Usually, the patient is stable, recovering or improving. The review and affirmation of the medical plan of care is required. Physicians typically spend 30 minutes at the bedside and on the patient's facility floor or unit.

99302 Evaluation and management of a new or established patient involving a nursing facility assessment which requires these three key components:

- a detailed interval history;
- a comprehensive examination; and
- medical decision making of moderate to high complexity.

Counseling and/or coordination of care with other providers or agencies are provided consistent with the nature of the problem(s) and the patient's and/or family's needs.

Usually, the patient has developed a significant complication or a significant new problem and has had a major permanent change in status.

The creation of a new medical plan of care is required. Physicians typically spend 40 minutes at the bedside and on the patient's facility floor or unit.

99303 Evaluation and management of a new or established patient involving a nursing facility assessment at the time of initial admission or readmission to the facility, which requires these three key components:

- a comprehensive history;
- a comprehensive examination; and
- medical decision making of moderate to high complexity.

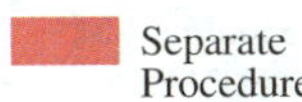
Separate
Procedure

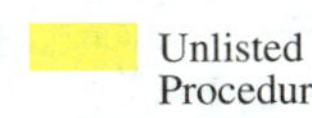
Unlisted
Procedure

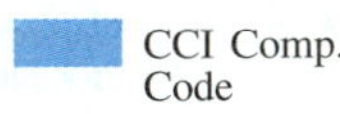
CCI Comp.
Code

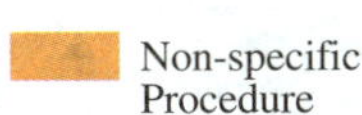
Non-specific
Procedure

185

Counseling and/or coordination of care with other providers or agencies are provided consistent with the nature of the problem(s) and the patient's and/or family's needs.

The creation of a medical plan of care is required. Physicians typically spend 50 minutes at the bedside and on the patient's facility floor or unit.

SUBSEQUENT NURSING FACILITY CARE

NEW OR ESTABLISHED PATIENT

99311 Subsequent nursing facility care, per day, for the evaluation and management of a new or established patient, which requires at least two of these three key components:

- a problem focused interval history;
- a problem focused examination;
- medical decision making that is straightforward or of low complexity.

Counseling and/or coordination of care with other providers or agencies are provided consistent with the nature of the problem(s) and the patient's and/or family's needs.

Usually, the patient is stable, recovering or improving. Physicians typically spend 15 minutes at the bedside and on the patient's facility floor or unit.

99312 Subsequent nursing facility care, per day, for the evaluation and management of a new or established patient, which requires at least two of these three key components:

- an expanded problem focused interval history;
- an expanded problem focused examination;
- medical decision making of moderate complexity.

Counseling and/or coordination of care with other providers or agencies are provided consistent with the nature of the problem(s) and the patient's and/or family's needs.

Usually, the patient is responding inadequately to therapy or has developed a minor complication. Physicians typically spend 25 minutes at the bedside and on the patient's facility floor or unit.

99313 Subsequent nursing facility care, per day, for the evaluation and management of a new or established patient, which requires at least two of these three key components:

- a detailed interval history;

● New Code   ▲ Revised Code   * Starred Procedure   + Add-On Code   ⊘ Modifier -51 Exempt

- a detailed examination;
- medical decision making of moderate to high complexity.

Counseling and/or coordination of care with other providers or agencies are provided consistent with the nature of the problem(s) and the patient's and/or family's needs.

Usually, the patient has developed a significant complication or a significant new problem. Physicians typically spend 35 minutes at the bedside and on the patient's facility floor or unit.

NURSING FACILITY DISCHARGE SERVICES

99315   Nursing facility discharge day management; 30 minutes or less

99316   more than 30 minutes

DOMICILIARY, REST HOME (eg, BOARDING HOME), OR CUSTODIAL CARE SERVICES

Evaluation and management service codes 99321-99333 are used to report services provided to new and established patients in domiciliary, rest home or custodial care facilities. The key coding issues are the extent of history obtained, the extent of examination performed, and the complexity of medical decision making. Additional reporting issues include counseling and/or coordination of care, the nature of presenting problem(s).

When reporting these CPT codes to Medicare include HCPCS modifier -SP or -MP to indicate single or multiple patients seen during the visit. Consult the local Medicare intermediary before using these modifiers.

NEW PATIENT

99321   Domiciliary or rest home visit for the evaluation and management of a new patient which requires these three key components:

- a problem focused history;
- a problem focused examination; and
- medical decision making that is straightforward or of low complexity.

Counseling and/or coordination of care with other providers or agencies are provided consistent with the nature of the problem(s) and the patient's and/or family's needs.

Usually, the presenting problem(s) are of low severity.

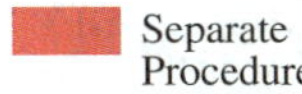

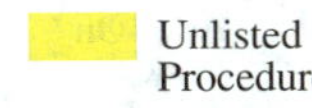

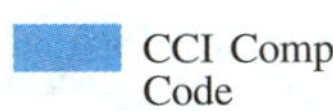

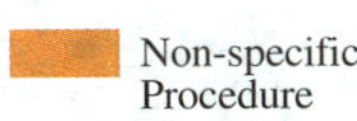

99322 Domiciliary or rest home visit for the evaluation and management of a new patient, which requires these three key components:

- an expanded problem focused history;
- an expanded problem focused examination; and
- medical decision making of moderate complexity.

Counseling and/or coordination of care with other providers or agencies are provided consistent with the nature of the problem(s) and the patient's and/or family's needs.

Usually, the presenting problem(s) are of moderate severity.

99323 Domiciliary or rest home visit for the evaluation and management of a new patient, which requires these three key components:

- a detailed history;
- a detailed examination; and
- medical decision making of high complexity.

Counseling and/or coordination of care with other providers or agencies are provided consistent with the nature of the problem(s) and the patient's and/or family's needs.

Usually, the presenting problem(s) are of high complexity.

ESTABLISHED PATIENT

99331 Domiciliary or rest home visit for the evaluation and management of an established patient, which requires at least two of these three key components:

- a problem focused interval history;
- a problem focused examination;
- medical decision making that is straightforward or of low complexity.

Counseling and/or coordination of care with other providers or agencies are provided consistent with the nature of the problem(s) and the patient's and/or family's needs.

Usually, the patient is stable, recovering or improving.

99332 Domiciliary or rest home visit for the evaluation and management of an established patient, which requires at least two of these three key components:

- an expanded problem focused interval history;
- an expanded problem focused examination;

■ medical decision making of moderate complexity.

Counseling and/or coordination of care with other providers or agencies are provided consistent with the nature of the problem(s) and the patient's and/or family's needs.

Usually, the patient is responding inadequately to therapy or has developed a minor complication.

99333 Domiciliary or rest home visit for the evaluation and management of an established patient, which requires at least two of these three key components:

■ a detailed interval history;
■ a detailed examination;
■ medical decision making of high complexity.

Counseling and/or coordination of care with other providers or agencies are provided consistent with the nature of the problem(s) and the patient's and/or family's needs.

Usually, the patient is unstable or has developed a significant complication or a significant new problem.

HOME SERVICES

Evaluation and management codes 99341-99353 are used to report services provided to new and established patients in the patient's home. The key coding issues are the extent of history obtained, the extent of examination performed, and the complexity of medical decision making. Additional reporting issues include counseling and/or coordination of care, and the nature of presenting problem(s).

NEW PATIENT

99341 Home visit for the evaluation and management of a new patient, which requires these three key components:

■ a problem focused history;
■ a problem focused examination; and
■ straightforward medical decision making.

Counseling and/or coordination of care with other providers or agencies are provided consistent with the nature of the problem(s) and the patient's and/or family's needs.

Usually, the presenting problem(s) are of low severity. Physicians typically spend 20 minutes face-to-face with the patient and/or family.

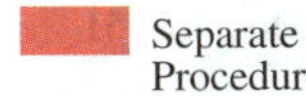

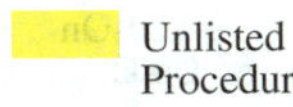

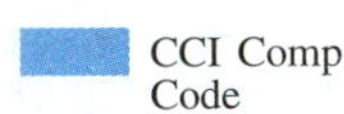

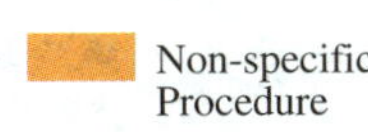

99342 Home visit for the evaluation and management of a new patient, which requires these three key components:

- an expanded problem focused history;
- an expanded problem focused examination; and
- medical decision making of low complexity.

Counseling and/or coordination of care with other providers or agencies are provided consistent with the nature of the problem(s) and the patient's and/or family's needs.

Usually, the presenting problem(s) are of moderate severity. Physicians typically spend 30 minutes face-to-face with the patient and/or family.

99343 Home visit for the evaluation and management of a new patient, which requires these three key components:

- a detailed history;
- a detailed examination; and
- medical decision making of moderate complexity.

Counseling and/or coordination of care with other providers or agencies are provided consistent with the nature of the problem(s) and the patient's and/or family's needs.

Usually, the presenting problem(s) are of moderate to high severity. Physicians typically spend 45 minutes face-to-face with the patient and/or family.

99344 Home visit for the evaluation and management of a new patient, which requires these three components:

- a comprehensive history;
- a comprehensive examination; and
- medical decision making of moderate complexity.

Counseling and/or coordination of care with other providers or agencies are provided consistent with the nature of the problem(s) and the patient's and/or family's needs.

Usually, the presenting problem(s) are of high severity. Physicians typically spend 60 minutes face-to-face with the patient and/or family.

99345 Home visit for the evaluation and management of a new patient, which requires these three key components:

- a comprehensive history;
- a comprehensive examination; and
- medical decision making of high complexity.

● New Code   ▲ Revised Code   ✱ Starred Procedure   + Add-On Code   ⊘ Modifier -51 Exempt

Counseling and/or coordination of care with other providers or agencies are provided consistent with the nature of the problem(s) and the patient's and/or family's needs.

Usually, the patient is unstable or has developed a significant new problem requiring immediate physician attention. Physicians typically spend 75 minutes face-to-face with the patient and/or family.

ESTABLISHED PATIENT

99347 Home visit for the evaluation and management of an established patient, which requires at least two of these three key components:

- a problem focused interval history;
- a problem focused examination;
- straightforward medical decision making.

Counseling and/or coordination of care with other providers or agencies are provided consistent with the nature of the problem(s) and the patient's and/or family's needs.

Usually, the presenting problem(s) are self-limited or minor. Physicians typically spend 15 minutes face-to-face with the patient and/or family.

99348 Home visit for the evaluation and management of an established patient, which requires at least two of these three key components:

- an expanded problem focused interval history;
- an expanded problem focused examination;
- medical decision making of low complexity.

Counseling and/or coordination of care with other providers or agencies are provided consistent with the nature of the problem(s) and the patient's and/or family's needs.

Usually, the presenting problem(s) are of low to moderate severity. Physicians typically spend 25 minutes face-to-face with the patient and/or family.

99349 Home visit for the evaluation and management of an established patient, which requires at least two of these three key components:

- a detailed interval history;
- a detailed examination;
- medical decision making of moderate complexity.

 Separate Procedure

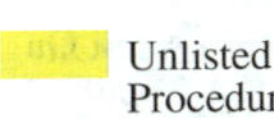 Unlisted Procedure

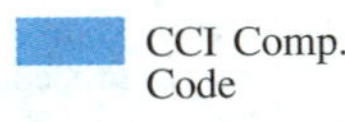 CCI Comp. Code

Non-specific Procedure

Counseling and/or coordination of care with other providers or agencies are provided consistent with the nature of the problem(s) and the patient's and/or family's needs.

Usually, the presenting problem(s) are moderate to high severity. Physicians typically spend 40 minutes face-to-face with the patient and/or family.

99350 Home visit for the evaluation and management of an established patient, which requires at least two of these three key components:

- a comprehensive interval history;
- a comprehensive examination;
- medical decision making of moderate to high complexity.

Counseling and/or coordination of care with other providers or agencies are provided consistent with the nature of the problem(s) and the patient's and/or family's needs.

Usually, the presenting problem(s) are of moderate to high severity. The patient may be unstable or may have developed a significant new problem requiring immediate physician attention. Physicians typically spend 60 minutes face-to-face with the patient and/or family.

PROLONGED SERVICES

Evaluation and management service CPT codes -99360 are used to report inpatient or outpatient services which include prolonged service or physician standby service that is beyond the usual service. The key coding issues are the location of the service, whether the service is direct (face-to-face) or not direct, and the total duration of the prolonged service.

CODING RULES

1. Prolonged services are reported in addition to other physician services.

2. Prolonged services involving direct (face-to-face) time is reported as cumulative time on a given date, even if the time is not continuous.

3. If the total duration of prolonged services is less than 30 minutes, the prolonged service is not reported.

● New Code	▲ Revised Code	* Starred Procedure	+ Add-On Code	⊘ Modifier -51 Exempt

CORRECT CODING CHART FOR PROLONGED SERVICES

DURATION OF PROLONGED SERVICE	CODE(S) TO REPORT
less than 30 minutes	not reported separately
30- 74 minutes	once
75-104 minutes	once and 99355 once
105-134 minutes	once and 99355 twice
135-164 minutes	once and 99355 three times
165-194 minutes	once and 99355 four times

PROLONGED PHYSICIAN SERVICE WITH DIRECT (FACE-TO-FACE) PATIENT CONTACT

+99354 Prolonged physician service in the office or other outpatient setting requiring direct (face-to-face) patient contact beyond the usual service (eg, prolonged care and treatment of an acute asthmatic patient in an outpatient setting); first hour (List separately in addition to code for office or other outpatient Evaluation and Management service)

(Use in conjunction with codes 99201-99215, 99241-99245, 99301-99350)

+99355 each additional 30 minutes (List separately in addition to code for prolonged physician service)

(Use 99355 in conjunction with codes)

+99356 Prolonged physician service in the inpatient setting, requiring direct (face-to-face) patient contact beyond the usual service (eg, maternal fetal monitoring for high risk delivery or other physiological monitoring, prolonged care of an acutely ill inpatient); first hour (List separately in addition to code for inpatient Evaluation and Management service)

(Use 99356 in conjunction with codes 99221-99233, 99251-99255, 99261-99263)

+99357 each additional 30 minutes (List separately in addition to code for prolonged physician service)

(Use 99357 in conjunction with code 99356)

Separate Procedure

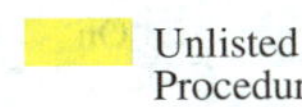
Unlisted Procedure

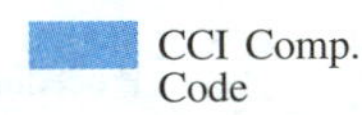
CCI Comp. Code

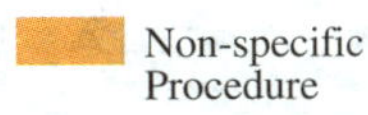
Non-specific Procedure

193

PROLONGED PHYSICIAN SERVICE WITHOUT DIRECT (FACE-TO-FACE) PATIENT CONTACT

+99358 Prolonged evaluation and management service before and/or after direct (face-to-face) patient care (eg, review of extensive records and tests, communication with other professionals and/or the patient/family); first hour (List separately in addition to code(s) for other physician service(s) and/or inpatient or outpatient Evaluation and Management service)

+99359 each additional 30 minutes (List separately in addition to code for prolonged physician service)

(Use 99359 in conjunction with code 99358)

(To report telephone calls, see 99371-99373)

PHYSICIAN STANDBY SERVICE

99360 Physician standby service, requiring prolonged physician attendance, each 30 minutes (eg, operative standby, standby for frozen section, for cesarean/high risk delivery, for monitoring EEG)

(99360 may be reported in addition to 99431, 99440 as appropriate)

(99360 may not be reported in addition to 99436)

CASE MANAGEMENT SERVICES

Case management is a process wherein a physician is responsible for direct care of the patient and has the additional responsibility of coordinating all other services provided to the patient. Case management services may be provided during medical conferences, or by telephone. The key coding issues are the type of service, the amount of time spent, and the level of service provided.

TEAM CONFERENCES

99361 Medical conference by a physician with interdisciplinary team of health professionals or representatives of community agencies to coordinate activities of patient care (patient not present); approximately 30 minutes

99362 approximately 60 minutes

● New Code   ▲ Revised Code   * Starred Procedure   + Add-On Code   ⊘ Modifier -51 Exempt

TELEPHONE CALLS

99371   Telephone call by a physician to patient or for consultation or medical management or for coordinating medical management with other health care professionals (eg, nurses, therapists, social workers, nutritionists, physicians, pharmacists); simple or brief (eg, to report on tests and/or laboratory results, to clarify or alter previous instructions, to integrate new information from other health professionals into the medical treatment plan, or to adjust therapy)

99372   intermediate (eg, to provide advice to an established patient on a new problem, to initiate therapy that can be handled by telephone, to discuss test results in detail, to coordinate medical management of a new problem in an established patient, to discuss and evaluate new information and details, or to initiate new plan of care)

99373   complex or lengthy (eg, lengthy counseling session with anxious or distraught patient, detailed or prolonged discussion with family members regarding seriously ill patient, lengthy communication necessary to coordinate complex services of several different health professionals working on different aspects of the total patient care plan)

CARE PLAN OVERSIGHT SERVICES

Care plans prepared and/or reviewed by a physician are frequently required for patients under the care of home health agencies, hospices, or residing in nursing facilities. Evaluation and management service codes 99374-99380 are used to report care plan oversight services. The key coding issues are the location of service, the complexity of the plan, and the amount of physician time provided within a 30-day period.

CODING RULES

1.   Evaluation and management services are not inclusive of care plan oversight services. Care plan oversight is coded separately.

2.   Care plan oversight services may be coded only by a single physician for each patient during a specific period of time.

▲ **99374**   Physician supervision of a patient under care of home health agency (patient not present) in home, domiciliary or equivalent environment (eg, Alzheimer's facility) requiring complex and multidisciplinary care modalities involving regular physician development and/or revision of care plans, review of subsequent reports of patient status, review of related laboratory and other

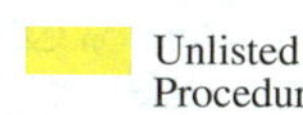

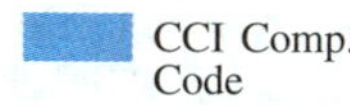

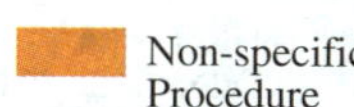

studies, communication (including telephone calls) for purposes of assessment or care decisions with health care professional(s), family member(s), surrogate decision maker(s) (eg., legal guardian) and/or key caregiver(s) involved in patient's care, integration of new information into the medical treatment plan and/or adjustment of medical therapy, within a calendar month; 15-29 minutes

99375   30 minutes or more

▲ **99377**   Physician supervision of a hospice patient (patient not present) requiring complex and multidisciplinary care modalities involving regular physician development and/or revision of care plans, review of subsequent reports of patient status, review of related laboratory and other studies, communication (including telephone calls) for purposes of assessment or care decisions with health care professional(s), family member(s), surrogate decision maker(s) (eg, legal guardian) and/or key caregiver(s) involved in patient's care, integration of new information into the medical treatment plan and/or adjustment of medical therapy, within a calendar month; 15-29 minutes

99378   30 minutes or more

▲ **99379**   Physician supervision of a nursing facility patient (patient not present) requiring complex and multidisciplinary care modalities involving regular physician development and/or revision of care plans, review of subsequent reports of patient status, review of related laboratory and other studies, communication (including telephone calls) for purposes of assessment or care decisions with health care professional(s), family member(s), surrogate decision maker(s) (eg, legal guardian) and/or key caregiver(s) involved in patient's care, integration of new information into the medical treatment plan and/or adjustment of medical therapy, within a calendar month; 15-29 minutes

99380   30 minutes or more

PREVENTIVE MEDICINE SERVICES

Preventive medicine services codes are used to report routine evaluation and management of adults and children in the absence of patient complaints or counseling and/or risk factor reduction intervention services to healthy individuals. The key coding issues are whether the patient is a new patient or established patient, the age of the patient, the circumstances of the examination, and the nature of any abnormalities encountered, and for counseling services, whether the service was provided to an individual or to a group and the amount of time spent counseling.

● New Code	▲ Revised Code	✳ Starred Procedure	✚ Add-On Code	⊘ Modifier -51 Exempt

CODING RULES

1. The selection of Preventive Medicine codes is mostly dependent upon the age of the patient.

2. Preventive medicine codes are coded only in the absence of illness. If illness, injury is discovered during provision of a preventive medicine service, office/outpatient evaluation and management codes are coded.

3. Immunizations and diagnostic studies involving laboratory or radiology, or other procedures are not included in the preventive medicine service and should be coded separately.

NEW PATIENT

▲ **99381**   Initial comprehensive preventive medicine evaluation and management of an individual including an age and gender appropriate history, examination, counseling/anticipatory guidance/risk factor reduction interventions, and the ordering of appropriate immunization(s), laboratory/diagnostic procedures, new patient; infant (age under 1 year)

99382   early childhood (age 1 through 4 years)

99383   late childhood (age 5 through 11 years)

99384   adolescent (age 12 through 17 years)

99385   18-39 years

99386   40-64 years

99387   65 years and over

ESTABLISHED PATIENT

▲ **99391**   Periodic comprehensive preventive medicine reevaluation and management of an individual including an age and gender appropriate history, examination, counseling/anticipatory guidance/risk factor reduction interventions, and the ordering of appropriate immunization(s), laboratory/diagnostic procedures, established patient; infant (age under 1 year)

99392   early childhood (age 1 through 4 years)

99393   late childhood (age 5 through 11 years)

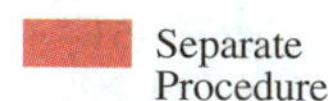 Separate Procedure

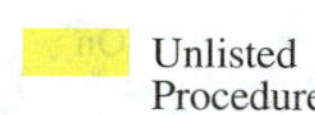 Unlisted Procedure

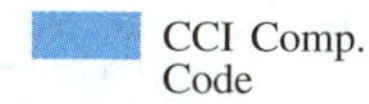 CCI Comp. Code

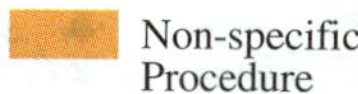 Non-specific Procedure

99394	adolescent (age 12 through 17 years)
99395	18-39 years
99396	40-64 years
99397	65 years and over

COUNSELING AND/OR RISK FACTOR REDUCTION INTERVENTION

NEW OR ESTABLISHED PATIENT

Preventive Medicine, Individual Counseling

99401 Preventive medicine counseling and/or risk factor reduction intervention(s) provided to an individual (separate procedure); approximately 15 minutes

99402 approximately 30 minutes

99403 approximately 45 minutes

99404 approximately 60 minutes

Preventive Medicine, Group Counseling

99411 Preventive medicine counseling and/or risk factor reduction intervention(s) provided to individuals in a group setting (separate procedure); approximately 30 minutes

99412 approximately 60 minutes

Other Preventive Medicine Services

99420 Administration and interpretation of health risk assessment instrument (eg, health hazard appraisal)

99429 Unlisted preventive medicine service

● New Code　　▲ Revised Code　　✱ Starred Procedure　　✚ Add-On Code　　⊘ Modifier -51 Exempt

NEWBORN CARE SERVICES

99431 History and examination of the normal newborn infant, initiation of diagnostic and treatment programs and preparation of hospital records. (This code should also be used for birthing room deliveries.)

99432 Normal newborn care in other than hospital or birthing room setting, including physical examination of baby and conference(s) with parent(s)

99433 Subsequent hospital care, for the evaluation and management of a normal newborn, per day

99435 History and examination of the normal newborn infant, including the preparation of medical records. (This code should only be used for newborns assessed and discharged from the hospital or birthing room on the same date.)

99436 Attendance at delivery (when requested by delivering physician) and initial stabilization of newborn

(99436 may be reported in addition to 99431)

(99436 may not be reported in addition to 99440)

99440 Newborn resuscitation: provision of positive pressure ventilation and/or chest compressions in the presence of acute inadequate ventilation and/or cardiac output

SPECIAL EVALUATION AND MANAGEMENT SERVICES

BASIC LIFE AND/OR DISABILITY EVALUATION SERVICES

99450 Basic life and/or disability examination that includes:

- measurement of height, weight and blood pressure;
- completion of a medical history following a life insurance pro forma;
- collection of blood sample and/or urinalysis complying with "chain of custody" protocols; and
- completion of necessary documentation/certificates.

Separate
Procedure

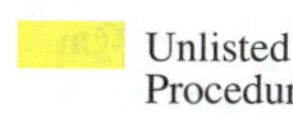
Unlisted
Procedure

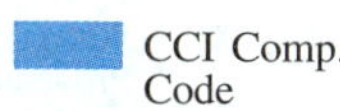
CCI Comp.
Code

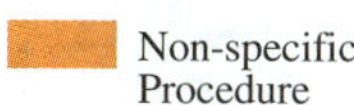
Non-specific
Procedure

WORK RELATED OR MEDICAL DISABILITY EVALUATION SERVICES

99455 Work related or medical disability examination by the treating physician that includes:

- completion of a medical history commensurate with the patient's condition;
- performance of an examination commensurate with the patient's condition;
- formulation of a diagnosis, assessment of capabilities and stability, and calculation of impairment;
- development of future medical treatment plan; and
- completion of necessary documentation/certificates and report.

99456 Work related or medical disability examination by other than the treating physician that includes:

- completion of a medical history commensurate with the patient's condition;
- performance of an examination commensurate with the patient's condition;
- formulation of a diagnosis, assessment of capabilities and stability, and calculation of impairment;
- development of future medical treatment plan; and
- completion of necessary documentation/certificates and report.

OTHER EVALUATION AND MANAGEMENT SERVICES

99499 Unlisted evaluation and management service

● New Code ▲ Revised Code ＊ Starred Procedure ＋ Add-On Code ⊘ Modifier -51 Exempt

ANESTHESIA OVERVIEW

The second section of the CPT coding system is the anesthesia section, which includes service codes for the delivery of anesthesia. Within each subsection, the CPT codes are arranged by anatomical site.

The Anesthesiologist provides pain relief and maintenance, or restoration, of a stable condition during and immediately following an operation, an obstetric or diagnostic procedure. The Anesthesiologist assesses the risk of the patient undergoing surgery and optimizes the patient's condition prior to, during, and after surgery.

Reporting of anesthesia services is dependent on the third party payer involved. Anesthesia services covered by Medicare are coded using codes from the ANESTHESIA section of the CPT coding system. For most other third party payers, anesthesia services are coded using codes from the SURGERY section of the CPT coding system to describe the major surgical procedure.

Anesthesia services may be coded by anesthesiologists or anesthetists working under the supervision of the anesthesiologist. Anesthesia services include pre- and post-op visits, anesthesia delivery, giving fluids and/or blood needed during a procedure, and monitoring. Anesthesia delivery includes general, regional, supplementing local anesthesia, and other supportive services.

KEY POINTS ABOUT ANESTHESIA CODING

1. Time recording for anesthesia services starts with patient preparation for anesthesia induction and ends until the anesthesiologist or anesthetist has completed his/her services and transfers responsibility for postoperative supervision.

2. Consultations and/or other evaluation and management services which are not included in the administration or supervising the administration of anesthesia, regardless of location provided, are reporting using CPT codes from the evaluation and management section of the CPT book.

3. Any supplies and/or materials provided by the anesthesiologist or anesthetist which are not considered to be included in the standard service may be coded separately.

 Separate Procedure

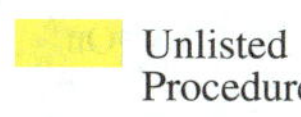 Unlisted Procedure

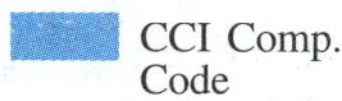 CCI Comp. Code

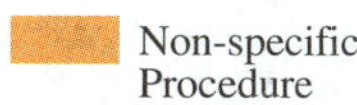 Non-specific Procedure

4. Multiple procedures provided on the same date of service should be coded separately.

5. Any service which may be considered rare, unusual, variable or not defined should be supported with a special report which clearly defines the need for the unusual service. These services are generally coded with an unlisted CPT code or by adding modifier -22 to the CPT code which defines the procedure.

ANESTHESIA SERVICE MODIFIERS

A physical status modifier must be added to all CPT codes when reporting anesthesia services. The physical status modifier defines the physical condition of the patient and ranges from a normal health patient to a declared brain-dead patient whose organs are being harvested for a transplant.

PHYSICAL STATUS MODIFIERS

-P1   A normal healthy patient.

-P2   A patient with a mild systemic disease.

-P3   A patient with severe systemic disease.

-P4   A patient with severe systemic disease that is a constant threat to life.

-P5   A moribund patient who is not expected to survive without the operation.

-P6   A declared brain-dead patient whose organs are being removed for donor purposes.

OTHER ANESTHESIA SERVICE MODIFIERS

Under certain circumstances, medical services and procedures may need to be further modified. Other CPT coding system and HCPCS Level II modifiers commonly used with ANESTHESIA services include:

-22   Unusual services

-23   anesthesia

-32   Mandated services

-51   Multiple procedures

-AA   Anesthesia by anesthesiologist

● New Code	▲ Revised Code	✳ Starred Procedure	✛ Add-On Code	⊘ Modifier -51 Exempt

-AB	Four or less concurrent services by CRNA or AA employed by anesthesiologist
-AC	Four or less concurrent services by CRNA not employed by anesthesiologist
-AD	Supervision of more than four concurrent anesthesia services by anesthesiologist
-AF	Anesthesia complicated by total body hypothermia
-AG	Anesthesia for emergency surgery on a patient who is moribund or who has an incapacitating systemic disease that is a constant threat to life
-QI	Medical direction of own employees by anesthesiologist (three concurrent procedures)
-OJ	Medical direction of own employees by anesthesiologist (four concurrent procedures)
-QK	Medical direction of other than own employees by anesthesiologist (two concurrent procedures)
-QL	Medical direction of other than own employees by anesthesiologist (three concurrent procedures)
-QM	Medical direction of other than own employees by anesthesiologist (four concurrent procedures)

QUALIFYING CIRCUMSTANCES FOR ANESTHESIA

In the case of difficult and/or extraordinary circumstances such as extreme youth or age, extraordinary condition of the patient, and/or unusual risk factors it may be appropriate to report one or more of the following qualifying circumstances in addition to the anesthesia services.

99100	Anesthesia for patient of extreme age, under one year and over seventy
99116	Anesthesia complicated by utilization of total body hypothermia
99135	Anesthesia complicated by utilization of controlled hypotension
99140	Anesthesia complicated by emergency conditions (specify)

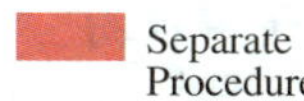 Separate Procedure

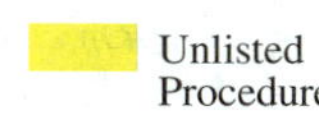 Unlisted Procedure

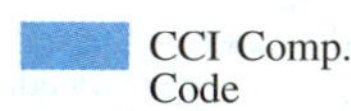 CCI Comp. Code

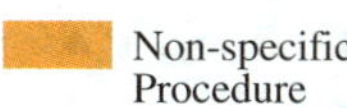 Non-specific Procedure

● New Code ▲ Revised Code ✱ Starred Procedure ✚ Add-On Code ⊘ Modifier -51 Exempt

ANESTHESIA CODES

<u>HEAD</u>

00100 Anesthesia for procedures on salivary glands, including biopsy

00102 Anesthesia for procedures on plastic repair of cleft lip

00103 Anesthesia for reconstructive procedures of eyelid (eg, blepharoplasty, ptosis surgery)

00104 Anesthesia for electroconvulsive therapy

00120 Anesthesia for procedures on external, middle, and inner ear including biopsy; not otherwise specified

00124 otoscopy

00126 tympanotomy

00140 Anesthesia for procedures on eye; not otherwise specified

00142 lens surgery

00144 corneal transplant

00145 vitreoretinal surgery

00147 iridectomy

00148 ophthalmoscopy

00160 Anesthesia for procedures on nose and accessory sinuses; not otherwise specified

00162 radical surgery

00164 biopsy, soft tissue

00170 Anesthesia for intraoral procedures, including biopsy; not otherwise specified

00172 repair of cleft palate

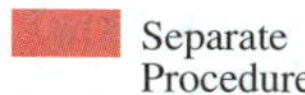 Separate Procedure

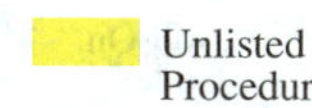 Unlisted Procedure

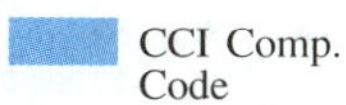 CCI Comp. Code

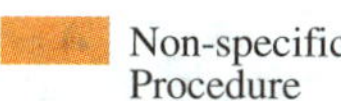 Non-specific Procedure

00174   excision of retropharyngeal tumor

00176   radical surgery

00190   Anesthesia for procedures on facial bones or skull; not otherwise specified

00192   radical surgery (including prognathism)

00210   Anesthesia for intracranial procedures; not otherwise specified

00212   subdural taps

00214   burr holes, including ventriculography

00215   cranioplasty or elevation of depressed skull fracture, extradural (simple or compound)

00216   vascular procedures

00218   procedures in sitting position

▲ **00220**   cerebrospinal fluid shunting procedures

00222   electrocoagulation of intracranial nerve

NECK

00300   Anesthesia for all procedures on the integumentary system, muscles and nerves of head, neck, and posterior trunk, not otherwise specified

00320   Anesthesia for all procedures on esophagus, thyroid, larynx, trachea and lymphatic system of neck; not otherwise specified

00322   needle biopsy of thyroid

(For procedures on cervical spine and cord, see 00600, 00604, 00670)

00350   Anesthesia for procedures on major vessels of neck; not otherwise specified

00352   simple ligation

● New Code   ▲ Revised Code   ✳ Starred Procedure   ✛ Add-On Code   ⊘ Modifier -51 Exempt

(For arteriography, use 01916)

THORAX (CHEST WALL AND SHOULDER GIRDLE)

00400   Anesthesia for procedures on the integumentary system on the extremities, anterior trunk and perineum; not otherwise specified

00402   reconstructive procedures on breast (eg, reduction or augmentation mammoplasty, muscle flaps)

00404   radical or modified radical procedures on breast

00406   radical or modified radical procedures on breast with internal mammary node dissection

00410   electrical conversion of arrhythmias

00450   Anesthesia for procedures on clavicle and scapula; not otherwise specified

00452   radical surgery

00454   biopsy of clavicle

00470   Anesthesia for partial rib resection; not otherwise specified

00472   thoracoplasty (any type)

00474   radical procedures (eg, pectus excavatum)

INTRATHORACIC

00500   Anesthesia for all procedures on esophagus

00520   Anesthesia for closed chest procedures; (including bronchoscopy) not otherwise specified

00522   needle biopsy of pleura

00524   pneumocentesis

00528   mediastinoscopy and diagnostic thoracoscopy

 Separate Procedure   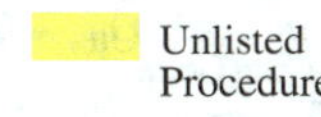 Unlisted Procedure   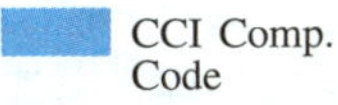 CCI Comp. Code   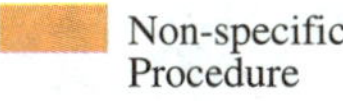 Non-specific Procedure

00530 Anesthesia for permanent transvenous pacemaker insertion

00532 Anesthesia for access to central venous circulation

00534 Anesthesia for transvenous insertion or replacement of pacing cardioverter/defibrillator

(For transthoracic approach, use 00560)

00537 Anesthesia for cardiac electrophysiologic procedures including radiofrequency ablation

00540 Anesthesia for thoracotomy procedures involving lungs, pleura, diaphragm, and mediastinum (including surgical thoracoscopy); not otherwise specified

00542 decortication

00544 pleurectomy

00546 pulmonary resection with thoracoplasty

00548 intrathoracic procedures on the trachea and bronchi

00550 Anesthesia for sternal debridement

▲ **00560** Anesthesia for procedures on heart, pericardial sac, and great vessels of chest; without pump oxygenator

00562 with pump oxygenator

00563 with pump oxygenator with hypothermic circulatory arrest

00566 Anesthesia for direct coronary artery bypass grafting without pump oxygenator

00580 Anesthesia for heart transplant or heart/lung transplant

SPINE AND SPINAL CORD

00600 Anesthesia for procedures on cervical spine and cord; not otherwise specified

(For myelography and diskography, see radiological procedures 01905)

●	New Code	▲ Revised Code	✻ Starred Procedure	✚ Add-On Code	⃠ Modifier -51 Exempt

00604   procedures with patient in the sitting position

00620   Anesthesia for procedures on thoracic spine and cord; not otherwise specified

00622   thoracolumbar sympathectomy

00630   Anesthesia for procedures in lumbar region; not otherwise specified

00632   lumbar sympathectomy

00634   chemonucleolysis

00635   diagnostic or therapeutic lumbar puncture

00670   Anesthesia for extensive spine and spinal cord procedures (eg, spinal instrumentation or vascular procedures)

UPPER ABDOMEN

00700   Anesthesia for procedures on upper anterior abdominal wall; not otherwise specified

00702   percutaneous liver biopsy

00730   Anesthesia for procedures on upper posterior abdominal wall

00740   Anesthesia for upper gastrointestinal endoscopic procedures, endoscope introduced proximal to duodenum

00750   Anesthesia for hernia repairs in upper abdomen; not otherwise specified

00752   lumbar and ventral (incisional) hernias and/or wound dehiscence

00754   omphalocele

00756   transabdominal repair of diaphragmatic hernia

00770   Anesthesia for all procedures on major abdominal blood vessels

00790   Anesthesia for intraperitoneal procedures in upper abdomen including laparoscopy; not otherwise specified

	Separate Procedure		Unlisted Procedure		CCI Comp. Code		Non-specific Procedure

00792   partial hepatectomy or management of liver hemorrhage (excluding liver biopsy)

00794   pancreatectomy, partial or total (eg, Whipple procedure)

00796   liver transplant (recipient)

(For harvesting of liver, use 01990)

● **00797**   gastric restrictive procedure for morbid obesity

LOWER ABDOMEN

00800   Anesthesia for procedures on lower anterior abdominal wall; not otherwise specified

00802   panniculectomy

00810   Anesthesia for lower intestinal endoscopic procedures, endoscope introduced distal to duodenum

00820   Anesthesia for procedures on lower posterior abdominal wall

00830   Anesthesia for hernia repairs in lower abdomen; not otherwise specified

00832   ventral and incisional hernias

00840   Anesthesia for intraperitoneal procedures in lower abdomen including laparoscopy; not otherwise specified

00842   amniocentesis

00844   abdominoperineal resection

00846   radical hysterectomy

00848   pelvic exenteration

(00850   deleted 2002 edition. To report, use 01961)

● **00851**   tubal ligation/transection

(00855   deleted 2002 edition. To report, use 01963)

● New Code   ▲ Revised Code   ✳ Starred Procedure   ✚ Add-On Code   ⊘ Modifier -51 Exempt

(00857   deleted 2002 edition. To report, use 01968, 01969)

00860   Anesthesia for extraperitoneal procedures in lower abdomen, including urinary tract; not otherwise specified

00862   renal procedures, including upper 1/3 of ureter, or donor nephrectomy

00864   total cystectomy

00865   radical prostatectomy (suprapubic, retropubic)

00866   adrenalectomy

00868   renal transplant (recipient)

(For donor nephrectomy, use 00862)

(For harvesting kidney from brain-dead patient, use 01990)

● 00869   vasectomy, unilateral/bilateral

00870   cystolithotomy

00872   Anesthesia for lithotripsy, extracorporeal shock wave; with water bath

00873   without water bath

00880   Anesthesia for procedures on major lower abdominal vessels; not otherwise specified

00882   inferior vena cava ligation

(00884   deleted 2002 edition. To report, use 01930)

PERINEUM

(00900   deleted 2001 edition. To report, see 00300, 00400)

00902   Anesthesia for; anorectal procedure

00904   radical perineal procedure

00906   vulvectomy

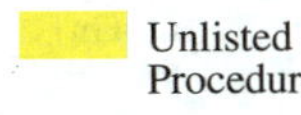

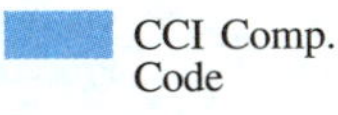

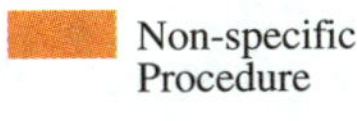

00908 perineal prostatectomy

00910 Anesthesia for transurethral procedures (including urethrocystoscopy); not otherwise specified

00912 transurethral resection of bladder tumor(s)

00914 transurethral resection of prostate

00916 post-transurethral resection bleeding

00918 with fragmentation, manipulation and/or removal of ureteral calculus

00920 Anesthesia for procedures on male genitalia (including open urethral procedures); not otherwise specified

00922 seminal vesicles

00924 undescended testis, unilateral or bilateral

00926 radical orchiectomy, inguinal

00928 radical orchiectomy, abdominal

00930 orchiopexy, unilateral or bilateral

00932 complete amputation of penis

00934 radical amputation of penis with bilateral inguinal lymphadenectomy

00936 radical amputation of penis with bilateral inguinal and iliac lymphadenectomy

00938 insertion of penile prosthesis (perineal approach)

00940 Anesthesia for vaginal procedures (including biopsy of labia, vagina, cervix or endometrium); not otherwise specified

▲ **00942** colpotomy, vaginectomy, colporrhaphy and open urethral procedures

00944 vaginal hysterectomy

(**00946** deleted 2002 edition. To report, use 01960)

212

● New Code ▲ Revised Code ∗ Starred Procedure ✛ Add-On Code ⊘ Modifier -51 Exempt

00948   cervical cerclage

00950   culdoscopy

00952   hysteroscopy and/or hysterosalpingography

(00955   deleted 2002 edition. To report, use 01967)

PELVIS

01112   Anesthesia for bone marrow aspiration and/or biopsy, anterior or posterior iliac crest

01120   Anesthesia for procedures on bony pelvis

01130   Anesthesia for body cast application or revision

01140   Anesthesia for interpelviabdominal (hindquarter) amputation

01150   Anesthesia for radical procedures for tumor of pelvis, except hindquarter amputation

01160   Anesthesia for closed procedures involving symphysis pubis or sacroiliac joint

01170   Anesthesia for open procedures involving symphysis pubis or sacroiliac joint

01180   Anesthesia for obturator neurectomy; extrapelvic

01190   intrapelvic

UPPER LEG (EXCEPT KNEE)

01200   Anesthesia for all closed procedures involving hip joint

01202   Anesthesia for arthroscopic procedures of hip joint

01210   Anesthesia for open procedures involving hip joint; not otherwise specified

01212   hip disarticulation

▲ **01214**   total hip arthroplasty

Separate Procedure	Unlisted Procedure	CCI Comp. Code	Non-specific Procedure

213

01215   revision of total hip arthroplasty

01220   Anesthesia for all closed procedures involving upper 2/3 of femur

01230   Anesthesia for open procedures involving upper 2/3 of femur; not otherwise specified

01232   amputation

01234   radical resection

01250   Anesthesia for all procedures on nerves, muscles, tendons, fascia, and bursae of upper leg

01260   Anesthesia for all procedures involving veins of upper leg, including exploration

01270   Anesthesia for procedures involving arteries of upper leg, including bypass graft; not otherwise specified

01272   femoral artery ligation

01274   femoral artery embolectomy

KNEE AND POPLITEAL AREA

01320   Anesthesia for all procedures on nerves, muscles, tendons, fascia, and bursae of knee and/or popliteal area

01340   Anesthesia for all closed procedures on lower 1/3 of femur

01360   Anesthesia for all open procedures on lower 1/3 of femur

01380   Anesthesia for all closed procedures on knee joint

01382   Anesthesia for arthroscopic procedures of knee joint

01390   Anesthesia for all closed procedures on upper ends of tibia, fibula, and/or patella

01392   Anesthesia for all open procedures on upper ends of tibia, fibula, and/or patella

  ● New Code   ▲ Revised Code   ＊ Starred Procedure   ✛ Add-On Code   ⊘ Modifier -51 Exempt

01400   Anesthesia for open procedures on knee joint; not otherwise specified

▲ **01402**   total knee arthroplasty

01404   disarticulation at knee

01420   Anesthesia for all cast applications, removal, or repair involving knee joint

01430   Anesthesia for procedures on veins of knee and popliteal area; not otherwise specified

01432   arteriovenous fistula

01440   Anesthesia for procedures on arteries of knee and popliteal area; not otherwise specified

01442   popliteal thromboendarterectomy, with or without patch graft

01444   popliteal excision and graft or repair for occlusion or aneurysm

LOWER LEG (BELOW KNEE, INCLUDES ANKLE AND FOOT)

01462   Anesthesia for all closed procedures on lower leg, ankle, and foot

01464   Anesthesia for arthroscopic procedures of ankle joint

01470   Anesthesia for procedures on nerves, muscles, tendons, and fascia of lower leg, ankle, and foot; not otherwise specified

01472   repair of ruptured Achilles tendon, with or without graft

01474   gastrocnemius recession (eg, Strayer procedure)

01480   Anesthesia for open procedures on bones of lower leg, ankle, and foot; not otherwise specified

01482   radical resection (including below knee amputation)

01484   osteotomy or osteoplasty of tibia and/or fibula

 Separate Procedure

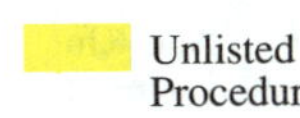 Unlisted Procedure

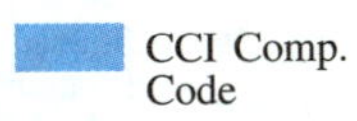 CCI Comp. Code

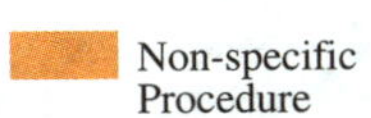 Non-specific Procedure

01486	total ankle replacement
01490	Anesthesia for lower leg cast application, removal, or repair
01500	Anesthesia for procedures on arteries of lower leg, including bypass graft; not otherwise specified
01502	embolectomy, direct or with catheter
01520	Anesthesia for procedures on veins of lower leg; not otherwise specified
01522	venous thrombectomy, direct or with catheter

SHOULDER AND AXILLA

(Includes humeral head and neck, sternoclavicular joint, acromioclavicular joint, and shoulder joint)

01610	Anesthesia for all procedures on nerves, muscles, tendons, fascia, and bursae of shoulder and axilla
01620	Anesthesia for all closed procedures on humeral head and neck, sternoclavicular joint, acromioclavicular joint, and shoulder joint
01622	Anesthesia for arthroscopic procedures of shoulder joint
01630	Anesthesia for open procedures on humeral head and neck, sternoclavicular joint, acromioclavicular joint, and shoulder joint; not otherwise specified
01632	radical resection
01634	shoulder disarticulation
01636	interthoracoscapular (forequarter) amputation
01638	total shoulder replacement
01650	Anesthesia for procedures on arteries of shoulder and axilla; not otherwise specified
01652	axillary-brachial aneurysm
01654	bypass graft

● New Code	▲ Revised Code	∗ Starred Procedure	+ Add-On Code	⊘ Modifier -51 Exempt

01656   axillary-femoral bypass graft

01670   Anesthesia for all procedures on veins of shoulder and axilla

01680   Anesthesia for shoulder cast application, removal or repair; not otherwise specified

01682   shoulder spica

UPPER ARM AND ELBOW

01710   Anesthesia for procedures on nerves, muscles, tendons, fascia, and bursae of upper arm and elbow; not otherwise specified

01712   tenotomy, elbow to shoulder, open

01714   tenoplasty, elbow to shoulder

01716   tenodesis, rupture of long tendon of biceps

01730   Anesthesia for all closed procedures on humerus and elbow

01732   Anesthesia for arthroscopic procedures of elbow joint

01740   Anesthesia for open procedures on humerus and elbow; not otherwise specified

01742   osteotomy of humerus

01744   repair of nonunion or malunion of humerus

01756   radical procedures

01758   excision of cyst or tumor of humerus

01760   total elbow replacement

01770   Anesthesia for procedures on arteries of upper arm and elbow; not otherwise specified

01772   embolectomy

01780   Anesthesia for procedures on veins of upper arm and elbow; not otherwise specified

---

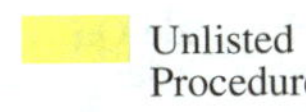

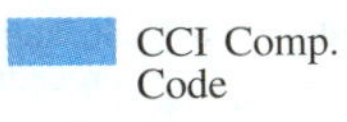

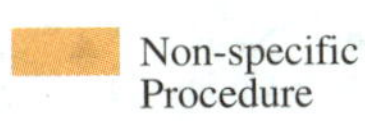

Non-specific
Procedure

217

| 01782 | phleborrhaphy |

(01784   deleted 2001 edition. To report, see 01770, 01780)

FOREARM, WRIST, AND HAND

| 01810 | Anesthesia for all procedures on nerves, muscles, tendons, fascia, and bursae of forearm, wrist, and hand |

| 01820 | Anesthesia for all closed procedures on radius, ulna, wrist, or hand bones |

| 01830 | Anesthesia for open procedures on radius, ulna, wrist, or hand bones; not otherwise specified |

| 01832 | total wrist replacement |

| 01840 | Anesthesia for procedures on arteries of forearm, wrist, and hand; not otherwise specified |

| 01842 | embolectomy |

| 01844 | Anesthesia for vascular shunt, or shunt revision, any type (eg, dialysis) |

| 01850 | Anesthesia for procedures on veins of forearm, wrist, and hand; not otherwise specified |

| 01852 | phleborrhaphy |

| 01860 | Anesthesia for forearm, wrist, or hand cast application, removal, or repair |

RADIOLOGICAL PROCEDURES

(01904   deleted 2002 edition. To report, use 01905)

● **01905**   Anesthesia for myelography, diskography, vertebroplasty

(01906   deleted 2002 edition. To report, use 01905)

(01908   deleted 2002 edition. To report, use 01905)

(01910   deleted 2002 edition. To report, use 01905)

● New Code   ▲ Revised Code   * Starred Procedure   + Add-On Code   ⊘ Modifier -51 Exempt

(01912   deleted 2002 edition. To report, use 01905)

(01914   deleted 2002 edition. To report, use 01905)

▲ **01916**   Anesthesia for diagnostic arteriography/venography

(Do not report 01916 in conjunction with therapeutic codes 01924-01926, 01930-01933)

(01918   deleted 2002 edition. To report, use 01916)

▲ **01920**   Anesthesia for cardiac catheterization including coronary angiography and ventriculography (not to include Swan-Ganz catheter)

(01921   deleted 2002 edition. To report, see 01924-01926)

01922   Anesthesia for non-invasive imaging or radiation therapy

● **01924**   Anesthesia for therapeutic interventional radiologic procedures involving the arterial system; not otherwise specified

● **01925**   carotid or coronary

● **01926**   intracranial, intracardiac, or aortic

● **01930**   Anesthesia for therapeutic interventional radiologic procedures involving the venous/lymphatic system (not to include access to the central circulation); not otherwise specified

● **01931**   intrahepatic or portal circulation (eg, transcutaneous porto-caval shunt (TIPS))

● **01932**   intrathoracic or jugular

● **01933**   intracranial

BURN EXCISIONS OR DEBRIDEMENT

▲ **01951**   Anesthesia for second and third degree burn excision or debridement with or without skin grafting, any site, for total body surface area (TBSA) treated during anesthesia and surgery; less than four percent total body surface area

▲ **01952**   between four and nine percent of total body surface area

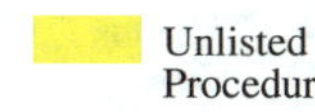
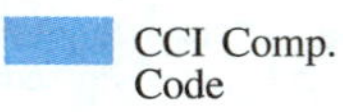
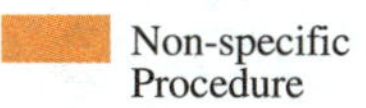

+01953 each additional nine percent total body surface area or part thereof (List separately in addition to code for primary procedure)

(Use 01953 in conjunction with code 01952)

OBSTETRIC

● **01960** Anesthesia for; vaginal delivery only

● **01961** cesarean delivery only

● **01962** urgent hysterectomy following delivery

● **01963** cesarean hysterectomy without any labor analgesia/anesthesia care

● **01964** abortion procedures

● **01967** Neuraxial labor analgesia/anesthesia for planned vaginal delivery (this includes any repeat subarachnoid needle placement and drug injection and/or any necessary replacement of an epidural catheter during labor)

●+**01968** Cesarean delivery following neuraxial labor analgesia/anasthesia (List separately in addition to code for primary procedure)

(Use 01968 in conjunction with code 01967)

●+**01969** Cesarean hysterectomy following neuraxial labor analgesia/anesthesia (List separately in addition to code for primary procedure)

(Use 01969 in conjunction with code 01967)

OTHER PROCEDURES

01990 Physiological support for harvesting of organ(s) from brain-dead patient

▲ **01995** Regional intravenous administration of local anesthetic agent or other medication (upper or lower extremity)

(For intra-arterial or intravenous therapy for pain management, see 90783, 90784)

● New Code   ▲ Revised Code   ✱ Starred Procedure   ✚ Add-On Code   ⊘ Modifier -51 Exempt

01996 Daily management of epidural or subarachnoid drug administration

01999 Unlisted anesthesia procedure(s)

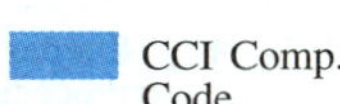

Separate Procedure	Unlisted Procedure	CCI Comp. Code	Non-specific Procedure

● New Code ▲ Revised Code ∗ Starred Procedure ✚ Add-On Code ⊘ Modifier -51 Exempt

SURGERY

SURGERY SECTION OVERVIEW

The third section of the CPT coding system is the surgery section, and it includes surgical procedure codes for all body areas. Within each subsection, the CPT codes are arranged by anatomical site.

It is essential to understand the organization of the CPT surgery section in order to locate the correct procedure code. Understanding other or alternative terms which may apply to a procedure, injury, illness or condition may also make the location of the appropriate procedure easier and faster.

All procedures listed in the surgery section of the CPT book include local, metacarpal/digital block or topical anesthesia if used, the surgical procedure, and normal uncomplicated follow-up care. For diagnostic surgical procedures, follow-up care includes only the care related to recovery from the diagnostic procedure. For therapeutic surgical procedures, follow-up care includes only the care which would usually be included in the surgical service. Any complications resulting in additional services are not considered to be included and should be coded separately.

KEY POINTS ABOUT SURGERY SERVICES

- Evaluation and management services provided by surgeons in the office, home or hospital, plus consultations and other medical services are coded using evaluation and management service codes.

- Any supplies and/or materials provided by the surgeon which are not considered to be included in the standard service may be coded separately.

GLOBAL SURGICAL PACKAGE

Third-party payers differ in their definition of a surgical or global surgical package concept. Medicare defines the global surgical package as follows:

- The surgeon's initial evaluation or consultation will be paid separately.

- There is a one day preoperative period covered under the global surgical package.

- Included in the package are all intraoperative services that are considered to be usual and necessary. Separate billing of these services would be considered unbundling.

Separate
Procedure

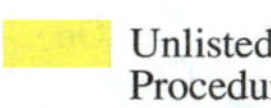
Unlisted
Procedure

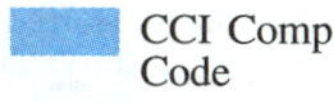
CCI Comp.
Code

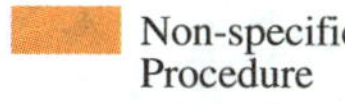
Non-specific
Procedure

223

■ Any treatment of complications by the surgeon not requiring a return to the operating room is included in the package.

■ The surgical package contains a standard 90-day postoperative period which includes all visits to the physician during that time unless the visit is for a totally different reason than that for the surgery.

■ In cases of organ transplant, immunosuppressive therapy is not included in the global package.

■ Minor surgical procedures are those with a 0 or 10-day postoperative period, and are excluded from the surgical package definition.

SPECIAL REPORT

Surgical procedures which are new, unusual or vary significantly from the standard definition may require a special report. When preparing reports to accompany health insurance claim forms the provider should include a description of the nature, extent, and need for the procedure, and the time, effort, and equipment necessary to provides the service. Try to keep these reports as brief and simple as possible. Additional items which may be needed are:

■ complexity of symptoms

■ final diagnosis

■ pertinent physical findings

■ diagnostic and therapeutic procedures

■ concurrent problems

■ follow-up care

MULTIPLE SURGICAL PROCEDURES

It is common for several surgical procedures to be performed at the same operative session. When multiple procedures are performed on the same day or at the same session, the "major" procedure or service is listed first followed by secondary, additional, or "lessor" procedures or services. CPT modifier -51 is added to all procedures following the first one.

Reporting multiple procedures incorrectly may have a serious impact on reimbursement from health insurance payers. An inexperienced health insurance biller may simply list the procedures on the health insurance claim form in the order dictated or described in the operative report.

● New Code ▲ Revised Code * Starred Procedure + Add-On Code ⊘ Modifier -51 Exempt

There are two critical decisions related to reporting multiple surgical procedures correctly; namely: 1) The order in which the procedures are listed on the health insurance claim form, and 2) whether or not to list the additional procedures with full or reduced fees.

ORDER OF LISTING MULTIPLE PROCEDURES

The first procedure to be listed when reporting services under the multiple procedure rule is the procedure with the highest fee. Additional procedures should be listed in descending order by fee. Modifier -51 should be added to each additional procedure.

21. DIAGNOSIS OR NATURE OF ILLNESS OR INJURY. (RELATE ITEMS 1,2,3 OR 4 TO ITEM 24E BY LINE)					
1. **952 . 10**			3.		
2.			4.		

24.	A DATE(S) OF SERVICE		B Place of Service	C Type of Service	D PROCEDURES, SERVICES, OR SUPPLIES (Explain Unusual Circumstances) CPT/HCPCS MODIFIER	E DIAGNOSIS CODE
	From MM DD YY	From MM DD YY				
1	06 15 02		21		63046	
2	06 15 02		21		62223 51	
3						
4						

All third party payers will reduce the allowance for the additional procedures, typically by 50 percent for the second procedure, and 50 to 75 percent for the third and subsequent procedures. Listing the procedures in descending order by fee minimizes the possibility of an incorrect reduction.

BILLING FULL VERSUS REDUCED FEES

The full fee should be listed for each procedure coded on the health insurance claim form as part of multiple surgical procedures. Third party payers will automatically reduce the allowances for the additional procedures by a specific formula. Listing all multiple procedures with full fees in descending fee order (the procedure with the highest fee first, the procedure with the next highest fee second, et cetera) will result in the maximum total allowable reimbursement for the provider or the insured.

After the maximum benefit has been paid by the health insurance company, the balance remaining, less any patient co-insurance or deductible requirements, should be written off. Note that billing practices vary in different areas of the country. Providers should continue to use the method that is customary or required by third party payers in the provider's practice location.

SEPARATE PROCEDURE

Some surgical procedures are considered to be an integral part of a more extensive surgical procedure. In this circumstance, the integral procedure is not coded. When the integral procedure is performed independently and is unrelated to other services, it should be listed as a "separate procedure."

SURGERY SUBSECTIONS

The SURGERY section of the CPT coding system is divided into 16 subsections:

Integumentary System	10040-19499
Musculoskeletal System	20000-29999
Respiratory System	30000-32999
Cardiovascular System	33000-37799
Hemic and Lymphatic Systems	38000-38999
Mediastinum and Diaphragm	39000-39599
Digestive System	40000-49999
Urinary System	50000-53899
Male Genital System	54000-55899
Intersex Surgery	55970-55980
Female Genital Surgery	56000-58999
Maternity Care and Delivery	59000-59899
Endocrine System	60000-60699
Nervous System	61000-64999
Eye and Ocular Adnexa	65000-68899
Auditory System	69000-69999

Each sub-section of the SURGERY section of the CPT coding system is divided into organs then into procedures involving anatomic sites. Each anatomic site is further separated into surgical processes such as incision, excision, repair, removal, amputation, etc.

SURGERY SECTION MODIFIERS

Due to various circumstances, surgical procedures may be considered to be modified in comparison to the full or complete procedure. Modified procedures are identified by reporting a two-digit modifier to the CPT procedure code(s). The following CPT modifiers may be coded with surgical procedures:

-20   Microsurgery

-22   Unusual Procedural Services

-26   Professional Component

● New Code   ▲ Revised Code   ✳ Starred Procedure   ✚ Add-On Code   ⊘ Modifier -51 Exempt

-32	Mandated Services
-47	Anesthesia by Surgeon
-50	Bilateral Procedure
-51	Multiple Procedures
-52	Reduced Services
-54	Surgical Care Only
-55	Postoperative Management Only
-56	Preoperative Management Only
-57	Decision for Surgery
-58	Staged or Related Procedure or Service by the Same Physician During the Postoperative Period
-62	Two Surgeons
-66	Surgical Team
-76	Repeat Procedure by Same Physician
-77	Repeat Procedure by Another Physician
-78	Return to the operating room for a related procedure during the post-operative period
-79	Unrelated procedure or service by the same physician during the post-operative period
-80	Assistant surgeon
-81	Minimum assistant surgeon
-82	Assistant surgeon (when qualified resident not available)
-90	Reference (Outside) Laboratory
-99	Multiple modifiers
-LT	Procedure performed on left side of body
-RT	Procedure performed on right side of body

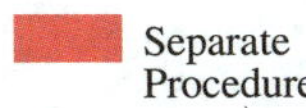 Separate Procedure   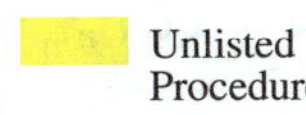 Unlisted Procedure   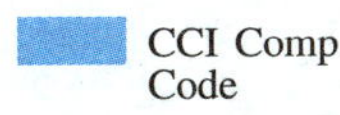 CCI Comp. Code   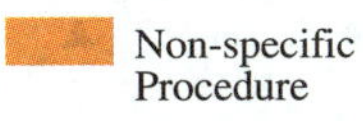 Non-specific Procedure

ADD-ON CODES

Many surgical procedures are performed secondary to primary surgical procedures. These procedures are classified as "additional" or "supplemental" procedures and are designated as "add-on" codes in the CPT coding system. "Add-on" CPT codes are identified in the CPT code book by a black plus sign "+" placed to the left of the code number.

Many of the CPT "Add-on" codes are further identified by phrases included within the descriptions of the definition of the CPT code or include the phrase "(List separately in addition to primary procedure)" following the definition. Examples of CPT codes identified as "add-on" codes in CPT 2002 include:

+11001 Debridement of extensive eczematous or infected skin; up to 10% of body surface, each additional 10% of the body surface (List separately in addition to code for primary procedure)

+33530 Re-operation, coronary artery bypass procedure or valve procedure, more than one month after original operation (List separately in addition to code for primary procedure)

STARRED PROCEDURES

There are numerous CPT codes which define minor surgical procedures without well-defined pre- and post-operative components. These procedures are exempt from the surgical package concept. Starred procedures are identified in the CPT code book by a star (*) following the procedure code number.

These procedures are identified in *CPT PLUS! 2002* by a star (*) <u>preceding</u> the procedure code number. When a star (*) precedes a surgical procedure code number, the following rules apply:

1. The starred procedure includes only the surgical procedure and does not include any pre-operative or post-operative services.

2. If the patient is a new patient, and the starred procedure is primary reason for the encounter, report CPT code 99025 instead of an customary evaluation and management visit code.

3. If the patient is an established patient, and the starred procedure is primary reason for the encounter, evaluation and management services are not usually coded.

● New Code   ▲ Revised Code   * Starred Procedure   + Add-On Code   ⊘ Modifier -51 Exempt

4. If the starred procedure is performed in the hospital, the customary hospital evaluation and management code should be coded in addition to the starred procedure.

Examples of CPT 2002 codes identified as starred procedures include:

✳20000   Incision of soft tissue abscess (eg, secondary to osteomyelitis); superficial

✳57150   Irrigation of vagina and/or application of medicament for treatment of bacterial, parasitic or fungoid disease

MEDICAL AND SURGICAL SUPPLIES

HCPCS Level II codes for medical and surgical supplies, A4000-A4999, may be used to report supplies and materials provided to Medicare patients if the supplies and materials are not considered to be included with or part of the basic service(s) or procedure(s).

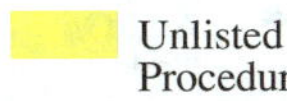 Separate Procedure   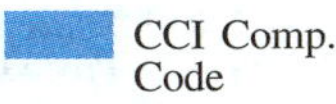 Unlisted Procedure   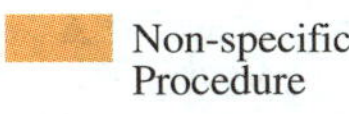 CCI Comp. Code   Non-specific Procedure

● New Code ▲ Revised Code ✱ Starred Procedure ✚ Add-On Code ⊘ Modifier -51 Exempt

SURGERY CODES

GENERAL

● **10021**   Fine needle aspiration; without imaging guidance

● **10022**   with imaging guidance

(For radiological supervision and interpretation, see 76003, 76360, 76942)

(For percutaneous needle biopsy, see 32405 for lung, 47000, 47001 for liver, 48102 for pancreas, 49180 for abdominal or retroperitoneal mass)

(For evaluation of fine needle aspirate, see 88172, 88173)

INTEGUMENTARY SYSTEM

SKIN, SUBCUTANEOUS AND ACCESSORY STRUCTURES

INCISION AND DRAINAGE SKIN

(For excision, see 11400, et seq)

***10040**   Acne surgery (eg, marsupialization, opening or removal of multiple milia, comedones, cysts, pustules)

***10060**   Incision and drainage of abscess (eg, carbuncle, suppurative hidradenitis, cutaneous or subcutaneous abscess, cyst, furuncle, or paronychia); simple or single

10061   complicated or multiple

***10080**   Incision and drainage of pilonidal cyst; simple

10081   complicated

(For excision of pilonidal cyst, see 11770-11772)

***10120**   Incision and removal of foreign body, subcutaneous tissues; simple

10121   complicated

Separate Procedure

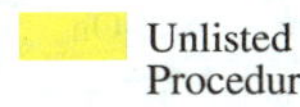
Unlisted Procedure

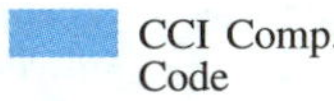
CCI Comp. Code

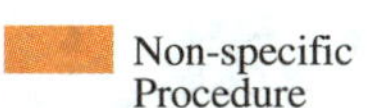
Non-specific Procedure

(To report wound exploration due to penetrating trauma without laparotomy or thoracotomy, see 20100-20103, as appropriate)

(To report debridement associated with open fracture(s) and/or dislocation(s), use 11010-11012, as appropriate)

***10140** Incision and drainage of hematoma, seroma or fluid collection

(If imaging guidance is performed, see 76360, 76393, 76942)

***10160** Puncture aspiration of abscess, hematoma, bulla, or cyst

(If imaging guidance is performed, see 76360, 76393, 76942)

10180 Incision and drainage, complex, postoperative wound infection

(For secondary closure of surgical wound, see 12020, 12021, 13160)

EXCISION-DEBRIDEMENT SKIN

(For dermabrasions, see 15780-15783)

(For nail debridement, see 11720-11721)

(For burn(s), see 16000-16035)

***11000** Debridement of extensive eczematous or infected skin; up to 10% of body surface

+11001 each additional 10% of the body surface (List separately in addition to code for primary procedure)

(Use 11001 in conjunction with code 11000)

11010 Debridement including removal of foreign material associated with open fracture(s) and/or dislocation(s); skin and subcutaneous tissues

11011 skin, subcutaneous tissue, muscle fascia, and muscle

11012 skin, subcutaneous tissue, muscle fascia, muscle, and bone

11040 Debridement; skin, partial thickness

11041 skin, full thickness

11042 skin, and subcutaneous tissue

● New Code   ▲ Revised Code   * Starred Procedure   + Add-On Code   ⊘ Modifier -51 Exempt

11043	skin, subcutaneous tissue, and muscle
11044	skin, subcutaneous tissue, muscle, and bone

(Do not report 11040-11044 in addition to 97601, 97602)

PARING OR CUTTING

11055	Paring or cutting of benign hyperkeratotic lesion (eg, corn or callus); single lesion
11056	two to four lesions
11057	more than four lesions

BIOPSY

11100	Biopsy of skin, subcutaneous tissue and/or mucous membrane (including simple closure), unless otherwise listed (separate procedure); single lesion
+11101	each separate/additional lesion (List separately in addition to code for primary procedure)

(Use 11101 in conjunction with code 11100)

(For biopsy of conjunctiva, use 68100; eyelid, use 67810)

REMOVAL OF SKIN TAGS

***11200**	Removal of skin tags, multiple fibrocutaneous tags, any area; up to and including 15 lesions
+11201	each additional ten lesions (List separately in addition to code for primary procedure)

(Use 11201 in conjunction with code 11200)

SHAVING OF EPIDERMAL OR DERMAL LESIONS

Many of the procedure codes listed in the integumentary system subsection of the CPT manual are designated in centimeters or square centimeters. Many physicians document sizes using inches or millimeters. Make sure to verify, and convert if necessary, measurements before assigning a code.

To be able to code lesion removal appropriately, the site, size in centimeters, method of removal and morphology must be documented in the medical record. Always code morphology from the pathology report.

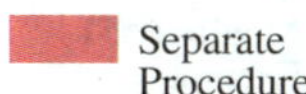 Separate Procedure
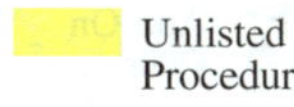 Unlisted Procedure
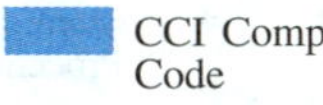 CCI Comp. Code
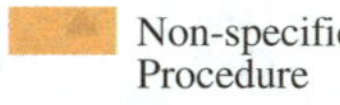 Non-specific Procedure

Excision of lesion codes are determined by the diameter of the actual lesion, not the specimen sent to pathology. However, the size of the specimen can be used when the size of the lesion cannot be located in the operative report or elsewhere in the medical record.

When more than one dimension of a lesion is provided in the documentation, select the code based on the largest size. For example, if the dimensions indicated are 3 cm x 2 cm x 1.5 cm, the lesion should be coded as 3 cm. Excision of benign and malignant lesions codes include simple repair of the defect site.

***11300**   Shaving of epidermal or dermal lesion, single lesion, trunk, arms or legs; lesion diameter 0.5 cm or less

11301   lesion diameter 0.6 to 1.0 cm

11302   lesion diameter 1.1 to 2.0 cm

11303   lesion diameter over 2.0 cm

***11305**   Shaving of epidermal or dermal lesion, single lesion, scalp, neck, hands, feet, genitalia; lesion diameter 0.5 cm or less

11306   lesion diameter 0.6 to 1.0 cm

11307   lesion diameter 1.1 to 2.0 cm

11308   lesion diameter over 2.0 cm

***11310**   Shaving of epidermal or dermal lesion, single lesion, face, ears, eyelids, nose, lips, mucous membrane; lesion diameter 0.5 cm or less

11311   lesion diameter 0.6 to 1.0 cm

11312   lesion diameter 1.1 to 2.0 cm

11313   lesion diameter over 2.0 cm

EXCISION OF BENIGN LESIONS

(For excision of benign lesions requiring more than simple closure, ie, requiring intermediate or complex closure, report 11400-11446 in addition to appropriate intermediate (12031-12057) or complex closure (13100-13153) codes. For reconstructive closure, see 14000-14300, 15000-15261, 15570-15770)

   ● New Code   ▲ Revised Code   * Starred Procedure   + Add-On Code   ⊘ Modifier -51 Exempt

(For electrosurgical and other methods, see 17000 et seq)

11400 Excision, benign lesion, except skin tag (unless listed elsewhere), trunk, arms or legs; lesion diameter 0.5 cm or less

11401 lesion diameter 0.6 to 1.0 cm

11402 lesion diameter 1.1 to 2.0 cm

11403 lesion diameter 2.1 to 3.0 cm

11404 lesion diameter 3.1 to 4.0 cm

11406 lesion diameter over 4.0 cm

(For unusual or complicated excision, add modifier -22)

11420 Excision, benign lesion, except skin tag (unless listed elsewhere), scalp, neck, hands, feet, genitalia; lesion diameter 0.5 cm or less

11421 lesion diameter 0.6 to 1.0 cm

11422 lesion diameter 1.1 to 2.0 cm

11423 lesion diameter 2.1 to 3.0 cm

11424 lesion diameter 3.1 to 4.0 cm

11426 lesion diameter over 4.0 cm

(For unusual or complicated excision, add modifier -22)

11440 Excision, other benign lesion (unless listed elsewhere), face, ears, eyelids, nose, lips, mucous membrane; lesion diameter 0.5 cm or less

11441 lesion diameter 0.6 to 1.0 cm

11442 lesion diameter 1.1 to 2.0 cm

11443 lesion diameter 2.1 to 3.0 cm

11444 lesion diameter 3.1 to 4.0 cm

11446 lesion diameter over 4.0 cm

Separate Procedure	Unlisted Procedure	CCI Comp. Code	Non-specific Procedure

235

(For unusual or complicated excision, add modifier -22)

(For eyelids involving more than skin, see also 67800 et seq)

11450 Excision of skin and subcutaneous tissue for hidradenitis, axillary; with simple or intermediate repair

11451 with complex repair

11462 Excision of skin and subcutaneous tissue for hidradenitis, inguinal; with simple or intermediate repair

11463 with complex repair

11470 Excision of skin and subcutaneous tissue for hidradenitis, perianal, perineal, or umbilical; with simple or intermediate repair

11471 with complex repair

(When skin graft or flap is used for closure, use appropriate procedure code in addition)

(For bilateral procedure, add modifier -50)

EXCISION OF MALIGNANT LESIONS

(For excision of malignant lesions requiring more than simple closure, i.e., requiring intermediate or complex closure, report 11600-11646 in addition to appropriate intermediate (12031-12057) or complex closure (13100-13153) codes. For reconstructive closure, see 14000-14300, 15000-15261, 15570-15770)

11600 Excision, malignant lesion, trunk, arms, or legs; lesion diameter 0.5 cm or less

11601 lesion diameter 0.6 to 1.0 cm

11602 lesion diameter 1.1 to 2.0 cm

11603 lesion diameter 2.1 to 3.0 cm

11604 lesion diameter 3.1 to 4.0 cm

11606 lesion diameter over 4.0 cm

• New Code   ▲ Revised Code   * Starred Procedure   + Add-On Code   ∅ Modifier -51 Exempt

11620	Excision, malignant lesion, scalp, neck, hands, feet, genitalia; lesion diameter 0.5 cm or less
11621	lesion diameter 0.6 to 1.0 cm
11622	lesion diameter 1.1 to 2.0 cm
11623	lesion diameter 2.1 to 3.0 cm
11624	lesion diameter 3.1 to 4.0 cm
11626	lesion diameter over 4.0 cm
11640	Excision, malignant lesion, face, ears, eyelids, nose, lips; lesion diameter 0.5 cm or less
11641	lesion diameter 0.6 to 1.0 cm
11642	lesion diameter 1.1 to 2.0 cm
11643	lesion diameter 2.1 to 3.0 cm
11644	lesion diameter 3.1 to 4.0 cm
11646	lesion diameter over 4.0 cm

(For eyelids involving more than skin, see also 67800 et seq)

NAILS

(For drainage of paronychia or onychia, see 10060, 10061)

11719	Trimming of nondystrophic nails, any number
11720	Debridement of nail(s) by any method(s); one to five
11721	six or more
***11730**	Avulsion of nail plate, partial or complete, simple; single
+11732	each additional nail plate (List separately in addition to code for primary procedure)

(Use 11732 in conjunction with code 11730)

11740	Evacuation of subungual hematoma

11750   Excision of nail and nail matrix, partial or complete, (eg, ingrown or deformed nail) for permanent removal;

11752   with amputation of tuft of distal phalanx

(For skin graft, if used, use 15050)

▲ **11755**   Biopsy of nail unit (eg, plate, bed, matrix, hyponychium, proximal and lateral nail folds) (separate procedure)

11760   Repair of nail bed

11762   Reconstruction of nail bed with graft

11765   Wedge excision of skin of nail fold (eg, for ingrown toenail)

(For incision of pilonidal cyst, see 10080, 10081)

11770   Excision of pilonidal cyst or sinus; simple

11771   extensive

11772   complicated

INTRODUCTION

***11900**   Injection, intralesional; up to and including seven lesions

***11901**   more than seven lesions

(11900, 11901 are not to be used for preoperative local anesthetic injection)

(For veins, see 36470, 36471)

(For intralesional chemotherapy administration, see 96405, 96406)

11920   Tattooing, intradermal introduction of insoluble opaque pigments to correct color defects of skin, including micropigmentation; 6.0 sq cm or less

11921   6.1 to 20.0 sq cm

+11922   each additional 20.0 sq cm (List separately in addition to code for primary procedure)

● New Code   ▲ Revised Code   * Starred Procedure   **+** Add-On Code   ⊘ Modifier -51 Exempt

(Use 11922 in conjunction with code 11921)

11950 Subcutaneous injection of filling material (eg, collagen); 1 cc or less

11951 1.1 to 5.0 cc

11952 5.1 to 10.0 cc

11954 over 10.0 cc

11960 Insertion of tissue expander(s) for other than breast, including subsequent expansion

(For breast reconstruction with tissue expander(s), use 19357)

11970 Replacement of tissue expander with permanent prosthesis

11971 Removal of tissue expander(s) without insertion of prosthesis

11975 Insertion, implantable contraceptive capsules

11976 Removal, implantable contraceptive capsules

11977 Removal with reinsertion, implantable contraceptive capsules

11980 Subcutaneous hormone pellet implantation (implantation of estradiol and/or testosterone pellets beneath the skin)

● **11981** Insertion, non-biodegradable drug delivery implant

● **11982** Removal, non-biodegradable drug delivery implant

● **11983** Removal with reinsertion, non-biodegradable drug delivery implant

REPAIR (CLOSURE)

To be able to code wound repair appropriately, the site, length of wound in centimeters and type of repair must be documented in the medical record. Review the definitions of simple, intermediate and complex repair in the current CPT coding system.

Multiple wound repairs from the same body site (category of codes) that were repaired using the same type of closure (simple, intermediate, or

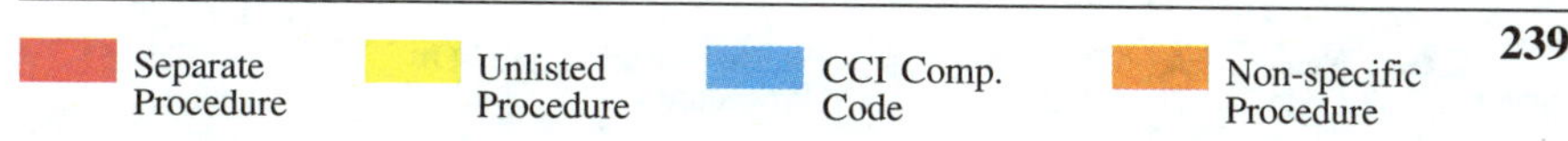

	Separate Procedure		Unlisted Procedure		CCI Comp. Code		Non-specific Procedure

complex) should be coded as one wound. Add the measurements of each wound and assign a single code for the repair.

Simple exploration of nerves, blood vessels or tendons exposed in an open wound are integral part of the wound repair treatment and should not be coded separately. If the wound requires enlargement, extension of dissection, debridement, removal of foreign body, ligation or coagulation of minor subcutaneous and/or muscular blood vessel(s), of the subcutaneous tissue, muscle fascia, and/or muscle, not requiring thoracotomy or laparotomy, use wound exploration codes (20100-20103), as appropriate.

REPAIR — SIMPLE

***12001**   Simple repair of superficial wounds of scalp, neck, axillae, external genitalia, trunk and/or extremities (including hands and feet); 2.5 cm or less

***12002**   2.6 cm to 7.5 cm

***12004**   7.6 cm to 12.5 cm

12005   12.6 cm to 20.0 cm

12006   20.1 cm to 30.0 cm

12007   over 30.0 cm

***12011**   Simple repair of superficial wounds of face, ears, eyelids, nose, lips and/or mucous membranes; 2.5 cm or less

***12013**   2.6 cm to 5.0 cm

12014   5.1 cm to 7.5 cm

12015   7.6 cm to 12.5 cm

12016   12.6 cm to 20.0 cm

12017   20.1 cm to 30.0 cm

12018   over 30.0 cm

12020   Treatment of superficial wound dehiscence; simple closure

12021   with packing

● New Code   ▲ Revised Code   * Starred Procedure   + Add-On Code   ⊘ Modifier -51 Exempt

(For extensive or complicated secondary wound closure, use 13160)

REPAIR — INTERMEDIATE

***12031**   Layer closure of wounds of scalp, axillae, trunk and/or extremities (excluding hands and feet); 2.5 cm or less

***12032**   2.6 cm to 7.5 cm

12034   7.6 cm to 12.5 cm

12035   12.6 cm to 20.0 cm

12036   20.1 cm to 30.0 cm

12037   over 30.0 cm

***12041**   Layer closure of wounds of neck, hands, feet and/or external genitalia; 2.5 cm or less

12042   2.6 cm to 7.5 cm

12044   7.6 cm to 12.5 cm

12045   12.6 cm to 20.0 cm

12046   20.1 cm to 30.0 cm

12047   over 30.0 cm

***12051**   Layer closure of wounds of face, ears, eyelids, nose, lips and/or mucous membranes; 2.5 cm or less

12052   2.6 cm to 5.0 cm

12053   5.1 cm to 7.5 cm

12054   7.6 cm to 12.5 cm

12055   12.6 cm to 20.0 cm

12056   20.1 cm to 30.0 cm

12057   over 30.0 cm

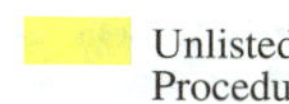
Separate Procedure

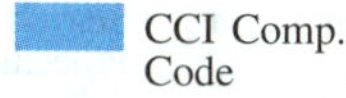
Unlisted Procedure

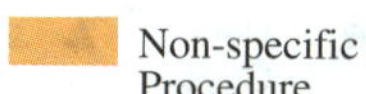
CCI Comp. Code

Non-specific Procedure

REPAIR — COMPLEX

(For full thickness repair of lip or eyelid, see respective anatomical subsections)

13100 Repair, complex, trunk; 1.1 cm to 2.5 cm

(For 1.0 cm or less, see simple or intermediate repairs)

13101 2.6 cm to 7.5 cm

+13102 each additional 5 cm or less (List separately in addition to code for primary procedure)

(Use 13102 in conjunction with code 13101)

13120 Repair, complex, scalp, arms, and/or legs; 1.1 cm to 2.5 cm

(For 1.0 cm or less, see simple or intermediate repairs)

13121 2.6 cm to 7.5 cm

+13122 each additional 5 cm or less (List separately in addition to code for primary procedure)

(Use 13122 in conjunction with 13121)

13131 Repair, complex, forehead, cheeks, chin, mouth, neck, axillae, genitalia, hands and/or feet; 1.1 cm to 2.5 cm

(For 1.0 cm or less, see simple or intermediate repairs)

13132 2.6 cm to 7.5 cm

+13133 each additional 5 cm or less (List separately in addition to code for primary procedure)

(Use 13133 in conjunction with 13132)

13150 Repair, complex, eyelids, nose, ears and/or lips; 1.0 cm or less

(See also 40650-40654, 67961-67975)

13151 1.1 cm to 2.5 cm

13152 2.6 cm to 7.5 cm

● New Code ▲ Revised Code ✻ Starred Procedure ✚ Add-On Code ⊘ Modifier -51 Exempt

+13153   each additional 5 cm or less (List separately in addition to code for primary procedure)

(Use 13153 in conjunction with code 13152)

13160   Secondary closure of surgical wound or dehiscence, extensive or complicated

(For packing or simple secondary wound closure, see 12020, 12021)

ADJACENT TISSUE TRANSFER OR REARRANGEMENT

Codes for adjacent tissuc transfer or rearrangement (14000-14350) are determined by the size and location of the defect site. Excision of lesions performed prior to an adjacent tissue transfer or rearrangement are included in codes 14000 to 14350.

14000   Adjacent tissue transfer or rearrangement, trunk; defect 10 sq cm or less

14001   defect 10.1 sq cm to 30.0 sq cm

14020   Adjacent tissue transfer or rearrangement, scalp, arms and/or legs; defect 10 sq cm or less

14021   defect 10.1 sq cm to 30.0 sq cm

14040   Adjacent tissue transfer or rearrangement, forehead, cheeks, chin, mouth, neck, axillae, genitalia, hands and/or feet; defect 10 sq cm or less

14041   defect 10.1 sq cm to 30.0 sq cm

14060   Adjacent tissue transfer or rearrangement, eyelids, nose, ears and/or lips; defect 10 sq cm or less

14061   defect 10.1 sq cm to 30.0 sq cm

(For eyelid, full thickness, see 67961 et seq)

14300   Adjacent tissue transfer or rcarrangement, more than 30 sq cm, unusual or complicated, any area

14350   Filleted finger or toe flap, including preparation of recipient site

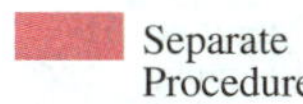
Separate
Procedure

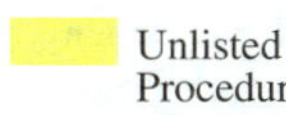
Unlisted
Procedure

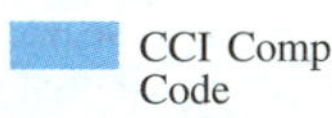
CCI Comp.
Code

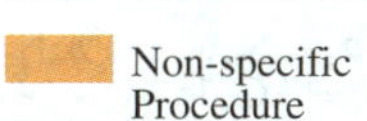
Non-specific
Procedure

FREE SKIN GRAFTS

When coding free skin grafts, the choice of CPT codes is based on the size and location of the defect (recipient area) and the type of graft to be used. The graft CPT codes include simple debridement of granulations or recent avulsion.

When a primary procedure such as orbitectomy, radical mastectomy or deep tumor removal requires skin graft for definite closure, use CPT codes from the appropriate anatomical subsection for the primary procedure and CPT codes from the series 15000-15416 for the skin graft. Note that the repair of a donor site requiring skin graft or local flaps should be coded as an additional procedure. HCPCS Level II codes for medical and surgical supplies, A4000-A4999, may be used to report supplies and materials provided to Medicare patients if the supplies and materials are not considered to be included with or part of the basic service(s) or procedure(s).

(Use 15000 for initial wound preparation)

(Use 15100-15261 for autogenous skin grafts)

(For microvascular flaps, see 15756-15758)

15000   Surgical preparation or creation of recipient site by excision of open wounds, burn eschar, or scar (including subcutaneous tissues); first 100 sq cm or one percent of body area of infants and children

(For appropriate skin grafts, see 15050-15261; list the free graft separately by its procedure number when the graft, immediate or delayed, is applied)

+15001   each additional 100 sq cm or each additional one percent of body area of infants and children (List separately in addition to code for primary procedure)

(Use code 15001 in conjunction with code 15000)

(For excision of benign lesions, see 11400-11471)

(For excision of malignant lesions, see 11600-11646)

(For excision with alloplastic dressing, use 15000 only)

(For excision with immediate skin grafting use 15050-15261 in addition to 15000)

(For excision with immediate allograft placement use 15350 in addition to 15000)

(For excision with immediate xenograft placement use 15400 in addition to 15000)

● New Code   ▲ Revised Code   ✳ Starred Procedure   + Add-On Code   ⊘ Modifier -51 Exempt

15050 Pinch graft, single or multiple, to cover small ulcer, tip of digit, or other minimal open area (except on face), up to defect size 2 cm diameter

15100 Split graft, trunk, arms, legs; first 100 sq cm or less, or one percent of body area of infants and children (except 15050)

+15101 each additional 100 sq cm, or each additional one percent of body area of infants and children, or part thereof (List separately in addition to code for primary procedure)

(Use 15101 in conjunction with code 15100)

15120 Split graft, face, scalp, eyelids, mouth, neck, ears, orbits, genitalia, hands, feet and/or multiple digits; first 100 sq cm or less, or one percent of body area of infants and children (except 15050)

+15121 each additional 100 sq cm, or each additional one percent of body area of infants and children, or part thereof (List separately in addition to code for primary procedure)

(Use 15121 in conjunction with code 15120)

(For eyelids, see also 67961 et seq)

15200 Full thickness graft, free, including direct closure of donor site, trunk; 20 sq cm or less

+15201 each additional 20 sq cm (List separately in addition to code for primary procedure)

(Use 15201 in conjunction with 15200)

15220 Full thickness graft, free, including direct closure of donor site, scalp, arms, and/or legs; 20 sq cm or less

+15221 each additional 20 sq cm (List separately in addition to code for primary procedure)

(Use 15221 in conjunction with 15220)

15240 Full thickness graft, free, including direct closure of donor site, forehead, cheeks, chin, mouth, neck, axillae, genitalia, hands, and/or feet; 20 sq cm or less

(For finger tip graft, use 15050)

 Separate Procedure
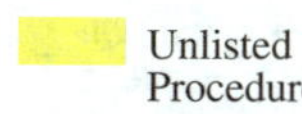 Unlisted Procedure
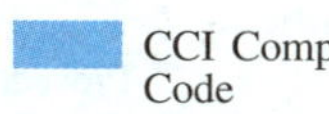 CCI Comp. Code
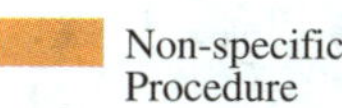 Non-specific Procedure

(For repair of syndactyly, fingers, see 26560-26562)

+15241   each additional 20 sq cm (List separately in addition to code for primary procedure)

(Use 15241 in conjunction with code 15240)

15260   Full thickness graft, free, including direct closure of donor site, nose, ears, eyelids, and/or lips; 20 sq cm or less

+15261   each additional 20 sq cm (List separately in addition to code for primary procedure)

(Use 15261 in conjunction with code 15260)

(For eyelids, see also 67961 et seq)

(Repair of donor site requiring skin graft or local flaps, to be added as additional separate procedure)

15342   Application of bilaminate skin substitute/neodermis; 25 sq cm

+15343   each additional 25 sq cm (List separately in addition to code for primary procedure)

(Use 15343 in conjunction with code 15342)

15350   Application of allograft, skin; 100 sq cm or less

(For staged tissue graft implantation, use modifier -58)

+15351   each additional 100 sq cm (List separately in addition to code for primary procedure)

(Use 15351 in conjunction with code 15350)

15400   Application of xenograft, skin; 100 sq cm or less

+15401   each additional 100 sq cm (List separately in addition to code for primary procedure)

(Use 15401 in conjunction with code 15400)

FLAPS (SKIN AND/OR DEEP TISSUES)

(For microvascular flaps, see 15756-15758)

15570   Formation of direct or tubed pedicle, with or without transfer; trunk

---

● New Code   ▲ Revised Code   * Starred Procedure   + Add-On Code   ⊘ Modifier -51 Exempt

15572   scalp, arms, or legs

15574   forehead, cheeks, chin, mouth, neck, axillae, genitalia, hands or feet

15576   eyelids, nose, ears, lips, or intraoral

15600   Delay of flap or sectioning of flap (division and inset); at trunk

15610   at scalp, arms, or legs

15620   at forehead, cheeks, chin, neck, axillae, genitalia, hands, or feet

15630   at eyelids, nose, ears, or lips

15650   Transfer, intermediate, of any pedicle flap (eg, abdomen to wrist, Walking tube), any location

(For eyelids, nose, ears, or lips, see also anatomical area)

(For revision, defatting or rearranging of transferred pedicle flap or skin graft, see 13100-14300)

(Procedures 15732-15738 are described by donor site of the muscle, myocutaneous, or fasciocutaneous flap)

▲ **15732**   Muscle, myocutaneous, or fasciocutaneous flap; head and neck (eg, temporalis, masseter muscle, sternocleidomastoid, levator scapulae)

15734   trunk

15736   upper extremity

15738   lower extremity

OTHER FLAPS AND GRAFTS

15740   Flap; island pedicle

15750   neurovascular pedicle

15756   Free muscle flap with or without skin with microvascular anastomosis

(Do not report code 69990 in addition to code 15756)

Separate Procedure   Unlisted Procedure   CCI Comp. Code   Non-specific Procedure

15757 Free skin flap with microvascular anastomosis

(Do not report code 69990 in addition to code 15757)

15758 Free fascial flap with microvascular anastomosis

(Do not report code 69990 in addition to code 15758)

15760 Graft; composite (eg, full thickness of external ear or nasal ala), including primary closure, donor area

15770 derma-fat-fascia

15775 Punch graft for hair transplant; 1 to 15 punch grafts

15776 more than 15 punch grafts

(For strip transplant, use 15220)

OTHER PROCEDURES

15780 Dermabrasion; total face (eg, for acne scarring, fine wrinkling, rhytids, general keratosis)

15781 segmental, face

15782 regional, other than face

15783 superficial, any site, (eg, tattoo removal)

***15786** Abrasion; single lesion (eg, keratosis, scar)

+15787 each additional four lesions or less (List separately in addition to code for primary procedure)

(Use 15787 in conjunction with code 15786)

15788 Chemical peel, facial; epidermal

15789 dermal

15792 Chemical peel, nonfacial; epidermal

15793 dermal

15810 Salabrasion; 20 sq cm or less

● New Code ▲ Revised Code * Starred Procedure **+** Add-On Code ⊘ Modifier -51 Exempt

15811   over 20 sq cm

15819 Cervicoplasty

15820 Blepharoplasty, lower eyelid;

15821   with extensive herniated fat pad

15822 Blepharoplasty, upper eyelid;

15823   with excessive skin weighting down lid

(For bilateral blepharoplasty, add modifier -50)

(See also 67916, 67917, 67923, 67924)

15824 Rhytidectomy; forehead

(For repair of brow ptosis, use 67900)

15825   neck with platysmal tightening (platysmal flap, P-flap)

15826   glabellar frown lines

15828   cheek, chin, and neck

15829   superficial musculoaponeurotic system (SMAS) flap

(For bilateral rhytidectomy, add modifier -50)

15831 Excision, excessive skin and subcutaneous tissue (including lipectomy); abdomen (abdominoplasty)

15832   thigh

15833   leg

15834   hip

15835   buttock

15836   arm

15837   forearm or hand

15838   submental fat pad

Separate Procedure   Unlisted Procedure   CCI Comp. Code   Non-specific Procedure

15839   other area

(For bilateral procedure, add modifier -50)

15840   Graft for facial nerve paralysis; free fascia graft (including obtaining fascia)

(For bilateral procedure, add modifier -50)

15841   free muscle graft (including obtaining graft)

15842   free muscle flap by microsurgical technique

(Do not report code 69990 in addition to code 15842)

15845   regional muscle transfer

(For intravenous fluorescein examination of blood flow in graft or flap, use 15860)

(For nerve transfers, decompression, or repair, see 64831-64876, 64905, 64907, 69720, 69725, 69740, 69745, 69955)

15850   Removal of sutures under anesthesia (other than local), same surgeon

15851   Removal of sutures under anesthesia (other than local), other surgeon

15852   Dressing change (for other than burns) under anesthesia (other than local)

▲ **15860**   Intravenous injection of agent (eg, fluorescein) to test vascular flow in flap or graft

15876   Suction assisted lipectomy; head and neck

15877   trunk

15878   upper extremity

15879   lower extremity

PRESSURE ULCERS (DECUBITUS ULCERS)

15920   Excision, coccygeal pressure ulcer, with coccygectomy; with primary suture

● New Code   ▲ Revised Code   ✳ Starred Procedure   ✚ Add-On Code   ⃠ Modifier -51 Exempt

15922   with flap closure

15931 Excision, sacral pressure ulcer, with primary suture;

15933   with ostectomy

15934 Excision, sacral pressure ulcer, with skin flap closure;

15935   with ostectomy

15936 Excision, sacral pressure ulcer, in preparation for muscle or myocutaneous flap or skin graft closure;

15937   with ostectomy

(For repair of defect using muscle or myocutaneous flap, use code(s) 15734 and/or 15738 in addition to 15936, 15937. For repair of defect using split skin graft, use codes 15100 and/or 15101 in addition to 15936, 15937)

15940 Excision, ischial pressure ulcer, with primary suture;

15941   with ostectomy (ischiectomy)

15944 Excision, ischial pressure ulcer, with skin flap closure;

15945   with ostectomy

15946 Excision, ischial pressure ulcer, with ostectomy, in preparation for muscle or myocutaneous flap or skin graft closure

(For repair of defect using muscle or myocutaneous flap, use code(s) 15734 and/or 15738 in addition to 15946. For repair of defect using split skin graft, use codes 15100 and/or 15101 in addition to 15946)

15950 Excision, trochanteric pressure ulcer, with primary suture;

15951   with ostectomy

15952 Excision, trochanteric pressure ulcer, with skin flap closure;

15953   with ostectomy

15956 Excision, trochanteric pressure ulcer, in preparation for muscle or myocutaneous flap or skin graft closure;

251

Separate Procedure	Unlisted Procedure	CCI Comp. Code	Non-specific Procedure

15958	with ostectomy

(For repair of defect using muscle or myocutaneous flap, use code(s) 15734 and/or 15738 in addition to 15956, 15958. For repair of defect using split skin graft, use codes 15100 and/or 15101 in addition to 15956, 15958)

15999 Unlisted procedure, excision pressure ulcer

(For free skin graft to close ulcer or donor site, see 15000 et seq)

BURNS, LOCAL TREATMENT

(For skin graft, see 15100-15650)

16000 Initial treatment, first degree burn, when no more than local treatment is required

16010 Dressings and/or debridement, initial or subsequent; under anesthesia, small

16015 under anesthesia, medium or large, or with major debridement

***16020** without anesthesia, office or hospital, small

***16025** without anesthesia, medium (eg, whole face or whole extremity)

16030 without anesthesia, large (eg, more than one extremity)

16035 Escharotomy; initial incision

+16036 each additional incision (List separately in addition to code for primary procedure)

(Use 16036 in conjunction with code 16035)

(For debridement, curettement of burn wound, see 16010-16030)

DESTRUCTION

(For destruction of lesion(s) in specific anatomic sites, see 40820, 46900-46917, 46924, 54050-54057, 54065, 56501, 56515, 57061, 57065, 67850, 68135)

(For paring or cutting of benign hyperkeratotic lesions (eg, corns or calluses), see 11055-11057)

● New Code   ▲ Revised Code   * Starred Procedure   + Add-On Code   ⊘ Modifier -51 Exempt

(For sharp removal or electrosurgical destruction of skin tags and fibrocutaneous tags, see 11200, 11201)

(For cryotherapy of acne, use 17340)

(For initiation or follow-up care of topical chemotherapy (eg, 5-FU or similar agents), see appropriate office visits)

(For shaving of epidermal or dermal lesions, see 11300-11313)

DESTRUCTION, BENIGN OR PREMALIGNANT LESIONS

▲*17000   Destruction (eg, laser surgery, electrosurgery, cryosurgery, chemosurgery, surgical curettement), all benign or premalignant lesions (eg, actinic keratoses) other than skin tags or cutaneous vascular proliferative lesions; first lesion

+17003   second through 14 lesions, each (List separately in addition to code for first lesion)

(Use 17003 in conjunction with 17000)

⊘▲17004   Destruction (eg, laser surgey, electrosurgery, cryosurgery, chemosurgery, surgical curettement), all benign or premalignant lesions (eg, actinic keratoses) other than skin tags or cutaneous vascular proliferative lesions; 15 or more lesions

(Do not report 17004 in conjunction with codes 17000-17003)

17106   Destruction of cutaneous vascular proliferative lesions (eg, laser technique); less than 10 sq cm

17107   10.0 - 50.0 sq cm

17108   over 50.0 sq cm

▲*17110   Destruction (eg, laser surgery, electrosurgery, cryosurgery, chemosurgery, surgical curettement), of flat warts, molluscum contagiosum, or milia; up to 14 lesions

17111   15 or more lesions

(For destruction of common or plantar warts, see 17000, 17003, 17004)

*17250   Chemical cauterization of granulation tissue (proud flesh, sinus or fistula)

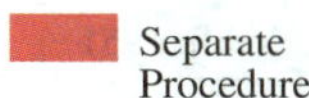 Separate Procedure 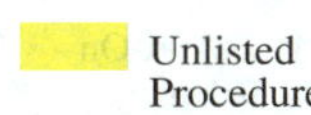 Unlisted Procedure 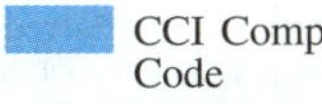 CCI Comp. Code 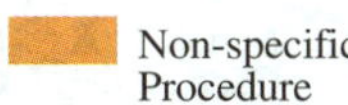 Non-specific Procedure

253

(17250 is not to be used with removal or excision codes for the same lesion)

DESTRUCTION, MALIGNANT LESIONS, ANY METHOD

▲*17260   Destruction, malignant lesion (eg, laser surgery, electrosurgery, cryosurgery, chemosurgery, surgical curettement), trunk, arms or legs; lesion diameter 0.5 cm or less

17261   lesion diameter 0.6 to 1.0 cm

17262   lesion diameter 1.1 to 2.0 cm

17263   lesion diameter 2.1 to 3.0 cm

17264   lesion diameter 3.1 to 4.0 cm

17266   lesion diameter over 4.0 cm

▲*17270   Destruction, malignant lesion (eg, laser surgery, electrosurgery, cryosurgery, chemosurgery, surgical curettement), scalp, neck, hands, feet, genitalia; lesion diameter 0.5 cm or less

17271   lesion diameter 0.6 to 1.0 cm

17272   lesion diameter 1.1 to 2.0 cm

17273   lesion diameter 2.1 to 3.0 cm

17274   lesion diameter 3.1 to 4.0 cm

17276   lesion diameter over 4.0 cm

▲*17280   Destruction, malignant lesion, (eg, laser surgery, electrosurgery, cryosurgery, chemosurgery, surgical curettement), face, ears, eyelids, nose, lips, mucous membrane; lesion diameter 0.5 cm or less

17281   lesion diameter 0.6 to 1.0 cm

17282   lesion diameter 1.1 to 2.0 cm

17283   lesion diameter 2.1 to 3.0 cm

17284   lesion diameter 3.1 to 4.0 cm

● New Code   ▲ Revised Code   * Starred Procedure   + Add-On Code   ⊘ Modifier -51 Exempt

17286   lesion diameter over 4.0 cm

MOHS MICROGRAPHIC SURGERY

⊘ **17304**   Chemosurgery (Mohs micrographic technique), including removal of all gross tumor, surgical excision of tissue specimens, mapping, color coding of specimens, microscopic examination of specimens by the surgeon, and complete histopathologic preparation; first stage, fresh tissue technique, up to 5 specimens

⊘ **17305**   second stage, fixed or fresh tissue, up to 5 specimens

⊘ **17306**   third stage, fixed or fresh tissue, up to 5 specimens

⊘ **17307**   additional stage(s), up to 5 specimens, each stage

⊘ **17310**   more than 5 specimens, fixed or fresh tissue, any stage

OTHER PROCEDURES

＊17340   Cryotherapy (CO2 slush, liquid N2) for acne

＊17360   Chemical exfoliation for acne (eg, acne paste, acid)

＊17380   Electrolysis epilation, each 1/2 hour

(For actinotherapy, use 96900)

17999   Unlisted procedure, skin, mucous membrane and subcutaneous tissue

BREAST

INCISION

＊19000   Puncture aspiration of cyst of breast;

+19001   each additional cyst (List separately in addition to code for primary procedure)

(Use 19001 in conjunction with code 19000)

(If imaging guidance is performed, see 76095, 76096, 76393, 76942)

19020   Mastotomy with exploration or drainage of abscess, deep

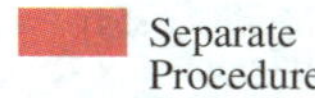

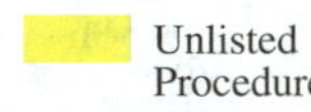

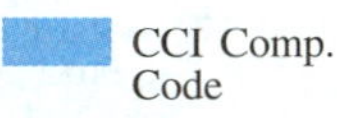

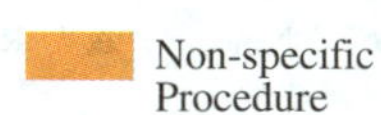

255

19030 Injection procedure only for mammary ductogram or galactogram

(For radiological supervision and interpretation, see 76086, 76088)

EXCISION

(All codes for bilateral procedures have been deleted. To report, add modifier -50)

**19100* Biopsy of breast; percutaneous, needle core, not using imaging guidance (separate procedure)

(For fine needle aspiration, use 10021)

(For image guided breast biopsy, see 19102, 19103, 10022)

19101 open, incisional

19102 percutaneous, needle core, using imaging guidance

(For placement of percutaneous localization clip, use 19295)

19103 percutaneous, automated vacuum assisted or rotating biopsy device, using imaging guidance

(For imaging guidance performed in conjunction with 19102, 19103, see 76095, 76096, 76360, 76393, 76942)

(For placement of percutaneous localization clip, use 19295)

19110 Nipple exploration, with or without excision of a solitary lactiferous duct or a papilloma lactiferous duct

19112 Excision of lactiferous duct fistula

19120 Excision of cyst, fibroadenoma, or other benign or malignant tumor, aberrant breast tissue, duct lesion, nipple or areolar lesion (except 19140), open, male or female, one or more lesions

19125 Excision of breast lesion identified by preoperative placement of radiological marker, open; single lesion

+19126 each additional lesion separately identified by a preoperative radiological marker (List separately in addition to code for primary procedure)

● New Code ▲ Revised Code * Starred Procedure + Add-On Code ⊘ Modifier -51 Exempt

(Use 19126 in conjunction with code 19125)

19140 Mastectomy for gynecomastia

19160 Mastectomy, partial;

19162   with axillary lymphadenectomy

19180 Mastectomy, simple, complete

(For immediate or delayed insertion of implant, use 19340 or 19342)

(For gynecomastia, use 19140)

19182 Mastectomy, subcutaneous

19200 Mastectomy, radical, including pectoral muscles, axillary lymph nodes

19220 Mastectomy, radical, including pectoral muscles, axillary and internal mammary lymph nodes (Urban type operation)

19240 Mastectomy, modified radical, including axillary lymph nodes, with or without pectoralis minor muscle, but excluding pectoralis major muscle

19260 Excision of chest wall tumor including ribs

19271 Excision of chest wall tumor involving ribs, with plastic reconstruction; without mediastinal lymphadenectomy

19272   with mediastinal lymphadenectomy

INTRODUCTION

19290 Preoperative placement of needle localization wire, breast;

+19291   each additional lesion (List separately in addition to code for primary procedure)

(Use 19291 in conjunction with code 19290)

(For radiological supervision and interpretation see 76095, 76096, 76942)

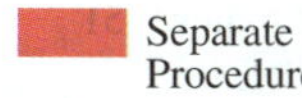 Separate Procedure
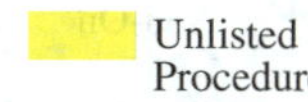 Unlisted Procedure
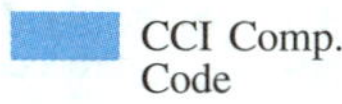 CCI Comp. Code
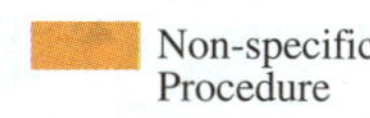 Non-specific Procedure

+19295   Image guided placement, metallic localization clip, percutaneous, during breast biopsy (List separately in addition to code for primary procedure)

(Use 19295 in conjunction with codes 19102, 19103)

REPAIR AND/OR RECONSTRUCTION

(All codes for bilateral procedures have been deleted. To report, add modifier -50)

19316   Mastopexy

19318   Reduction mammaplasty

19324   Mammaplasty, augmentation; without prosthetic implant

19325   with prosthetic implant

(For flap or graft, use also appropriate number)

19328   Removal of intact mammary implant

19330   Removal of mammary implant material

19340   Immediate insertion of breast prosthesis following mastopexy, mastectomy or in reconstruction

19342   Delayed insertion of breast prosthesis following mastopexy, mastectomy or in reconstruction

(For supply of implant, use 99070)

(For preparation of custom breast implant, use 19396)

19350   Nipple/areola reconstruction

19355   Correction of inverted nipples

19357   Breast reconstruction, immediate or delayed, with tissue expander, including subsequent expansion

19361   Breast reconstruction with latissimus dorsi flap, with or without prosthetic implant

19364   Breast reconstruction with free flap

● New Code   ▲ Revised Code   ✳ Starred Procedure   + Add-On Code   ⊘ Modifier -51 Exempt

(Do not report code 69990 in addition to code 19364)

(19364 includes harvesting of the flap, microvascular transfer, closure of the donor site, and inset shaping the flap into a breast)

19366 Breast reconstruction with other technique

(For operating microscope, use 69990)

(For insertion of prosthesis, use also 19340 or 19342)

19367 Breast reconstruction with transverse rectus abdominis myocutaneous flap (TRAM), single pedicle, including closure of donor site;

19368   with microvascular anastomosis (supercharging)

(Do not report code 69990 in addition to code 19368)

19369 Breast reconstruction with transverse rectus abdominis myocutaneous flap (TRAM), double pedicle, including closure of donor site

19370 Open periprosthetic capsulotomy, breast

19371 Periprosthetic capsulectomy, breast

19380 Revision of reconstructed breast

19396 Preparation of moulage for custom breast implant

OTHER PROCEDURES

19499 Unlisted procedure, breast

Separate Procedure   Unlisted Procedure   CCI Comp. Code   Non-specific Procedure

MUSCULOSKELETAL SYSTEM

Musculoskeletal procedure codes include the application and removal of the initial cast or traction device. Use codes in range 29000 to 29799 to report subsequent cast or traction-device applications. Review the instructional notes under the "Application of Casts and Strapping" to identify other uses for these codes.

The procedures and services listed in this section of the CPT coding system include the application and removal of the first cast or traction device only. Subsequent replacement of the cast and/or traction device may be coded using the cast and strapping procedure CPT codes appearing at the end of the section.

MISCELLANEOUS CODING RULES

Most bone, cartilage and fascia graft procedures include obtaining of the graft by the operating surgeon. When a surgical associate obtains the graft for the operating surgeon, the additional service should be coded and coded separately using CPT codes from the 20900-20926 range. In addition, a surgical modifier for assistant surgeon or co-surgeon should be included when reporting the associates services.

CPT codes 20100-20103 relate to treatment of wounds resulting from penetrating trauma (e.g., gunshot, stab wound). Use these codes for wound explorations only if the procedure does not require a thoracotomy or laparotomy and/or repairs to major structure(s) or major blood vessels.

The term "complicated" appears in some narratives in the musculoskeletal subsection. This term implies that an infection occurred, treatment was delayed, or the surgery took longer than usual to perform. Send supporting documentation when the codes containing this descriptor are assigned.

An intermediate repair associated with a musculoskeletal surgery is an integral portion of the surgery and should not be coded separately.

Code the injection codes according to the location of the joint injected or aspirated. Example: small joint = fingers, toes; intermediate joint = wrist, elbow; and major joint = shoulder, hip, or knee.

When removing a foreign body or performing soft tissue biopsy, determine the site and whether or not the foreign body/biopsy is superficial or deep.

FRACTURES

Remember to differentiate between the type of fracture and the type of treatment when coding fractures. Review the meanings of open and closed treatment of fractures. Dislocations must also be coded with emphasis on whether the treatment is open or closed.

| ● New Code | ▲ Revised Code | ✳ Starred Procedure | ✚ Add-On Code | ⊘ Modifier -51 Exempt |

When coding the re-reduction of a fracture and/or dislocation performed by the primary physician, add modifier -76 to the procedure code. If the re-reduction were performed by another physician, then modifier -77 would be added to the procedure code.

STARRED PROCEDURES

There are numerous starred (*) procedures in this section of the CPT coding system indicating the opportunity of reporting an appropriate visit code in addition to the surgical procedure.

GENERAL

INCISION

***20000** Incision of soft tissue abscess (eg, secondary to osteomyelitis); superficial

20005 deep or complicated

WOUND EXPLORATION - TRAUMA (EG, PENETRATING GUNSHOT, STAB WOUND)

20100 Exploration of penetrating wound (separate procedure); neck

20101 chest

20102 abdomen/flank/back

20103 extremity

EXCISION

20150 Excision of epiphyseal bar, with or without autogenous soft tissue graft obtained through same fascial incision

(For aspiration of bone marrow, use 38220)

20200 Biopsy, muscle; superficial

20205 deep

***20206** Biopsy, muscle, percutaneous needle

(If imaging guidance is performed, see 76360, 76393, 76942)

(For fine needle aspiration, use 10021 or 10022)

(For evaluation of fine needle aspirate, see 88172-88173)

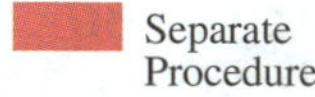

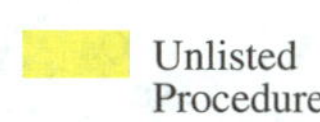

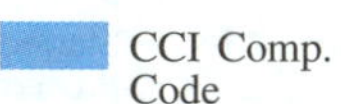

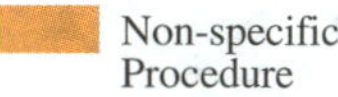

(For excision of muscle tumor, deep, see specific anatomic section)

20220 Biopsy, bone, trocar, or needle; superficial (eg, ilium, sternum, spinous process, ribs)

▲ **20225** deep (eg, vertebral body, femur)

(For bone marrow biopsy, use 38221)

(For radiologic supervision and interpretation, see 76003, 76360, 76393)

20240 Biopsy, bone, excisional; superficial (eg, ilium, sternum, spinous process, ribs, trochanter of femur)

20245 deep (eg, humerus, ischium, femur)

20250 Biopsy, vertebral body, open; thoracic

20251 lumbar or cervical

(For sequestrectomy, osteomyelitis or drainage of bone abscess, see anatomical area)

INTRODUCTION OR REMOVAL

(For injection procedure for arthrography, see anatomical area)

***20500** Injection of sinus tract; therapeutic (separate procedure)

***20501** diagnostic (sinogram)

(For radiological supervision and interpretation, use 76080)

***20520** Removal of foreign body in muscle or tendon sheath; simple

20525 deep or complicated

● **20526** Injection, therapeutic (eg, local anesthetic, corticosteroid), carpal tunnel

▲ ***20550** Injection; tendon sheath, ligament, ganglion cyst

(If imaging guidance is performed, see 76003, 76393, 76942)

● **20551** tendon origin/insertion

● **20552** single or multiple trigger point(s), one or two muscle group(s)

● **20553** single or multiple trigger point(s), three or more muscle group(s)

***20600** Arthrocentesis, aspiration and/or injection; small joint, bursa or ganglion cyst (eg, fingers, toes)

***20605** intermediate joint, bursa or ganglion cyst (eg, temporomandibular, acromioclavicular, wrist, elbow or ankle, olecranon bursa)

***20610** major joint or bursa (eg, shoulder, hip, knee joint, subacromial bursa)

(If imaging guidance is performed, see 76003, 76360, 76393, 76942)

20615 Aspiration and injection for treatment of bone cyst

***20650** Insertion of wire or pin with application of skeletal traction, including removal (separate procedure)

⊘ **20660** Application of cranial tongs, caliper, or stereotactic frame, including removal (separate procedure)

20661 Application of halo, including removal; cranial

20662 pelvic

20663 femoral

20664 Application of halo, including removal, cranial, 6 or more pins placed, for thin skull osteology (eg, pediatric patients, hydrocephalus, osteogenesis imperfecta), requiring general anesthesia

***20665** Removal of tongs or halo applied by another physician

***20670** Removal of implant; superficial, (eg, buried wire, pin or rod) (separate procedure)

20680 deep (eg, buried wire, pin, screw, metal band, nail,rod or plate)

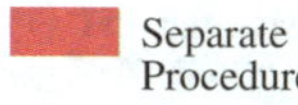 Separate Procedure

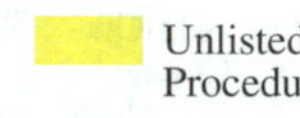 Unlisted Procedure

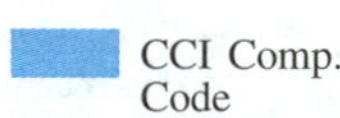 CCI Comp. Code

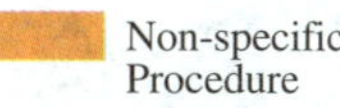 Non-specific Procedure

⊘ **20690** Application of a uniplane (pins or wires in one plane), unilateral, external fixation system

⊘ **20692** Application of a multiplane (pins or wires in more than one plane), unilateral, external fixation system (eg, Ilizarov, Monticelli type)

20693 Adjustment or revision of external fixation system requiring anesthesia (eg, new pin(s) or wire(s) and/or new ring(s) or bar(s))

20694 Removal, under anesthesia, of external fixation system

REPLANTATION

20802 Replantation, arm (includes surgical neck of humerus through elbow joint), complete amputation

20805 Replantation, forearm (includes radius and ulna to radial carpal joint), complete amputation

20808 Replantation, hand (includes hand through metacarpophalangeal joints), complete amputation

20816 Replantation, digit, excluding thumb (includes metacarpophalangeal joint to insertion of flexor sublimis tendon), complete amputation

20822 Replantation, digit, excluding thumb (includes distal tip to sublimis tendon insertion), complete amputation

20824 Replantation, thumb (includes carpometacarpal joint to MP joint), complete amputation

20827 Replantation, thumb (includes distal tip to MP joint), complete amputation

20838 Replantation, foot, complete amputation

GRAFTS OR IMPLANTS

(For spinal surgery bone graft(s) see codes 20930-20938)

⊘ **20900** Bone graft, any donor area; minor or small (eg, dowel or button)

⊘ **20902** major or large

● New Code   ▲ Revised Code   ✳ Starred Procedure   ✛ Add-On Code   ⊘ Modifier -51 Exempt

○ **20910** Cartilage graft; costochondral

○ **20912**   nasal septum

(For ear cartilage, use 21235)

○ **20920** Fascia lata graft; by stripper

○ **20922**   by incision and area exposure, complex or sheet

○ **20924** Tendon graft, from a distance (eg, palmaris, toe extensor, plantaris)

○ **20926** Tissue grafts, other (eg, paratenon, fat, dermis)

(Codes 20930-20938 are reported in addition to codes for the definitive procedure(s) without modifier -51)

○ **20930** Allograft for spine surgery only; morselized

○ **20931**   structural

○ **20936** Autograft for spine surgery only (includes harvesting the graft); local (eg, ribs, spinous process, or laminar fragments) obtained from same incision

○ **20937**   morselized (through separate skin or fascial incision)

○ **20938**   structural, bicortical or tricortical (through separate skin or fascial incision)

(For needle aspiration of bone marrow for the purpose of bone grafting, use 38220)

OTHER PROCEDURES

20950 Monitoring of interstitial fluid pressure (includes insertion of device,eg, wick catheter technique, needle manometer technique) in detection of muscle compartment syndrome

20955 Bone graft with microvascular anastomosis; fibula

20956   iliac crest

20957   metatarsal

20962		other than fibula, iliac crest, or metatarsal

(Do not report code 69990 in addition to codes 20955-20962)

20969 Free osteocutaneous flap with microvascular anastomosis; other than iliac crest, metatarsal, or great toe

20970 iliac crest

20972 metatarsal

20973 great toe with web space

(Do not report code 69990 in addition to codes 20969-20973)

(For great toe, wrap-around procedure, use 26551)

⊘ **20974** Electrical stimulation to aid bone healing; noninvasive (nonoperative)

⊘ **20975** invasive (operative)

20979 Low intensity ultrasound stimulation to aid bone healing, noninvasive (nonoperative)

20999 Unlisted procedure, musculoskeletal system, general

HEAD

INCISION

(For drainage of superficial abscess and hematoma, use 20000)

(For removal of embedded foreign body from dentoalveolar structure, see 41805, 41806)

21010 Arthrotomy, temporomandibular joint

EXCISION

(For biopsy, see 20220, 20240)

21015 Radical resection of tumor (eg, malignant neoplasm), soft tissue of face or scalp

21025 Excision of bone (eg, for osteomyelitis or bone abscess); mandible

● New Code ▲ Revised Code ✳ Starred Procedure ✚ Add-On Code ⊘ Modifier -51 Exempt

21026   facial bone(s)

21029   Removal by contouring of benign tumor of facial bone (eg, fibrous dysplasia)

21030   Excision of benign tumor or cyst of facial bone other than mandible

21031   Excision of torus mandibularis

21032   Excision of maxillary torus palatinus

21034   Excision of malignant tumor of facial bone other than mandible

21040   Excision of benign cyst or tumor of mandible; simple

21041   complex

21044   Excision of malignant tumor of mandible;

21045   radical resection

(For bone graft, use 21215)

21050   Condylectomy, temporomandibular joint (separate procedure)

21060   Meniscectomy, partial or complete, temporomandibular joint (separate procedure)

21070   Coronoidectomy (separate procedure)

INTRODUCTION OR REMOVAL

21076   Impression and custom preparation; surgical obturator prosthesis

21077   orbital prosthesis

21079   interim obturator prosthesis

21080   definitive obturator prosthesis

21081   mandibular resection prosthesis

21082   palatal augmentation prosthesis

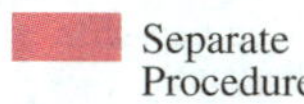 Separate Procedure

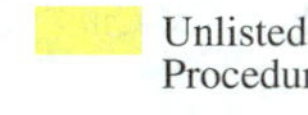 Unlisted Procedure

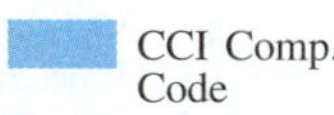 CCI Comp. Code

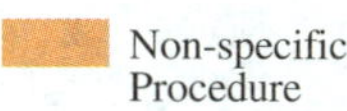 Non-specific Procedure

| **21083** | palatal lift prosthesis |

| **21084** | speech aid prosthesis |

| **21085** | oral surgical splint |

| **21086** | auricular prosthesis |

| **21087** | nasal prosthesis |

| **21088** | facial prosthesis |

21089 Unlisted maxillofacial prosthetic procedure

***21100** Application of halo type appliance for maxillofacial fixation, includes removal (separate procedure)

21110 Application of interdental fixation device for conditions other than fracture or dislocation, includes removal

(For removal of interdental fixation by another physician, see 20670-20680)

21116 Injection procedure for temporomandibular joint arthrography

(For radiological supervision and interpretation, use 70332. Do not report 76003 in addition to 70332)

REPAIR, REVISION AND/OR RECONSTRUCTION

(For cranioplasty, see 21179, 21180 and 62116, 62120, 62140-62147)

21120 Genioplasty; augmentation (autograft, allograft, prosthetic material)

21121 sliding osteotomy, single piece

21122 sliding osteotomies, two or more osteotomies (eg, wedge excision or bone wedge reversal for asymmetrical chin)

21123 sliding, augmentation with interpositional bone grafts (includes obtaining autografts)

21125 Augmentation, mandibular body or angle; prosthetic material

---

● New Code   ▲ Revised Code   * Starred Procedure   + Add-On Code   ⊘ Modifier -51 Exempt

21127   with bone graft, onlay or interpositional (includes obtaining autograft)

21137   Reduction forehead; contouring only

21138   contouring and application of prosthetic material or bone graft (includes obtaining autograft)

21139   contouring and setback of anterior frontal sinus wall

21141   Reconstruction midface, LeFort I; single piece, segment movement in any direction (eg, for Long Face Syndrome), without bone graft

21142   two pieces, segment movement in any direction, without bone graft

21143   three or more pieces, segment movement in any direction, without bone graft

21145   single piece, segment movement in any direction, requiring bone grafts (includes obtaining autografts)

21146   two pieces, segment movement in any direction, requiring bone grafts (includes obtaining autografts) (eg, ungrafted unilateral alveolar cleft)

21147   three or more pieces, segment movement in any direction, requiring bone grafts (includes obtaining autografts) (eg, ungrafted bilateral alveolar cleft or multiple osteotomies)

21150   Reconstruction midface, LeFort II; anterior intrusion (eg, Treacher-Collins Syndrome)

21151   any direction, requiring bone grafts (includes obtaining autografts)

21154   Reconstruction midface, LeFort III (extracranial), any type, requiring bone grafts (includes obtaining autografts); without LeFort I

21155   with LeFort I

21159   Reconstruction midface, LeFort III (extra and intracranial) with forehead advancement (eg, mono bloc), requiring bone grafts (includes obtaining autografts); without LeFort I

269

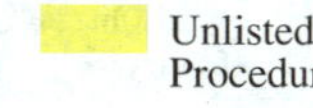
Separate Procedure

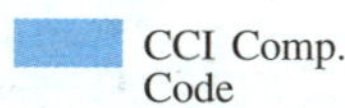
Unlisted Procedure

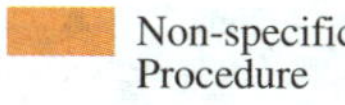
CCI Comp. Code

Non-specific Procedure

21160　　　with LeFort I

21172　Reconstruction superior-lateral orbital rim and lower forehead, advancement or alteration, with or without grafts (includes obtaining autografts)

(For frontal or parietal craniotomy performed for craniosynostosis, use 61556)

21175　Reconstruction, bifrontal, superior-lateral orbital rims and lower forehead, advancement or alteration (eg, plagiocephaly, trigonocephaly, brachycephaly), with or without grafts (includes obtaining autografts)

(For bifrontal craniotomy performed for craniosynostosis, use 61557)

21179　Reconstruction, entire or majority of forehead and/or supraorbital rims; with grafts (allograft or prosthetic material)

21180　　　with autograft (includes obtaining grafts)

(For extensive craniectomy for multiple suture craniosynostosis, use only 61558 or 61559)

21181　Reconstruction by contouring of benign tumor of cranial bones (eg, fibrous dysplasia), extracranial

▲ **21182**　Reconstruction of orbital walls, rims, forehead, nasoethmoid complex following intra- and extracranial excision of benign tumor of cranial bone (eg, fibrous dysplasia), with multiple autografts (includes obtaining grafts); total area of bone grafting less than 40 sq cm

▲ **21183**　　　total area of bone grafting greater than 40 sq cm but less than 80 sq cm

▲ **21184**　　　total area of bone grafting greater than 80 sq cm

(For excision of benign tumor of cranial bones, see 61563, 61564)

21188　Reconstruction midface, osteotomies (other than LeFort type) and bone grafts (includes obtaining autografts)

21193　Reconstruction of mandibular rami, horizontal, vertical, C, or L osteotomy; without bone graft

---

● New Code　　▲ Revised Code　　✻ Starred Procedure　　✛ Add-On Code　　⊘ Modifier -51 Exempt

21194   with bone graft (includes obtaining graft)

21195 Reconstruction of mandibular rami and/or body, sagittal split; without internal rigid fixation

21196   with internal rigid fixation

21198 Osteotomy, mandible, segmental;

21199   with genioglossus advancement

21206 Osteotomy, maxilla, segmental (eg, Wassmund or Schuchard)

21208 Osteoplasty, facial bones; augmentation (autograft, allograft, or prosthetic implant)

21209   reduction

21210 Graft, bone; nasal, maxillary or malar areas (includes obtaining graft)

(For cleft palate repair, see 42200-42225)

21215   mandible (includes obtaining graft)

21230 Graft; rib cartilage, autogenous, to face, chin, nose or ear (includes obtaining graft)

21235   ear cartilage, autogenous, to nose or ear (includes obtaining graft)

21240 Arthroplasty, temporomandibular joint, with or without autograft (includes obtaining graft)

21242 Arthroplasty, temporomandibular joint, with allograft

21243 Arthroplasty, temporomandibular joint, with prosthetic joint replacement

21244 Reconstruction of mandible, extraoral, with transosteal bone plate (eg, mandibular staple bone plate)

21245 Reconstruction of mandible or maxilla, subperiosteal implant; partial

21246   complete

Separate Procedure	Unlisted Procedure	CCI Comp. Code	Non-specific Procedure

21247 Reconstruction of mandibular condyle with bone and cartilage autografts (includes obtaining grafts) (eg, for hemifacial microsomia)

21248 Reconstruction of mandible or maxilla, endosteal implant (eg, blade, cylinder); partial

21249 complete

21255 Reconstruction of zygomatic arch and glenoid fossa with bone and cartilage (includes obtaining autografts)

21256 Reconstruction of orbit with osteotomies (extracranial) and with bone grafts (includes obtaining autografts) (eg, micro-ophthalmia)

21260 Periorbital osteotomies for orbital hypertelorism, with bone grafts; extracranial approach

21261 combined intra- and extracranial approach

21263 with forehead advancement

21267 Orbital repositioning, periorbital osteotomies, unilateral, with bone grafts; extracranial approach

21268 combined intra- and extracranial approach

21270 Malar augmentation, prosthetic material

(For malar augmentation with bone graft, use 21210)

21275 Secondary revision of orbitocraniofacial reconstruction

21280 Medial canthopexy (separate procedure)

(For medial canthoplasty, use 67950)

21282 Lateral canthopexy

21295 Reduction of masseter muscle and bone (eg, for treatment of benign masseteric hypertrophy); extraoral approach

21296 intraoral approach

OTHER PROCEDURES

21299 Unlisted craniofacial and maxillofacial procedure

FRACTURE AND/OR DISLOCATION

21300 Closed treatment of skull fracture without operation

(For operative repair, see 62000-62010)

21310 Closed treatment of nasal bone fracture without manipulation

***21315** Closed treatment of nasal bone fracture; without stabilization

21320 with stabilization

21325 Open treatment of nasal fracture; uncomplicated

21330 complicated, with internal and/or external skeletal fixation

21335 with concomitant open treatment of fractured septum

21336 Open treatment of nasal septal fracture, with or without stabilization

21337 Closed treatment of nasal septal fracture, with or without stabilization

21338 Open treatment of nasoethmoid fracture; without external fixation

21339 with external fixation

21340 Percutaneous treatment of nasoethmoid complex fracture, with splint, wire or headcap fixation, including repair of canthal ligaments and/or the nasolacrimal apparatus

21343 Open treatment of depressed frontal sinus fracture

21344 Open treatment of complicated (eg, comminuted or involving posterior wall) frontal sinus fracture, via coronal or multiple approaches

21345 Closed treatment of nasomaxillary complex fracture (LeFort II type), with interdental wire fixation or fixation of denture or splint

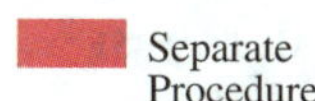

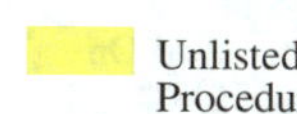

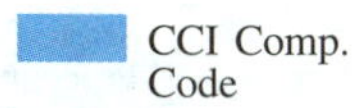

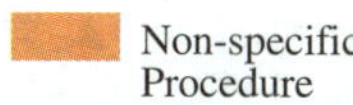

273

21346	Open treatment of nasomaxillary complex fracture (LeFort II type); with wiring and/or local fixation
21347	requiring multiple open approaches
21348	with bone grafting (includes obtaining graft)
***21355**	Percutaneous treatment of fracture of malar area, including zygomatic arch and malar tripod, with manipulation
21356	Open treatment of depressed zygomatic arch fracture (eg, Gillies approach)
21360	Open treatment of depressed malar fracture, including zygomatic arch and malar tripod
21365	Open treatment of complicated (eg, comminuted or involving cranial nerve foramina) fracture(s) of malar area, including zygomatic arch and malar tripod; with internal fixation and multiple surgical approaches
21366	with bone grafting (includes obtaining graft)
21385	Open treatment of orbital floor blowout fracture; transantral approach (Caldwell-Luc type operation)
21386	periorbital approach
21387	combined approach
21390	periorbital approach, with alloplastic or other implant
21395	periorbital approach with bone graft (includes obtaining graft)
21400	Closed treatment of fracture of orbit, except blowout; without manipulation
21401	with manipulation
21406	Open treatment of fracture of orbit, except blowout; without implant
21407	with implant
21408	with bone grafting (includes obtaining graft)

● New Code   ▲ Revised Code   * Starred Procedure   ✛ Add-On Code   ⊘ Modifier -51 Exempt

21421 Closed treatment of palatal or maxillary fracture (LeFort I type), with interdental wire fixation or fixation of denture or splint

21422 Open treatment of palatal or maxillary fracture (LeFort I type);

21423 complicated (comminuted or involving cranial nerve foramina), multiple approaches

21431 Closed treatment of craniofacial separation (LeFort III type) using interdental wire fixation of denture or splint

21432 Open treatment of craniofacial separation (LeFort III type); with wiring and/or internal fixation

21433 complicated (eg, comminuted or involving cranial nerve foramina), multiple surgical approaches

21435 complicated, utilizing internal and/or external fixation techniques (eg, head cap, halo device, and/or intermaxillary fixation)

(For removal of internal or external fixation device, use 20670)

21436 complicated, multiple surgical approaches, internal fixation, with bone grafting (includes obtaining graft)

21440 Closed treatment of mandibular or maxillary alveolar ridge fracture (separate procedure)

21445 Open treatment of mandibular or maxillary alveolar ridge fracture (separate procedure)

21450 Closed treatment of mandibular fracture; without manipulation

21451 with manipulation

21452 Percutaneous treatment of mandibular fracture, with external fixation

21453 Closed treatment of mandibular fracture with interdental fixation

21454 Open treatment of mandibular fracture with external fixation

---

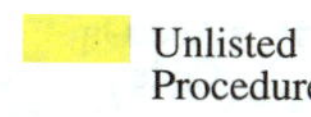
Separate
Procedure

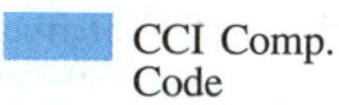
Unlisted
Procedure

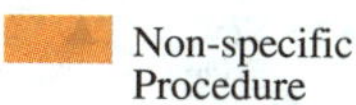
CCI Comp.
Code

Non-specific
Procedure

275

21461 Open treatment of mandibular fracture; without interdental fixation

21462 with interdental fixation

21465 Open treatment of mandibular condylar fracture

21470 Open treatment of complicated mandibular fracture by multiple surgical approaches including internal fixation, interdental fixation, and/or wiring of dentures or splints

21480 Closed treatment of temporomandibular dislocation; initial or subsequent

21485 complicated (eg, recurrent requiring intermaxillary fixation or splinting), initial or subsequent

21490 Open treatment of temporomandibular dislocation

(For interdental wire fixation, use 21497)

21493 Closed treatment of hyoid fracture; without manipulation

21494 with manipulation

21495 Open treatment of hyoid fracture

(For treatment of fracture of larynx, see 31584-31586)

21497 Interdental wiring, for condition other than fracture

OTHER PROCEDURES

21499 Unlisted musculoskeletal procedure, head

(For unlisted craniofacial or maxillofacial procedure, use 21299)

NECK (SOFT TISSUES) AND THORAX

(For cervical spine and back, see 21920 et seq)

(For injection of fracture site or trigger point, use 20550)

INCISION

(For incision and drainage of abscess or hematoma, superficial, see 10060, 10140)

● New Code　　▲ Revised Code　　✱ Starred Procedure　　＋ Add-On Code　　⊘ Modifier -51 Exempt

21501   Incision and drainage, deep abscess or hematoma, soft tissues of neck or thorax;

21502   with partial rib ostectomy

21510   Incision, deep, with opening of bone cortex (eg, for osteomyelitis or bone abscess), thorax

EXCISION

(For bone biopsy, see 20220-20251)

21550   Biopsy, soft tissue of neck or thorax

(For needle biopsy of soft tissue, use 20206)

21555   Excision tumor, soft tissue of neck or thorax; subcutaneous

21556   deep, subfascial, intramuscular

21557   Radical resection of tumor (eg, malignant neoplasm), soft tissue of neck or thorax

21600   Excision of rib, partial

(For radical resection of chest wall and rib cage for tumor, use 19260)

(For radical debridement of chest wall and rib cage for injury, see 11040-11044)

21610   Costotransversectomy (separate procedure)

21615   Excision first and/or cervical rib;

21616   with sympathectomy

21620   Ostectomy of sternum, partial

21627   Sternal debridement

(For debridement and closure, use 21750)

21630   Radical resection of sternum;

21632   with mediastinal lymphadenectomy

Separate Procedure

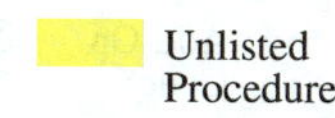
Unlisted Procedure

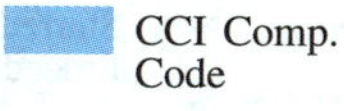
CCI Comp. Code

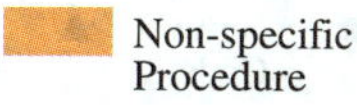
Non-specific Procedure

REPAIR, REVISION, AND/OR RECONSTRUCTION

(For superficial wound, see Integumentary System section under Repair—Simple)

21700 Division of scalenus anticus; without resection of cervical rib

21705   with resection of cervical rib

21720 Division of sternocleidomastoid for torticollis, open operation; without cast application

(For transection of spinal accessory and cervical nerves, see 63191, 64722)

21725   with cast application

21740 Reconstructive repair of pectus excavatum or carinatum

▲ **21750** Closure of median sternotomy separation with or without debridement (separate procedure)

FRACTURE AND/OR DISLOCATION

21800 Closed treatment of rib fracture, uncomplicated, each

21805 Open treatment of rib fracture without fixation, each

21810 Treatment of rib fracture requiring external fixation (flail chest)

21820 Closed treatment of sternum fracture

21825 Open treatment of sternum fracture with or without skeletal fixation

(For sternoclavicular dislocation, see 23520-23532)

OTHER PROCEDURES

21899 Unlisted procedure, neck or thorax

BACK AND FLANK

EXCISION

21920 Biopsy, soft tissue of back or flank; superficial

● New Code   ▲ Revised Code   ✳ Starred Procedure   ✚ Add-On Code   ⊘ Modifier -51 Exempt

21925   deep

(For needle biopsy of soft tissue, use 20206)

21930   Excision, tumor, soft tissue of back or flank

21935   Radical resection of tumor (eg, malignant neoplasm), soft tissue of back or flank

SPINE (VERTEBRAL COLUMN)

(Do not append modifier -62 to bone graft code 20931)

(For injection procedure for myelography, use 62284)

(For injection procedure for diskography, see 62290, 62291)

(For injection procedure, chemonucleolysis, single or multiple leveles, use 62292)

(For injection procedure for facet joints, see 64470-64476, 64622-64627)

(For needle or trocar biopsy, see 20220-20225)

EXCISION

(For bone biopsy, see 20220-20251)

22100   Partial excision of posterior vertebral component (eg, spinous process, lamina or facet) for intrinsic bony lesion, single vertebral segment; cervical

22101   thoracic

22102   lumbar

+22103   each additional segment (List separately in addition to code for primary procedure)

(Use 22103 in conjunction with codes 22100, 22101, 22102)

22110   Partial excision of vertebral body, for intrinsic bony lesion, without decompression of spinal cord or nerve root(s), single vertebral segment; cervical

22112   thoracic

22114   lumbar

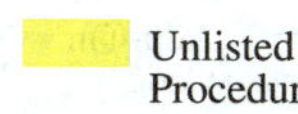

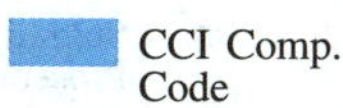

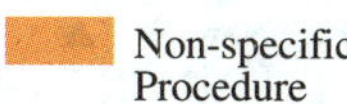

+22116   each additional vertebral segment (List separately in addition to code for primary procedure)

(Use 22116 in conjunction with codes 22110, 22112, 22114)

OSTEOTOMY

22210   Osteotomy of spine, posterior or posterolateral approach, one vertebral segment; cervical

22212   thoracic

22214   lumbar

+22216   each additional vertebral segment (List separately in addition to primary procedure)

(Use 22216 in conjunction with codes 22210, 22212, 22214)

22220   Osteotomy of spine, including diskectomy, anterior approach, single vertebral segment; cervical

22222   thoracic

22224   lumbar

+22226   each additional vertebral segment (List separately in addition to code for primary procedure)

(Use 22226 in conjunction with codes 22220, 22222, 22224)

FRACTURE AND/OR DISLOCATION

22305   Closed treatment of vertebral process fracture(s)

22310   Closed treatment of vertebral body fracture(s), without manipulation, requiring and including casting or bracing

22315   Closed treatment of vertebral fracture(s) and/or dislocation(s) requiring casting or bracing, with and including casting and/or bracing, with or without anesthesia, by manipulation or traction

(For spinal subluxation, use 97140)

22318   Open treatment and/or reduction of odontoid fracture(s) and or dislocation(s) (including os odontoideum), anterior approach, including placement of internal fixation; without grafting

---

   ● New Code   ▲ Revised Code   ✳ Starred Procedure   **+** Add-On Code   ⊘ Modifier -51 Exempt

22319   with grafting

22325   Open treatment and/or reduction of vertebral fracture(s) and/or dislocation(s), posterior approach, one fractured vertebrae or dislocated segment; lumbar

22326   cervical

22327   thoracic

+22328   each additional fractured vertebrae or dislocated segment (List separately in addition to code for primary procedure)

(Use 22328 in conjunction with codes 22325, 22326, 22327)

(For treatment of vertebral fracture by the anterior approach, see corpectomy 63081-63091, and appropriate arthrodesis, bone graft and instrument codes)

MANIPULATION

22505   Manipulation of spine requiring anesthesia, any region

VERTEBRAL BODY, EMBOLIZATION OR INJECTION

22520   Percutaneous vertebroplasty, one vertebral body, unilateral or bilateral injection; thoracic

22521   lumbar

+22522   each additional thoracic or lumbar body (List separately in addition to code for primary procedure)

(Use 22522 in conjunction with codes 22520, 22521 as appropriate)

(For radiological supervision and interpretation, see 76012, 76013)

ARTHRODESIS

Anterior or Anterolateral Approach Technique

22548   Arthrodesis, anterior transoral or extraoral technique, clivus-C1-C2 (atlas-axis), with or without excision of odontoid process

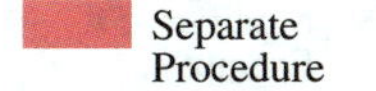 Separate Procedure

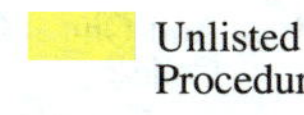 Unlisted Procedure

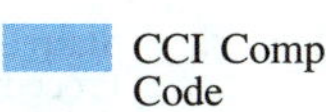 CCI Comp. Code

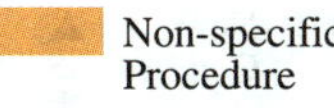 Non-specific Procedure

22554 Arthrodesis, anterior interbody technique, including minimal diskectomy to prepare interspace (other than for decompression); cervical below C2

22556 thoracic

22558 lumbar

+22585 each additional interspace (List separately in addition to code for primary procedure)

(Use 22585 in conjunction with codes 22554, 22556, 22558)

Posterior, Posterolateral or Lateral Transverse Process Technique

22590 Arthrodesis, posterior technique, craniocervical (occiput-C2)

22595 Arthrodesis, posterior technique, atlas-axis (C1-C2)

22600 Arthrodesis, posterior or posterolateral technique, single level; cervical below C2 segment

22610 thoracic (with or without lateral transverse technique)

22612 lumbar (with or without lateral transverse technique)

+22614 each additional vertebral segment (List separately in addition to code for primary procedure)

(Use 22614 in conjunction with codes 22600, 22610, 22612)

22630 Arthrodesis, posterior interbody technique, including laminectomy and/or diskectomy to prepare interspace (other than for decompression), single interspace; lumbar

+22632 each additional interspace (List separately in addition to code for primary procedure)

(Use 22632 in conjunction with code 22630)

SPINE DEFORMITY (eg, SCOLIOSIS, KYPHOSIS)

22800 Arthrodesis, posterior, for spinal deformity, with or without cast; up to 6 vertebral segments

22802 7 to 12 vertebral segments

282

  ● New Code   ▲ Revised Code   ✳ Starred Procedure   + Add-On Code   ⊘ Modifier -51 Exempt

22804   13 or more vertebral segments

22808   Arthrodesis, anterior, for spinal deformity, with or without cast; 2 to 3 vertebral segments

22810   4 to 7 vertebral segments

22812   8 or more vertebral segments

22818   Kyphectomy, circumferential exposure of spine and resection of vertebral segment(s) (including body and posterior elements); single or 2 segments

22819   3 or more segments

(To report arthrodesis, see 22800-22804 and add modifier -51)

EXPLORATION

22830   Exploration of spinal fusion

SPINAL INSTRUMENTATION

(List codes 22840-22848, 22851 separately, in addition to code for fracture, dislocation, or arthrodesis of the spine, 22325, 22326, 22327, 22548-22812)

⊘ **22840**   Posterior non-segmental instrumentation (eg, Harrington rod technique, pedicle fixation across one interspace, atlantoaxial transarticular screw fixation, sublaminar wiring at C1, facet screw fixation)

⊘ **22841**   Internal spinal fixation by wiring of spinous processes

⊘ **22842**   Posterior segmental instrumentation (eg, pedicle fixation, dual rods with multiple hooks and sublaminar wires); 3 to 6 vertebral segments

⊘ **22843**   7 to 12 vertebral segments

⊘ **22844**   13 or more vertebral segments

⊘ **22845**   Anterior instrumentation; 2 to 3 vertebral segments

⊘ **22846**   4 to 7 vertebral segments

⊘ **22847**   8 or more vertebral segments

 Separate Procedure

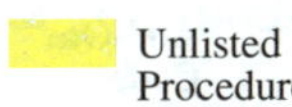 Unlisted Procedure

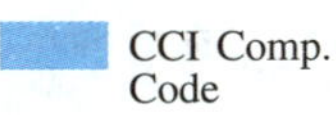 CCI Comp. Code

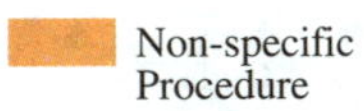 Non-specific Procedure

283

⊘ **22848** Pelvic fixation (attachment of caudal end of instrumentation to pelvic bony structures) other than sacrum

22849 Reinsertion of spinal fixation device

22850 Removal of posterior nonsegmental instrumentation (eg, Harrington rod)

⊘ **22851** Application of intervertebral biomechanical device(s) (eg, synthetic cage(s), threaded bone dowel(s), methylmethacrylate) to vertebral defector interspace

22852 Removal of posterior segmental instrumentation

22855 Removal of anterior instrumentation

OTHER PROCEDURES

22899 Unlisted procedure, spine

ABDOMEN

EXCISION

22900 Excision, abdominal wall tumor, subfascial (eg, desmoid)

OTHER PROCEDURES

22999 Unlisted procedure, abdomen, musculoskeletal system

SHOULDER

INCISION

▲ **23000** Removal of subdeltoid calcareous deposits, open

23020 Capsular contracture release (eg, Sever type procedure)

(For incision and drainage procedures, superficial, see 10040-10160)

23030 Incision and drainage, shoulder area; deep abscess or hematoma

23031   infected bursa

23035	Incision, bone cortex (eg, osteomyelitis or bone abscess), shoulder area
23040	Arthrotomy, glenohumeral joint, including exploration, drainage, or removal of foreign body
23044	Arthrotomy, acromioclavicular, sternoclavicular joint, including exploration, drainage, or removal of foreign body

EXCISION

23065	Biopsy, soft tissue of shoulder area; superficial
23066	deep

(For needle biopsy of soft tissue, use 20206)

23075	Excision, soft tissue tumor, shoulder area; subcutaneous
23076	deep, subfascial, or intramuscular
23077	Radical resection of tumor (eg, malignant neoplasm), soft tissue of shoulder area
23100	Arthrotomy, glenohumeral joint, including biopsy
23101	Arthrotomy, acromioclavicular joint or sternoclavicular joint, including biopsy and/or excision of torn cartilage
23105	Arthrotomy; glenohumeral joint, with synovectomy, with or without biopsy
23106	sternoclavicular joint, with synovectomy, with or without biopsy
23107	Arthrotomy, glenohumeral joint, with joint exploration, with or without removal of loose or foreign body
23120	Claviculectomy; partial

(For arthroscopic procedure, use 29824)

23125	total
23130	Acromioplasty or acromionectomy, partial, with or without coracoacromial ligament release

285

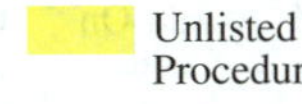

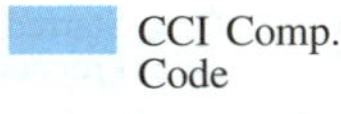

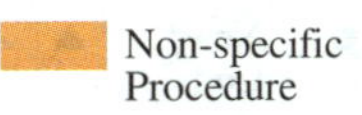

Non-specific
Procedure

23140 Excision or curettage of bone cyst or benign tumor of clavicle or scapula;

23145   with autograft (includes obtaining graft)

23146   with allograft

23150 Excision or curettage of bone cyst or benign tumor of proximal humerus;

23155   with autograft (includes obtaining graft)

23156   with allograft

23170 Sequestrectomy (eg, for osteomyelitis or bone abscess), clavicle

23172 Sequestrectomy (eg, for osteomyelitis or bone abscess), scapula

23174 Sequestrectomy (eg, for osteomyelitis or bone abscess), humeral head to surgical neck

23180 Partial excision (craterization, saucerization, or diaphysectomy) bone (eg, osteomyelitis), clavicle

23182 Partial excision (craterization, saucerization, or diaphysectomy) bone (eg, osteomyelitis), scapula

23184 Partial excision (craterization, saucerization, or diaphysectomy) bone (eg, osteomyelitis), proximal humerus

23190 Ostectomy of scapula, partial (eg, superior medial angle)

23195 Resection, humeral head

(For replacement with implant, use 23470)

23200 Radical resection for tumor; clavicle

23210   scapula

23220 Radical resection of bone tumor, proximal humerus;

23221   with autograft (includes obtaining graft)

23222   with prosthetic replacement

● New Code   ▲ Revised Code   * Starred Procedure   + Add-On Code   ⊘ Modifier -51 Exempt

INTRODUCTION OR REMOVAL

(For arthrocentesis or needling of bursa, use 20610)

(For K-wire or pin insertion or removal, see 20650, 20670, 20680)

23330 Removal of foreign body, shoulder; subcutaneous

23331 deep (eg, Neer hemiarthroplasty removal)

23332 complicated (eg, total shoulder)

▲ **23350** Injection procedure for shoulder arthrography or enhanced CT/MRI shoulder arthrography

(For radiological supervision and interpretation for arthrography, use 73040)

(For radiographic arthrography, radiological supervision and interpretation, use 73040. Fluoroscopy (76003) is inclusive of radiographic arthrography)

(When fluoroscopic guided injection is performed for enhanced CT arthrography, use codes 23350, 76003, and 73201 or 73202)

(When fluoroscopic guided injection is performed for enhanced MR arthrography, use codes 23350, 76003, and 73222 or 73223)

(For enhanced CT or enhanced MRI arthrography, use 76003 and either 73201, 73202, 73222 or 73223)

REPAIR, REVISION AND/OR RECONSTRUCTION

23395 Muscle transfer, any type, shoulder or upper arm; single

23397 multiple

23400 Scapulopexy (eg, Sprengels deformity or for paralysis)

23405 Tenotomy, shoulder area; single tendon

23406 multiple tendons through same incision

23410 Repair of ruptured musculotendinous cuff (eg, rotator cuff); acute

23412 chronic

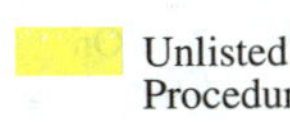

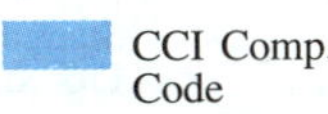

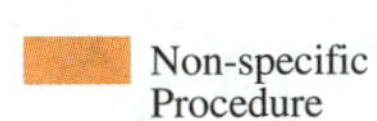

23415   Coracoacromial ligament release, with or without acromioplasty

(For arthroscopic procedure, use 29826)

23420   Reconstruction of complete shoulder (rotator) cuff avulsion, chronic (includes acromioplasty)

23430   Tenodesis of long tendon of biceps

23440   Resection or transplantation of long tendon of biceps

23450   Capsulorrhaphy, anterior; Putti-Platt procedure or Magnuson type operation

(To report arthroscopic thermal capsulorrhaphy, use 29999)

23455   with labral repair (eg, Bankart procedure)

(For arthroscopic procedure, use 29807)

23460   Capsulorrhaphy, anterior, any type; with bone block

23462   with coracoid process transfer

(To report open thermal capsulorrhaphy, use 23929)

23465   Capsulorrhaphy, glenohumeral joint, posterior, with or without bone block

(For sternoclavicular and acromioclavicular reconstruction, see 23530, 23550)

23466   Capsulorrhaphy, glenohumeral joint, any type multi-directional instability

23470   Arthroplasty, glenohumeral joint; hemiarthroplasty

23472   total shoulder (glenoid and proximal humeral replacement (eg, total shoulder))

(For removal of total shoulder implants, see 23331, 23332)

(For osteotomy, proximal humerus, use 24400)

23480   Osteotomy, clavicle, with or without internal fixation;

23485   with bone graft for nonunion or malunion (includes obtaining graft and/or necessary fixation)

23490 Prophylactic treatment (nailing, pinning, plating or wiring) with or without methylmethacrylate; clavicle

23491   proximal humerus

FRACTURE AND/OR DISLOCATION

23500 Closed treatment of clavicular fracture; without manipulation

23505   with manipulation

23515 Open treatment of clavicular fracture, with or without internal or external fixation

23520 Closed treatment of sternoclavicular dislocation; without manipulation

23525   with manipulation

23530 Open treatment of sternoclavicular dislocation, acute or chronic;

23532   with fascial graft (includes obtaining graft)

23540 Closed treatment of acromioclavicular dislocation; without manipulation

23545   with manipulation

23550 Open treatment of acromioclavicular dislocation, acute or chronic;

23552   with fascial graft (includes obtaining graft)

23570 Closed treatment of scapular fracture; without manipulation

23575   with manipulation, with or without skeletal traction (with or without shoulder joint involvement)

23585 Open treatment of scapular fracture (body, glenoid or acromion) with or without internal fixation

23600 Closed treatment of proximal humeral (surgical or anatomical neck) fracture; without manipulation

---

23605   with manipulation, with or without skeletal traction

23615   Open treatment of proximal humeral (surgical or anatomical neck) fracture, with or without internal or external fixation, with or without repair of tuberosity(-ies);

23616   with proximal humeral prosthetic replacement

23620   Closed treatment of greater humeral tuberosity fracture; without manipulation

23625   with manipulation

23630   Open treatment of greater humeral tuberosity fracture, with or without internal or external fixation

23650   Closed treatment of shoulder dislocation, with manipulation; without anesthesia

23655   requiring anesthesia

23660   Open treatment of acute shoulder dislocation

(Repairs for recurrent dislocations, see 23450-23466)

23665   Closed treatment of shoulder dislocation, with fracture of greater humeral tuberosity, with manipulation

23670   Open treatment of shoulder dislocation, with fracture of greater humeral tuberosity, with or without internal or external fixation

23675   Closed treatment of shoulder dislocation, with surgical or anatomical neck fracture, with manipulation

23680   Open treatment of shoulder dislocation, with surgical or anatomical neck fracture, with or without internal or external fixation

MANIPULATION

✷23700   Manipulation under anesthesia, shoulder joint, including application of fixation apparatus (dislocation excluded)

ARTHRODESIS

23800   Arthrodesis, glenohumeral joint;

● New Code   ▲ Revised Code   ✷ Starred Procedure   + Add-On Code   ⊘ Modifier -51 Exempt

23802   with autogenous graft (includes obtaining graft)

AMPUTATION

23900 Interthoracoscapular amputation (forequarter)

23920 Disarticulation of shoulder;

23921   secondary closure or scar revision

OTHER PROCEDURES

23929 Unlisted procedure, shoulder

HUMERUS (UPPER ARM) AND ELBOW

INCISION

(For incision and drainage procedures, superficial, see 10040-10160)

23930 Incision and drainage, upper arm or elbow area; deep abscess or hematoma

23931   bursa

23935 Incision, deep, with opening of bone cortex (eg, for osteomyelitis or bone abscess), humerus or elbow

24000 Arthrotomy, elbow, including exploration, drainage, or removal of foreign body

24006 Arthrotomy of the elbow, with capsular excision for capsular release (separate procedure)

EXCISION

24065 Biopsy, soft tissue of upper arm or elbow area; superficial

24066   deep (subfascial or intramuscular)

(For needle biopsy of soft tissue, use 20206)

▲ **24075** Excision, tumor, soft tissue of upper arm or elbow area; subcutaneous

24076   deep (subfascial or intramuscular)

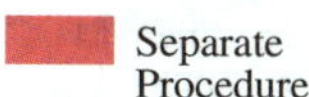 Separate Procedure

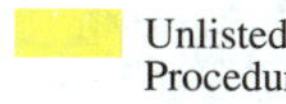 Unlisted Procedure

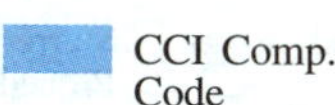 CCI Comp. Code

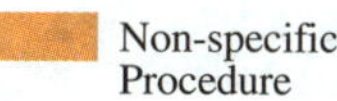 Non-specific Procedure

24077 Radical resection of tumor (eg, malignant neoplasm), soft tissue of upper arm or elbow area

24100 Arthrotomy, elbow; with synovial biopsy only

24101 with joint exploration, with or without biopsy, with or without removal of loose or foreign body

24102 with synovectomy

24105 Excision, olecranon bursa

24110 Excision or curettage of bone cyst or benign tumor, humerus;

24115 with autograft (includes obtaining graft)

24116 with allograft

24120 Excision or curettage of bone cyst or benign tumor of head or neck of radius or olecranon process;

24125 with autograft (includes obtaining graft)

24126 with allograft

24130 Excision, radial head

(For replacement with implant, use 24366)

24134 Sequestrectomy (eg, for osteomyelitis or bone abscess), shaft or distal humerus

24136 Sequestrectomy (eg, for osteomyelitis or bone abscess), radial head or neck

24138 Sequestrectomy (eg, for osteomyelitis or bone abscess), olecranon process

24140 Partial excision (craterization, saucerization, or diaphysectomy) bone (eg, osteomyelitis), humerus

24145 Partial excision (craterization, saucerization, or diaphysectomy) bone (eg, osteomyelitis), radial head or neck

24147 Partial excision (craterization, saucerization, or diaphysectomy) bone (eg, osteomyelitis), olecranon process

---

292

● New Code   ▲ Revised Code   ✳ Starred Procedure   ✛ Add-On Code   ⊘ Modifier -51 Exempt

24149 Radical resection of capsule, soft tissue, and heterotopic bone, elbow, with contracture release (separate procedure)

(For capsular and soft tissue release only, use 24006)

24150 Radical resection for tumor, shaft or distal humerus;

24151 with autograft (includes obtaining graft)

24152 Radical resection for tumor, radial head or neck;

24153 with autograft (includes obtaining graft)

24155 Resection of elbow joint (arthrectomy)

INTRODUCTION OR REMOVAL

(For K-wire or pin insertion or removal, see 20650, 20670, 20680)

(For arthrocentesis or needling of bursa or joint, use 20605)

24160 Implant removal; elbow joint

24164 radial head

24200 Removal of foreign body, upper arm or elbow area; subcutaneous

24201 deep (subfascial or intramuscular)

24220 Injection procedure for elbow arthrography

(For radiological supervision and interpretation, use 73085. Do not report 76003 in addition to 73085)

(For injection of tennis elbow, use 20550)

REPAIR, REVISION, AND/OR RECONSTRUCTION

● **24300** Manipulation, elbow, under anesthesia

(For application of external fixation, see 20690 or 20692)

24301 Muscle or tendon transfer, any type, upper arm or elbow, single (excluding 24320-24331)

24305 Tendon lengthening, upper arm or elbow, each tendon

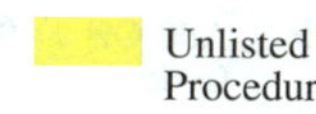

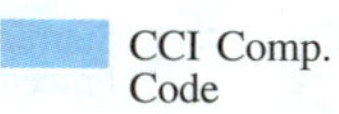

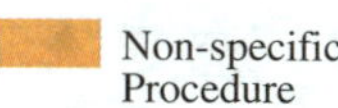

24310   Tenotomy, open, elbow to shoulder, each tendon

24320   Tenoplasty, with muscle transfer, with or without free graft, elbow to shoulder, single (Seddon-Brookes type procedure)

24330   Flexor-plasty, elbow (eg, Steindler type advancement);

24331   with extensor advancement

● **24332**   Tenolysis, triceps

24340   Tenodesis of biceps tendon at elbow (separate procedure)

24341   Repair, tendon or muscle, upper arm or elbow, each tendon or muscle, primary or secondary (excludes rotator cuff)

24342   Reinsertion of ruptured biceps or triceps tendon, distal, with or without tendon graft

● **24343**   Repair lateral collateral ligament, elbow, with local tissue

● **24344**   Reconstruction lateral collateral ligament, elbow, with tendon graft (includes harvesting of graft)

● **24345**   Repair medial collateral ligament, elbow, with local tissue

● **24346**   Reconstruction medial collateral ligament, elbow, with tendon graft (includes harvesting of graft)

24350   Fasciotomy, lateral or medial (eg, tennis elbow or epicondylitis);

24351   with extensor origin detachment

24352   with annular ligament resection

24354   with stripping

24356   with partial ostectomy

24360   Arthroplasty, elbow; with membrane (eg, fascial)

24361   with distal humeral prosthetic replacement

24362   with implant and fascia lata ligament reconstruction

● New Code   ▲ Revised Code   * Starred Procedure   + Add-On Code   ⊘ Modifier -51 Exempt

24363   with distal humerus and proximal ulnar prosthetic replacement (eg, total elbow)

24365   Arthroplasty, radial head;

24366   with implant

24400   Osteotomy, humerus, with or without internal fixation

24410   Multiple osteotomies with realignment on intramedullary rod, humeral shaft (Sofield type procedure)

24420   Osteoplasty, humerus (eg, shortening or lengthening) (excluding 64876)

24430   Repair of nonunion or malunion, humerus; without graft (eg, compression technique)

24435   with iliac or other autograft (includes obtaining graft)

(For proximal radius and/or ulna, see 25400-25420)

24470   Hemiepiphyseal arrest (eg, cubitus varus or valgus, distal humerus)

24495   Decompression fasciotomy, forearm, with brachial artery exploration

24498   Prophylactic treatment (nailing, pinning, plating or wiring), with or without methylmethacrylate, humeral shaft

FRACTURE AND/OR DISLOCATION

24500   Closed treatment of humeral shaft fracture; without manipulation

24505   with manipulation, with or without skeletal traction

24515   Open treatment of humeral shaft fracture with plate/screws, with or without cerclage

24516   Open treatment of humeral shaft fracture, with insertion of intramedullary implant, with or without cerclage and/or locking screws

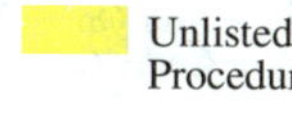

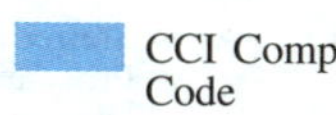

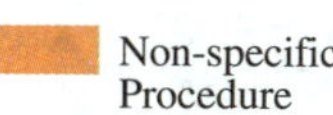

Non-specific
Procedure

24530 Closed treatment of supracondylar or transcondylar humeral fracture, with or without intercondylar extension; without manipulation

24535 with manipulation, with or without skin or skeletal traction

24538 Percutaneous skeletal fixation of supracondylar or transcondylar humeral fracture, with or without intercondylar extension

24545 Open treatment of humeral supracondylar or transcondylar fracture, with or without internal or external fixation; without intercondylar extension

24546 with intercondylar extension

24560 Closed treatment of humeral epicondylar fracture, medial or lateral; without manipulation

24565 with manipulation

24566 Percutaneous skeletal fixation of humeral epicondylar fracture, medial or lateral, with manipulation

24575 Open treatment of humeral epicondylar fracture, medial or lateral, with or without internal or external fixation

24576 Closed treatment of humeral condylar fracture, medial or lateral; without manipulation

24577 with manipulation

24579 Open treatment of humeral condylar fracture, medial or lateral, with or without internal or external fixation

24582 Percutaneous skeletal fixation of humeral condylar fracture, medial or lateral, with manipulation

24586 Open treatment of periarticular fracture and/or dislocation of the elbow (fracture distal humerus and proximal ulna and/or proximal radius);

24587 with implant arthroplasty

(See also 24361)

24600 Treatment of closed elbow dislocation; without anesthesia

---

● New Code   ▲ Revised Code   ✳ Starred Procedure   ✚ Add-On Code   ⊘ Modifier -51 Exempt

24605   requiring anesthesia

24615   Open treatment of acute or chronic elbow dislocation

24620   Closed treatment of Monteggia type of fracture dislocation at elbow (fracture proximal end of ulna with dislocation of radial head), with manipulation

24635   Open treatment of Monteggia type of fracture dislocation at elbow (fracture proximal end of ulna with dislocation of radial head), with or without internal or external fixation

∗24640   Closed treatment of radial head subluxation in child, nursemaid elbow, with manipulation

24650   Closed treatment of radial head or neck fracture; without manipulation

24655   with manipulation

24665   Open treatment of radial head or neck fracture, with or without internal fixation or radial head excision;

24666   with radial head prosthetic replacement

24670   Closed treatment of ulnar fracture, proximal end (olecranon process); without manipulation

24675   with manipulation

24685   Open treatment of ulnar fracture proximal end (olecranon process), with or without internal or external fixation

ARTHRODESIS

24800   Arthrodesis, elbow joint; local

24802   with autogenous graft (includes obtaining graft)

AMPUTATION

24900   Amputation, arm through humerus; with primary closure

24920   open, circular (guillotine)

24925   secondary closure or scar revision

Separate Procedure   Unlisted Procedure   CCI Comp. Code   Non-specific Procedure

24930   re-amputation

24931   with implant

24935   Stump elongation, upper extremity

24940   Cineplasty, upper extremity, complete procedure

OTHER PROCEDURES

24999   Unlisted procedure, humerus or elbow

FOREARM AND WRIST

INCISION

25000   Incision, extensor tendon sheath, wrist (eg, deQuervains disease)

(For decompression median nerve or for carpal tunnel syndrome, use 64721)

● **25001**   Incision, flexor tendon sheath, wrist (eg, flexor carpi radialis)

▲ **25020**   Decompression fasciotomy, forearm and/or wrist, flexor OR extensor compartment; without debridement of nonviable muscle and/or nerve

25023   with debridement of nonviable muscle and/or nerve

(For decompression fasciotomy with brachial artery exploration, use 24495)

(For incision and drainage procedures, superficial, see 10040-10160)

(For debridement, see also 11000-11044)

● **25024**   Decompression fasciotomy, forearm and/or wrist, flexor AND extensor compartment; without debridement of nonviable muscle and/or nerve

● **25025**   with debridement of nonviable muscle and/or nerve

25028   Incision and drainage, forearm and/or wrist; deep abscess or hematoma

---

298   ● New Code   ▲ Revised Code   ✱ Starred Procedure   ✚ Add-On Code   ⊘ Modifier -51 Exempt

25031   bursa

25035   Incision, deep, bone cortex, forearm and/or wrist (eg, osteomyelitis or bone abscess)

25040   Arthrotomy, radiocarpal or midcarpal joint, with exploration, drainage, or removal of foreign body

EXCISION

25065   Biopsy, soft tissue of forearm and/or wrist; superficial

25066   deep (subfascial or intramuscular)

(For needle biopsy of soft tissue, use 20206)

▲ **25075**   Excision, tumor, soft tissue of forearm and/or wrist area; subcutaneous

25076   deep (subfascial or intramuscular)

25077   Radical resection of tumor (eg, malignant neoplasm), soft tissue of forearm and/or wrist area

25085   Capsulotomy, wrist (eg, contracture)

25100   Arthrotomy, wrist joint; with biopsy

25101   with joint exploration, with or without biopsy, with or without removal of loose or foreign body

25105   with synovectomy

25107   Arthrotomy, distal radioulnar joint including repair of triangular cartilage, complex

25110   Excision, lesion of tendon sheath, forearm and/or wrist

25111   Excision of ganglion, wrist (dorsal or volar); primary

25112   recurrent

(For hand or finger, use 26160)

 Separate Procedure

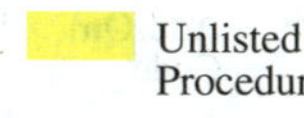 Unlisted Procedure

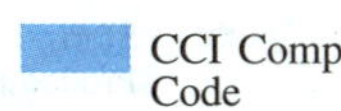 CCI Comp. Code

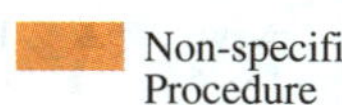 Non-specific Procedure

25115 Radical excision of bursa, synovia of wrist, or forearm tendon sheaths (eg, tenosynovitis, fungus, Tbc, or other granulomas, rheumatoid arthritis); flexors

25116 extensors, with or without transposition of dorsal retinaculum

(For finger synovectomies, use 26145)

25118 Synovectomy, extensor tendon sheath, wrist, single compartment;

25119 with resection of distal ulna

25120 Excision or curettage of bone cyst or benign tumor of radius or ulna (excluding head or neck of radius and olecranon process);

(For head or neck of radius or olecranon process, see 24120-24126)

25125 with autograft (includes obtaining graft)

25126 with allograft

25130 Excision or curettage of bone cyst or benign tumor of carpal bones;

25135 with autograft (includes obtaining graft)

25136 with allograft

25145 Sequestrectomy (eg, for osteomyelitis or bone abscess), forearm and/or wrist

25150 Partial excision (craterization, saucerization, or diaphysectomy) of bone (eg, for osteomyelitis); ulna

25151 radius

(For head or neck of radius or olecranon process, see 24145, 24147)

25170 Radical resection for tumor, radius or ulna

25210 Carpectomy; one bone

(For carpectomy with implant, see 25441-25445)

● New Code   ▲ Revised Code   ✳ Starred Procedure   ✚ Add-On Code   ⊘ Modifier -51 Exempt

25215   all bones of proximal row

25230 Radial styloidectomy (separate procedure)

25240 Excision distal ulna partial or complete (eg, Darrach type or matched resection)

(For implant replacement, distal ulna, use 25442)

(For obtaining fascia for interposition, see 20920, 20922)

INTRODUCTION OR REMOVAL

(For K-wire, pin or rod insertion or removal, see 20650, 20670, 20680)

25246 Injection procedure for wrist arthrography

(For radiological supervision and interpretation, use 73115. Do not report 76003 in addition to 73115)

(For foreign body removal, superficial use 20520)

25248 Exploration with removal of deep foreign body, forearm or wrist

25250 Removal of wrist prosthesis; (separate procedure)

25251   complicated, including total wrist

● **25259** Manipulation, wrist, under anesthesia

(For application of external fixation, see 20690 or 20692)

REPAIR, REVISION, AND/OR RECONSTRUCTION

25260 Repair, tendon or muscle, flexor, forearm and/or wrist; primary, single, each tendon or muscle

25263   secondary, single, each tendon or muscle

25265   secondary, with free graft (includes obtaining graft), each tendon or muscle

25270 Repair, tendon or muscle, extensor, forearm and/or wrist; primary, single, each tendon or muscle

25272   secondary, single, each tendon or muscle

	Separate Procedure		Unlisted Procedure		CCI Comp. Code		Non-specific Procedure

301

▲ **25274** secondary, with free graft (includes obtaining graft), each tendon or muscle

● **25275** Repair, tendon sheath, extensor, forearm and/or wrist, with free graft (includes obtaining graft) (eg, for extensor carpi ulnaris subluxation)

25280 Lengthening or shortening of flexor or extensor tendon, forearm and/or wrist, single, each tendon

25290 Tenotomy, open, flexor or extensor tendon, forearm and/or wrist, single, each tendon

25295 Tenolysis, flexor or extensor tendon, forearm and/or wrist, single, each tendon

25300 Tenodesis at wrist; flexors of fingers

25301 extensors of fingers

25310 Tendon transplantation or transfer, flexor or extensor, forearm and/or wrist, single; each tendon

25312 with tendon graft(s) (includes obtaining graft), each tendon

25315 Flexor origin slide (eg, for cerebral palsy, Volkmann contracture), forearm and/or wrist;

25316 with tendon(s) transfer

25320 Capsulorrhaphy or reconstruction, wrist, any method (eg, capsulodesis, ligament repair, tendon transfer or graft) (includes synovectomy, capsulotomy and open reduction) for carpal instability

25332 Arthroplasty, wrist, with or without interposition, with or without external or internal fixation

(For obtaining fascia for interposition, see 20920, 20922)

(For prosthetic replacement arthroplasty, see 25441-25446)

25335 Centralization of wrist on ulna (eg, radial club hand)

25337 Reconstruction for stabilization of unstable distal ulna or distal radioulnar joint, secondary by soft tissue stabilization (eg,

---

● New Code	▲ Revised Code	∗ Starred Procedure	+ Add-On Code	⊘ Modifier -51 Exempt

tendon transfer, tendon graft or weave, or tenodesis) with or without open reduction of distal radioulnar joint

(For harvesting of fascia lata graft, see 20920, 20922)

25350 Osteotomy, radius; distal third

25355 middle or proximal third

25360 Osteotomy; ulna

25365 radius AND ulna

25370 Multiple osteotomies, with realignment on intramedullary rod (Sofield type procedure); radius OR ulna

25375 radius AND ulna

25390 Osteoplasty, radius OR ulna; shortening

25391 lengthening with autograft

25392 Osteoplasty, radius AND ulna; shortening (excluding 64876)

25393 lengthening with autograft

● **25394** Osteoplasty, carpal bone, shortening

25400 Repair of nonunion or malunion, radius OR ulna; without graft (eg, compression technique)

▲ **25405** with autograft (includes obtaining graft)

25415 Repair of nonunion or malunion, radius AND ulna; without graft (eg, compression technique)

▲ **25420** with autograft (includes obtaining graft)

25425 Repair of defect with autograft; radius OR ulna

25426 radius AND ulna

● **25430** Insertion of vascular pedicle into carpal bone (eg, Harii procedure)

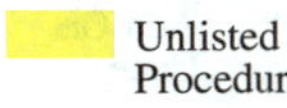 Separate Procedure
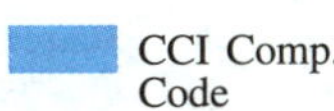 Unlisted Procedure
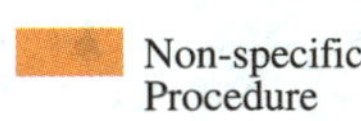 CCI Comp. Code
Non-specific Procedure

● **25431**   Repair of nonunion of carpal bone (excluding carpal scaphoid (navicular) (includes obtaining graft and necessary fixation), each bone

▲ **25440**   Repair of nonunion, scaphoid carpal (navicular) bone, with or without radial styloidectomy (includes obtaining graft and necessary fixation)

25441   Arthroplasty with prosthetic replacement; distal radius

25442   distal ulna

▲ **25443**   scaphoid carpal (navicular)

25444   lunate

25445   trapezium

25446   distal radius and partial or entire carpus (total wrist)

25447   Arthroplasty, interposition, intercarpal or carpometacarpal joints

(For wrist arthroplasty, use 25332)

25449   Revision of arthroplasty, including removal of implant, wrist joint

25450   Epiphyseal arrest by epiphysiodesis or stapling; distal radius OR ulna

25455   distal radius AND ulna

25490   Prophylactic treatment (nailing, pinning, plating or wiring) with or without methylmethacrylate; radius

25491   ulna

25492   radius AND ulna

FRACTURE AND/OR DISLOCATION

25500   Closed treatment of radial shaft fracture; without manipulation

25505   with manipulation

25515 Open treatment of radial shaft fracture, with or without internal or external fixation

▲ **25520** Closed treatment of radial shaft fracture and closed treatment of dislocation of distal radioulnar joint (Galeazzi fracture/dislocation)

25525 Open treatment of radial shaft fracture, with internal and/or external fixation and closed treatment of dislocation of distal radioulnar joint (Galeazzi fracture/dislocation), with or without percutaneous skeletal fixation

▲ **25526** Open treatment of radial shaft fracture, with internal and/or external fixation and open treatment, with or without internal or external fixation of distal radioulnar joint (Galeazzi fracture/dislocation), includes repair of triangular fibrocartilage complex

25530 Closed treatment of ulnar shaft fracture; without manipulation

25535   with manipulation

25545 Open treatment of ulnar shaft fracture, with or without internal or external fixation

25560 Closed treatment of radial and ulnar shaft fractures; without manipulation

25565   with manipulation

25574 Open treatment of radial AND ulnar shaft fractures, with internal or external fixation; of radius OR ulna

25575   of radius AND ulna

25600 Closed treatment of distal radial fracture (eg, Colles or Smith type) or epiphyseal separation, with or without fracture of ulnar styloid; without manipulation

25605   with manipulation

25611 Percutaneous skeletal fixation of distal radial fracture (eg, Colles or Smith type) or epiphyseal separation, with or without fracture of ulnar styloid, requiring manipulation, with or without external fixation

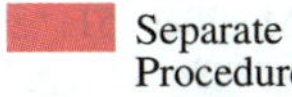
Separate Procedure

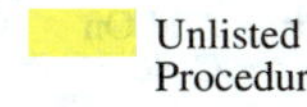
Unlisted Procedure

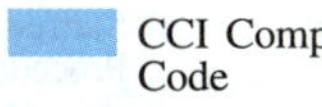
CCI Comp. Code

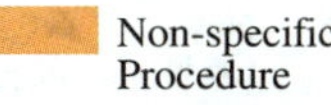
Non-specific Procedure

305

25620 Open treatment of distal radial fracture (eg, Colles or Smith type) or epiphyseal separation, with or without fracture of ulnar styloid, with or without internal or external fixation

25622 Closed treatment of carpal scaphoid (navicular) fracture; without manipulation

25624   with manipulation

25628 Open treatment of carpal scaphoid (navicular) fracture, with or without internal or external fixation

25630 Closed treatment of carpal bone fracture (excluding carpal scaphoid (navicular)); without manipulation, each bone

25635   with manipulation, each bone

▲ **25645** Open treatment of carpal bone fracture (other than carpal scaphoid (navicular)), each bone

25650 Closed treatment of ulnar styloid fracture

● **25651** Percutaneous skeletal fixation of ulnar styloid fracture

● **25652** Open treatment of ulnar styloid fracture

25660 Closed treatment of radiocarpal or intercarpal dislocation, one or more bones, with manipulation

25670 Open treatment of radiocarpal or intercarpal dislocation, one or more bones

● **25671** Percutaneous skeletal fixation of distal radioulnar dislocation

25675 Closed treatment of distal radioulnar dislocation with manipulation

25676 Open treatment of distal radioulnar dislocation, acute or chronic

25680 Closed treatment of trans-scaphoperilunar type of fracture dislocation, with manipulation

25685 Open treatment of trans-scaphoperilunar type of fracture dislocation

---

● New Code   ▲ Revised Code   * Starred Procedure   + Add-On Code   ⊘ Modifier -51 Exempt

25690 Closed treatment of lunate dislocation, with manipulation

25695 Open treatment of lunate dislocation

ARTHRODESIS

25800 Arthrodesis, wrist; complete, without bone graft (includes radiocarpal and/or intercarpal and/or carpometacarpal joints)

25805 with sliding graft

25810 with iliac or other autograft (includes obtaining graft)

25820 Arthrodesis, wrist; limited, without bone graft (eg, intercarpal or radiocarpal)

25825 with autograft (includes obtaining graft)

25830 Arthrodesis, distal radioulnar joint with segmental resection of ulna, with or without bone graft (eg, Sauve-Kapandji procedure)

AMPUTATION

25900 Amputation, forearm, through radius and ulna;

25905 open, circular (guillotine)

25907 secondary closure or scar revision

25909 re-amputation

25915 Krukenberg procedure

25920 Disarticulation through wrist;

25922 secondary closure or scar revision

25924 re-amputation

25927 Transmetacarpal amputation;

25929 secondary closure or scar revision

25931 re-amputation

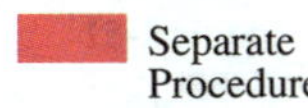

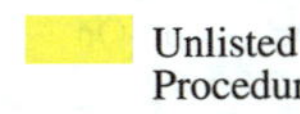

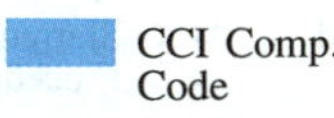

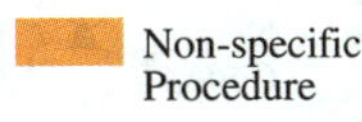

OTHER PROCEDURES

25999 Unlisted procedure, forearm or wrist

HAND AND FINGERS

INCISION

***26010** Drainage of finger abscess; simple

***26011** complicated (eg, felon)

26020 Drainage of tendon sheath, digit and/or palm, each

26025 Drainage of palmar bursa; single, bursa

26030 multiple bursa

26034 Incision, bone cortex, hand or finger (eg, osteomyelitis or bone abscess)

26035 Decompression fingers and/or hand, injection injury (eg, grease gun)

26037 Decompressive fasciotomy, hand (excludes 26035)

(For injection injury, use 26035)

26040 Fasciotomy, palmar (eg, Dupuytren's contracture); percutaneous

26045 open, partial

(For fasciectomy, see 26121-26125)

26055 Tendon sheath incision (eg, for trigger finger)

26060 Tenotomy, percutaneous, single, each digit

26070 Arthrotomy, with exploration, drainage, or removal of loose or foreign body; carpometacarpal joint

26075 metacarpophalangeal joint, each

26080 interphalangeal joint, each

● New Code   ▲ Revised Code   * Starred Procedure   ✛ Add-On Code   ⊘ Modifier -51 Exempt

EXCISION

26100   Arthrotomy with biopsy; carpometacarpal joint, each

26105   metacarpophalangeal joint, each

26110   interphalangeal joint, each

▲ **26115**   Excision, tumor or vascular malformation, soft tissue of hand or finger; subcutaneous

▲ **26116**   deep (subfascial or intramuscular)

26117   Radical resection of tumor (eg, malignant neoplasm), soft tissue of hand or finger

26121   Fasciectomy, palm only, with or without Z-plasty, other local tissue rearrangement, or skin grafting (includes obtaining graft)

26123   Fasciectomy, partial palmar with release of single digit including proximal interphalangeal joint, with or without Z-plasty, other local tissue rearrangement, or skin grafting (includes obtaining graft);

+26125   each additional digit (List separately in addition to code for primary procedure)

(Use 26125 in conjunction with code 26123)

(For fasciotomy, see 26040, 26045)

26130   Synovectomy, carpometacarpal joint

26135   Synovectomy, metacarpophalangeal joint including intrinsic release and extensor hood reconstruction, each digit

26140   Synovectomy, proximal interphalangeal joint, including extensor reconstruction, each interphalangeal joint

26145   Synovectomy, tendon sheath, radical (tenosynovectomy), flexor tendon, palm and/or finger, each tendon

(For tendon sheath synovectomies at wrist, see 25115, 25116)

▲ **26160**   Excision of lesion of tendon sheath or joint capsule (eg, cyst, mucous cyst, or ganglion), hand or finger

---

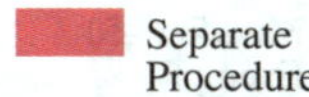 Separate Procedure   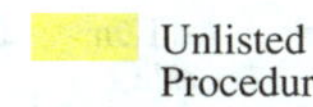 Unlisted Procedure   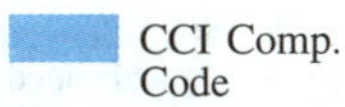 CCI Comp. Code   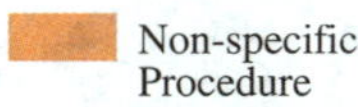 Non-specific Procedure

(For wrist ganglion, see 25111, 25112)

(For trigger digit, use 26055)

26170 Excision of tendon, palm, flexor, single (separate procedure), each

26180 Excision of tendon, finger, flexor (separate procedure), each tendon

26185 Sesamoidectomy, thumb or finger (separate procedure)

26200 Excision or curettage of bone cyst or benign tumor of metacarpal;

26205   with autograft (includes obtaining graft)

26210 Excision or curettage of bone cyst or benign tumor of proximal, middle, or distal phalanx of finger;

26215   with autograft (includes obtaining graft)

26230 Partial excision (craterization, saucerization, or diaphysectomy) bone (eg, osteomyelitis); metacarpal

26235   proximal or middle phalanx of finger

26236   distal phalanx of finger

26250 Radical resection, metacarpal (eg, tumor);

26255   with autograft (includes obtaining graft)

26260 Radical resection, proximal or middle phalanx of finger (eg, tumor);

26261   with autograft (includes obtaining graft)

26262 Radical resection, distal phalanx of finger (eg, tumor)

INTRODUCTION OR REMOVAL

26320 Removal of implant from finger or hand

(For removal of foreign body in hand or finger, see 20520, 20525)

● New Code   ▲ Revised Code   * Starred Procedure   ✛ Add-On Code   ⊘ Modifier -51 Exempt

REPAIR, REVISION, AND/OR RECONSTRUCTION

● **26340**   Manipulation, finger joint, under anesthesia, each joint

(For application of external fixation, see 20690 or 20692)

▲ **26350**   Repair or advancement, flexor tendon, not in zone 2 digital flexor tendon sheath (eg, no man's land); primary or secondary without free graft, each tendon

26352   secondary with free graft (includes obtaining graft), each tendon

▲ **26356**   Repair or advancement, flexor tendon, in zone 2 digital flexor tendon sheath (eg, no man's land); primary or secondary without free graft, each tendon

26357   secondary, each tendon

26358   secondary with free graft (includes obtaining graft), each tendon

26370   Repair or advancement of profundus tendon, with intact superficialis tendon; primary, each tendon

26372   secondary with free graft (includes obtaining graft), each tendon

26373   secondary without free graft, each tendon

▲ **26390**   Excision flexor tendon, with implantation of synthetic rod for delayed tendon graft, hand or finger, each rod

▲ **26392**   Removal of synthetic rod and insertion of flexor tendon graft, hand or finger (includes obtaining graft), each rod

26410   Repair, extensor tendon, hand, primary or secondary; without free graft, each tendon

26412   with free graft (includes obtaining graft), each tendon

▲ **26415**   Excision of extensor tendon, with implantation of synthetic rod for delayed tendon graft, hand or finger, each rod

▲ **26416**   Removal of synthetic rod and insertion of extensor tendon graft (includes obtaining graft), hand or finger, each rod

Separate
Procedure

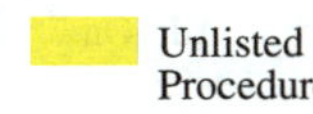
Unlisted
Procedure

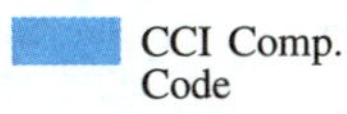
CCI Comp.
Code

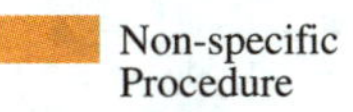
Non-specific
Procedure

26418 Repair, extensor tendon, finger, primary or secondary; without free graft, each tendon

26420   with free graft (includes obtaining graft) each tendon

▲ **26426** Repair of extensor tendon, central slip, secondary (eg, boutonniere deformity); using local tissue(s), including lateral band(s), each finger

▲ **26428**   with free graft (includes obtaining graft), each finger

26432 Closed treatment of distal extensor tendon insertion, with or without percutaneous pinning (eg, mallet finger)

26433 Repair of extensor tendon, distal insertion, primary or secondary; without graft (eg, mallet finger)

26434   with free graft (includes obtaining graft)

(for tenovaginotomy for trigger finger, use 26055)

26437 Realignment of extensor tendon, hand, each tendon

26440 Tenolysis, flexor tendon; palm OR finger; each tendon

26442   palm AND finger, each tendon

▲ **26445** Tenolysis, extensor tendon, hand OR finger; each tendon

26449 Tenolysis, complex, extensor tendon, finger, including forearm, each tendon

26450 Tenotomy, flexor, palm, open, each tendon

26455 Tenotomy, flexor, finger, open, each tendon

26460 Tenotomy, extensor, hand or finger, open, each tendon

26471 Tenodesis; of proximal interphalangeal joint, each joint

26474   of distal joint, each joint

26476 Lengthening of tendon, extensor, hand or finger, each tendon

26477 Shortening of tendon, extensor, hand or finger, each tendon

● New Code   ▲ Revised Code   * Starred Procedure   + Add-On Code   ⊘ Modifier -51 Exempt

26478   Lengthening of tendon, flexor, hand or finger, each tendon

26479   Shortening of tendon, flexor, hand or finger, each tendon

26480   Transfer or transplant of tendon, carpometacarpal area or dorsum of hand; without free graft, each tendon

26483   with free tendon graft (includes obtaining graft), each tendon

26485   Transfer or transplant of tendon, palmar; without free tendon graft, each tendon

26489   with free tendon graft (includes obtaining graft), each tendon

26490   Opponensplasty; superficialis tendon transfer type, each tendon

26492   tendon transfer with graft (includes obtaining graft), each tendon

26494   hypothenar muscle transfer

26496   other methods

(For thumb fusion in opposition, use 26820)

26497   Transfer of tendon to restore intrinsic function; ring and small finger

26498   all four fingers

26499   Correction claw finger, other methods

26500   Reconstruction of tendon pulley, each tendon; with local tissues (separate procedure)

26502   with tendon or fascial graft (includes obtaining graft) (separate procedure)

26504   with tendon prosthesis (separate procedure)

26508   Release of thenar muscle(s) (eg, thumb contracture)

▲ **26510**   Cross intrinsic transfer, each tendon

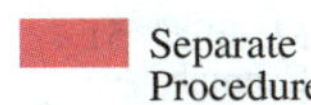
Separate Procedure

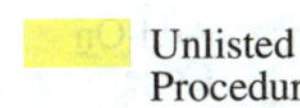
Unlisted Procedure

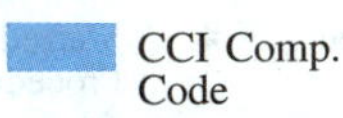
CCI Comp. Code

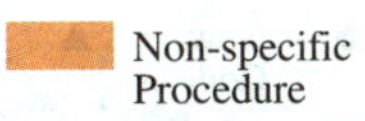
Non-specific Procedure

26516 Capsulodesis, metacarpophalangeal joint; single digit

26517 two digits

26518 three or four digits

26520 Capsulectomy or capsulotomy; metacarpophalangeal joint, each joint

26525 interphalangeal joint, each joint

26530 Arthroplasty, metacarpophalangeal joint; each joint

26531 with prosthetic implant, each joint

26535 Arthroplasty, interphalangeal joint; each joint

26536 with prosthetic implant, each joint

26540 Repair of collateral ligament, metacarpophalangeal or interphalangeal joint

26541 Reconstruction, collateral ligament, metacarpophalangeal joint, single; with tendon or fascial graft (includes obtaining graft)

26542 with local tissue (eg, adductor advancement)

26545 Reconstruction, collateral ligament, interphalangeal joint, single, including graft, each joint

26546 Repair non-union, metacarpal or phalanx, (includes obtaining bone graft with or without external or internal fixation)

26548 Repair and reconstruction, finger, volar plate, interphalangeal joint

26550 Pollicization of a digit

26551 Transfer, toe-to-hand with microvascular anastomosis; great toe wrap-around with bone graft

(For great toe with web space, use 20973)

26553 other than great toe, single

26554 other than great toe, double

(Do not report code 69990 in addition to codes 26551-26554)

26555 Transfer, finger to another position without microvascular anastomosis

26556 Transfer, free toe joint, with microvascular anastomosis

(Do not report code 69990 in addition to code 26556)

26560 Repair of syndactyly (web finger) each web space; with skin flaps

26561 with skin flaps and grafts

26562 complex (eg, involving bone, nails)

26565 Osteotomy; metacarpal, each

26567 phalanx of finger, each

26568 Osteoplasty, lengthening, metacarpal or phalanx

26580 Repair cleft hand

(**26585** deleted 2002 edition. To report, use 26587)

▲ **26587** Reconstruction of polydactylous digit, soft tissue and bone

(For excision of polydactylous digit, soft tissue only, use 11200)

▲ **26590** Repair macrodactylia, each digit

26591 Repair, intrinsic muscles of hand, each muscle

26593 Release, intrinsic muscles of hand, each muscle

26596 Excision of constricting ring of finger, with multiple Z-plasties

(**26597** deleted 2002 edition. To report, see 11041-11042, 14040-14041, or 15120, 15240)

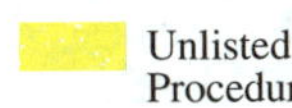
Separate
Procedure

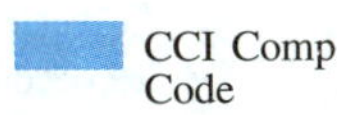
Unlisted
Procedure

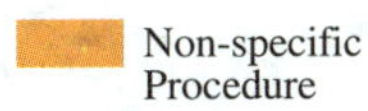
CCI Comp.
Code

Non-specific
Procedure

FRACTURE AND/OR DISLOCATION

26600   Closed treatment of metacarpal fracture, single; without manipulation, each bone

26605   with manipulation, each bone

▲ **26607**   Closed treatment of metacarpal fracture, with manipulation, with external fixation, each bone

26608   Percutaneous skeletal fixation of metacarpal fracture, each bone

26615   Open treatment of metacarpal fracture, single, with or without internal or external fixation, each bone

26641   Closed treatment of carpometacarpal dislocation, thumb, with manipulation

26645   Closed treatment of carpometacarpal fracture dislocation, thumb (Bennett fracture), with manipulation

26650   Percutaneous skeletal fixation of carpometacarpal fracture dislocation, thumb (Bennett fracture), with manipulation, with or without external fixation

26665   Open treatment of carpometacarpal fracture dislocation, thumb (Bennett fracture), with or without internal or external fixation

▲ **26670**   Closed treatment of carpometacarpal dislocation, other than thumb, with manipulation, each joint; without anesthesia

26675   requiring anesthesia

▲ **26676**   Percutaneous skeletal fixation of carpometacarpal dislocation, other than thumb, with manipulation, each joint

▲ **26685**   Open treatment of carpometacarpal dislocation, other than thumb; with or without internal or external fixation, each joint

26686   complex, multiple or delayed reduction

26700   Closed treatment of metacarpophalangeal dislocation, single, with manipulation; without anesthesia

26705   requiring anesthesia

● New Code   ▲ Revised Code   ✳ Starred Procedure   ✛ Add-On Code   ⊘ Modifier -51 Exempt

26706 Percutaneous skeletal fixation of metacarpophalangeal dislocation, single, with manipulation

26715 Open treatment of metacarpophalangeal dislocation, single, with or without internal or external fixation

26720 Closed treatment of phalangeal shaft fracture, proximal or middle phalanx, finger or thumb; without manipulation, each

26725 with manipulation, with or without skin or skeletal traction, each

26727 Percutaneous skeletal fixation of unstable phalangeal shaft fracture, proximal or middle phalanx, finger or thumb, with manipulation, each

26735 Open treatment of phalangeal shaft fracture, proximal or middle phalanx, finger or thumb, with or without internal or external fixation, each

26740 Closed treatment of articular fracture, involving metacarpophalangeal or interphalangeal joint; without manipulation, each

26742 with manipulation, each

26746 Open treatment of articular fracture, involving metacarpophalangeal or interphalangeal joint, with or without internal or external fixation, each

26750 Closed treatment of distal phalangeal fracture, finger or thumb; without manipulation, each

26755 with manipulation, each

26756 Percutaneous skeletal fixation of distal phalangeal fracture, finger or thumb, each

26765 Open treatment of distal phalangeal fracture, finger or thumb, with or without internal or external fixation, each

26770 Closed treatment of interphalangeal joint dislocation, single, with manipulation; without anesthesia

26775 requiring anesthesia

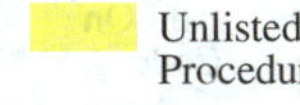 Separate Procedure

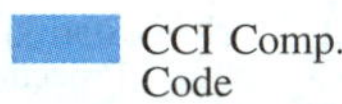 Unlisted Procedure

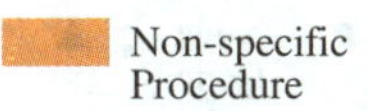 CCI Comp. Code

Non-specific Procedure

26776 Percutaneous skeletal fixation of interphalangeal joint dislocation, single, with manipulation

26785 Open treatment of interphalangeal joint dislocation, with or without internal or external fixation, single

ARTHRODESIS

26820 Fusion in opposition, thumb, with autogenous graft (includes obtaining graft)

26841 Arthrodesis, carpometacarpal joint, thumb, with or without internal fixation;

26842 with autograft (includes obtaining graft)

▲ **26843** Arthrodesis, carpometacarpal joint, digit, other than thumb, each;

26844 with autograft (includes obtaining graft)

26850 Arthrodesis, metacarpophalangeal joint, with or without internal fixation;

26852 with autograft (includes obtaining graft)

26860 Arthrodesis, interphalangeal joint, with or without internal fixation;

+26861 each additional interphalangeal joint (List separately in addition to code for primary procedure)

(Use 26861 in conjunction with code 26860)

26862 with autograft (includes obtaining graft)

+26863 with autograft (includes obtaining graft), each additional joint (List separately in addition to code for primary procedure)

(Use 26863 in conjunction with code 26862)

AMPUTATION

(For hand through metacarpal bones, use 25927)

26910 Amputation, metacarpal, with finger or thumb (ray amputation), single, with or without interosseous transfer

● New Code ▲ Revised Code ✳ Starred Procedure ✛ Add-On Code ⊘ Modifier -51 Exempt

(For repositioning see 26550, 26555)

26951 Amputation, finger or thumb, primary or secondary, any joint or phalanx, single, including neurectomies; with direct closure

26952   with local advancement flaps (V-Y, hood)

(For repair of soft tissue defect requiring split or full thickness graft or other pedicle flaps, see 15050-15758)

OTHER PROCEDURES

26989 Unlisted procedure, hands or fingers

PELVIS AND HIP JOINT

INCISION

(For incision and drainage procedures, superficial, see 10040-10160)

26990 Incision and drainage, pelvis or hip joint area; deep abscess or hematoma

26991   infected bursa

26992 Incision, bone cortex, pelvis and/or hip joint (eg, osteomyelitis or bone abscess)

27000 Tenotomy, adductor of hip, percutaneous (separate procedure)

27001 Tenotomy, adductor of hip, open

27003 Tenotomy, adductor, subcutaneous, open, with obturator neurectomy

27005 Tenotomy, hip flexor(s), open (separate procedure)

27006 Tenotomy, abductors and/or extensor(s) of hip, open (separate procedure)

27025 Fasciotomy, hip or thigh, any type

27030 Arthrotomy, hip, with drainage (eg, infection)

27033 Arthrotomy, hip, including exploration or removal of loose or foreign body

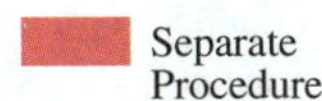
Separate Procedure

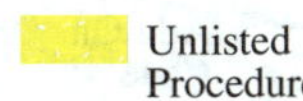
Unlisted Procedure

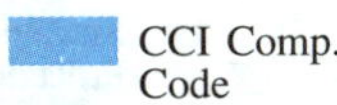
CCI Comp. Code

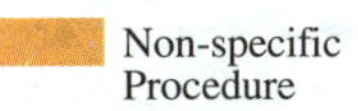
Non-specific Procedure

27035 Denervation, hip joint, intrapelvic or extrapelvic intra-articular branches of sciatic, femoral, or obturator nerves

(For obturator neurectomy, see 64763, 64766)

27036 Capsulectomy or capsulotomy, hip, with or without excision of heterotopic bone, with release of hip flexor muscles (ie, gluteus medius, gluteus minimus, tensor fascia latae, rectus femoris, sartorius, iliopsoas)

EXCISION

27040 Biopsy, soft tissue of pelvis and hip area; superficial

27041 deep, subfascial or intramuscular

(For needle biopsy of soft tissue, use 20206)

27047 Excision, tumor, pelvis and hip area; subcutaneous tissue

27048 deep, subfascial, intramuscular

27049 Radical resection of tumor, soft tissue of pelvis and hip area (eg, malignant neoplasm)

27050 Arthrotomy, with biopsy; sacroiliac joint

27052 hip joint

27054 Arthrotomy with synovectomy, hip joint

27060 Excision; ischial bursa

27062 trochanteric bursa or calcification

(For arthrocentesis or needling of bursa, use 20610)

27065 Excision of bone cyst or benign tumor; superficial (wing of ilium, symphysis pubis, or greater trochanter of femur) with or without autograft

27066 deep, with or without autograft

27067 with autograft requiring separate incision

● New Code   ▲ Revised Code   ✳ Starred Procedure   ✚ Add-On Code   ⊘ Modifier -51 Exempt

27070 Partial excision (craterization, saucerization) (eg, osteomyelitis or bone abscess); superficial (eg, wing of ilium, symphysis pubis, or greater trochanter of femur)

27071 deep (subfascial or intramuscular)

27075 Radical resection of tumor or infection; wing of ilium, one pubic or ischial ramus or symphysis pubis

27076 ilium, including acetabulum, both pubic rami, or ischium and acetabulum

27077 innominate bone, total

27078 ischial tuberosity and greater trochanter of femur

27079 ischial tuberosity and greater trochanter of femur, with skin flaps

27080 Coccygectomy, primary

(For pressure (decubitus) ulcer, see 15920, 15922 and 15931-15958)

INTRODUCTION OR REMOVAL

***27086** Removal of foreign body, pelvis or hip; subcutaneous tissue

27087 deep (subfascial or intramuscular)

27090 Removal of hip prosthesis; (separate procedure)

27091 complicated, including total hip prosthesis, methylmethacrylate with or without insertion of spacer

27093 Injection procedure for hip arthrography; without anesthesia

(For radiological supervision and interpretation, use 73525. Do not report 76003 in addition to 73525)

27095 with anesthesia

(For radiological supervision and interpretation, use 73525. Do not report 76003 in addition to 73525)

27096 Injection procedure for sacroiliac joint, arthrography and/or anesthetic/steroid

	Separate Procedure		Unlisted Procedure		CCI Comp. Code		Non-specific Procedure

(27096 is to be used only with imaging confirmation of intra-articular needle positioning)

(For radiological supervision and interpretation of sacroiliac joint arthrography, use 73542)

(For fluoroscopic guidance without formal arthrography, use 76005)

(Code 27096 is a unilateral procedure. For bilateral procedure, use modifier -50)

REPAIR, REVISION, AND/OR RECONSTRUCTION

27097 Release or recession, hamstring, proximal

27098 Transfer, adductor to ischium

27100 Transfer external oblique muscle to greater trochanter including fascial or tendon extension (graft)

27105 Transfer paraspinal muscle to hip (includes fascial or tendon extension graft)

▲ **27110** Transfer iliopsoas; to greater trochanter of femur

27111   to femoral neck

27120 Acetabuloplasty; (eg, Whitman, Colonna, Haygroves, or cup type)

27122   resection, femoral head (eg, Girdlestone procedure)

27125 Hemiarthroplasty, hip, partial (eg, femoral stem prosthesis, bipolar arthroplasty)

(For prosthetic replacement following fracture of the hip, use 27236)

▲ **27130** Arthroplasty, acetabular and proximal femoral prosthetic replacement (total hip arthroplasty), with or without autograft or allograft

▲ **27132** Conversion of previous hip surgery to total hip arthroplasty, with or without autograft or allograft

27134 Revision of total hip arthroplasty; both components, with or without autograft or allograft

● New Code   ▲ Revised Code   ✻ Starred Procedure   ✚ Add-On Code   ⊘ Modifier -51 Exempt

27137 acetabular component only, with or without autograft or allograft

27138 femoral component only, with or without allograft

▲ **27140** Osteotomy and transfer of greater trochanter of femur (separate procedure)

27146 Osteotomy, iliac, acetabular or innominate bone;

27147 with open reduction of hip

27151 with femoral osteotomy

27156 with femoral osteotomy and with open reduction of hip

27158 Osteotomy, pelvis, bilateral (eg, congenital malformation)

27161 Osteotomy, femoral neck (separate procedure)

27165 Osteotomy, intertrochanteric or subtrochanteric including internal or external fixation and/or cast

27170 Bone graft, femoral head, neck, intertrochanteric or subtrochanteric area (includes obtaining bone graft)

27175 Treatment of slipped femoral epiphysis; by traction, without reduction

27176 by single or multiple pinning, in situ

27177 Open treatment of slipped femoral epiphysis; single or multiple pinning or bone graft (includes obtaining graft)

27178 closed manipulation with single or multiple pinning

27179 osteoplasty of femoral neck (Heyman type procedure)

27181 osteotomy and internal fixation

▲ **27185** Epiphyseal arrest by epiphysiodesis or stapling, greater trochanter of femur

Separate
Procedure

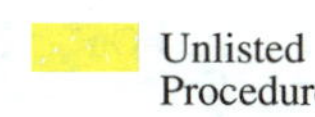
Unlisted
Procedure

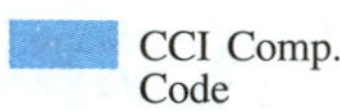
CCI Comp.
Code

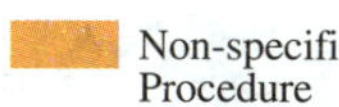
Non-specific
Procedure

27187 Prophylactic treatment (nailing, pinning, plating or wiring) with or without methylmethacrylate, femoral neck and proximal femur

FRACTURE AND/OR DISLOCATION

27193 Closed treatment of pelvic ring fracture, dislocation, diastasis or subluxation; without manipulation

27194   with manipulation, requiring more than local anesthesia

27200 Closed treatment of coccygeal fracture

27202 Open treatment of coccygeal fracture

27215 Open treatment of iliac spine(s), tuberosity avulsion, or iliac wing fracture(s) (eg, pelvic fracture(s) which do not disrupt the pelvic ring), with internal fixation

27216 Percutaneous skeletal fixation of posterior pelvic ring fracture and/or dislocation (includes ilium, sacroiliac joint and/or sacrum)

27217 Open treatment of anterior ring fracture and/or dislocation with internal fixation (includes pubic symphysis and/or rami)

27218 Open treatment of posterior ring fracture and/or dislocation with internal fixation (includes ilium, sacroiliac joint and/or sacrum)

27220 Closed treatment of acetabulum (hip socket) fracture(s); without manipulation

27222   with manipulation, with or without skeletal traction

27226 Open treatment of posterior or anterior acetabular wall fracture, with internal fixation

27227 Open treatment of acetabular fracture(s) involving anterior or posterior (one) column, or a fracture running transversely across the acetabulum, with internal fixation

27228 Open treatment of acetabular fracture(s) involving anterior and posterior (two) columns, includes T-fracture and both column fracture with complete articular detachment, or single column

● New Code   ▲ Revised Code   ✱ Starred Procedure   ✚ Add-On Code   ⊘ Modifier -51 Exempt

or transverse fracture with associated acetabular wall fracture, with internal fixation

27230 Closed treatment of femoral fracture, proximal end, neck; without manipulation

27232 with manipulation, with or without skeletal traction

27235 Percutaneous skeletal fixation of femoral fracture, proximal end, neck, undisplaced, mildly displaced, or impacted fracture

27236 Open treatment of femoral fracture, proximal end, neck, internal fixation or prosthetic replacement

27238 Closed treatment of intertrochanteric, pertrochanteric, or subtrochanteric femoral fracture; without manipulation

27240 with manipulation, with or without skin or skeletal traction

27244 Open treatment of intertrochanteric, pertrochanteric or subtrochanteric femoral fracture; with plate/screw type implant, with or without cerclage

27245 with intramedullary implant, with or without interlocking screws and/or cerclage

27246 Closed treatment of greater trochanteric fracture, without manipulation

27248 Open treatment of greater trochanteric fracture, with or without internal or external fixation

27250 Closed treatment of hip dislocation, traumatic; without anesthesia

27252 requiring anesthesia

27253 Open treatment of hip dislocation, traumatic, without internal fixation

27254 Open treatment of hip dislocation, traumatic, with acetabular wall and femoral head fracture, with or without internal or external fixation

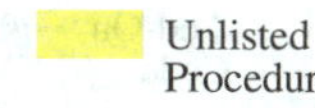 Separate Procedure   Unlisted Procedure   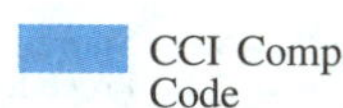 CCI Comp. Code   Non-specific Procedure

***27256** Treatment of spontaneous hip dislocation (developmental, including congenital or pathological), by abduction, splint or traction; without anesthesia, without manipulation

***27257** with manipulation, requiring anesthesia

27258 Open treatment of spontaneous hip dislocation (developmental, including congenital or pathological), replacement of femoral head in acetabulum (including tenotomy, etc);

27259 with femoral shaft shortening

27265 Closed treatment of post hip arthroplasty dislocation; without anesthesia

27266 requiring regional or general anesthesia

MANIPULATION

***27275** Manipulation, hip joint, requiring general anesthesia

ARTHRODESIS

27280 Arthrodesis, sacroiliac joint (including obtaining graft)

27282 Arthrodesis, symphysis pubis (including obtaining graft)

27284 Arthrodesis, hip joint (including obtaining graft);

27286 with subtrochanteric osteotomy

AMPUTATION

27290 Interpelviabdominal amputation (hindquarter amputation)

27295 Disarticulation of hip

OTHER PROCEDURES

27299 Unlisted procedure, pelvis or hip joint

● New Code   ▲ Revised Code   * Starred Procedure   ✚ Add-On Code   ⊘ Modifier -51 Exempt

FEMUR (THIGH REGION) AND KNEE JOINT

INCISION

(For incision and drainage of abscess or hematoma, superficial, see 10040-10160)

27301 Incision and drainage, deep abscess, bursa, or hematoma, thigh or knee region

27303 Incision, deep, with opening of bone cortex, femur or knee (eg, osteomyelitis or bone abscess)

27305 Fasciotomy, iliotibial (tenotomy), open

(For combined Ober-Yount fasciotomy, use 27025)

27306 Tenotomy, percutaneous, adductor or hamstring; single tendon (separate procedure)

27307   multiple tendons

27310 Arthrotomy, knee, with exploration, drainage, or removal of foreign body(eg, infection)

27315 Neurectomy, hamstring muscle

27320 Neurectomy, popliteal (gastrocnemius)

EXCISION

27323 Biopsy, soft tissue of thigh or knee area; superficial

27324   deep (subfascial or intramuscular)

(For needle biopsy of soft tissue, use 20206)

27327 Excision, tumor, thigh or knee area; subcutaneous

27328   deep, subfascial, or intramuscular

27329 Radical resection of tumor (eg, malignant neoplasm), soft tissue of thigh or knee area

27330 Arthrotomy, knee; with synovial biopsy only

27331	including joint exploration, biopsy, or removal of loose or foreign bodies
27332	Arthrotomy, with excision of semilunar cartilage (meniscectomy) knee; medial OR lateral
27333	medial AND lateral
27334	Arthrotomy, with synovectomy, knee; anterior OR posterior
27335	anterior AND posterior including popliteal area
27340	Excision, prepatellar bursa
27345	Excision of synovial cyst of popliteal space (eg, Baker's cyst)
27347	Excision of lesion of meniscus or capsule (eg, cyst, ganglion), knee
27350	Patellectomy or hemipatellectomy
27355	Excision or curettage of bone cyst or benign tumor of femur;
27356	with allograft
27357	with autograft (includes obtaining graft)
+27358	with internal fixation (List in addition to code for primary procedure)

(Use 27358 in conjunction with codes 27355, 27356 or 27357)

27360	Partial excision (craterization, saucerization, or diaphysectomy) bone, femur, proximal tibia and/or fibula (eg, osteomyelitis or bone abscess)
27365	Radical resection of tumor, bone, femur or knee

(For radical resection of tumor, soft tissue, use 27329)

INTRODUCTION OR REMOVAL

27370	Injection procedure for knee arthrography

(For radiological supervision and interpretation, use 73580. Do not report 76003 in addition to 73580)

● New Code   ▲ Revised Code   * Starred Procedure   + Add-On Code   ⊘ Modifier -51 Exempt

27372   Removal of foreign body, deep, thigh region or knee area

(For removal of knee prosthesis including "total knee," use 27488)

REPAIR, REVISION, AND/OR RECONSTRUCTION

27380   Suture of infrapatellar tendon; primary

27381   secondary reconstruction, including fascial or tendon graft

27385   Suture of quadriceps or hamstring muscle rupture; primary

27386   secondary reconstruction, including fascial or tendon graft

27390   Tenotomy, open, hamstring, knee to hip; single tendon

27391   multiple tendons, one leg

27392   multiple tendons, bilateral

27393   Lengthening of hamstring tendon; single tendon

27394   multiple tendons, one leg

27395   multiple tendons, bilateral

27396   Transplant, hamstring tendon to patella; single tendon

27397   multiple tendons

27400   Transfer, tendon or muscle, hamstrings to femur (eg, Egger's type procedure)

27403   Arthrotomy with meniscus repair, knee

(For arthroscopic repair, use 29882)

27405   Repair, primary, torn ligament and/or capsule, knee; collateral

27407   cruciate

27409   collateral and cruciate ligaments

27418   Anterior tibial tubercleplasty (eg, Maquet type procedure)

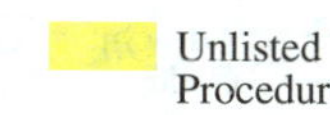

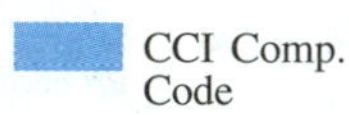

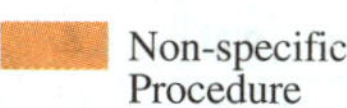

Non-specific Procedure

27420	Reconstruction of dislocating patella; (eg, Hauser type procedure)
27422	with extensor realignment and/or muscle advancement or release (eg, Campbell, Goldwaite type procedure)
27424	with patellectomy
27425	Lateral retinacular release (any method)
27427	Ligamentous reconstruction (augmentation), knee; extra-articular
27428	intra-articular (open)
27429	intra-articular (open) and extra-articular

(For primary repair of ligament(s) performed in addition to reconstruction, report 27405, 27407 or 27409 in addition to code 27427, 27428 or 27429)

27430	Quadricepsplasty (eg, Bennett or Thompson type)
27435	Capsulotomy, posterior capsular release, knee
27437	Arthroplasty, patella; without prosthesis
27438	with prosthesis
27440	Arthroplasty, knee, tibial plateau;
27441	with debridement and partial synovectomy
27442	Arthroplasty, femoral condyles or tibial plateau(s), knee;
27443	with debridement and partial synovectomy
27445	Arthroplasty, knee, hinge prosthesis (eg, Walldius type)
27446	Arthroplasty, knee, condyle and plateau; medial OR lateral compartment
▲ **27447**	medial AND lateral compartments with or without patella resurfacing (total knee arthroplasty)

(For revision of total knee arthroplasty, use 27487)

● New Code   ▲ Revised Code   ✳ Starred Procedure   ✚ Add-On Code   ⊘ Modifier -51 Exempt

(For removal of total knee prosthesis, use 27488)

27448 Osteotomy, femur, shaft or supracondylar; without fixation

27450 with fixation

27454 Osteotomy, multiple, with realignment on intramedullary rod, femoral shaft (eg, Sofield type procedure)

27455 Osteotomy, proximal tibia, including fibular excision or osteotomy (includes correction of genu varus (bowleg) or genu valgus (knock-knee)); before epiphyseal closure

27457 after epiphyseal closure

27465 Osteoplasty, femur; shortening (excluding 64876)

27466 lengthening

27468 combined, lengthening and shortening with femoral segment transfer

27470 Repair, nonunion or malunion, femur, distal to head and neck; without graft (eg, compression technique)

27472 with iliac or other autogenous bone graft (includes obtaining graft)

27475 Arrest, epiphyseal, any method (eg, epiphysiodesis); distal femur

27477 tibia and fibula, proximal

27479 combined distal femur, proximal tibia and fibula

27485 Arrest, hemiepiphyseal, distal femur or proximal tibia or fibula (eg, genu varus or valgus)

27486 Revision of total knee arthroplasty, with or without allograft; one component

27487 femoral and entire tibial component

27488 Removal of prosthesis, including total knee prosthesis, methylmethacrylate with or without insertion of spacer, knee

Separate
Procedure

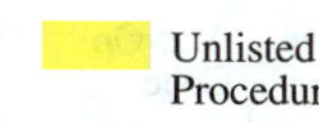
Unlisted
Procedure

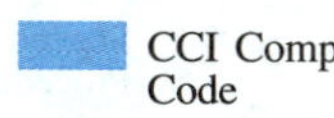
CCI Comp.
Code

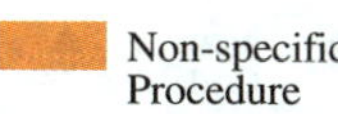
Non-specific
Procedure

331

27495	Prophylactic treatment (nailing, pinning, plating or wiring) with or without methylmethacrylate, femur
27496	Decompression fasciotomy, thigh and/or knee, one compartment (flexor or extensor or adductor);
27497	with debridement of nonviable muscle and/or nerve
27498	Decompression fasciotomy, thigh and/or knee, multiple compartments;
27499	with debridement of nonviable muscle and/or nerve

FRACTURE/DISLOCATION

(For arthroscopic treatment of intercondylar spine(s) and tuberosity fracture(s) of the knee, see 29850, 29851)

(For arthroscopic treatment of tibial fracture, see 29855, 29856)

27500	Closed treatment of femoral shaft fracture, without manipulation
27501	Closed treatment of supracondylar or transcondylar femoral fracture with or without intercondylar extension, without manipulation
27502	Closed treatment of femoral shaft fracture, with manipulation, with or without skin or skeletal traction
27503	Closed treatment of supracondylar or transcondylar femoral fracture with or without intercondylar extension, with manipulation, with or without skin or skeletal traction
27506	Open treatment of femoral shaft fracture, with or without external fixation, with insertion of intramedullary implant, with or without cerclage and/or locking screws
27507	Open treatment of femoral shaft fracture with plate/screws, with or without cerclage
27508	Closed treatment of femoral fracture, distal end, medial or lateral condyle, without manipulation
27509	Percutaneous skeletal fixation of femoral fracture, distal end, medial or lateral condyle, or supracondylar or transcondylar,

---

● New Code   ▲ Revised Code   ✱ Starred Procedure   ✚ Add-On Code   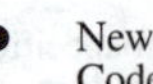 Modifier -51 Exempt with or without intercondylar extension, or distal femoral epiphyseal separation

27510 Closed treatment of femoral fracture, distal end, medial or lateral condyle, with manipulation

27511 Open treatment of femoral supracondylar or transcondylar fracture without intercondylar extension, with or without internal or external fixation

27513 Open treatment of femoral supracondylar or transcondylar fracture with intercondylar extension, with or without internal or external fixation

27514 Open treatment of femoral fracture, distal end, medial or lateral condyle, with or without internal or external fixation

27516 Closed treatment of distal femoral epiphyseal separation; without manipulation

27517   with manipulation, with or without skin or skeletal traction

27519 Open treatment of distal femoral epiphyseal separation, with or without internal or external fixation

27520 Closed treatment of patellar fracture, without manipulation

27524 Open treatment of patellar fracture, with internal fixation and/or partial or complete patellectomy and soft tissue repair

27530 Closed treatment of tibial fracture, proximal (plateau); without manipulation

27532   with or without manipulation, with skeletal traction

(For arthroscopic treatment, see 29855, 29856)

27535 Open treatment of tibial fracture, proximal (plateau); unicondylar, with or without internal or external fixation

27536   bicondylar, with or without internal fixation

(For arthroscopic treatment, see 29855, 29856)

27538 Closed treatment of intercondylar spine(s) and/or tuberosity fracture(s) of knee, with or without manipulation

---

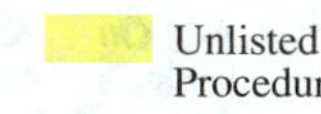

Separate
Procedure

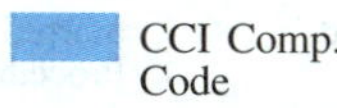

Unlisted
Procedure

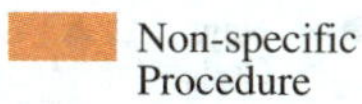

CCI Comp.
Code

Non-specific
Procedure

333

(For arthroscopic treatment, see 29850, 29851)

27540 Open treatment of intercondylar spine(s) and/or tuberosity fracture(s) of the knee, with or without internal or external fixation

27550 Closed treatment of knee dislocation; without anesthesia

27552 requiring anesthesia

27556 Open treatment of knee dislocation, with or without internal or external fixation; without primary ligamentous repair or augmentation/reconstruction

27557 with primary ligamentous repair

27558 with primary ligamentous repair, with augmentation/ reconstruction

27560 Closed treatment of patellar dislocation; without anesthesia

(For recurrent dislocation, see 27420-27424)

27562 requiring anesthesia

27566 Open treatment of patellar dislocation, with or without partial or total patellectomy

MANIPULATION

***27570** Manipulation of knee joint under general anesthesia (includes application of traction or other fixation devices)

ARTHRODESIS

27580 Arthrodesis, knee, any technique

AMPUTATION

27590 Amputation, thigh, through femur, any level;

27591 immediate fitting technique including first cast

27592 open, circular (guillotine)

27594 secondary closure or scar revision

● New Code   ▲ Revised Code   * Starred Procedure   + Add-On Code   ⊘ Modifier -51 Exempt

27596   re-amputation

27598   Disarticulation at knee

OTHER PROCEDURES

27599   Unlisted procedure, femur or knee

LEG (TIBIA AND FIBULA) AND ANKLE JOINT

INCISION

27600   Decompression fasciotomy, leg; anterior and/or lateral compartments only

27601   posterior compartment(s) only

27602   anterior and/or lateral, and posterior compartment(s)

(For incision and drainage procedures, superficial, see 10040-10160)

(For decompression fasciotomy with debridement, see 27892-27894)

27603   Incision and drainage, leg or ankle; deep abscess or hematoma

27604   infected bursa

***27605**   Tenotomy, percutaneous, Achilles tendon (separate procedure); local anesthesia

27606   general anesthesia

27607   Incision (eg, osteomyelitis or bone abscess), leg or ankle

27610   Arthrotomy, ankle, including exploration, drainage, or removal of foreign body

27612   Arthrotomy, posterior capsular release, ankle, with or without Achilles tendon lengthening

(See also 27685)

EXCISION

27613   Biopsy, soft tissue of leg or ankle area; superficial

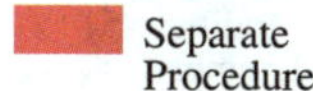 Separate Procedure

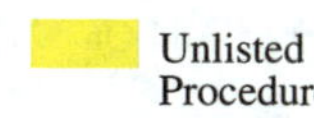 Unlisted Procedure

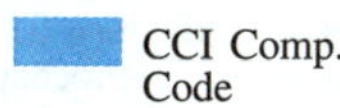 CCI Comp. Code

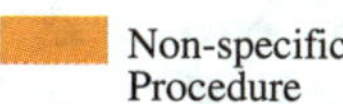 Non-specific Procedure

335

27614	deep (subfascial or intramuscular)

(For needle biopsy of soft tissue, use 20206)

27615 Radical resection of tumor (eg, malignant neoplasm), soft tissue of leg or ankle area

27618 Excision, tumor, leg or ankle area; subcutaneous tissue

27619 deep (subfascial or intramuscular)

27620 Arthrotomy, ankle, with joint exploration, with or without biopsy, with or without removal of loose or foreign body

27625 Arthrotomy, with synovectomy, ankle;

27626 including tenosynovectomy

27630 Excision of lesion of tendon sheath or capsule (eg, cyst or ganglion), leg and/or ankle

27635 Excision or curettage of bone cyst or benign tumor, tibia or fibula;

27637 with autograft (includes obtaining graft)

27638 with allograft

27640 Partial excision (craterization, saucerization, or diaphysectomy) bone (eg, osteomyelitis or exostosis); tibia

27641 fibula

27645 Radical resection of tumor, bone; tibia

27646 fibula

27647 talus or calcaneus

INTRODUCTION OR REMOVAL

27648 Injection procedure for ankle arthrography

(For radiological supervision and interpretation use 73615. Do not report 76003 in addition to 73615)

(For ankle arthroscopy, see 29894-29898)

REPAIR, REVISION, AND/OR RECONSTRUCTION

27650 Repair, primary, open or percutaneous, ruptured Achilles tendon;

27652 with graft (includes obtaining graft)

27654 Repair, secondary, Achilles tendon, with or without graft

27656 Repair, fascial defect of leg

27658 Repair, flexor tendon, leg; primary, without graft, each tendon

27659 secondary, with or without graft, each tendon

27664 Repair, extensor tendon, leg; primary, without graft, each tendon

27665 secondary, with or without graft, each tendon

27675 Repair, dislocating peroneal tendons; without fibular osteotomy

27676 with fibular osteotomy

27680 Tenolysis, flexor or extensor tendon, leg and/or ankle; single, each tendon

27681 multiple tendons (through separate incision(s))

27685 Lengthening or shortening of tendon, leg or ankle; single tendon (separate procedure)

27686 multiple tendons (through same incision), each

27687 Gastrocnemius recession (eg, Strayer procedure)

(Toe extensors are considered as a group to be single tendon when transplanted into midfoot)

27690 Transfer or transplant of single tendon (with muscle redirection or rerouting); superficial (eg, anterior tibial extensors into midfoot)

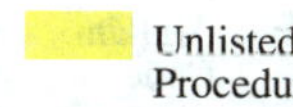 Separate Procedure

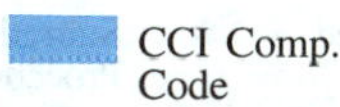 Unlisted Procedure

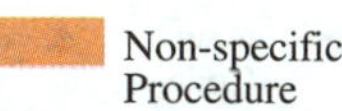 CCI Comp. Code

Non-specific Procedure

337

27691	deep (eg, anterior tibial or posterior tibial through interosseous space, flexor digitorum longus, flexor hallucis longus, or peroneal tendon to midfoot or hind foot)
+27692	each additional tendon (List separately in addition to code for primary procedure)

(Use 27692 in conjunction with codes 27690, 27691)

27695	Repair, primary, disrupted ligament, ankle; collateral
27696	both collateral ligaments
27698	Repair, secondary disrupted ligament, ankle, collateral (eg, Watson-Jones procedure)
27700	Arthroplasty, ankle;
27702	with implant (total ankle)
27703	revision, total ankle
27704	Removal of ankle implant
27705	Osteotomy; tibia
27707	fibula
27709	tibia and fibula
27712	multiple, with realignment on intramedullary rod (eg, Sofield type procedure)

(For osteotomy to correct genu varus (bowleg) or genu valgus (knock-knee), see 27455-27457)

27715	Osteoplasty, tibia and fibula, lengthening or shortening
27720	Repair of nonunion or malunion, tibia; without graft, (eg, compression technique)
27722	with sliding graft
27724	with iliac or other autograft (includes obtaining graft)
27725	by synostosis, with fibula, any method

● New Code   ▲ Revised Code   ＊ Starred Procedure   ＋ Add-On Code   ⊘ Modifier -51 Exempt

27727   Repair of congenital pseudarthrosis, tibia

27730   Arrest, epiphyseal (epiphysiodesis), any method; distal tibia

27732   distal fibula

27734   distal tibia and fibula

27740   Arrest, epiphyseal (epiphysiodesis), any method, combined, proximal and distal tibia and fibula;

27742   and distal femur

(For epiphyseal arrest of proximal tibia and fibula, use 27477)

27745   Prophylactic treatment (nailing, pinning, plating or wiring) with or without methylmethacrylate, tibia

FRACTURE AND/OR DISLOCATION

27750   Closed treatment of tibial shaft fracture (with or without fibular fracture); without manipulation

27752   with manipulation, with or without skeletal traction

27756   Percutaneous skeletal fixation of tibial shaft fracture (with or without fibular fracture) (eg, pins or screws)

27758   Open treatment of tibial shaft fracture, (with or without fibular fracture) with plate/screws, with or without cerclage

27759   Open treatment of tibial shaft fracture (with or without fibular fracture) by intramedullary implant, with or without interlocking screws and/or cerclage

27760   Closed treatment of medial malleolus fracture; without manipulation

27762   with manipulation, with or without skin or skeletal traction

27766   Open treatment of medial malleolus fracture, with or without internal or external fixation

27780   Closed treatment of proximal fibula or shaft fracture; without manipulation

Separate Procedure

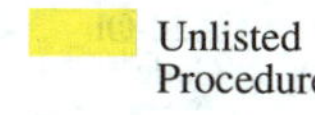
Unlisted Procedure

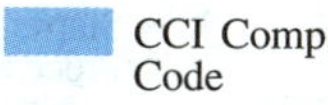
CCI Comp. Code

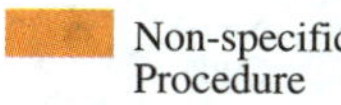
Non-specific Procedure

339

27781   with manipulation

27784   Open treatment of proximal fibula or shaft fracture, with or without internal or external fixation

27786   Closed treatment of distal fibular fracture (lateral malleolus); without manipulation

27788   with manipulation

27792   Open treatment of distal fibular fracture (lateral malleolus), with or without internal or external fixation

27808   Closed treatment of bimalleolar ankle fracture, (including Potts); without manipulation

27810   with manipulation

27814   Open treatment of bimalleolar ankle fracture, with or without internal or external fixation

27816   Closed treatment of trimalleolar ankle fracture; without manipulation

27818   with manipulation

27822   Open treatment of trimalleolar ankle fracture, with or without internal or external fixation, medial and/or lateral malleolus; without fixation of posterior lip

27823   with fixation of posterior lip

27824   Closed treatment of fracture of weight bearing articular portion of distal tibia (eg, pilon or tibial plafond), with or without anesthesia; without manipulation

27825   with skeletal traction and/or requiring manipulation

27826   Open treatment of fracture of weight bearing articular surface/portion of distal tibia (eg, pilon or tibial plafond), with internal or external fixation; of fibula only

27827   of tibia only

27828   of both tibia and fibula

340

● New Code   ▲ Revised Code   * Starred Procedure   + Add-On Code   ⊘ Modifier -51 Exempt

27829 Open treatment of distal tibiofibular joint (syndesmosis) disruption, with or without internal or external fixation

27830 Closed treatment of proximal tibiofibular joint dislocation; without anesthesia

27831 requiring anesthesia

27832 Open treatment of proximal tibiofibular joint dislocation, with or without internal or external fixation, or with excision of proximal fibula

27840 Closed treatment of ankle dislocation; without anesthesia

27842 requiring anesthesia, with or without percutaneous skeletal fixation

27846 Open treatment of ankle dislocation, with or without percutaneous skeletal fixation; without repair or internal fixation

27848 with repair or internal or external fixation

MANIPULATION

∗27860 Manipulation of ankle under general anesthesia (includes application of traction or other fixation apparatus)

ARTHRODESIS

27870 Arthrodesis, ankle, any method

27871 Arthrodesis, tibiofibular joint, proximal or distal

AMPUTATION

27880 Amputation, leg, through tibia and fibula;

27881 with immediate fitting technique including application of first cast

27882 open, circular (guillotine)

27884 secondary closure or scar revision

27886 re-amputation

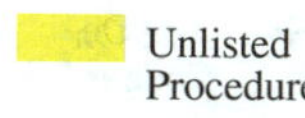

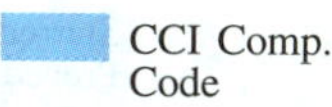

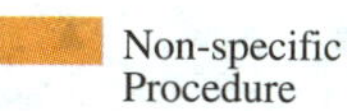

27888   Amputation, ankle, through malleoli of tibia and fibula (eg, Syme, Pirogoff type procedures), with plastic closure and resection of nerves

27889   Ankle disarticulation

OTHER PROCEDURES

27892   Decompression fasciotomy, leg; anterior and/or lateral compartments only, with debridement of nonviable muscle and/or nerve

(For decompression fasciotomy of the leg without debridement, use 27600)

27893   posterior compartment(s) only, with debridement of nonviable muscle and/or nerve

(For decompession fasciotomy of the leg without debridement, use 27601)

27894   anterior and/or lateral, and posterior compartment(s), with debridement of nonviable muscle and/or nerve

(For decompression fasciotomy of the leg without debridement, use 27602)

27899   Unlisted procedure, leg or ankle

FOOT AND TOES

INCISION

(For incision and drainage procedures, superficial, see 10040-10160)

∗28001   Incision and drainage, bursa, foot

∗28002   Incision and drainage below fascia, with or without tendon sheath involvement, foot; single bursal space

28003   multiple areas

28005   Incision, bone cortex (eg, osteomyelitis or bone abscess), foot

28008   Fasciotomy, foot and/or toe

(See also 28060, 28062, 28250)

28010 Tenotomy, percutaneous, toe; single tendon

28011   multiple tendons

(For open tenotomy, see 28230-28234)

28020 Arthrotomy, including exploration, drainage, or removal of loose or foreign body; intertarsal or tarsometatarsal joint

28022   metatarsophalangeal joint

28024   interphalangeal joint

28030 Neurectomy, intrinsic musculature of foot

28035 Release, tarsal tunnel (posterior tibial nerve decompression)

(For other nerve entrapments, see 64704, 64722)

EXCISION

28043 Excision, tumor, foot; subcutaneous tissue

28045   deep, subfascial, intramuscular

28046 Radical resection of tumor (eg, malignant neoplasm), soft tissue of foot

28050 Arthrotomy with biopsy; intertarsal or tarsometatarsal joint

28052   metatarsophalangeal joint

28054   interphalangeal joint

28060 Fasciectomy, plantar fascia; partial (separate procedure)

28062   radical (separate procedure)

(For plantar fasciotomy, see 28008, 28250)

28070 Synovectomy; intertarsal or tarsometatarsal joint, each

28072   metatarsophalangeal joint, each

28080 Excision, interdigital (Morton) neuroma, single, each

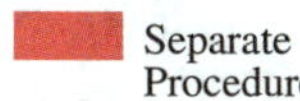
Separate
Procedure

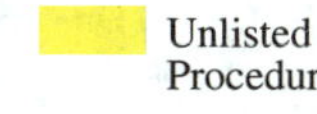
Unlisted
Procedure

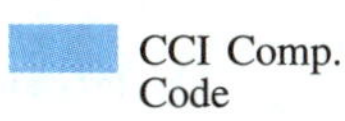
CCI Comp.
Code

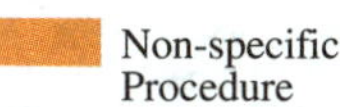
Non-specific
Procedure

28086	Synovectomy, tendon sheath, foot; flexor
28088	extensor
28090	Excision of lesion, tendon, tendon sheath, or capsule (including synovectomy) (eg, cyst or ganglion); foot
28092	toe(s), each
28100	Excision or curettage of bone cyst or benign tumor, talus or calcaneus;
28102	with iliac or other autograft (includes obtaining graft)
28103	with allograft
▲ **28104**	Excision or curettage of bone cyst or benign tumor, tarsal or metatarsal, except talus or calcaneus;
28106	with iliac or other autograft (includes obtaining graft)
28107	with allograft
28108	Excision or curettage of bone cyst or benign tumor, phalanges of foot

(For ostectomy, partial (eg, hallux valgus, Silver type procedure), use 28290)

28110	Ostectomy, partial excision, fifth metatarsal head (bunionette) (separate procedure)
28111	Ostectomy, complete excision; first metatarsal head
28112	other metatarsal head (second, third or fourth)
28113	fifth metatarsal head
28114	all metatarsal heads, with partial proximal phalangectomy, excluding first metatarsal (eg, Clayton type procedure)
28116	Ostectomy, excision of tarsal coalition
28118	Ostectomy, calcaneus;

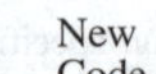 New Code 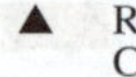 Revised Code  Starred Procedure 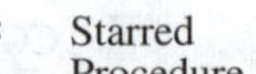 Add-On Code 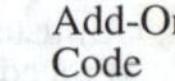 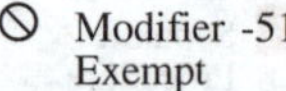 Modifier -51 Exempt

28119	for spur, with or without plantar fascial release
28120	Partial excision (craterization, saucerization, sequestrectomy, or diaphysectomy) bone (eg, osteomyelitis or bossing); talus or calcaneus
28122	tarsal or metatarsal bone, except talus or calcaneus

(For partial excision of talus or calcaneus, use 28120)

(For cheilectomy for hallux rigidus, use 28289)

28124	phalanx of toe
28126	Resection, partial or complete, phalangeal base, each toe
28130	Talectomy (astragalectomy)
28140	Metatarsectomy
28150	Phalangectomy, toe, each toe
28153	Resection, condyle(s), distal end of phalanx, each toe
28160	Hemiphalangectomy or interphalangeal joint excision, toe, proximal end of phalanx, each
28171	Radical resection of tumor, bone; tarsal (except talus or calcaneus)
28173	metatarsal
28175	phalanx of toe

(For talus or calcaneus, use 27647)

INTRODUCTION OR REMOVAL

***28190**	Removal of foreign body, foot; subcutaneous
28192	deep
28193	complicated

REPAIR, REVISION, AND/OR RECONSTRUCTION

28200 Repair, tendon, flexor, foot; primary or secondary, without free graft, each tendon

28202 secondary with free graft, each tendon (includes obtaining graft)

28208 Repair, tendon, extensor, foot; primary or secondary, each tendon

28210 secondary with free graft, each tendon (includes obtaining graft)

28220 Tenolysis, flexor, foot; single tendon

28222 multiple tendons

28225 Tenolysis, extensor, foot; single tendon

28226 multiple tendons

28230 Tenotomy, open, tendon flexor; foot, single or multiple tendon(s) (separate procedure)

28232 toe, single tendon (separate procedure)

28234 Tenotomy, open, extensor, foot or toe, each tendon

▲ **28238** Reconstruction (advancement), posterior tibial tendon with excision of accessory tarsal navicular bone (eg, Kidner type procedure)

(For subcutaneous tenotomy, see 28010, 28011)

(For transfer or transplant of tendon with muscle redirection or rerouting, see 27690-27692)

(For extensor hallucis longus transfer with great toe IP fusion (Jones procedure), use 28760)

28240 Tenotomy, lengthening, or release, abductor hallucis muscle

28250 Division of plantar fascia and muscle (eg, Steindler stripping) (separate procedure)

28260 Capsulotomy, midfoot; medial release only (separate procedure)

● New Code ▲ Revised Code * Starred Procedure + Add-On Code ⊘ Modifier -51 Exempt

28261   with tendon lengthening

28262   extensive, including posterior talotibial capsulotomy and tendon(s) lengthening (eg, resistant clubfoot deformity)

28264   Capsulotomy, midtarsal (eg, Heyman type procedure)

28270   Capsulotomy; metatarsophalangeal joint, with or without tenorrhaphy, each joint (separate procedure)

28272   interphalangeal joint, each joint (separate procedure)

28280   Syndactylization, toes (eg, webbing or Kelikian type procedure)

28285   Correction, hammertoe (eg, interphalangeal fusion, partial or total phalangectomy)

28286   Correction, cock-up fifth toe, with plastic skin closure (eg, Ruiz-Mora type procedure)

28288   Ostectomy, partial, exostectomy or condylectomy, metatarsal head, each metatarsal head

28289   Hallux rigidus correction with cheilectomy, debridement and capsular release of the first metatarsophalangeal joint

28290   Correction, hallux valgus (bunion), with or without sesamoidectomy; simple exostectomy (eg, Silver type procedure)

28292   Keller, McBride, or Mayo type procedure

28293   resection of joint with implant

28294   with tendon transplants (eg, Joplin type procedure)

28296   with metatarsal osteotomy (eg, Mitchell, Chevron, or concentric type procedures)

28297   Lapidus type procedure

28298   by phalanx osteotomy

▲ **28299**   by double osteotomy

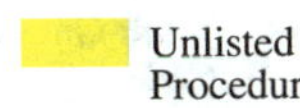
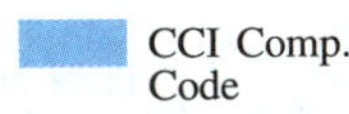
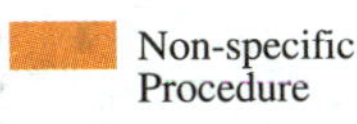

28300 Osteotomy; calcaneus (eg, Dwyer or Chambers type procedure), with or without internal fixation

28302 talus

28304 Osteotomy, tarsal bones, other than calcaneus or talus;

28305 with autograft (includes obtaining graft) (eg, Fowler type)

28306 Osteotomy, with or without lengthening, shortening or angular correction, metatarsal; first metatarsal

28307 first metatarsal with autograft (other than first toe)

28308 other than first metatarsal, each

28309 multiple (eg, Swanson type cavus foot procedure)

28310 Osteotomy, shortening, angular or rotational correction; proximal phalanx, first toe (separate procedure)

28312 other phalanges, any toe

28313 Reconstruction, angular deformity of toe, soft tissue procedures only (eg, overlapping second toe, fifth toe, curly toes)

28315 Sesamoidectomy, first toe (separate procedure)

28320 Repair, nonunion or malunion; tarsal bones

28322 metatarsal, with or without bone graft (includes obtaining graft)

28340 Reconstruction, toe, macrodactyly; soft tissue resection

28341 requiring bone resection

28344 Reconstruction, toe(s); polydactyly

28345 syndactyly, with or without skin graft(s), each web

28360 Reconstruction, cleft foot

● New Code　　▲ Revised Code　　✳ Starred Procedure　　✚ Add-On Code　　⊘ Modifier -51 Exempt

FRACTURE AND/OR DISLOCATION

28400 Closed treatment of calcaneal fracture; without manipulation

28405   with manipulation

28406 Percutaneous skeletal fixation of calcaneal fracture, with manipulation

28415 Open treatment of calcaneal fracture, with or without internal or external fixation;

28420   with primary iliac or other autogenous bone graft (includes obtaining graft)

28430 Closed treatment of talus fracture; without manipulation

28435   with manipulation

28436 Percutaneous skeletal fixation of talus fracture, with manipulation

28445 Open treatment of talus fracture, with or without internal or external fixation

28450 Treatment of tarsal bone fracture (except talus and calcaneus); without manipulation, each

28455   with manipulation, each

28456 Percutaneous skeletal fixation of tarsal bone fracture (except talus and calcaneus), with manipulation, each

28465 Open treatment of tarsal bone fracture (except talus and calcaneus), with or without internal or external fixation, each

28470 Closed treatment of metatarsal fracture; without manipulation, each

28475   with manipulation, each

28476 Percutaneous skeletal fixation of metatarsal fracture, with manipulation, each

28485 Open treatment of metatarsal fracture, with or without internal or external fixation, each

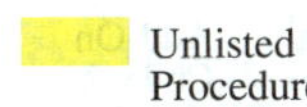
Separate Procedure

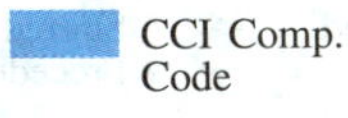
Unlisted Procedure

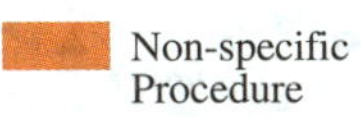
CCI Comp. Code

Non-specific Procedure

28490 Closed treatment of fracture great toe, phalanx or phalanges; without manipulation

28495 with manipulation

28496 Percutaneous skeletal fixation of fracture great toe, phalanx or phalanges, with manipulation

28505 Open treatment of fracture great toe, phalanx or phalanges, with or without internal or external fixation

28510 Closed treatment of fracture, phalanx or phalanges, other than great toe; without manipulation, each

28515 with manipulation, each

28525 Open treatment of fracture, phalanx or phalanges, other than great toe, with or without internal or external fixation, each

28530 Closed treatment of sesamoid fracture

28531 Open treatment of sesamoid fracture, with or without internal fixation

28540 Closed treatment of tarsal bone dislocation, other than talotarsal; without anesthesia

28545 requiring anesthesia

28546 Percutaneous skeletal fixation of tarsal bone dislocation, other than talotarsal, with manipulation

28555 Open treatment of tarsal bone dislocation, with or without internal or external fixation

28570 Closed treatment of talotarsal joint dislocation; without anesthesia

28575 requiring anesthesia

28576 Percutaneous skeletal fixation of talotarsal joint dislocation, with manipulation

28585 Open treatment of talotarsal joint dislocation, with or without internal or external fixation

● New Code   ▲ Revised Code   * Starred Procedure   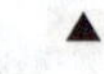 Add-On Code   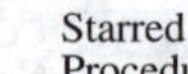 Modifier -51 Exempt

| 28600 | Closed treatment of tarsometatarsal joint dislocation; without anesthesia |

| 28605 | requiring anesthesia |

| 28606 | Percutaneous skeletal fixation of tarsometatarsal joint dislocation, with manipulation |

| 28615 | Open treatment of tarsometatarsal joint dislocation, with or without internal or external fixation |

| *28630 | Closed treatment of metatarsophalangeal joint dislocation; without anesthesia |

| *28635 | requiring anesthesia |

| 28636 | Percutaneous skeletal fixation of metatarsophalangeal joint dislocation, with manipulation |

| 28645 | Open treatment of metatarsophalangeal joint dislocation, with or without internal or external fixation |

| *28660 | Closed treatment of interphalangeal joint dislocation; without anesthesia |

| *28665 | requiring anesthesia |

| 28666 | Percutaneous skeletal fixation of interphalangeal joint dislocation, with manipulation |

| 28675 | Open treatment of interphalangeal joint dislocation, with or without internal or external fixation |

ARTHRODESIS

| 28705 | Arthrodesis; pantalar |

| 28715 | triple |

| 28725 | subtalar |

| 28730 | Arthrodesis, midtarsal or tarsometatarsal, multiple or transverse; |

| 28735 | with osteotomy (eg, flatfoot correction) |

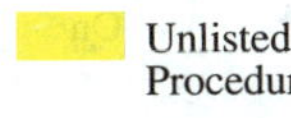

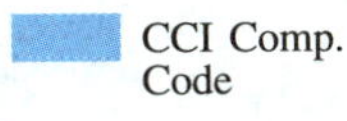

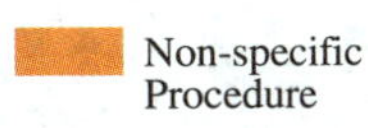

▲ **28737** Arthrodesis, with tendon lengthening and advancement, midtarsal, tarsal navicular-cuneiform (eg, Miller type procedure)

28740 Arthrodesis, midtarsal or tarsometatarsal, single joint

28750 Arthrodesis, great toe; metatarsophalangeal joint

28755 interphalangeal joint

28760 Arthrodesis, with extensor hallucis longus transfer to first metatarsal neck, great toe, interphalangeal joint (eg, Jones type procedure)

(For hammertoe operation or interphalangeal fusion, use 28285)

AMPUTATION

28800 Amputation, foot; midtarsal (eg, Chopart type procedure)

28805 transmetatarsal

28810 Amputation, metatarsal, with toe, single

28820 Amputation, toe; metatarsophalangeal joint

28825 interphalangeal joint

(For amputation of tuft of distal phalanx, use 11752)

OTHER PROCEDURES

(For extracorporeal shock wave therapy involving musculoskeletal system, or plantar fascia, see Category III codes 0019T, 0020T)

28899 Unlisted procedure, foot or toes

APPLICATION OF CASTS AND STRAPPING

CPT codes in this section are used only when the cast application or strapping is a replacement procedure performed during or after the period of follow-up care. An additional evaluation and management service code, dependent on location, is reportable only if significant identifiable other services are provided at the time of the cast application or strapping.

For coding cast or strap application in situations not involving surgery, for example, casting of a sprained ankle or knee, use the appropriate level of

● New Code   ▲ Revised Code   * Starred Procedure   + Add-On Code   ⊘ Modifier -51 Exempt

evaluation and management services code plus code 99070 or equivalent HCPCS Level II code to report casting materials.

APPLICATION OF CASTS AND STRAPPING

(For orthotics fitting and training, use 97504)

BODY AND UPPER EXTREMITY

Casts

29000	Application of halo type body cast (see 20661-20663 for insertion)
29010	Application of Risser jacket, localizer, body; only
29015	including head
29020	Application of turnbuckle jacket, body; only
29025	including head
29035	Application of body cast, shoulder to hips;
29040	including head, Minerva type
29044	including one thigh
29046	including both thighs
▲ **29049**	Application, cast; figure-of-eight
29055	shoulder spica
29058	plaster Velpeau
29065	shoulder to hand (long arm)
29075	elbow to finger (short arm)
29085	hand and lower forearm (gauntlet)
● **29086**	finger (eg, contracture)

Splints

29105   Application of long arm splint (shoulder to hand)

29125   Application of short arm splint (forearm to hand); static

29126   dynamic

29130   Application of finger splint; static

29131   dynamic

Strapping - Any Age

29200   Strapping; thorax

29220   low back

29240   shoulder (eg, Velpeau)

29260   elbow or wrist

29280   hand or finger

LOWER EXTREMITY

Casts

29305   Application of hip spica cast; one leg

29325   one and one-half spica or both legs

       (For hip spica (body) cast, including thighs only, use 29046)

29345   Application of long leg cast (thigh to toes);

29355   walker or ambulatory type

29358   Application of long leg cast brace

29365   Application of cylinder cast (thigh to ankle)

29405   Application of short leg cast (below knee to toes);

29425   walking or ambulatory type

29435 Application of patellar tendon bearing (PTB) cast

29440 Adding walker to previously applied cast

29445 Application of rigid total contact leg cast

29450 Application of clubfoot cast with molding or manipulation, long or short leg

Splints

29505 Application of long leg splint (thigh to ankle or toes)

29515 Application of short leg splint (calf to foot)

Strapping - Any Age

29520 Strapping; hip

29530 knee

29540 ankle

29550 toes

29580 Unna boot

29590 Denis-Browne splint strapping

REMOVAL OR REPAIR

29700 Removal or bivalving; gauntlet, boot or body cast

29705 full arm or full leg cast

29710 shoulder or hip spica, Minerva, or Risser jacket, etc.

29715 turnbuckle jacket

29720 Repair of spica, body cast or jacket

29730 Windowing of cast

29740 Wedging of cast (except clubfoot casts)

 Separate Procedure   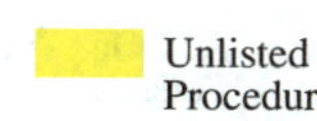 Unlisted Procedure   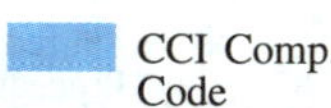 CCI Comp. Code   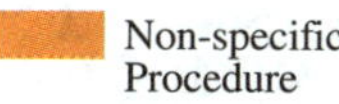 Non-specific Procedure

| 29750 | Wedging of clubfoot cast |

OTHER PROCEDURES

| 29799 | Unlisted procedure, casting or strapping |

ENDOSCOPY/ARTHROSCOPY

Surgical arthroscopy always includes a diagnostic arthroscopy and is therefore never reported in addition to the surgical procedure. However, there are several arthroscopy procedures defined as separate procedures, indicating that the codes may be reported if the diagnostic arthroscopy is the only procedure performed.

| 29800 | Arthroscopy, temporomandibular joint, diagnostic, with or without synovial biopsy (separate procedure) |

| 29804 | Arthroscopy, temporomandibular joint, surgical |

(For open procedure, use 21010)

● **29805**   Arthroscopy, shoulder, diagnostic, with or without synovial biopsy (separate procedure)

(For open procedure, see 23065-23066, 23100-23101)

● **29806**   Arthroscopy, shoulder, surgical; capsulorrhaphy

(For open procedure, see 23450-23466)

(To report thermal capsulorrhaphy, use 29999)

● **29807**   repair of slap lesion

(29815   deleted 2002 edition. To report, use 29805)

| 29819 | Arthroscopy, shoulder, surgical; with removal of loose body or foreign body |

(For open procedure, see 23040-23044, 23107)

| 29820 | synovectomy, partial |

(For open procedure, see 23105)

| 29821 | synovectomy, complete |

● New Code   ▲ Revised Code   ✳ Starred Procedure   ✚ Add-On Code   ⊘ Modifier -51 Exempt

(For open procedure, see 23105)

29822   debridement, limited

(For open procedure, see specific open shoulder procedure performed)

29823   debridement, extensive

(For open procedure, see specific open shoulder procedure performed)

● **29824**   distal claviculectomy including distal articular surface (Mumford procedure)

(For open procedure, use 23120)

29825   with lysis and resection of adhesions, with or without manipulation

(For open procedure, see specific open shoulder procedure performed)

29826   decompression of subacromial space with partial acromioplasty, with or without coracoacromial release

(For open procedure, use 23130 or 23415)

29830   Arthroscopy, elbow, diagnostic, with or without synovial biopsy (separate procedure)

29834   Arthroscopy, elbow, surgical; with removal of loose body or foreign body

29835   synovectomy, partial

29836   synovectomy, complete

29837   debridement, limited

29838   debridement, extensive

29840   Arthroscopy, wrist, diagnostic, with or without synovial biopsy (separate procedure)

29843   Arthroscopy, wrist, surgical; for infection, lavage and drainage

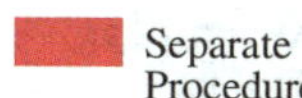 Separate Procedure   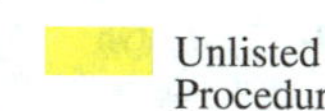 Unlisted Procedure   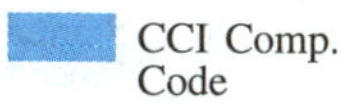 CCI Comp. Code   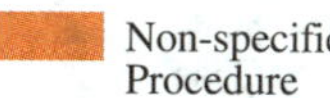 Non-specific Procedure

29844   synovectomy, partial

29845   synovectomy, complete

29846   excision and/or repair of triangular fibrocartilage and/or joint debridement

29847   internal fixation for fracture or instability

29848   Endoscopy, wrist, surgical, with release of transverse carpal ligament

(For open procedure, use 64721)

29850   Arthroscopically aided treatment of intercondylar spine(s) and/or tuberosity fracture(s) of the knee, with or without manipulation; without internal or external fixation (includes arthroscopy)

29851   with internal or external fixation (includes arthroscopy)

(For bone graft, use 20900, 20902)

29855   Arthroscopically aided treatment of tibial fracture, proximal (plateau); nicondylar, with or without internal or external fixation (includes arthroscopy)

29856   bicondylar, with or without internal or external fixation (includes arthroscopy)

(For bone graft, use 20900, 20902)

29860   Arthroscopy, hip, diagnostic with or without synovial biopsy (separate procedure)

29861   Arthroscopy, hip, surgical; with removal of loose body or foreign body

29862   with debridement/shaving of articular cartilage (chondroplasty), abrasion arthroplasty, and/or resection of labrum

29863   with synovectomy

29870   Arthroscopy, knee, diagnostic, with or without synovial biopsy (separate procedure)

● New Code   ▲ Revised Code   ✱ Starred Procedure   + Add-On Code   ⦰ Modifier -51 Exempt

(For surgical arthroscopy of the knee with implantation of osteochondral graft for treatment of articular surface defect, see Category III codes 0012T, 0013T)

(For meniscal transplantation, medial or lateral, knee, use Category III code 0014T)

29871 Arthroscopy, knee, surgical; for infection, lavage and drainage

29874 for removal of loose body or foreign body (eg, osteochondritis dissecans fragmentation, chondral fragmentation)

29875 synovectomy, limited (eg, plica or shelf resection) (separate procedure)

29876 synovectomy, major, two or more compartments (eg, medial or lateral)

29877 debridement/shaving of articular cartilage (chondroplasty)

29879 abrasion arthroplasty (includes chondroplasty where necessary) or multiple drilling or microfracture

29880 with meniscectomy (medial AND lateral, including any meniscal shaving)

29881 with meniscectomy (medial OR lateral, including any meniscal shaving)

29882 with meniscus repair (medial OR lateral)

29883 with meniscus repair (medial AND lateral)

29884 with lysis of adhesions, with or without manipulation (separate procedure)

29885 drilling for osteochondritis dissecans with bone grafting, with or without internal fixation (including debridement of base of lesion)

29886 drilling for intact osteochondritis dissecans lesion

29887 drilling for intact osteochondritis dissecans lesion with internal fixation

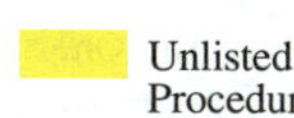 Separate Procedure

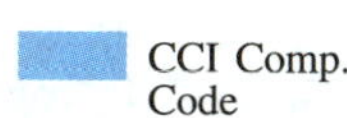 Unlisted Procedure

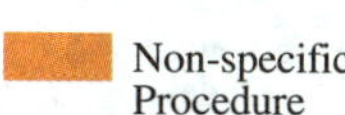 CCI Comp. Code

Non-specific Procedure

29888   Arthroscopically aided anterior cruciate ligament repair/augmentation or reconstruction

29889   Arthroscopically aided posterior cruciate ligament repair/augmentation or reconstruction

(Procedures 29888 and 29889 should not be used with reconstruction procedures 27427-27429)

29891   Arthroscopy, ankle, surgical; excision of osteochondral defect of talus and/or tibia, including drilling of the defect

29892   Arthroscopically aided repair of large osteochondritis dissecans lesion, talar dome fracture, or tibial plafond fracture, with or without internal fixation (includes arthroscopy)

29893   Endoscopic plantar fasciotomy

29894   Arthroscopy, ankle (tibiotalar and fibulotalar joints), surgical; with removal of loose body or foreign body

29895   synovectomy, partial

29897   debridement, limited

29898   debridement, extensive

● **29900**   Arthroscopy, metacarpophalangeal joint, diagnostic, includes synovial biopsy

(Do not report 29900 with 29901, 29902)

● **29901**   Arthroscopy, metacarpophalangeal joint, surgical; with debridement

● **29902**   with reduction of displaced ulnar collateral ligament (eg, Stenar lesion)

(29909   deleted 2002 edition. To report, use 29999)

● **29999**   Unlisted procedure, arthroscopy

● New Code   ▲ Revised Code   * Starred Procedure   + Add-On Code   ⊘ Modifier -51 Exempt

RESPIRATORY SYSTEM

CPT codes from this section of the CPT coding system are used to report invasive and surgical procedures performed on the nose, sinuses, larynx, trachea and bronchi, and the lungs and pleura.

MISCELLANEOUS CODING RULES

Functional Endoscopic Sinus Surgery (FESS) codes are coded based on the procedures described in the operative report or on the nasal sinus endoscopy report. Each FESS code represents a unilateral procedure. To express that a procedure was performed bilaterally requires the application of the modifier -50, bilateral procedure.

Indirect laryngoscopy involves the visualization of the larynx using a warm laryngeal mirror positioned at the back of the throat. Direct laryngoscopy involves the visualization using a rigid or fiberoptic endoscope. Operative direct laryngoscopy involves an endoscopic examination under general anesthesia.

To code nasal hemorrhages appropriately, documentation needs to substantiate whether the hemorrhage is anterior or posterior and how the hemorrhage is controlled. Control of anterior nasal hemorrhage typically involves the insertion of gauze packing, or anterior packing or performance of cauterization. Control of posterior nasal hemorrhage most likely requires the insertion of nasal stents, tampons, balloon catheters, or posterior packing.

STARRED PROCEDURES

There are numerous starred (*) procedures in this section of the CPT coding system indicating the possibility of reporting an appropriate evaluation and management service code in addition to the surgical procedure. When coding endoscopic procedures from this section of the CPT coding system, code the appropriate endoscopy of each anatomic site examined.

NOSE

INCISION

***30000** Drainage abscess or hematoma, nasal, internal approach

(For external approach, see 10060, 10140)

***30020** Drainage abscess or hematoma, nasal septum

(For lateral rhinotomy, see specific application (eg, 30118, 30320))

 Separate Procedure

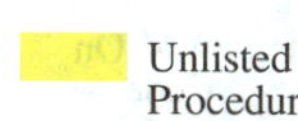 Unlisted Procedure

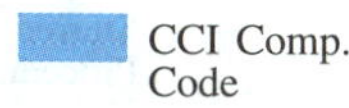 CCI Comp. Code

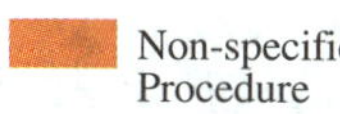 Non-specific Procedure

361

EXCISION

30100   Biopsy, intranasal

(For biopsy skin of nose, see 11100, 11101)

30110   Excision, nasal polyp(s), simple

(30110 would normally be completed in an office setting)

30115   Excision, nasal polyp(s), extensive

(30115 would normally require the facilities available in a hospital setting)

▲ **30117**   Excision or destruction (eg, laser), intranasal lesion; internal approach

30118   external approach (lateral rhinotomy)

30120   Excision or surgical planing of skin of nose for rhinophyma

30124   Excision dermoid cyst, nose; simple, skin, subcutaneous

30125   complex, under bone or cartilage

30130   Excision turbinate, partial or complete, any method

30140   Submucous resection turbinate, partial or complete, any method

(For submucous resection of nasal septum, use 30520)

(For reduction of turbinates, use 30140 with modifier -52)

30150   Rhinectomy; partial

30160   total

(For closure and/or reconstruction, primary or delayed, see Integumentary System, 13150-13160, 14060-14300, 15120, 15121, 15260, 15261, 15760, 20900-20912)

INTRODUCTION

***30200**   Injection into turbinate(s), therapeutic

***30210**   Displacement therapy (Proetz type)

● New Code   ▲ Revised Code   * Starred Procedure   ＋ Add-On Code   ⊘ Modifier -51 Exempt

30220 Insertion, nasal septal prosthesis (button)

REMOVAL OF FOREIGN BODY

***30300** Removal foreign body, intranasal; office type procedure

30310 requiring general anesthesia

30320 by lateral rhinotomy

REPAIR

(For obtaining tissues for graft, see 20900-20926, 21210)

30400 Rhinoplasty, primary; lateral and alar cartilages and/or elevation of nasal tip

(For columellar reconstruction, see 13150 et seq)

30410 complete, external parts including bony pyramid, lateral and alar cartilages, and/or elevation of nasal tip

30420 including major septal repair

30430 Rhinoplasty, secondary; minor revision (small amount of nasal tip work)

30435 intermediate revision (bony work with osteotomies)

30450 major revision (nasal tip work and osteotomies)

30460 Rhinoplasty for nasal deformity secondary to congenital cleft lip and/or palate, including columellar lengthening; tip only

30462 tip, septum, osteotomies

30465 Repair of nasal vestibular stenosis (eg, spreader grafting, lateral nasal wall reconstruction)

(30465 excludes obtaining graft. For graft procedure, see 20900-20926, 21210)

(30465 is used to report a bilateral procedure. For unilateral procedure, use modifier -52)

30520 Septoplasty or submucous resection, with or without cartilage scoring, contouring or replacement with graft

---

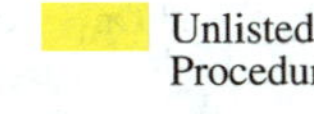

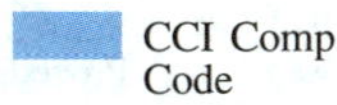

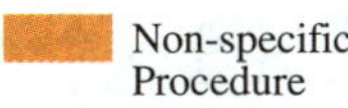

Non-specific
Procedure

363

(For submucous resection of turbinates, use 30140)

30540 Repair choanal atresia; intranasal

30545 transpalatine

***30560** Lysis intranasal synechia

30580 Repair fistula; oromaxillary (combine with 31030 if antrotomy is included)

30600 oronasal

30620 Septal or other intranasal dermatoplasty (does not include obtaining graft)

30630 Repair nasal septal perforations

DESTRUCTION

▲ ***30801** Cautery and/or ablation, mucosa of turbinates, unilateral or bilateral, any method, (separate procedure); superficial

30802 intramural

OTHER PROCEDURES

***30901** Control nasal hemorrhage, anterior, simple (limited cautery and/or packing) any method

***30903** Control nasal hemorrhage, anterior, complex (extensive cautery and/or packing) any method

▲ ***30905** Control nasal hemorrhage, posterior, with posterior nasal packs and/or cautery, any method; initial

***30906** subsequent

30915 Ligation arteries; ethmoidal

30920 internal maxillary artery, transantral

(For ligation external carotid artery, use 37600)

30930 Fracture nasal turbinate(s), therapeutic

● New Code   ▲ Revised Code   * Starred Procedure   + Add-On Code   ⊘ Modifier -51 Exempt

30999   Unlisted procedure, nose

ACCESSORY SINUSES

INCISION

***31000**   Lavage by cannulation; maxillary sinus (antrum puncture or natural ostium)

***31002**   sphenoid sinus

31020   Sinusotomy, maxillary (antrotomy); intranasal

31030   radical (Caldwell-Luc) without removal of antrochoanal polyps

31032   radical (Caldwell-Luc) with removal of antrochoanal polyps

31040   Pterygomaxillary fossa surgery, any approach

(For transantral ligation of internal maxillary artery, use 30920)

31050   Sinusotomy, sphenoid, with or without biopsy;

31051   with mucosal stripping or removal of polyp(s)

31070   Sinusotomy frontal; external, simple (trephine operation)

31075   transorbital, unilateral (for mucocele or osteoma, Lynch type)

31080   obliterative without osteoplastic flap, brow incision (includes ablation)

31081   obliterative, without osteoplastic flap, coronal incision (includes ablation)

31084   obliterative, with osteoplastic flap, brow incision

31085   obliterative, with osteoplastic flap, coronal incision

31086   nonobliterative, with osteoplastic flap, brow incision

31087   nonobliterative, with osteoplastic flap, coronal incision

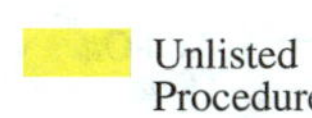 Separate Procedure   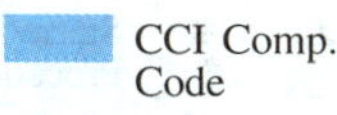 Unlisted Procedure   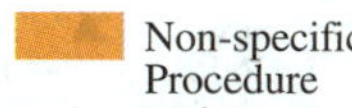 CCI Comp. Code   Non-specific Procedure

365

31090	Sinusotomy, unilateral, three or more paranasal sinuses (frontal, maxillary, ethmoid, sphenoid)

EXCISION

31200	Ethmoidectomy; intranasal, anterior
31201	intranasal, total
31205	extranasal, total
31225	Maxillectomy; without orbital exenteration
31230	with orbital exenteration (en bloc)

(For orbital exenteration only, see 65110 et seq)

(For skin graft, see 15120 et seq)

ENDOSCOPY

31231	Nasal endoscopy, diagnostic, unilateral or bilateral (separate procedure)
31233	Nasal/sinus endoscopy, diagnostic with maxillary sinusoscopy (via inferior meatus or canine fossa puncture)
31235	Nasal/sinus endoscopy, diagnostic with sphenoid sinusoscopy (via puncture of sphenoidal face or cannulation of ostium)
31237	Nasal/sinus endoscopy, surgical; with biopsy, polypectomy or debridement (separate procedure)
▲ **31238**	with control of nasal hemorrhage
31239	with dacryocystorhinostomy
31240	with concha bullosa resection
31254	with ethmoidectomy, partial (anterior)
31255	with ethmoidectomy, total (anterior andposterior)
31256	Nasal/sinus endoscopy, surgical, with maxillary antrostomy;
31267	with removal of tissue from maxillary sinus

● New Code ▲ Revised Code ✱ Starred Procedure ✚ Add-On Code ⊘ Modifier -51 Exempt

31276   Nasal/sinus endoscopy, surgical with frontal sinus exploration, with or without removal of tissue from frontal sinus

31287   Nasal/sinus endoscopy, surgical, with sphenoidotomy;

31288   with removal of tissue from the sphenoid sinus

31290   Nasal/sinus endoscopy, surgical, with repair of cerebrospinal fluid leak; ethmoid region

31291   sphenoid region

31292   Nasal/sinus endoscopy, surgical; with medial or inferior orbital wall decompression

31293   with medial orbital wall and inferior orbital wall decompression

31294   with optic nerve decompression

OTHER PROCEDURES

(For hypophysectomy, transantral or transeptal approach, use 61548)

(For transcranial hypophysectomy, use 61546)

31299   Unlisted procedure, accessory sinuses

LARYNX

EXCISION

31300   Laryngotomy (thyrotomy, laryngofissure); with removal of tumor or laryngocele, cordectomy

31320   diagnostic

31360   Laryngectomy; total, without radical neck dissection

31365   total, with radical neck dissection

31367   subtotal supraglottic, without radical neck dissection

31368   subtotal supraglottic, with radical neck dissection

31370   Partial laryngectomy (hemilaryngectomy); horizontal

31375 laterovertical

31380 anterovertical

31382 antero-latero-vertical

31390 Pharyngolaryngectomy, with radical neck dissection; without reconstruction

31395 with reconstruction

31400 Arytenoidectomy or arytenoidopexy, external approach

(For endoscopic arytenoidecomy, use 31560)

31420 Epiglottidectomy

INTRODUCTION

⊘ **31500** Intubation, endotracheal, emergency procedure

(For injection procedure for bronchography, see 31656, 31708, 31710)

31502 Tracheotomy tube change prior to establishment of fistula tract

ENDOSCOPY

31505 Laryngoscopy, indirect; diagnostic (separate procedure)

31510 with biopsy

31511 with removal of foreign body

31512 with removal of lesion

31513 with vocal cord injection

31515 Laryngoscopy direct, with or without tracheoscopy; for aspiration

31520 diagnostic, newborn

31525 diagnostic, except newborn

31526 diagnostic, with operating microscope

● New Code   ▲ Revised Code   ✳ Starred Procedure   ＋ Add-On Code   ⊘ Modifier -51 Exempt

(Do not report code 69990 in addition to code 31526)

31527   with insertion of obturator

▲ **31528**   with dilation, initial

▲ **31529**   with dilation, subsequent

31530   Laryngoscopy, direct, operative, with foreign body removal;

31531   with operating microscope

(Do not report code 69990 in addition to code 31531)

31535   Laryngoscopy, direct, operative, with biopsy;

31536   with operating microscope

(Do not report code 69990 in addition to code 31536)

31540   Laryngoscopy, direct, operative, with excision of tumor and/or strippingof vocal cords or epiglottis;

31541   with operating microscope

(Do not report code 69990 in addition to code 31541)

31560   Laryngoscopy, direct, operative, with arytenoidectomy;

31561   with operating microscope

(Do not report code 69990 in addition to code 31561)

31570   Laryngoscopy, direct, with injection into vocal cord(s), therapeutic;

31571   with operating microscope

(Do not report code 69990 in addition to code 31571)

31575   Laryngoscopy, flexible fiberoptic; diagnostic

31576   with biopsy

31577   with removal of foreign body

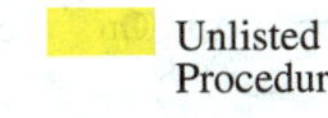

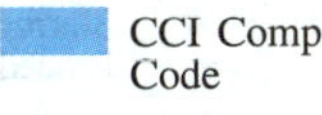

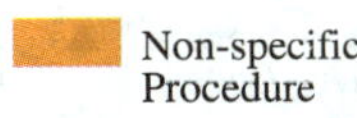

31578   with removal of lesion

31579   Laryngoscopy, flexible or rigid fiberoptic, with stroboscopy

REPAIR

31580   Laryngoplasty; for laryngeal web, two stage, with keel insertion and removal

31582   for laryngeal stenosis, with graft or core mold, including tracheotomy

31584   with open reduction of fracture

31585   Treatment of closed laryngeal fracture; without manipulation

31586   with closed manipulative reduction

31587   Laryngoplasty, cricoid split

31588   Laryngoplasty, not otherwise specified (eg, for burns, reconstruction after partial laryngectomy)

31590   Laryngeal reinnervation by neuromuscular pedicle

DESTRUCTION

31595   Section recurrent laryngeal nerve, therapeutic (separate procedure), unilateral

OTHER PROCEDURES

31599   Unlisted procedure, larynx

TRACHEA AND BRONCHI

INCISION

31600   Tracheostomy, planned (separate procedure);

31601   under two years

31603   Tracheostomy, emergency procedure; transtracheal

31605   cricothyroid membrane

● New Code   ▲ Revised Code   * Starred Procedure   + Add-On Code   ⊘ Modifier -51 Exempt

31610 Tracheostomy, fenestration procedure with skin flaps

(For endotracheal intubation, use 31500)

(For tracheal aspiration under direct vision, use 31515)

31611 Construction of tracheoesophageal fistula and subsequent insertion of an alaryngeal speech prosthesis (eg, voice button, Blom-Singer prosthesis)

31612 Tracheal puncture, percutaneous with transtracheal aspiration and/or injection

31613 Tracheostoma revision; simple, without flap rotation

31614 complex, with flap rotation

ENDOSCOPY

(For tracheoscopy, see laryngoscopy codes 31515-31578)

31615 Tracheobronchoscopy through established tracheostomy incision

31622 Bronchoscopy, (rigid or flexible); diagnostic, with or without cell washing (separate procedure)

31623 with brushing or protected brushings

31624 with bronchial alveolar lavage

31625 with biopsy

31628 with transbronchial lung biopsy, with or without fluoroscopic guidance

31629 with transbronchial needle aspiration biopsy

31630 with tracheal or bronchial dilation or closed reduction of fracture

31631 with tracheal dilation and placement of tracheal stent

31635 with removal of foreign body

31640 with excision of tumor

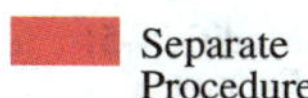
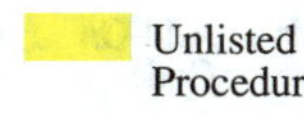
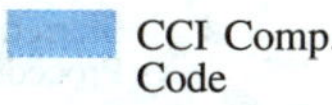
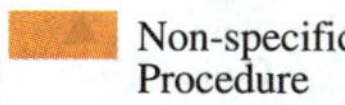

371

▲ **31641** Bronchoscopy, (rigid or flexible); with destruction of tumor or relief of stenosis by any method other than excision (eg, laser therapy, cryotherapy)

(For bronchoscopic photodynamic therapy, report 31641 in addition to 96570, 96571 as appropriate)

31643 with placement of catheter(s) for intracavitary radioelement application

(For intracavitary radioelement application, see 77761-77763, 77781-77784)

31645 with therapeutic aspiration of tracheobronchial tree, initial (eg, drainage of lung abscess)

31646 with therapeutic aspiration of tracheobronchial tree, subsequent

(For catheter aspiration of tracheobronchial tree at bedside, use 31725)

31656 with injection of contrast material for segmental bronchography (fiberscope only)

(For radiological supervision and interpretation, see 71040, 71060)

INTRODUCTION

(For endotracheal intubation, use 31500)

(For tracheal aspiration under direct vision, see 31515)

31700 Catheterization, transglottic (separate procedure)

31708 Instillation of contrast material for laryngography or bronchography, without catheterization

(For radiological supervision and interpretation, see 70373, 71040, 71060)

31710 Catheterization for bronchography, with or without instillation of contrast material

(For bronchoscopic catheterization for bronchography, fiberscope only, use 31656)

(For radiological supervision and interpretation, see 71040, 71060)

● New Code   ▲ Revised Code   ✻ Starred Procedure   ✛ Add-On Code   ⊘ Modifier -51 Exempt

31715   Transtracheal injection for bronchography

(For radiological supervision and interpretation, see 71040, 71060)

(For prolonged services, see 99354-99360)

31717   Catheterization with bronchial brush biopsy

31720   Catheter aspiration (separate procedure); nasotracheal

31725   tracheobronchial with fiberscope, bedside

31730   Transtracheal (percutaneous) introduction of needle wire dilator/stent or indwelling tube for oxygen therapy

REPAIR

31750   Tracheoplasty; cervical

31755   tracheopharyngeal fistulization, each stage

31760   intrathoracic

31766   Carinal reconstruction

31770   Bronchoplasty; graft repair

31775   excision stenosis and anastomosis

(For lobectomy and bronchoplasty, use 32501)

31780   Excision tracheal stenosis and anastomosis; cervical

31781   cervicothoracic

31785   Excision of tracheal tumor or carcinoma; cervical

31786   thoracic

31800   Suture of tracheal wound or injury; cervical

31805   intrathoracic

31820   Surgical closure tracheostomy or fistula; without plastic repair

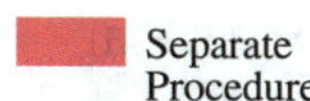 Separate Procedure   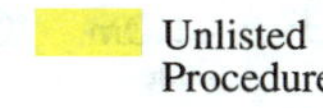 Unlisted Procedure   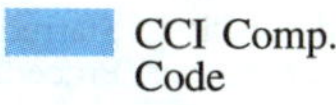 CCI Comp. Code   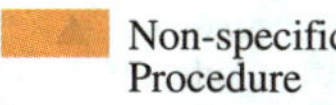 Non-specific Procedure

31825	with plastic repair

(For repair tracheoesophageal fistula, see 43305, 43312)

31830	Revision of tracheostomy scar

OTHER PROCEDURES

31899	Unlisted procedure, trachea, bronchi

LUNGS AND PLEURA

INCISION

⊘*32000	Thoracentesis, puncture of pleural cavity for aspiration, initial or subsequent

(If imaging guidance is performed, see 76003, 76360, 76942)

⊘ 32002	Thoracentesis with insertion of tube with or without water seal (eg, for pneumothorax) (separate procedure)

(If imaging guidance is performed, see 76003, 76360, 76942)

32005	Chemical pleurodesis (eg, for recurrent or persistent pneumothorax)

⊘ 32020	Tube thoracostomy with or without water seal (eg, for abscess, hemothorax, empyema) (separate procedure)

(If imaging guidance is performed, use 75989)

32035	Thoracostomy; with rib resection for empyema

32036	with open flap drainage for empyema

32095	Thoracotomy, limited, for biopsy of lung or pleura

(To report wound exploration due to penetrating trauma without thoractomy, use 20102)

32100	Thoracotomy, major; with exploration and biopsy

32110	with control of traumatic hemorrhage and/or repair of lung tear

32120	for postoperative complications

● New Code   ▲ Revised Code   * Starred Procedure   + Add-On Code   ⊘ Modifier -51 Exempt

32124	with open intrapleural pneumonolysis
32140	with cyst(s) removal, with or without a pleural procedure
32141	with excision-plication of bullae, with or without any pleural procedure

(For lung volume reduction, use 32491)

32150	with removal of intrapleural foreign body or fibrin deposit
32151	with removal of intrapulmonary foreign body
32160	with cardiac massage

(For segmental or other resections of lung, see 32480-32525)

32200	Pneumonostomy; with open drainage of abscess or cyst
32201	with percutaneous drainage of abscess or cyst

(For radiological supervision and interpretation, use 75989)

32215	Pleural scarification for repeat pneumothorax
32220	Decortication, pulmonary (separate procedure); total
32225	partial

EXCISION

32310	Pleurectomy, parietal (separate procedure)
32320	Decortication and parietal pleurectomy
***32400**	Biopsy, pleura; percutaneous needle

(If imaging guidance is performed, see 76003, 76360, 76393, 76942)

(For fine needle aspiration, use 10021 or 10022)

(For evaluation of fine needle aspirate, see 88172, 88173)

32402	open
32405	Biopsy, lung or mediastinum, percutaneous needle

■ Separate Procedure	■ Unlisted Procedure	■ CCI Comp. Code	■ Non-specific Procedure

(For radiological supervision and interpretation, see 76003, 76360, 76393, 76942)

(For fine needle aspiration, use 10022)

(For evaluation of fine needle aspirate, see 88172, 88173)

▲ *32420   Pneumocentesis, puncture of lung for aspiration

32440   Removal of lung, total pneumonectomy;

32442   with resection of segment of trachea followed by broncho-tracheal anastomosis (sleeve pneumonectomy)

32445   extrapleural

32480   Removal of lung, other than total pneumonectomy; single lobe (lobectomy)

32482   two lobes (bilobectomy)

32484   single segment (segmentectomy)

32486   with circumferential resection of segment of bronchus followed by broncho-bronchial anastomosis (sleeve lobectomy)

32488   all remaining lung following previous removal of a portion of lung (completion pneumonectomy)

32491   excision-plication of emphysematous lung(s) (bullous or non-bullous) for lung volume reduction, sternal split or transthoracic approach, with or without any pleural procedure

32500   wedge resection, single or multiple

+32501   Resection and repair of portion of bronchus (bronchoplasty) when performed at time of lobectomy or segmentectomy (List separately in addition to code for primary procedure)

(Use 32501 in conjunction with codes 32480, 32482, 32484)

(32501 is to be used when a portion of the bronchus to preserved lung is removed and requires plastic closure to preserve function of that preserved lung. It is not to be used for closure for the proximal end of a resected bronchus.)

● New Code   ▲ Revised Code   ✳ Starred Procedure   ✚ Add-On Code   ⊘ Modifier -51 Exempt

| 32520 | Resection of lung; with resection of chest wall |

| 32522 | with reconstruction of chest wall, without prosthesis |

| 32525 | with major reconstruction of chest wall, with prosthesis |

| 32540 | Extrapleural enucleation of empyema (empyemectomy) |

ENDOSCOPY

| 32601 | Thoracoscopy, diagnostic (separate procedure); lungs and pleural space, without biopsy |

| 32602 | lungs and pleural space, with biopsy |

| 32603 | pericardial sac, without biopsy |

| 32604 | pericardial sac, with biopsy |

| 32605 | mediastinal space, without biopsy |

| 32606 | mediastinal space, with biopsy |

(Surgical thoracoscopy always includes diagnostic thoracoscopy)

| ▲ 32650 | Thoracoscopy, surgical; with pleurodesis (eg, mechanical or chemical) |

| 32651 | with partial pulmonary decortication |

| 32652 | with total pulmonary decortication, including intrapleural pneumonolysis |

| 32653 | with removal of intrapleural foreign body or fibrin deposit |

| 32654 | with control of traumatic hemorrhage |

| 32655 | with excision-plication of bullae, including any pleural procedure |

| 32656 | with parietal pleurectomy |

| 32657 | with wedge resection of lung, single or multiple |

| 32658 | with removal of clot or foreign body from pericardial sac |

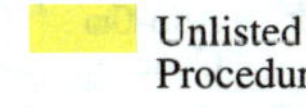
Separate
Procedure

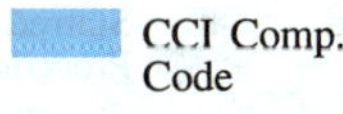
Unlisted
Procedure

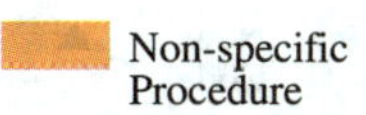
CCI Comp.
Code

Non-specific
Procedure

377

32659	with creation of pericardial window or partial resection of pericardial sac for drainage
32660	with total pericardiectomy
32661	with excision of pericardial cyst, tumor, or mass
32662	with excision of mediastinal cyst, tumor, or mass
32663	with lobectomy, total or segmental
32664	with thoracic sympathectomy
32665	with esophagomyotomy (Heller type)

REPAIR

32800	Repair lung hernia through chest wall
32810	Closure of chest wall following open flap drainage for empyema (Clagett type procedure)
32815	Open closure of major bronchial fistula
32820	Major reconstruction, chest wall (posttraumatic)

LUNG TRANSPLANTATION

32850	Donor pneumonectomy(ies) with preparation and maintenance of allograft (cadaver)
32851	Lung transplant, single; without cardiopulmonary bypass
32852	with cardiopulmonary bypass
32853	Lung transplant, double (bilateral sequential or en bloc); without cardiopulmonary bypass
32854	with cardiopulmonary bypass

SURGICAL COLLAPSE THERAPY; THORACOPLASTY

(See also 32520-32525)

32900	Resection of ribs, extrapleural, all stages

● New Code   ▲ Revised Code   ✳ Starred Procedure   ✚ Add-On Code   ⊘ Modifier -51 Exempt

32905   Thoracoplasty, Schede type or extrapleural (all stages);

32906   with closure of bronchopleural fistula

(For open closure of major bronchial fistula, use 32815)

(For resection of first rib for thoracic outlet compression, see 21615, 21616)

32940   Pneumonolysis, extraperiosteal, including filling or packing procedures

***32960**   Pneumothorax, therapeutic, intrapleural injection of air

OTHER PROCEDURES

32997   Total lung lavage (unilateral)

(For bronchoscopic bronchial alveolar lavage, use 31624)

32999   Unlisted procedure, lungs and pleura

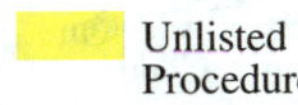

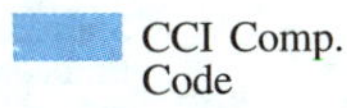

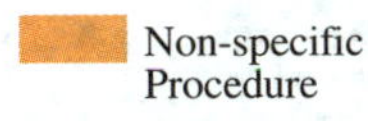

Non-specific
Procedure

CARDIOVASCULAR SYSTEM

CPT codes from this section of the CPT coding system are used to report invasive and surgical procedures performed on the heart and pericardium, including pacemakers or defibrillators; cardiac valves; coronary arteries; aorta; and arteries and veins.

For coding services such as monitoring, operation of pump and other non-surgical services performed during cardiovascular surgery, see the Special Services CPT codes 99150, 99151, 99160-99162 or CPT codes 99291-99292 and 99190-99192 from the evaluation and management section of the CPT coding system.

MISCELLANEOUS CODING RULES

A pacemaker system includes a pulse generator containing electronics and a battery, and one or more electrodes (leads) inserted one of several ways. Pulse generators may be placed in a subcutaneous "pocket" created in either a subclavicular or intra-abdominal site. Electrodes may be inserted through a vein (transvenous) or on the surface of the heart (epicardial). A single chamber system includes a pulse generator and one electrode inserted into either the atrium or ventricle. A dual chamber system includes a pulse generator and one electrode inserted in the atrium and one electrode inserted in the ventricle.

Assign two CPT codes when a pacemaker or cardioverter-defibrillator "battery"/pulse generator is replaced. One code should describe the removal of the old pulse generator and the other should describe the insertion of the new pulse generator.

Cardiac catheterization codes are classified in the Medicine Section of the CPT coding system. Insertion of a dilator into a vein prior to the placement of a catheter should not be separately coded.

STARRED PROCEDURES

There are a few starred (*) procedures in this section of the CPT coding system indicating the possibility of reporting an appropriate evaluation and management service code in addition to the surgical procedure. In addition, the complexity of procedures in this section would frequently require the presence of multiple assistant surgeons, co-surgeons and/or surgical teams.

(For monitoring, operation of pump and other nonsurgical services, see 99190-99192, 99291, 99292, 99354-99360)

(For other medical or laboratory related services, see appropriate section)

(For radiological supervision and interpretation, see 75600-75978)

● New Code　　▲ Revised Code　　✳ Starred Procedure　　✚ Add-On Code　　⊘ Modifier -51 Exempt

HEART AND PERICARDIUM

PERICARDIUM

***33010** Pericardiocentesis; initial

(For radiological supervision and interpretation, use 76930)

***33011** subsequent

(For radiological supervision and interpretation, use 76930)

33015 Tube pericardiostomy

33020 Pericardiotomy for removal of clot or foreign body (primary procedure)

33025 Creation of pericardial window or partial resection for drainage

33030 Pericardiectomy, subtotal or complete; without cardiopulmonary bypass

33031 with cardiopulmonary bypass

33050 Excision of pericardial cyst or tumor

CARDIAC TUMOR

33120 Excision of intracardiac tumor, resection with cardiopulmonary bypass

33130 Resection of external cardiac tumor

TRANSMYOCARDIAL REVASCULARIZATION

33140 Transmyocardial laser revascularization, by thoracotomy (separate procedure)

+33141 performed at the time of other open cardiac procedure(s) (List separately in addition to code for primary procedure)

(Use 33141 in conjunction with codes 33400-33496, 33510-33536)

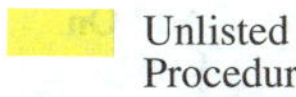
Separate Procedure

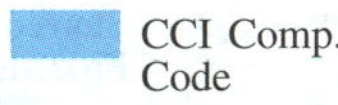
Unlisted Procedure

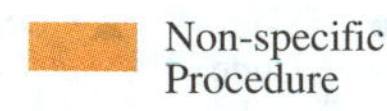
CCI Comp. Code

Non-specific Procedure

PACEMAKER OR PACING CARDIOVERTER-DEFIBRILLATOR

(For electronic, telephonic analysis of internal pacemaker system, see 93731-93736)

(For radiological supervision and interpretation with insertion of pacemaker, use 71090)

33200 Insertion of permanent pacemaker with epicardial electrode(s); by thoracotomy

33201 by xiphoid approach

33206 Insertion or replacement of permanent pacemaker with transvenous electrode(s); atrial

33207 ventricular

33208 atrial and ventricular

(Codes 33206-33208 include subcutaneous insertion of the pulse generator and transvenous placement of electrode(s))

33210 Insertion or replacement of temporary transvenous single chamber cardiac electrode or pacemaker catheter (separate procedure)

33211 Insertion or replacement of temporary transvenous dual chamber pacing electrodes (separate procedure)

33212 Insertion or replacement of pacemaker pulse generator only; single chamber, atrial or ventricular

33213 dual chamber

33214 Upgrade of implanted pacemaker system, conversion of single chamber system to dual chamber system (includes removal of previously placed pulse generator, testing of existing lead, insertion of new lead, insertion of new pulse generator)

33216 Insertion or repositioning of a transvenous electrode (15 days or more after initial insertion); single chamber (one electrode) permanent pacemaker or single chamber pacing cardioverter-defibrillator

33217 dual chamber (two electrodes) permanent pacemaker or dual chamber pacing cardioverter-defibrillator

● New Code   ▲ Revised Code   ∗ Starred Procedure   + Add-On Code   ⊘ Modifier -51 Exempt

(Do not report 33216-33217 in conjunction with code 33214)

33218 Repair of single transvenous electrode for a single chamber, permanent pacemaker or single chamber pacing cardioverter-defibrillator

33220 Repair of two transvenous electrodes for a dual chamber permanent pacemaker or dual chamber pacing cardioverter-defibrillator

33222 Revision or relocation of skin pocket for pacemaker

33223 Revision of skin pocket for single or dual chamber pacing cardioverter-defibrillator

33233 Removal of permanent pacemaker pulse generator

33234 Removal of transvenous pacemaker electrode(s); single lead system, atrial or ventricular

33235   dual lead system

33236 Removal of permanent epicardial pacemaker and electrodes by thoracotomy; single lead system, atrial or ventricular

33237   dual lead system

33238 Removal of permanent transvenous electrode(s) by thoracotomy

33240 Insertion of single or dual chamber pacing cardioverter-defibrillator pulse generator

33241 Subcutaneous removal of single or dual chamber pacing cardioverter-defibrillator pulse generator

(For removal of electrode(s) by thoracotomy, use 33243 in conjunction with code 33241)

(For removal of electrode(s) by transvenous extraction, use 33244 in conjunction with code 33241)

(For removal and reinsertion of a pacing cardioverter-defibrillator system (pulse generator and electrodes), report 33241 and 33243 or 33244 and 33249)

33243 Removal of single or dual chamber pacing cardioverter-defibrillator electrode(s); by thoracotomy

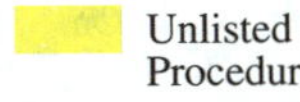

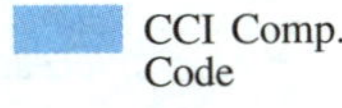

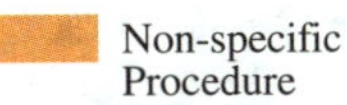

Non-specific
Procedure

383

33244   by transvenous extraction

(For subcutaneous removal of the pulse generator, use 33241 in conjunction with code 33243 or 33244)

33245   Insertion of epicardial single or dual chamber pacing cardioverter-defibrillator electrodes by thoracotomy;

33246   with insertion of pulse generator

33249   Insertion or repositioning of electrode lead(s) for single or dual chamber pacing cardioverter-defibrillator and insertion of pulse generator

(For removal and reinsertion of a pacing cardioverter-defibrillator system (pulse generator and electrodes), report 33241 and 33243 or 33244 and 33249)

ELECTROPHYSIOLOGIC OPERATIVE PROCEDURES

▲ **33250**   Operative ablation of supraventricular arrhythmogenic focus or pathway (eg, Wolff-Parkinson-White, atrioventricular node re-entry), tract(s) and/or focus (foci); without cardiopulmonary bypass

33251   with cardiopulmonary bypass

33253   Operative incisions and reconstruction of atria for treatment of atrial fibrillation or atrial flutter (eg, maze procedure)

33261   Operative ablation of ventricular arrhythmogenic focus with cardiopulmonary bypass

PATIENT-ACTIVATED EVENT RECORDER

33282   Implantation of patient-activated cardiac event recorder

(Initial implantation includes programming. For subsequent electronic analysis and/or reprogramming, use 93727)

33284   Removal of an implantable, patient-activated cardiac event recorder

WOUNDS OF THE HEART AND GREAT VESSELS

33300   Repair of cardiac wound; without bypass

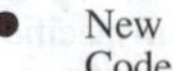

● New Code   ▲ Revised Code   * Starred Procedure   + Add-On Code   ⊘ Modifier -51 Exempt

| **33305** | with cardiopulmonary bypass |

| **33310** | Cardiotomy, exploratory (includes removal of foreign body); without bypass |

| **33315** | with cardiopulmonary bypass |

| **33320** | Suture repair of aorta or great vessels; without shunt or cardiopulmonary bypass |

| **33321** | with shunt bypass |

| **33322** | with cardiopulmonary bypass |

| **33330** | Insertion of graft, aorta or great vessels; without shunt, or cardiopulmonary bypass |

| **33332** | with shunt bypass |

| **33335** | with cardiopulmonary bypass |

CARDIAC VALVES

Aortic Valve

| **33400** | Valvuloplasty, aortic valve; open, with cardiopulmonary bypass |

| **33401** | open, with inflow occlusion |

| **33403** | using transventricular dilation, with cardiopulmonary bypass |

| **33404** | Construction of apical-aortic conduit |

| **33405** | Replacement, aortic valve, with cardiopulmonary bypass; with prosthetic valve other than homograft or stentless valve |

| ▲ **33406** | with allograft valve (freehand) |

| **33410** | with stentless tissue valve |

| **33411** | Replacement, aortic valve; with aortic annulus enlargement, noncoronary cusp |

| **33412** | with transventricular aortic annulus enlargement (Konno procedure) |

385

▲ **33413**   by translocation of autologous pulmonary valve with allograft replacement of pulmonary valve (Ross procedure)

33414   Repair of left ventricular outflow tract obstruction by patch enlargement of the outflow tract

33415   Resection or incision of subvalvular tissue for discrete subvalvular aortic stenosis

33416   Ventriculomyotomy (-myectomy) for idiopathic hypertrophic subaortic stenosis (eg, asymmetric septal hypertrophy)

33417   Aortoplasty (gusset) for supravalvular stenosis

Mitral Valve

33420   Valvotomy, mitral valve; closed heart

33422   open heart, with cardiopulmonary bypass

33425   Valvuloplasty, mitral valve, with cardiopulmonary bypass;

33426   with prosthetic ring

33427   radical reconstruction, with or without ring

33430   Replacement, mitral valve, with cardiopulmonary bypass

Tricuspid Valve

33460   Valvectomy, tricuspid valve, with cardiopulmonary bypass

33463   Valvuloplasty, tricuspid valve; without ring insertion

33464   with ring insertion

33465   Replacement, tricuspid valve, with cardiopulmonary bypass

33468   Tricuspid valve repositioning and plication for Ebstein anomaly

Pulmonary Valve

33470   Valvotomy, pulmonary valve, closed heart; transventricular

33471   via pulmonary artery

● New Code   ▲ Revised Code   ✱ Starred Procedure   ✚ Add-On Code   ⊘ Modifier -51 Exempt

(To report percutaneous valvuloplasty of pulmonary valve, use 92990)

33472 Valvotomy, pulmonary valve, open heart; with inflow occlusion

33474   with cardiopulmonary bypass

33475 Replacement, pulmonary valve

33476 Right ventricular resection for infundibular stenosis, with or without commissurotomy

33478 Outflow tract augmentation (gusset), with or without commissurotomy or infundibular resection

OTHER VALVULAR PROCEDURES

33496 Repair of non-structural prosthetic valve dysfunction with cardiopulmonary bypass (separate procedure)

(For reoperation, use 33530 in addition to 33496)

CORONARY ARTERY ANOMALIES

33500 Repair of coronary arteriovenous or arteriocardiac chamber fistula; with cardiopulmonary bypass

33501   without cardiopulmonary bypass

33502 Repair of anomalous coronary artery; by ligation

33503   by graft, without cardiopulmonary bypass

33504   by graft, with cardiopulmonary bypass

33505   with construction of intrapulmonary artery tunnel (Takeuchi procedure)

33506   by translocation from pulmonary artery to aorta

VENOUS GRAFTING ONLY FOR CORONARY ARTERY BYPASS

33510 Coronary artery bypass, vein only; single coronary venous graft

33511   two coronary venous grafts

Separate Procedure

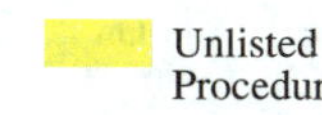
Unlisted Procedure

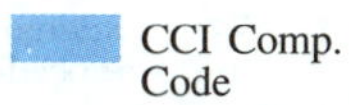
CCI Comp. Code

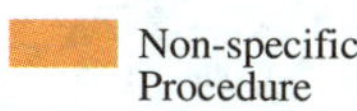
Non-specific Procedure

387

33512	three coronary venous grafts
33513	four coronary venous grafts
33514	five coronary venous grafts
33516	six or more coronary venous grafts

COMBINED ARTERIAL-VENOUS GRAFTING FOR CORONARY BYPASS

⊘ **33517** Coronary artery bypass, using venous graft(s) and arterial graft(s); single vein graft (List separately in addition to code for arterial graft)

⊘ **33518** two venous grafts (List separately in addition to code for arterial graft)

⊘ **33519** three venous grafts (List separately in addition to code for arterial graft)

⊘ **33521** four venous grafts (List separately in addition to code for arterial graft)

⊘ **33522** five venous grafts (List separately in addition to code for arterial graft)

⊘ **33523** six or more venous grafts (List separately in addition to code for arterial graft)

+**33530** Reoperation, coronary artery bypass procedure or valve procedure, more than one month after original operation (List separately in addition to code for primary procedure)

(Use 33530 in conjunction with codes 33400-33496; 33510-33536, 33863)

ARTERIAL GRAFTING FOR CORONARY ARTERY BYPASS

33533 Coronary artery bypass, using arterial graft(s); single arterial graft

33534 two coronary arterial grafts

33535 three coronary arterial grafts

33536 four or more coronary arterial grafts

388

• New Code	▲ Revised Code	✳ Starred Procedure	✚ Add-On Code	⊘ Modifier -51 Exempt

33542   Myocardial resection (eg, ventricular aneurysmectomy)

33545   Repair of postinfarction ventricular septal defect, with or without myocardial resection

CORONARY ENDARTERECTOMY

+33572   Coronary endarterectomy, open, any method, of left anterior descending, circumflex, or right coronary artery performed in conjunction with coronary artery bypass graft procedure, each vessel (List separately in addition to primary procedure)

(Use 33572 in conjunction with 33510-33516, 33533-33536)

SINGLE VENTRICLE AND OTHER COMPLEX CARDIAC ANOMALIES

33600   Closure of atrioventricular valve (mitral or tricuspid) by suture or patch

33602   Closure of semilunar valve (aortic or pulmonary) by suture or patch

33606   Anastomosis of pulmonary artery to aorta (Damus-Kaye-Stansel procedure)

33608   Repair of complex cardiac anomaly other than pulmonary atresia with ventricular septal defect by construction or replacement of conduit from right or left ventricle to pulmonary artery

(For repair of pulmonary atresia with ventricular septal defect, see 33918, 33919, 33920)

▲ **33610**   Repair of complex cardiac anomalies (eg, single ventricle with subaortic obstruction) by surgical enlargement of ventricular septal defect

33611   Repair of double outlet right ventricle with intraventricular tunnel repair;

33612   with repair of right ventricular outflow tract obstruction

33615   Repair of complex cardiac anomalies (eg, tricuspid atresia) by closure of atrial septal defect and anastomosis of atria or vena cava to pulmonary artery (simple Fontan procedure)

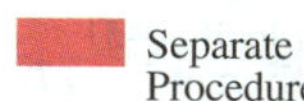
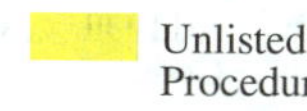
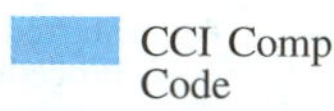
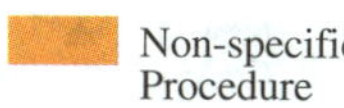

Separate Procedure   Unlisted Procedure   CCI Comp. Code   Non-specific Procedure

33617 Repair of complex cardiac anomalies (eg, single ventricle) by modified Fontan procedure

33619 Repair of single ventricle with aortic outflow obstruction and aortic arch hypoplasia (hypoplastic left heart syndrome) (eg, Norwood procedure)

SEPTAL DEFECT

33641 Repair atrial septal defect, secundum, with cardiopulmonary bypass, with or without patch

33645 Direct or patch closure, sinus venosus, with or without anomalous pulmonary venous drainage

33647 Repair of atrial septal defect and ventricular septal defect, with direct or patch closure

33660 Repair of incomplete or partial atrioventricular canal (ostium primum atrial septal defect), with or without atrioventricular valve repair

33665 Repair of intermediate or transitional atrioventricular canal, with or without atrioventricular valve repair

33670 Repair of complete atrioventricular canal, with or without prosthetic valve

33681 Closure of ventricular septal defect, with or without patch;

33684   with pulmonary valvotomy or infundibular resection (acyanotic)

33688   with removal of pulmonary artery band, with or without gusset

33690 Banding of pulmonary artery

33692 Complete repair tetralogy of Fallot without pulmonary atresia;

33694   with transannular patch

33697 Complete repair tetralogy of Fallot with pulmonary atresia including construction of conduit from right ventricle to pulmonary artery and closure of ventricular septal defect

---

390   ● New Code   ▲ Revised Code   ✳ Starred Procedure   ✚ Add-On Code   ⊘ Modifier -51 Exempt

SINUS OF VALSALVA

33702 Repair sinus of Valsalva fistula, with cardiopulmonary bypass;

33710 with repair of ventricular septal defect

33720 Repair sinus of Valsalva aneurysm, with cardiopulmonary bypass

33722 Closure of aortico-left ventricular tunnel

TOTAL ANOMALOUS PULMONARY VENOUS DRAINAGE

33730 Complete repair of anomalous venous return (supracardiac, intracardiac, or infracardiac types)

(For partial anomalous return, see atrial septal defect)

33732 Repair of cor triatriatum or supravalvular mitral ring by resection of left atrial membrane

SHUNTING PROCEDURES

33735 Atrial septectomy or septostomy; closed heart (Blalock-Hanlon type operation)

33736 open heart with cardiopulmonary bypass

33737 open heart, with inflow occlusion

33750 Shunt; subclavian to pulmonary artery (Blalock-Taussig type operation)

33755 ascending aorta to pulmonary artery (Waterston type operation)

33762 descending aorta to pulmonary artery (Potts-Smith type operation)

33764 central, with prosthetic graft

33766 superior vena cava to pulmonary artery for flow to one lung (classical Glenn procedure)

33767 superior vena cava to pulmonary artery for flow to both lungs (bidirectional Glenn procedure)

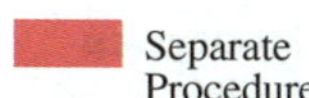 Separate Procedure 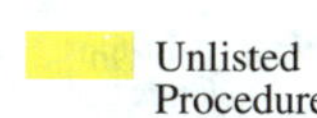 Unlisted Procedure 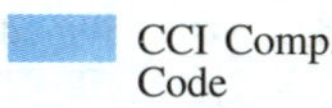 CCI Comp. Code 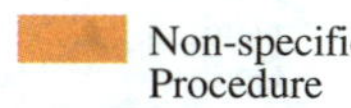 Non-specific Procedure

TRANSPOSITION OF THE GREAT VESSELS

33770 Repair of transposition of the great arteries with ventricular septal defect and subpulmonary stenosis; without surgical enlargement of ventricular septal defect

33771 with surgical enlargement of ventricular septal defect

33774 Repair of transposition of the great arteries, atrial baffle procedure (eg, Mustard or Senning type) with cardiopulmonary bypass;

33775 with removal of pulmonary band

33776 with closure of ventricular septal defect

33777 with repair of subpulmonic obstruction

33778 Repair of transposition of the great arteries, aortic pulmonary artery reconstruction (eg, Jatene type);

33779 with removal of pulmonary band

33780 with closure of ventricular septal defect

33781 with repair of subpulmonic obstruction

TRUNCUS ARTERIOSUS

33786 Total repair, truncus arteriosus (Rastelli type operation)

33788 Reimplantation of an anomalous pulmonary artery

(For pulmonary artery band, use 33690)

AORTIC ANOMALIES

33800 Aortic suspension (aortopexy) for tracheal decompression (eg, for tracheomalacia) (separate procedure)

33802 Division of aberrant vessel (vascular ring);

33803 with reanastomosis

33813 Obliteration of aortopulmonary septal defect; without cardiopulmonary bypass

---

● New Code   ▲ Revised Code   ✳ Starred Procedure   ✚ Add-On Code   ⊘ Modifier -51 Exempt

33814   with cardiopulmonary bypass

33820   Repair of patent ductus arteriosus; by ligation

33822   by division, under 18 years

33824   by division, 18 years and older

33840   Excision of coarctation of aorta, with or without associated patent ductus arteriosus; with direct anastomosis

33845   with graft

33851   repair using either left subclavian artery or prosthetic material as gusset for enlargement

33852   Repair of hypoplastic or interrupted aortic arch using autogenous or prosthetic material; without cardiopulmonary bypass

33853   with cardiopulmonary bypass

THORACIC AORTIC ANEURYSM

33860   Ascending aorta graft, with cardiopulmonary bypass, with or without valve suspension;

33861   with coronary reconstruction

33863   with aortic root replacement using composite prosthesis and coronary reconstruction

33870   Transverse arch graft, with cardiopulmonary bypass

33875   Descending thoracic aorta graft, with or without bypass

33877   Repair of thoracoabdominal aortic aneurysm with graft, with or without cardiopulmonary bypass

PULMONARY ARTERY

33910   Pulmonary artery embolectomy; with cardiopulmonary bypass

33915   without cardiopulmonary bypass

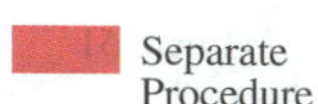 Separate Procedure

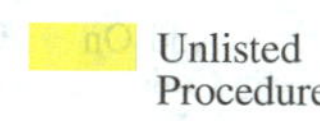 Unlisted Procedure

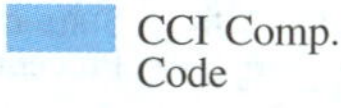 CCI Comp. Code

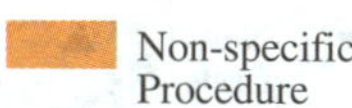 Non-specific Procedure

33916 Pulmonary endarterectomy, with or without embolectomy, with cardiopulmonary bypass

33917 Repair of pulmonary artery stenosis by reconstruction with patch or graft

33918 Repair of pulmonary atresia with ventricular septal defect, by unifocalization of pulmonary arteries; without cardiopulmonary bypass

33919   with cardiopulmonary bypass

33920 Repair of pulmonary atresia with ventricular septal defect, by construction or replacement of conduit from right or left ventricle to pulmonary artery

(For repair of other complex cardiac anomalies by construction or replacement of right or left ventricle to pulmonary artery conduit, use 33608)

33922 Transection of pulmonary artery with cardiopulmonary bypass

+33924 Ligation and takedown of a systemic-to-pulmonary artery shunt, performed in conjunction with a congenital heart procedure (List separately in addition to code for primary procedure)

(Use 33924 in conjunction with 33470-33475, 33600-33619, 33684-33688, 33692-33697, 33735-33767, 33770-33781, 33786, 33918-33922)

HEART/LUNG TRANSPLANTATION

33930 Donor cardiectomy-pneumonectomy, with preparation and maintenance of allograft

33935 Heart-lung transplant with recipient cardiectomy-pneumonectomy

33940 Donor cardiectomy, with preparation and maintenance of allograft

33945 Heart transplant, with or without recipient cardiectomy

CARDIAC ASSIST

33960 Prolonged extracorporeal circulation for cardiopulmonary insufficiency; initial 24 hours

---

● New Code ▲ Revised Code ✱ Starred Procedure ＋ Add-On Code ⊘ Modifier -51 Exempt

+33961	each additional 24 hours (List separately in addition to code for primary procedure)

(Use 33961 in conjunction with code 33960)

(For insertion of cannula for prolonged extracorporeal circulation, use 36822)

● **33967**   Insertion of intra-aortic balloon assist device, percutaneous

33968   Removal of intra-aortic balloon assist device, percutaneous

33970   Insertion of intra-aortic balloon assist device through the femoral artery, open approach

33971   Removal of intra-aortic balloon assist device including repair of femoral artery, with or without graft

33973   Insertion of intra-aortic balloon assist device through the ascending aorta

33974   Removal of intra-aortic balloon assist device from the ascending aorta, including repair of the ascending aorta, with or without graft

▲ **33975**   Insertion of ventricular assist device; extracorporeal, single ventricle

▲ **33976**   extracorporeal, biventricular

▲ **33977**   Removal of ventricular assist device; extracorporeal, single ventricle

▲ **33978**   extracorporeal, biventricular

● **33979**   Insertion of ventricular assist device, implantable intracorporeal, single ventricle

● **33980**   Removal of ventricular assist device, implantable intracorporeal, single ventricle

OTHER PROCEDURES, CARDIAC SURGERY

33999   Unlisted procedure, cardiac surgery

Separate Procedure

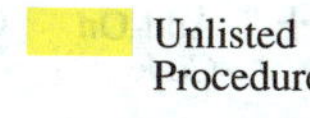
Unlisted Procedure

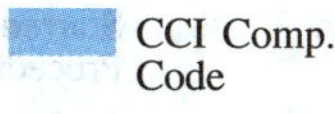
CCI Comp. Code

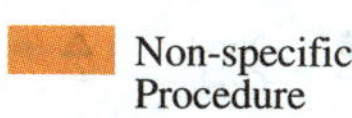
Non-specific Procedure

ARTERIES AND VEINS

EMBOLECTOMY/THROMBECTOMY

Arterial, With or Without Catheter

34001 Embolectomy or thrombectomy, with or without catheter; carotid, subclavian or innominate artery, by neck incision

34051 innominate, subclavian artery, by thoracic incision

34101 axillary, brachial, innominate, subclavian artery, by arm incision

34111 radial or ulnar artery, by arm incision

34151 renal, celiac, mesentery, aortoiliac artery, by abdominal incision

34201 femoropopliteal, aortoiliac artery, by leg incision

34203 popliteal-tibio-peroneal artery, by leg incision

Venous, Direct or With Catheter

34401 Thrombectomy, direct or with catheter; vena cava, iliac vein, by abdominal incision

34421 vena cava, iliac, femoropopliteal vein, by leg incision

34451 vena cava, iliac, femoropopliteal vein, by abdominal and leg incision

34471 subclavian vein, by neck incision

34490 axillary and subclavian vein, by arm incision

VENOUS RECONSTRUCTION

34501 Valvuloplasty, femoral vein

34502 Reconstruction of vena cava, any method

34510 Venous valve transposition, any vein donor

34520 Cross-over vein graft to venous system

34530 Saphenopopliteal vein anastomosis

ENDOVASCULAR REPAIR OF ABDOMINAL AORTIC ANEURYSM

34800 Endovascular repair of infrarenal abdominal aortic aneurysm or dissection; using aorto-aortic tube prosthesis

34802 using modular bifurcated prosthesis (one docking limb)

(For endovascular repair of infrarenal abdominal aortic aneurysm or dissection using a modular bifurcated prosthesis (two docking limbs), use Category III code 0001T)

34804 using unibody bifurcated prosthesis

(For endovascular repair of infrarenal abdominal aortic aneurysm or dissection using an aorto-uniiliac or aorto-unifemoral prosthesis, use Category III code 0002T)

+34808 Endovascular placement of iliac artery occlusion device (List separately in addition to code for primary procedure)

(Use 34808 in conjunction with codes 34800, 34813, 34825, 34826)

(For radiological supervision and interpretation, use 75952 in conjunction with 34800, 34802, 34804, 34808)

(For open approach, report codes 34812-34820 in addition to codes 34800, 34802, 34804, 34808 as appropriate)

34812 Open femoral artery exposure for delivery of aortic endovascular prosthesis, by groin incision, unilateral

(For bilateral procedure, use modifier -50)

+34813 Placement of femoral-femoral prosthetic graft during endovascular aortic aneurysm report (List separately in addition to code for primary procedure)

(Use 34813 in conjunction with code 34812)

(For femoral artery grafting, see 35521, 35533, 35546, 35551-35558, 35621, 35646, 35651-35661, 35666, 35700)

34820 Open iliac artery exposure for delivery of endovascular prosthesis or iliac occlusion during endovascular therapy, by abdominal or retroperitoneal incision, unilateral

---

Separate Procedure

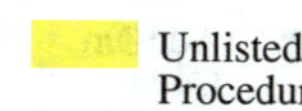
Unlisted Procedure

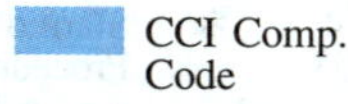
CCI Comp. Code

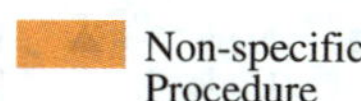
Non-specific Procedure

397

(For bilateral procedure, use modifier -50)

34825 Placement of proximal or distal extension prosthesis for endovascular repair of infrarenal abdominal aortic aneurysm; initial vessel

+34826 each additional vessel (List separately in addition to code for primary procedure)

(Use 34826 in conjunction with code 34825)

(Use 34825, 34826 in addition to codes 34800-34808 as appropriate)

(For staged procedure, use modifier -58)

(For radiological supervision and interpretation, use 75953)

34830 Open repair of infrarenal aortic aneurysm or dissection, plus repair of associated arterial trauma, following unsuccessful endovascular repair; tube prosthesis

34831 aorto-bi-iliac prosthesis

34832 aorto-bifemoral prosthesis

DIRECT REPAIR OF ANEURYSM OR EXCISION (PARTIAL OR TOTAL) AND GRAFT INSERTION FOR ANEURYSM, FALSE ANEURYSM, RUPTURED ANEURYSM, AND ASSOCIATED OCCLUSIVE DISEASE

(For direct repairs associated with occlusive disease only, see 35201-35286)

(For intracranial aneurysm, see 61700 et seq)

(For thoracic aortic aneurysm, see 33860-33875)

▲ 35001 Direct repair of aneurysm, pseudoaneurysm, or excision (partial or total) and graft insertion, with or without patch graft; for aneurysm and associated occlusive disease, carotid, subclavian artery, by neck incision

35002 for ruptured aneurysm, carotid, subclavian artery, by neck incision

▲ 35005 for aneurysm, pseudoaneurysm, and associated occlusive disease, vertebral artery

● New Code	▲ Revised Code	* Starred Procedure	+ Add-On Code	⊘ Modifier -51 Exempt

35011	for aneurysm and associated occlusive disease, axillary-brachial artery, by arm incision
35013	for ruptured aneurysm, axillary-brachial artery, by arm incision
▲ **35021**	for aneurysm, pseudoaneurysm, and associated occlusive disease, innominate, subclavian artery, by thoracic incision
35022	for ruptured aneurysm, innominate, subclavian artery, by thoracic incision
▲ **35045**	for aneurysm, pseudoaneurysm, and associated occlusive disease, radial or ulnar artery
▲ **35081**	for aneurysm, pseudoaneurysm, and associated occlusive disease, abdominal aorta
35082	for ruptured aneurysm, abdominal aorta
▲ **35091**	for aneurysm, pseudoaneurysm, and associated occlusive disease, abdominal aorta involving visceral vessels (mesenteric, celiac, renal)
35092	for ruptured aneurysm, abdominal aorta involving visceral vessels (mesenteric, celiac, renal)
▲ **35102**	for aneurysm, pseudoaneurysm, and associated occlusive disease, abdominal aorta involving iliac vessels (common, hypogastric, external)
35103	for ruptured aneurysm, abdominal aorta involving iliac vessels (common, hypogastric, external)
▲ **35111**	for aneurysm, pseudoaneurysm, and associated occlusive disease, splenic artery
35112	for ruptured aneurysm, splenic artery
▲ **35121**	for aneurysm, pseudoaneurysm, and associated occlusive disease, hepatic, celiac, renal, or mesenteric artery
35122	for ruptured aneurysm, hepatic, celiac, renal, or mesenteric artery
▲ **35131**	for aneurysm, pseudoaneurysm, and associated occlusive disease, iliac artery (common, hypogastric, external)

35132	for ruptured aneurysm, iliac artery (common, hypogastric, external)
▲ **35141**	for aneurysm, pseudoaneurysm, and associated occlusive disease, common femoral artery (profunda femoris, superficial femoral)
35142	for ruptured aneurysm, common femoral artery (profunda femoris, superficial femoral)
▲ **35151**	for aneurysm, pseudoaneurysm, and associated occlusive disease, popliteal artery
35152	for ruptured aneurysm, popliteal artery
▲ **35161**	for aneurysm, pseudoaneurysm, and associated occlusive disease, other arteries
35162	for ruptured aneurysm, other arteries

REPAIR ARTERIOVENOUS FISTULA

35180	Repair, congenital arteriovenous fistula; head and neck
35182	thorax and abdomen
35184	extremities
35188	Repair, acquired or traumatic arteriovenous fistula; head and neck
35189	thorax and abdomen
35190	extremities

REPAIR BLOOD VESSEL OTHER THAN FOR FISTULA, WITH OR WITHOUT PATCH ANGIOPLASTY

(For AV fistula repair, see 35180-35190)

35201	Repair blood vessel, direct; neck
35206	upper extremity
35207	hand, finger
35211	intrathoracic, with bypass

● New Code ▲ Revised Code * Starred Procedure ✛ Add-On Code ⊘ Modifier -51 Exempt

35216	intrathoracic, without bypass
35221	intra-abdominal
35226	lower extremity
35231	Repair blood vessel with vein graft; neck
35236	upper extremity
35241	intrathoracic, with bypass
35246	intrathoracic, without bypass
35251	intra-abdominal
35256	lower extremity
35261	Repair blood vessel with graft other than vein; neck
35266	upper extremity
35271	intrathoracic, with bypass
35276	intrathoracic, without bypass
35281	intra-abdominal
35286	lower extremity

THROMBOENDARTERECTOMY

(For coronary artery, see 33510-33536 and 33572)

35301	Thromboendarterectomy, with or without patch graft; carotid, vertebral, subclavian, by neck incision
35311	subclavian, innominate, by thoracic incision
35321	axillary-brachial
35331	abdominal aorta
35341	mesenteric, celiac, or renal
35351	iliac

35355   iliofemoral

35361   combined aortoiliac

35363   combined aortoiliofemoral

35371   common femoral

35372   deep (profunda) femoral

35381   femoral and/or popliteal, and/or tibioperoneal

+35390   Reoperation, carotid, thromboendarterectomy, more than one month after original operation (List separately in addition to code for primary procedure)

(Use 35390 in conjunction with code 35301)

ANGIOSCOPY

+35400   Angioscopy (non-coronary vessels or grafts) during therapeutic intervention (List separately in addition to code for primary procedure)

TRANSLUMINAL ANGIOPLASTY

(For radiological supervision and interpretation, see 75962-75968 and 75978)

Open

35450   Transluminal balloon angioplasty, open; renal or other visceral artery

35452   aortic

35454   iliac

35456   femoral-popliteal

35458   brachiocephalic trunk or branches, each vessel

35459   tibioperoneal trunk and branches

35460   venous

Percutaneous

35470   Transluminal balloon angioplasty, percutaneous; tibioperoneal trunk or branches, each vessel

35471   renal or visceral artery

35472   aortic

35473   iliac

35474   femoral-popliteal

35475   brachiocephalic trunk or branches, each vessel

35476   venous

(For radiological supervision and interpretation, use 75978)

TRANSLUMINAL ATHERECTOMY

(For radiological supervision and interpretation, see 75992-75996)

Open

35480   Transluminal peripheral atherectomy, open; renal or other visceral artery

35481   aortic

35482   iliac

35483   femoral-popliteal

35484   brachiocephalic trunk or branches, each vessel

35485   tibioperoneal trunk and branches

Percutaneous

35490   Transluminal peripheral atherectomy, percutaneous; renal or other visceral artery

35491   aortic

35492   iliac

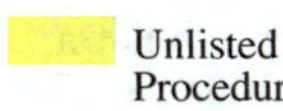

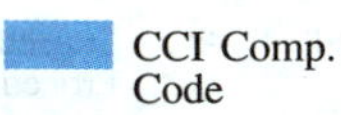

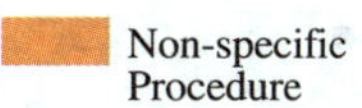

35493	femoral-popliteal
35494	brachiocephalic trunk or branches, each vessel
35495	tibioperoneal trunk and branches

BYPASS GRAFT

Vein

+35500   Harvest of upper extremity vein, one segment, for lower extremity or coronary artery bypass procedure (List separately in addition to code for primary procedure)

(Use 35500 in conjunction with codes 33510-33536, 35556, 35566, 35571, 35583-35587)

(For harvest of more than one vein segment, see 35682, 35683)

35501	Bypass graft, with vein; carotid
35506	carotid-subclavian
35507	subclavian-carotid
35508	carotid-vertebral
35509	carotid-carotid
35511	subclavian-subclavian
35515	subclavian-vertebral
35516	subclavian-axillary
35518	axillary-axillary
35521	axillary-femoral

(For bypass graft performed with synthetic graft, use 35621)

35526	aortosubclavian or carotid

(For bypass graft performed with synthetic graft, use 35626)

35531	aortoceliac or aortomesenteric

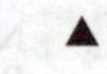

● New Code	▲ Revised Code	✳ Starred Procedure	✛ Add-On Code	⊘ Modifier -51 Exempt

35533	axillary-femoral-femoral

(For bypass graft performed with synthetic graft, use 35654)

35536	splenorenal
35541	aortoiliac or bi-iliac

(For bypass graft performed with synthetic graft, use 35641)

35546	aortofemoral or bifemoral

(For bypass graft performed with synthetic graft, use 35646)

35548	aortoiliofemoral, unilateral

(For bypass graft performed with synthetic graft, use 37799)

35549	aortoiliofemoral, bilateral

(For bypass graft performed with synthetic graft, use 37799)

35551	aortofemoral-popliteal
35556	femoral-popliteal
35558	femoral-femoral
35560	aortorenal
35563	ilioiliac
35565	iliofemoral
35566	femoral-anterior tibial, posterior tibial, peroneal artery or other distal vessels
35571	popliteal-tibial, -peroneal artery or other distal vessels

In-Situ Vein

35582	In-situ vein bypass; aortofemoral-popliteal (only femoral-popliteal portion in-situ)
35583	femoral-popliteal
35585	femoral-anterior tibial, posterior tibial, or peroneal artery

| 35587 | popliteal-tibial, peroneal |

Other Than Vein

⊘ **35600**   Harvest of upper extremity artery, one segment, for coronary artery bypass procedure

35601	Bypass graft, with other than vein; carotid
35606	carotid-subclavian
35612	subclavian-subclavian
35616	subclavian-axillary
35621	axillary-femoral
35623	axillary-popliteal or -tibial
35626	aortosubclavian or carotid
35631	aortoceliac, aortomesenteric, aortorenal
35636	splenorenal (splenic to renal arterial anastomosis)
35641	aortoiliac or bi-iliac
35642	carotid-vertebral
35645	subclavian-vertebral

▲ **35646**   aortobifemoral

● **35647**   aortofemoral

35650	axillary-axillary
35651	aortofemoral-popliteal
35654	axillary-femoral-femoral
35656	femoral-popliteal
35661	femoral-femoral

● New Code   ▲ Revised Code   ✳ Starred Procedure   ✛ Add-On Code   ⊘ Modifier -51 Exempt

35663	ilioiliac
35665	iliofemoral
35666	femoral-anterior tibial, posterior tibial, or peroneal artery
35671	popliteal-tibial or -peroneal artery

COMPOSITE GRAFTS

+35681 Bypass graft; composite, prosthetic and vein (List separately in addition to code for primary procedure)

(Do not report 35681 in addition to 35682, 35683)

+35682 autogenous composite, two segments of veins from two locations (List separately in addition to code for primary procedure)

(Do not report 35682 in addition to 35681, 35683)

+35683 autogenous composite, three or more segments of vein from two or more locations (List separately in addition to code for primary procedure)

(Do not report 35683 in addition to 35681, 35682)

ADJUVANT TECHNIQUES

(For composite graft(s), see 35681-35683)

●+35685 Placement of vein patch or cuff at distal anastomosis of bypass graft, synthetic conduit (List separately in addition to code for primary procedure)

(Use 35685 in conjunction with codes 35656, 35666 or 35671)

●+35686 Creation of distal arteriovenous fistula during lower extremity bypass surgery (non-hemodialysis) (List separately in addition to code for primary procedure)

(Use 35686 in conjunction with codes 35556, 35566, 35571, 35583-35587, 35623, 35656, 35666, 35671)

ARTERIAL TRANSPOSITION

35691 Transposition and/or reimplantation; vertebral to carotid artery

---

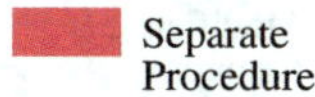 Separate Procedure

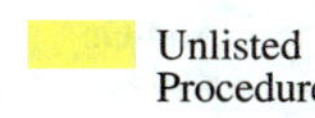 Unlisted Procedure

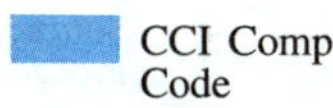 CCI Comp. Code

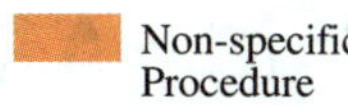 Non-specific Procedure

407

35693	vertebral to subclavian artery
35694	subclavian to carotid artery
35695	carotid to subclavian artery

EXPLORATION/REVISION

+35700 Reoperation, femoral-popliteal or femoral (popliteal)-anterior tibial, posterior tibial, peroneal artery or other distal vessels, more than one month after original operation (List separately in addition to code for primary procedure)

(Use 35700 in conjunction with codes 35556, 35566, 35571, 35583, 35585, 35587, 35656, 35666, 35671)

35701 Exploration (not followed by surgical repair), with or without lysis of artery; carotid artery

35721 femoral artery

35741 popliteal artery

35761 other vessels

35800 Exploration for postoperative hemorrhage, thrombosis or infection; neck

35820 chest

35840 abdomen

35860 extremity

35870 Repair of graft-enteric fistula

35875 Thrombectomy of arterial or venous graft (other than hemodialysis graft or fistula);

35876 with revision of arterial or venous graft

(For thrombectomy of hemodialysis graft or fistula, see 36831, 36833)

35879 Revision, lower extremity arterial bypass, without thrombectomy, open; with vein patch angioplasty

● New Code   ▲ Revised Code   ✳ Starred Procedure   ✚ Add-On Code   ⊘ Modifier -51 Exempt

35881   with segmental vein interposition

35901   Excision of infected graft; neck

35903   extremity

35905   thorax

35907   abdomen

VASCULAR INJECTION PROCEDURES

When using CPT codes from this section, note that the listed procedures include local anesthesia, introduction of needles or catheter, injection of contrast medium with or without automatic power injection, and pre- and post-injection care specifically related to the injection procedure.

Note that catheters, drugs and contrast media are not included in CPT codes listed in this section. These should be coded using CPT code 99070 or the appropriate HCPCS Level II code for Medicare patients.

CPT codes listed in this section do not cover radiological vascular injections, injection procedures for cardiac catheterization or chemotherapy. Refer to the RADIOLOGY or MEDICINE sections of CPT for the appropriate CPT codes for these procedures.

> (For radiological supervision and interpretation, see RADIOLOGY)
>
> (For injection procedures in conjunction with cardiac catheterization, see 93541-93545)
>
> (For chemotherapy of malignant disease, see 96400-96549)

INTRAVENOUS

***36000**   Introduction of needle or intracatheter, vein

● **36002**   Injection procedures (eg, thrombin) for percutaneous treatment of extremity pseudoaneurysm

> (For imaging guidance, see 76003, 76360, 76393, or 76942)
>
> (For ultrasound guided compression repair of pseudoaneurysms, use 76936)
>
> (Do not report 36002 for vascular sealant of an arteriotomy site)

 Separate Procedure

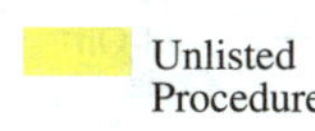 Unlisted Procedure

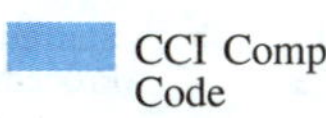 CCI Comp. Code

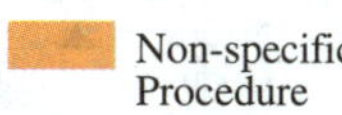 Non-specific Procedure

▲ **36005** Injection procedure for extremity venography (including introduction of needle or intracatheter)

(For radiological supervision and interpretation, see 75820, 75822)

36010 Introduction of catheter, superior or inferior vena cava

36011 Selective catheter placement, venous system; first order branch (eg, renal vein, jugular vein)

36012 second order, or more selective, branch (eg, left adrenal vein, petrosal sinus)

36013 Introduction of catheter, right heart or main pulmonary artery

36014 Selective catheter placement, left or right pulmonary artery

36015 Selective catheter placement, segmental or subsegmental pulmonary artery

(For insertion of flow directed catheter (eg, Swan-Ganz), use 93503)

(For venous catheterization for selective organ blood sampling, use 36500)

INTRA-ARTERIAL/INTRA-AORTIC

(For radiological supervision and interpretation, see RADIOLOGY)

36100 Introduction of needle or intracatheter, carotid or vertebral artery

36120 Introduction of needle or intracatheter; retrograde brachial artery

36140 extremity artery

36145 arteriovenous shunt created for dialysis (cannula, fistula, or graft)

(For insertion of arteriovenous cannula, see 36810-36821)

36160 Introduction of needle or intracatheter, aortic, translumbar

36200 Introduction of catheter, aorta

● New Code ▲ Revised Code * Starred Procedure + Add-On Code ⊘ Modifier -51 Exempt

36215 Selective catheter placement, arterial system; each first order thoracic or brachiocephalic branch, within a vascular family

(For catheter placement for coronary angiography, use 93508)

36216 initial second order thoracic or brachiocephalic branch, within a vascular family

36217 initial third order or more selective thoracic or brachiocephalic branch, within a vascular family

+36218 additional second order, third order, and beyond, thoracic or brachiocephalic branch, within a vascular family (List in addition to code for initial second or third order vessel as appropriate)

(Use 36218 in conjunction with codes 36216, 36217)

(For angiography, see 75600-75790)

(For angioplasty, see 35470-35475)

(For transcatheter therapies, see 37200-37208, 61624, 61626)

36245 Selective catheter placement, arterial system; each first order abdominal, pelvic, or lower extremity artery branch, within a vascular family

36246 initial second order abdominal, pelvic, or lower extremity artery branch, within a vascular family

36247 initial third order or more selective abdominal, pelvic, or lower extremity artery branch, within a vascular family

+36248 additional second order, third order, and beyond, abdominal, pelvic, or lower extremity artery branch, within a vascular family (List in addition to code for initial second or third order vessel as appropriate)

(Use 36248 in conjunction with codes 36246, 36247)

36260 Insertion of implantable intra-arterial infusion pump (eg, for chemotherapy of liver)

36261 Revision of implanted intra-arterial infusion pump

36262 Removal of implanted intra-arterial infusion pump

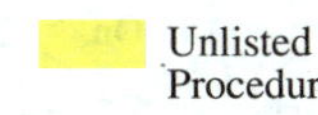 Separate Procedure

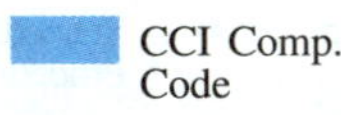 Unlisted Procedure

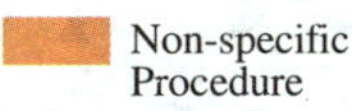 CCI Comp. Code

Non-specific Procedure

36299 Unlisted procedure, vascular injection

VENOUS

▲ **36400** Venipuncture, under age 3 years; femoral or jugular

***36405** scalp vein

36406 other vein

***36410** Venipuncture, child over age 3 years or adult, necessitating physician's skill (separate procedure), for diagnostic or therapeutic purposes. Not to be used for routine venipuncture.

***36415** Routine venipuncture or finger/heel/ear stick for collection of specimen(s)

36420 Venipuncture, cutdown; under age 1 year

36425 age 1 or over

36430 Transfusion, blood or blood components

***36440** Push transfusion, blood, 2 years or under

36450 Exchange transfusion, blood; newborn

36455 other than newborn

36460 Transfusion, intrauterine, fetal

(For radiological supervision and interpretation, use 76941)

36468 Single or multiple injections of sclerosing solutions, spider veins (telangiectasia); limb or trunk

36469 face

***36470** Injection of sclerosing solution; single vein

***36471** multiple veins, same leg

36481 Percutaneous portal vein catheterization by any method

(For radiological supervision and interpretation, see 75885, 75887)

● New Code   ▲ Revised Code   * Starred Procedure   + Add-On Code   ⊘ Modifier -51 Exempt

⊘*36488   Placement of central venous catheter (subclavian, jugular, or other vein) (eg, for central venous pressure, hyperalimentation, hemodialysis,or chemotherapy); percutaneous, age 2 years or under

⊘*36489   percutaneous, over age 2

(If imaging guidance is performed, see 76000, 76003, 76942)

⊘*36490   cutdown, age 2 years or under

⊘*36491   cutdown, over age 2

(For examination of patient and instruction to patient, review of prescription of fluids for long-term or permanent hyperalimentation, use Evaluation and Management codes for office or hospital inpatient category or follow-up inpatient consultation codes as appropriate)

36493   Repositioning of previously placed central venous catheter under fluoroscopic guidance

(For fluoroscopic guidance, use 76000)

36500   Venous catheterization for selective organ blood sampling

(For catheterization in superior or inferior vena cava, use 36010)

(For radiological supervision and interpretation, use 75893)

*36510   Catheterization of umbilical vein for diagnosis or therapy, newborn

36520   Therapeutic apheresis; plasma and/or cell exchange

36521   with extracorporeal affinity column adsorption and plasma reinfusion

36522   Photopheresis, extracorporeal

36530   Insertion of implantable intravenous infusion pump

(If imaging guidance is performed, see 76000, 76003, 76942)

36531   Revision of implantable intravenous infusion pump

36532   Removal of implantable intravenous infusion pump

413

Separate Procedure   Unlisted Procedure   CCI Comp. Code   Non-specific Procedure

(If imaging guidance is performed, use 76000)

36533   Insertion of implantable venous access device, with or without subcutaneous reservoir

(For removal, use 36535)

(If imaging guidance is performed, see 76000, 76003, 76942)

(For refilling and maintenance of an implantable venous access device reservoir, use 96530)

36534   Revision of implantable venous access device, and/or subcutaneous reservoir

(For removal, use 36535)

36535   Removal of implantable venous access device, and/or subcutaneous reservoir

(Use 36535 in conjunction with codes 36533, 36534, as appropriate)

(Do not use 36535 in conjunction with codes 36488-36491)

(If imaging guidance is performed, use 76000)

36540   Collection of blood specimen from a partially or completely implantable venous access device

36550   Declotting by thrombolytic agent of implanted vascular access device or catheter

ARTERIAL

***36600**   Arterial puncture, withdrawal of blood for diagnosis

⊘ **36620**   Arterial catheterization or cannulation for sampling, monitoring or transfusion (separate procedure); percutaneous

36625   cutdown

36640   Arterial catheterization for prolonged infusion therapy (chemotherapy), cutdown

(See also 96420-96425)

(For arterial catheterization for occlusion therapy, see 75894)

● New Code   ▲ Revised Code   * Starred Procedure   ✛ Add-On Code   ⊘ Modifier -51 Exempt

⊘*36660 Catheterization, umbilical artery, newborn, for diagnosis or therapy

INTRAOSSEOUS

36680 Placement of needle for intraosseous infusion

HEMODIALYSIS ACCESS, INTERVASCULAR CANNULIZATION FOR EXTRACORPOREAL CIRCULATION, OR SHUNT INSERTION

36800 Insertion of cannula for hemodialysis, other purpose (separate procedure); vein to vein

36810 arteriovenous, external (Scribner type)

36815 arteriovenous, external revision, or closure

▲ **36819** Arteriovenous anastomosis, open; by upper arm basilic vein transposition

● **36820** by forearm vein transposition

36821 direct, any site (eg, Cimino type) (separate procedure)

36822 Insertion of cannula(s) for prolonged extracorporeal circulation for cardiopulmonary insufficiency (ECMO) (separate procedure)

(For maintenance of prolonged extracorporeal circulation, use 33960)

▲ **36823** Insertion of arterial and venous cannula(s) for isolated extracorporeal circulation including regional chemotherapy perfusion to an extremity, with or without hyperthermia, with removal of cannula(s) and repair of arteriotomy and venotomy sites

(36823 includes chemotherapy perfusion supported by a membrane oxygenator/perfusion pump. Do not report 96408-96425 in conjunction with 36823)

36825 Creation of arteriovenous fistula by other than direct arteriovenous anastomosis (separate procedure); autogenous graft

(For direct arteriovenous anastomosis, use 36821)

36830 nonautogenous graft

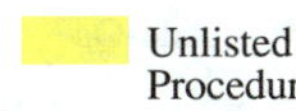

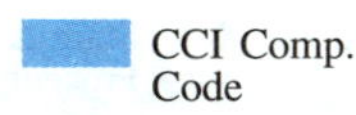

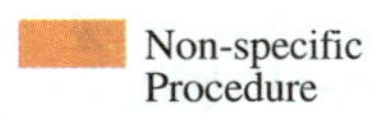

(For direct arteriovenous anastomosis, use 36821)

36831 Thrombectomy, open, arteriovenous fistula without revision, autogenous or nonautogenous dialysis graft (separate procedure)

36832 Revision, open, arteriovenous fistula; without thrombectomy, autogenous or nonautogenous dialysis graft (separate procedure)

36833 with thrombectomy, autogenous or nonautogenous dialysis graft (separate procedure)

36834 Plastic repair of arteriovenous aneurysm (separate procedure)

36835 Insertion of Thomas shunt (separate procedure)

36860 External cannula declotting (separate procedure); without balloon catheter

36861 with balloon catheter

(If imaging guidance is performed, use 76000)

36870 Thrombectomy, percutaneous, arteriovenous fistula, autogenous or nonautogenous graft (includes mechanical thrombus extraction and intro-graft thrombolysis)

(Do not report 36550 in conjunction with code 36870)

(For catheterization, use 36145)

(For radiological supervision and interpretation, use 75790)

PORTAL DECOMPRESSION PROCEDURES

37140 Venous anastomosis; portocaval

(For peritoneal-venous shunt, use 49425)

37145 renoportal

37160 caval-mesenteric

37180 splenorenal, proximal

37181 splenorenal, distal (selective decompression of esophagogastric varices, any technique)

● New Code ▲ Revised Code * Starred Procedure ✛ Add-On Code ⊘ Modifier -51 Exempt

TRANSCATHETER PROCEDURES

37195 Thrombolysis, cerebral, by intravenous infusion

37200 Transcatheter biopsy

(For radiological supervision and interpretation, use 75970)

37201 Transcatheter therapy, infusion for thrombolysis other than coronary

(For radiological supervision and interpretation, use 75896)

37202 Transcatheter therapy, infusion other than for thrombolysis, any type (eg, spasmolytic, vasoconstrictive)

(For thrombolysis of coronary vessels, see 92975, 92977)

(For radiological supervision and interpretation, use 75896)

37203 Transcatheter retrieval, percutaneous, of intravascular foreign body (eg, fractured venous or arterial catheter)

(For radiological supervision and interpretation, use 75961)

37204 Transcatheter occlusion or embolization (eg, for tumor destruction, to achieve hemostasis, to occlude a vascular malformation), percutaneous, any method, non-central nervous system, non-head or neck

(See also 61624, 61626)

(For radiological supervision and interpretation, use 75894)

37205 Transcatheter placement of an intravascular stent(s), (non-coronary vessel), percutaneous; initial vessel

(For radiological supervision and interpretation, use 75960)

+37206   each additional vessel (List separately in addition to code for primary procedure)

(Use 37206 in conjunction with 37205)

(For transcatheter placement of extracranial cerebrovascular artery stent(s), see Category III codes 0005T, 0006T)

(For radiological supervision and interpretation, use 75960)

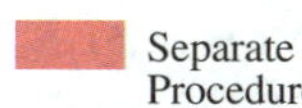

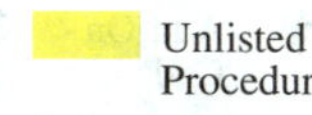

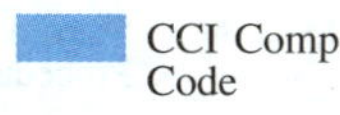

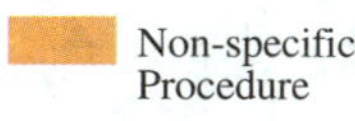

37207   Transcatheter placement of an intravascular stent(s), (non-coronary vessel), open; initial vessel

+37208   each additional vessel (List separately in addition to code for primary procedure)

(Use 37208 in conjunction with 37207)

(For radiological supervision and interpretation, use 75960)

(For catheterizations, see 36215-36248)

(For transcatheter placement of intracoronary stent(s), see 92980, 92981)

37209   Exchange of a previously placed arterial catheter during thrombolytic therapy

(For radiological supervision and interpretation, use 75900)

INTRAVASCULAR ULTRASOUND SERVICES

+37250   Intravascular ultrasound (non-coronary vessel) during diagnostic evaluation and/or therapeutic intervention; initial vessel (List separately in addition to code for primary procedure)

+37251   each additional vessel (List separately in addition to code for primary procedure)

(Use 37251 in conjunction with 37250)

(For catheterizations, see 36215-36248)

(For transcatheter therapies, see 37200-37208, 61624, 61626)

(For radiological supervision and interpretation, see 75945, 75946)

LIGATION AND OTHER PROCEDURES

37565   Ligation, internal jugular vein

37600   Ligation; external carotid artery

37605   internal or common carotid artery

37606   internal or common carotid artery, with gradual occlusion, as with Selverstone or Crutchfield clamp

(For ligation treatment of intracranial aneurysm, use 61703)

37607 Ligation or banding of angioaccess arteriovenous fistula

37609 Ligation or biopsy, temporal artery

37615 Ligation, major artery (eg, post-traumatic, rupture); neck

37616   chest

37617   abdomen

37618   extremity

37620 Interruption, partial or complete, of inferior vena cava by suture, ligation, plication, clip, extravascular, intravascular (umbrella device)

(For radiological supervision and interpretation, use 75940)

37650 Ligation of femoral vein

37660 Ligation of common iliac vein

37700 Ligation and division of long saphenous vein at saphenofemoral junction, or distal interruptions

37720 Ligation and division and complete stripping of long or short saphenous veins

37730 Ligation and division and complete stripping of long and short saphenous veins

37735 Ligation and division and complete stripping of long or short saphenous veins with radical excision of ulcer and skin graft and/or interruption of communicating veins of lower leg, with excision of deep fascia

37760 Ligation of perforators, subfascial, radical (Linton type), with or without skin graft

37780 Ligation and division of short saphenous vein at saphenopopliteal junction (separate procedure)

37785 Ligation, division, and/or excision of recurrent or secondary varicose veins (clusters), one leg

37788 Penile revascularization, artery, with or without vein graft

37790 Penile venous occlusive procedure

37799 Unlisted procedure, vascular surgery

● New Code   ▲ Revised Code   ✱ Starred Procedure   ✚ Add-On Code   ⊘ Modifier -51 Exempt

HEMIC AND LYMPHATIC SYSTEMS

CPT codes from this section of CPT are used to report invasive and surgical procedures performed on the spleen and lymph nodes. Bone marrow transplants are reported using CPT codes 38230-38241 from this section.

SPLEEN

EXCISION

38100   Splenectomy; total (separate procedure)

38101   partial (separate procedure)

+38102   total, en bloc for extensive disease, in conjunction with other procedure (List in addition to code for primary procedure)

REPAIR

38115   Repair of ruptured spleen (splenorrhaphy) with or without partial splenectomy

LAPAROSCOPY

38120   Laparoscopy, surgical, splenectomy

38129   Unlisted laparoscopy procedure, spleen

INTRODUCTION

38200   Injection procedure for splenoportography

(For radiological supervision and interpretation, use 75810)

GENERAL

BONE MARROW OR STEM CELL SERVICES/PROCEDURES

● **38220**   Bone marrow aspiration

● **38221**   Bone marrow biopsy, needle or trocar

(For bone marrow biopsy interpretation, use 88305)

38230   Bone marrow harvesting for transplantation

 Separate Procedure

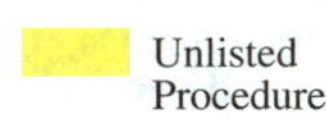 Unlisted Procedure

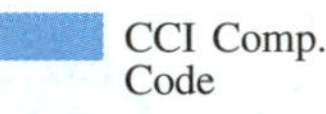 CCI Comp. Code

 Non-specific Procedure

421

38231   Blood-derived peripheral stem cell harvesting for transplantation, per collection

38240   Bone marrow or blood-derived peripheral stem cell transplantation; allogenic

38241   autologous

(For bone marrow aspiration, use 38220)

(For modification, treatment, and processing of bone marrow or blood-derived stem cell specimens for transplantation, use 86915)

(For cryopreservation, freezing and storage of blood-derived stem cells for transplantation, use 88240)

(For thawing and expansion of blood-derived stem cells for transplantation, use 88241)

(For compatibility studies, see 86812-86822)

LYMPH NODES AND LYMPHATIC CHANNELS

INCISION

***38300**   Drainage of lymph node abscess or lymphadenitis; simple

38305   extensive

38308   Lymphangiotomy or other operations on lymphatic channels

38380   Suture and/or ligation of thoracic duct; cervical approach

38381   thoracic approach

38382   abdominal approach

EXCISION

(For injection for sentinel node identification, use 38792)

38500   Biopsy or excision of lymph node(s); open, superficial

(Do not report 38500 with 38700-38780)

38505   by needle, superficial (eg, cervical, inguinal, axillary)

(If imaging guidance is performed, see 76360, 76393, 76942)

(For fine needle aspiration, use 10021 or 10022)

(For evaluation of fine needle aspirate, see 88172, 88173)

38510   open, deep cervical node(s)

38520   open, deep cervical node(s) with excision scalene fat pad

38525   open, deep axillary node(s)

38530   open, internal mammary node(s)

(Do not report 38530 with 38720-38746)

(For percutaneous needle biopsy, retroperitoneal lymph node or mass, use 49180. For fine needle aspiration, use 10022)

38542 Dissection, deep jugular node(s)

(For radical cervical neck dissection, use 38720)

38550 Excision of cystic hygroma, axillary or cervical; without deep neurovascular dissection

38555   with deep neurovascular dissection

LIMITED LYMPHADENECTOMY FOR STAGING

38562 Limited lymphadenectomy for staging (separate procedure); pelvic and para-aortic

(When combined with prostatectomy, use 55812 or 55842)

(When combined with insertion of radioactive substance into prostate, use 55862)

38564   retroperitoneal (aortic and/or splenic)

LAPAROSCOPY

38570 Laparoscopy, surgical; with retroperitoneal lymph node sampling (biopsy), single or multiple

38571   with bilateral total pelvic lymphadenectomy

38572   with bilateral total pelvic lymphadenectomy and peri-aortic lymph node sampling (biopsy), single or multiple

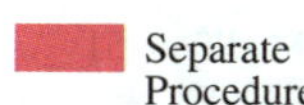 Separate Procedure

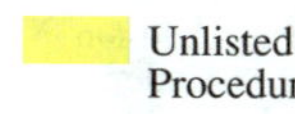 Unlisted Procedure

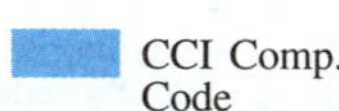 CCI Comp. Code

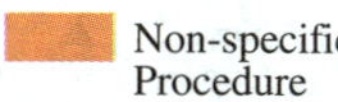 Non-specific Procedure

(For drainage of lymphocele to peritoneal cavity, use 49323)

38589 Unlisted laparoscopy procedure, lymphatic system

RADICAL LYMPHADENECTOMY (RADICAL RESECTION OF LYMPH NODES)

(For limited pelvic and retroperitoneal lymphadenectomies, see 38562, 38564)

38700 Suprahyoid lymphadenectomy

38720 Cervical lymphadenectomy (complete)

38724 Cervical lymphadenectomy (modified radical neck dissection)

38740 Axillary lymphadenectomy; superficial

38745   complete

+38746 Thoracic lymphadenectomy, regional, including mediastinal and peritracheal nodes (List separately in addition to code for primary procedure)

+38747 Abdominal lymphadenectomy, regional, including celiac, gastric, portal, peripancreatic, with or without para-aortic and vena caval nodes (List separately in addition to code for primary procedure)

38760 Inguinofemoral lymphadenectomy, superficial, including Cloquets node (separate procedure)

38765 Inguinofemoral lymphadenectomy, superficial, in continuity with pelvic lymphadenectomy, including external iliac, hypogastric, and obturator nodes (separate procedure)

38770 Pelvic lymphadenectomy, including external iliac, hypogastric, and obturator nodes (separate procedure)

38780 Retroperitoneal transabdominal lymphadenectomy, extensive, including pelvic, aortic, and renal nodes (separate procedure)

(For excision and repair of lymphedematous skin and subcutaneous tissue, see 15000, 15570-15650)

● New Code   ▲ Revised Code   ＊ Starred Procedure   ✚ Add-On Code   ⊘ Modifier -51 Exempt

INTRODUCTION

38790 Injection procedure; lymphangiography

(For radiological supervision and interpretation, see 75801-75807)

⊘ **38792** for identification of sentinel node

(For excision of sentinel node, see 38500-38542)

(For nuclear medicine lymphatics and lymph gland imaging, use 78195)

38794 Cannulation, thoracic duct

OTHER PROCEDURES

38999 Unlisted procedure, hemic or lymphatic system

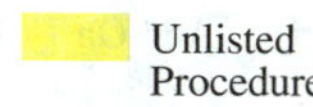
Separate Procedure

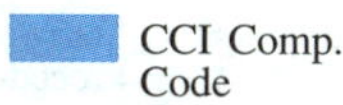
Unlisted Procedure

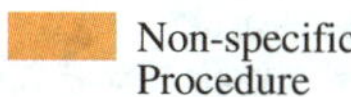
CCI Comp. Code

Non-specific Procedure

425

MEDIASTINUM AND DIAPHRAGM

CPT codes from this section of CPT are used to report invasive and surgical procedures performed on the mediastinum and the diaphragm.

MEDIASTINUM

INCISION

39000 Mediastinotomy with exploration, drainage, removal of foreign body, or biopsy; cervical approach

39010 transthoracic approach, including either transthoracic or median sternotomy

EXCISION

39200 Excision of mediastinal cyst

39220 Excision of mediastinal tumor

(For substernal thyroidectomy, use 60270)

(For thymectomy, use 60520)

ENDOSCOPY

39400 Mediastinoscopy, with or without biopsy

OTHER PROCEDURES

39499 Unlisted procedure, mediastinum

DIAPHRAGM

REPAIR

39501 Repair, laceration of diaphragm, any approach

39502 Repair, paraesophageal hiatus hernia, transabdominal, with or without fundoplasty, vagotomy, and/or pyloroplasty, except neonatal

39503 Repair, neonatal diaphragmatic hernia, with or without chest tube insertion and with or without creation of ventral hernia

39520 Repair, diaphragmatic hernia (esophageal hiatal); transthoracic

---

426   ● New Code   ▲ Revised Code   ✱ Starred Procedure   ✚ Add-On Code   ⊘ Modifier -51 Exempt

39530   combined, thoracoabdominal

39531   combined, thoracoabdominal, with dilation of stricture (with or without gastroplasty)

39540   Repair, diaphragmatic hernia (other than neonatal), traumatic; acute

39541   chronic

39545   Imbrication of diaphragm for eventration, transthoracic or transabdominal, paralytic or nonparalytic

39560   Resection, diaphragm; with simple repair (eg, primary suture)

39561   with complex repair (eg, prosthetic material, local muscle flap)

OTHER PROCEDURES

39599   Unlisted procedure, diaphragm

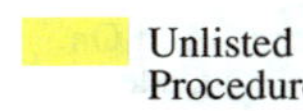
Separate Procedure

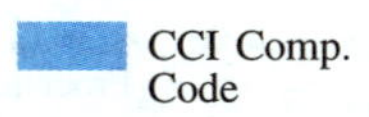
Unlisted Procedure

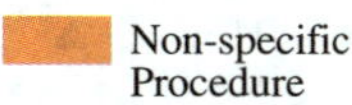
CCI Comp. Code

Non-specific Procedure

427

DIGESTIVE SYSTEM

CPT codes from this section of the CPT coding system are used to invasive and surgical procedures performed on the lips; mouth; tongue; dentoalveolar structures; palate; salivary gland; pharynx, adenoids and tonsils; esophagus; stomach; intestines; rectum; anus; liver; biliary tract; pancreas; and the abdomen, peritoneum, and omentum.

MISCELLANEOUS CODING RULES

Gastrointestinal endoscopy codes should be assigned based on the extent of visualization performed. HCFA's official guidelines for excision or destruction of a lesion are:

1. use only the biopsy code if a single lesion is biopsied but not excised;

2. code only for the excision if a lesion is biopsied and the remaining portion is excised;

3. use the biopsy code once even if multiple biopsies are performed and none are excised; and

4. use both a biopsy and excision code if each lesion is taken from different sites.

If the phrase "with or without biopsy" appears in the excision code's narrative, do not use a separate biopsy code. Diagnostic endoscopies are included in surgical endoscopies.

For upper gastrointestinal endoscopies, choose the appropriate code from documentation indicating whether the procedure was a simple exam, a diagnostic procedure or surgical procedure. Remember that code selection is based on the procedure(s) performed and the anatomical sites the scope passes through. For example, if the scope is passed to the esophagus only, the code would be chosen from endoscopy codes beginning with 43200. If the scope is passed through the esophagus to the stomach, duodenum and/or the jejunum, the code selection would begin at 43235.

HERNIA REPAIR

Review the patient's age, the kind of hernia, the clinical presentation of the hernia, and method of repair documented in the medical record before assigning a hernia repair code.

APPENDECTOMY

To code appendectomies appropriately, review the documentation for an indicated purpose for the removal. If there is none, then it is probably incidental to a more serious surgery and should not be coded.

428

● New Code	▲ Revised Code	✳ Starred Procedure	✛ Add-On Code	⊘ Modifier -51 Exempt

STARRED PROCEDURES

There are numerous starred (*) procedures in this section of the CPT coding system indicating the possibility of reporting an appropriate visit code in addition to the surgical procedure. When coding esophagoscopy procedures, code the appropriate endoscopy of each anatomic site examined.

LIPS

(For procedures on skin of lips, see 10040 et seq)

EXCISION

40490 Biopsy of lip

40500 Vermilionectomy (lip shave), with mucosal advancement

40510 Excision of lip; transverse wedge excision with primary closure

40520 V-excision with primary direct linear closure

(For excision of mucous lesions, see 40810-40816)

40525 full thickness, reconstruction with local flap (eg, Estlander or fan)

40527 full thickness, reconstruction with cross lip flap (Abbe-Estlander)

40530 Resection of lip, more than one-fourth, without reconstruction

(For reconstruction, see 13131 et seq)

REPAIR (CHEILOPLASTY)

40650 Repair lip, full thickness; vermilion only

40652 up to half vertical height

40654 over one-half vertical height, or complex

40700 Plastic repair of cleft lip/nasal deformity; primary, partial or complete, unilateral

40701 primary bilateral, one stage procedure

40702 primary bilateral, one of two stages

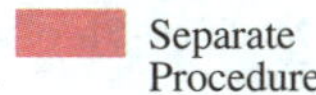
Separate
Procedure

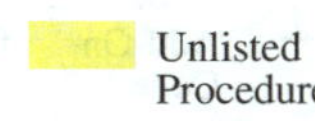
Unlisted
Procedure

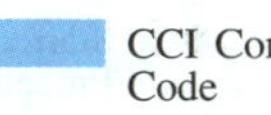
CCI Comp.
Code

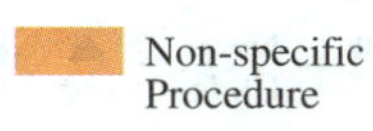
Non-specific
Procedure

429

40720	secondary, by recreation of defect and reclosure

(To report rhinoplasty only for nasal deformity secondary to congenital cleft lip, see 30460, 30462)

40761	with cross lip pedicle flap (Abbe-Estlander type), including sectioning and inserting of pedicle

(For repair cleft palate, see 42200 et seq)

(For other reconstructive procedures, see 14060, 14061, 15120-15261, 15574, 15576, 15630)

OTHER PROCEDURES

40799 Unlisted procedure, lips

VESTIBULE OF MOUTH

INCISION

***40800** Drainage of abscess, cyst, hematoma, vestibule of mouth; simple

40801 complicated

***40804** Removal of embedded foreign body, vestibule of mouth; simple

40805 complicated

40806 Incision of labial frenum (frenotomy)

EXCISION, DESTRUCTION

40808 Biopsy, vestibule of mouth

40810 Excision of lesion of mucosa and submucosa, vestibule of mouth; without repair

40812 with simple repair

40814 with complex repair

40816 complex, with excision of underlying muscle

40818 Excision of mucosa of vestibule of mouth as donor graft

● New Code	▲ Revised Code	* Starred Procedure	＋ Add-On Code	⊘ Modifier -51 Exempt

40819 Excision of frenum, labial or buccal (frenumectomy, frenulectomy, frenectomy)

40820 Destruction of lesion or scar of vestibule of mouth by physical methods (eg, laser, thermal, cryo, chemical)

REPAIR

40830 Closure of laceration, vestibule of mouth; 2.5 cm or less

40831 over 2.5 cm or complex

40840 Vestibuloplasty; anterior

40842 posterior, unilateral

40843 posterior, bilateral

40844 entire arch

40845 complex (including ridge extension, muscle repositioning)

(For skin grafts, see 15000 et seq)

OTHER PROCEDURES

40899 Unlisted procedure, vestibule of mouth

TONGUE AND FLOOR OF MOUTH

INCISION

***41000** Intraoral incision and drainage of abscess, cyst, or hematoma of tongue or floor of mouth; lingual

***41005** sublingual, superficial

41006 sublingual, deep, supramylohyoid

41007 submental space

41008 submandibular space

41009 masticator space

41010 Incision of lingual frenum (frenotomy)

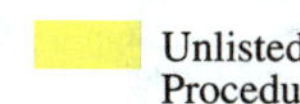

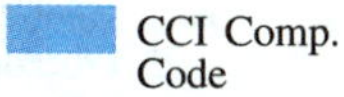

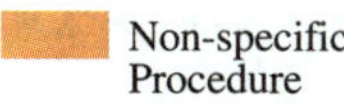

41015   Extraoral incision and drainage of abscess, cyst, or hematoma of floor of mouth; sublingual

41016   submental

41017   submandibular

41018   masticator space

(For frenoplasty, use 41520)

EXCISION

41100   Biopsy of tongue; anterior two-thirds

41105   posterior one-third

41108   Biopsy of floor of mouth

41110   Excision of lesion of tongue without closure

41112   Excision of lesion of tongue with closure; anterior two-thirds

41113   posterior one-third

41114   with local tongue flap

(List 41114 in addition to code 41112 or 41113)

41115   Excision of lingual frenum (frenectomy)

41116   Excision, lesion of floor of mouth

41120   Glossectomy; less than one-half tongue

41130   hemiglossectomy

41135   partial, with unilateral radical neck dissection

41140   complete or total, with or without tracheostomy, without radical neck dissection

41145   complete or total, with or without tracheostomy, with unilateral radical neck dissection

---

432

● New Code   ▲ Revised Code   * Starred Procedure   + Add-On Code   ○ Modifier -51 Exempt

41150   composite procedure with resection floor of mouth and mandibular resection, without radical neck dissection

41153   composite procedure with resection floor of mouth, with suprahyoid neck dissection

41155   composite procedure with resection floor of mouth, mandibular resection, and radical neck dissection (Commando type)

REPAIR

***41250**   Repair of laceration 2.5 cm or less; floor of mouth and/or anterior two-thirds of tongue

***41251**   posterior one-third of tongue

***41252**   Repair of laceration of tongue, floor of mouth, over 2.6 cm or complex

OTHER PROCEDURES

41500   Fixation of tongue, mechanical, other than suture (eg, K-wire)

41510   Suture of tongue to lip for micrognathia (Douglas type procedure)

41520   Frenoplasty (surgical revision of frenum, eg, with Z-plasty)

(For frenotomy, see 40806, 41010)

41599   Unlisted procedure, tongue, floor of mouth

DENTOALVEOLAR STRUCTURES

INCISION

***41800**   Drainage of abscess, cyst, hematoma from dentoalveolar structures

41805   Removal of embedded foreign body from dentoalveolar structures; soft tissues

41806   bone

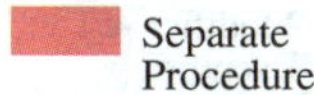
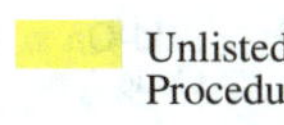
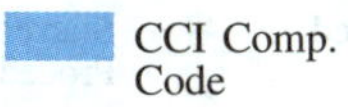
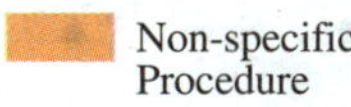

Separate Procedure   Unlisted Procedure   CCI Comp. Code   Non-specific Procedure

433

EXCISION, DESTRUCTION

41820 Gingivectomy, excision gingiva, each quadrant

41821 Operculectomy, excision pericoronal tissues

41822 Excision of fibrous tuberosities, dentoalveolar structures

41823 Excision of osseous tuberosities, dentoalveolar structures

41825 Excision of lesion or tumor (except listed above), dentoalveolar structures; without repair

41826 with simple repair

41827 with complex repair

(For nonexcisional destruction, use 41850)

41828 Excision of hyperplastic alveolar mucosa, each quadrant (specify)

41830 Alveolectomy, including curettage of osteitis or sequestrectomy

41850 Destruction of lesion (except excision), dentoalveolar structures

OTHER PROCEDURES

41870 Periodontal mucosal grafting

41872 Gingivoplasty, each quadrant (specify)

41874 Alveoloplasty, each quadrant (specify)

(For closure of lacerations, see 40830, 40831)

(For segmental osteotomy, use 21206)

(For reduction of fractures, see 21421-21490)

41899 Unlisted procedure, dentoalveolar structures

● New Code ▲ Revised Code * Starred Procedure + Add-On Code ⊘ Modifier -51 Exempt

PALATE AND UVULA

INCISION

***42000** Drainage of abscess of palate, uvula

EXCISION, DESTRUCTION

42100 Biopsy of palate, uvula

42104 Excision, lesion of palate, uvula; without closure

42106 with simple primary closure

42107 with local flap closure

(For skin graft, see 14040-14300)

(For mucosal graft, use 40818)

42120 Resection of palate or extensive resection of lesion

(For reconstruction of palate with extraoral tissue, see 14040-14300, 15050, 15120, 15240, 15576)

42140 Uvulectomy, excision of uvula

42145 Palatopharyngoplasty (eg, uvulopalatopharyngoplasty, uvulopharyngoplasty)

42160 Destruction of lesion, palate or uvula (thermal, cryo or chemical)

REPAIR

42180 Repair, laceration of palate; up to 2 cm

42182 over 2 cm or complex

42200 Palatoplasty for cleft palate, soft and/or hard palate only

42205 Palatoplasty for cleft palate, with closure of alveolar ridge; soft tissue only

42210 with bone graft to alveolar ridge (includes obtaining graft)

42215 Palatoplasty for cleft palate; major revision

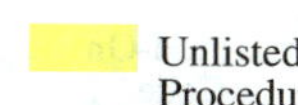

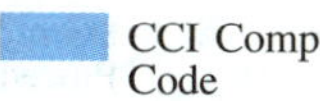

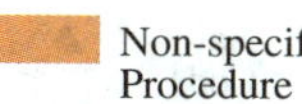

435

42220	secondary lengthening procedure
42225	attachment pharyngeal flap
42226	Lengthening of palate, and pharyngeal flap
42227	Lengthening of palate, with island flap
42235	Repair of anterior palate, including vomer flap
42260	Repair of nasolabial fistula

(For repair of cleft lip, see 40700 et seq)

| 42280 | Maxillary impression for palatal prosthesis |
| 42281 | Insertion of pin-retained palatal prosthesis |

OTHER PROCEDURES

| 42299 | Unlisted procedure, palate, uvula |

SALIVARY GLAND AND DUCTS

INCISION

*42300	Drainage of abscess; parotid, simple
42305	parotid, complicated
*42310	submaxillary or sublingual, intraoral
*42320	submaxillary, external
42325	Fistulization of sublingual salivary cyst (ranula);
42326	with prosthesis
42330	Sialolithotomy; submandibular (submaxillary), sublingual or parotid, uncomplicated, intraoral
42335	submandibular (submaxillary), complicated, intraoral
42340	parotid, extraoral or complicated intraoral

● New Code ▲ Revised Code * Starred Procedure + Add-On Code ⊘ Modifier -51 Exempt

EXCISION

***42400** Biopsy of salivary gland; needle

42405 incisional

(If imaging guidance is performed, see 76003, 76360, 76393, 76942)

42408 Excision of sublingual salivary cyst (ranula)

42409 Marsupialization of sublingual salivary cyst (ranula)

(For fistulization of sublingual salivary cyst, use 42325)

42410 Excision of parotid tumor or parotid gland; lateral lobe, without nerve dissection

42415 lateral lobe, with dissection and preservation of facial nerve

42420 total, with dissection and preservation of facial nerve

42425 total, en bloc removal with sacrifice of facial nerve

42426 total, with unilateral radical neck dissection

(For suture or grafting of facial nerve, see 64864, 64865, 69740, 69745)

42440 Excision of submandibular (submaxillary) gland

42450 Excision of sublingual gland

REPAIR

42500 Plastic repair of salivary duct, sialodochoplasty; primary or simple

42505 secondary or complicated

42507 Parotid duct diversion, bilateral (Wilke type procedure);

42508 with excision of one submandibular gland

42509 with excision of both submandibular glands

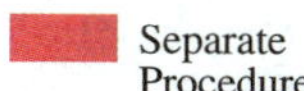
Separate Procedure

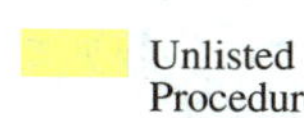
Unlisted Procedure

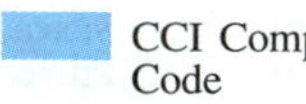
CCI Comp. Code

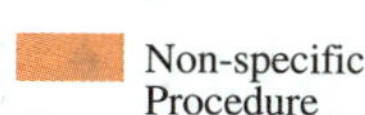
Non-specific Procedure

437

42510	with ligation of both submandibular (Wharton's) ducts

OTHER PROCEDURES

42550	Injection procedure for sialography

(For radiological supervision and interpretation, use 70390)

42600	Closure salivary fistula
∗42650	Dilation salivary duct
∗42660	Dilation and catheterization of salivary duct, with or without injection
42665	Ligation salivary duct, intraoral
42699	Unlisted procedure, salivary glands or ducts

PHARYNX, ADENOIDS, AND TONSILS

INCISION

∗42700	Incision and drainage abscess; peritonsillar
42720	retropharyngeal or parapharyngeal, intraoral approach
42725	retropharyngeal or parapharyngeal, external approach

EXCISION, DESTRUCTION

42800	Biopsy; oropharynx
42802	hypopharynx
42804	nasopharynx, visible lesion, simple
42806	nasopharynx, survey for unknown primary lesion

(For laryngoscopic biopsy, see 31510, 31535, 31536)

42808	Excision or destruction of lesion of pharynx, any method
42809	Removal of foreign body from pharynx

438

● New Code	▲ Revised Code	∗ Starred Procedure	✚ Add-On Code	⊘ Modifier -51 Exempt

42810 Excision branchial cleft cyst or vestige, confined to skin and subcutaneous tissues

42815 Excision branchial cleft cyst, vestige, or fistula, extending beneath subcutaneous tissues and/or into pharynx

42820 Tonsillectomy and adenoidectomy; under age 12

42821   age 12 or over

42825 Tonsillectomy, primary or secondary; under age 12

42826   age 12 or over

42830 Adenoidectomy, primary; under age 12

42831   age 12 or over

42835 Adenoidectomy, secondary; under age 12

42836   age 12 or over

42842 Radical resection of tonsil, tonsillar pillars, and/or retromolar trigone; without closure

42844   closure with local flap (eg, tongue, buccal)

42845   closure with other flap

(For closure with other flap(s), use appropriate number for flap(s))

(When combined with radical neck dissection, use also 38720)

42860 Excision of tonsil tags

42870 Excision or destruction lingual tonsil, any method (separate procedure)

42890 Limited pharyngectomy

42892 Resection of lateral pharyngeal wall or pyriform sinus, direct closure by advancement of lateral and posterior pharyngeal walls

(When combined with radical neck dissection, use also 38720)

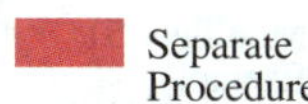

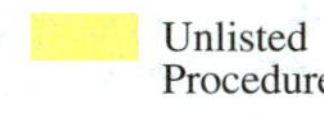

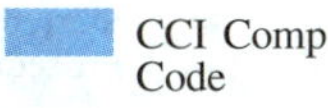

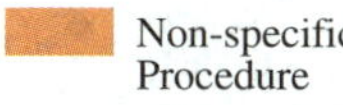

42894 Resection of pharyngeal wall requiring closure with myocutaneous flap

(When combined with radical neck dissection, use also 38720)

REPAIR

42900 Suture pharynx for wound or injury

42950 Pharyngoplasty (plastic or reconstructive operation on pharynx)

(For pharyngeal flap, use 42225)

42953 Pharyngoesophageal repair

(For closure with myocutaneous or other flap, use appropriate number in addition)

OTHER PROCEDURES

42955 Pharyngostomy (fistulization of pharynx, external for feeding)

42960 Control oropharyngeal hemorrhage, primary or secondary (eg, post-tonsillectomy); simple

42961 complicated, requiring hospitalization

42962 with secondary surgical intervention

▲ **42970** Control of nasopharyngeal hemorrhage, primary or secondary (eg, postadenoidectomy); simple, with posterior nasal packs, with or without anterior packs and/or cautery

42971 complicated, requiring hospitalization

42972 with secondary surgical intervention

42999 Unlisted procedure, pharynx, adenoids, or tonsils

ESOPHAGUS

INCISION

(For esophageal intubation with laparotomy, use 43510)

43020 Esophagotomy, cervical approach, with removal of foreign body

● New Code   ▲ Revised Code   * Starred Procedure   + Add-On Code   ⊘ Modifier -51 Exempt

43030 Cricopharyngeal myotomy

43045 Esophagotomy, thoracic approach, with removal of foreign body

EXCISION

(For gastrointestinal reconstruction for previous esophagectomy, see 43360, 43361)

43100 Excision of lesion, esophagus, with primary repair; cervical approach

43101 thoracic or abdominal approach

43107 Total or near total esophagectomy, without thoracotomy; with pharyngogastrostomy or cervical esophagogastrostomy, with or without pyloroplasty (transhiatal)

▲ **43108** with colon interposition or small intestine reconstruction, including intestine mobilization, preparation and anastomosis(es)

43112 Total or near total esophagectomy, with thoracotomy; with pharyngogastrostomy or cervical esophagogastrostomy, with or without pyloroplasty

▲ **43113** with colon interposition or small intestine reconstruction, including intestine mobilization, preparation, and anastomosis(es)

43116 Partial esophagectomy, cervical, with free intestinal graft, including microvascular anastomosis, obtaining the graft and intestinal reconstruction

(Do not report code 69990 in addition to code 43116)

(Report 43116 with the modifier -52 appended if intestinal or free jejunal graft with microvascular anastomosis is performed by another physician)

(For free jejunal graft with microvascular anastomosis performed by another physician, use 43496)

43117 Partial esophagectomy, distal two-thirds, with thoracotomy and separate abdominal incision, with or without proximal gastrectomy; with thoracic esophagogastrostomy, with or without pyloroplasty (Ivor Lewis)

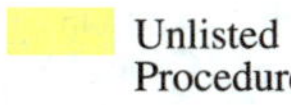

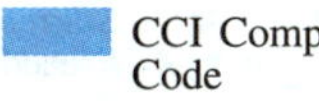

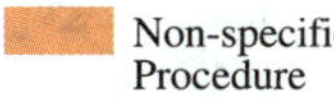

Non-specific
Procedure

▲ **43118**   with colon interposition or small intestine reconstruction, including intestine mobilization, preparation, and anastomosis(es)

43121   Partial esophagectomy, distal two-thirds, with thoracotomy only, with or without proximal gastrectomy, with thoracic esophagogastrostomy, with or without pyloroplasty

43122   Partial esophagectomy, thoracoabdominal or abdominal approach, with or without proximal gastrectomy; with esophagogastrostomy, with or without pyloroplasty

▲ **43123**   with colon interposition or small intestine reconstruction, including intestine mobilization, preparation, and anastomosis(es)

43124   Total or partial esophagectomy, without reconstruction (any approach), with cervical esophagostomy

43130   Diverticulectomy of hypopharynx or esophagus, with or without myotomy; cervical approach

43135   thoracic approach

ENDOSCOPY

43200   Esophagoscopy, rigid or flexible; diagnostic, with or without collection of specimen(s) by brushing or washing (separate procedure)

43202   with biopsy, single or multiple

43204   with injection sclerosis of esophageal varices

43205   with band ligation of esophageal varices

43215   with removal of foreign body

(For radiological supervision and interpretation, use 74235)

43216   with removal of tumor(s), polyp(s), or other lesion(s) by hot biopsy forceps or bipolar cautery

43217   with removal of tumor(s), polyp(s), or other lesion(s) by snare technique

43219   with insertion of plastic tube or stent

43220   with balloon dilation (less than 30 mm diameter)

(If imaging guidance is performed, use 74360)

(For endoscopic dilation with balloon 30 mm diameter or larger, use 43458)

(For dilation without visualization, see 43450-43453)

43226   with insertion of guide wire followed by dilation over guide wire

(For radiological supervision and interpretation, use 74360)

▲ **43227**   with control of bleeding (eg, injection, bipolar cautery, unipolar cautery, laser, heater probe, stapler, plasma coagulator)

43228   with ablation of tumor(s), polyp(s), or other lesion(s), not amenable to removal by hot biopsy forceps, bipolar cautery or snare technique

(For esophagoscopic photodynamic therapy, report 43228 in addition to 96570, 96571 as appropriate)

43231   with endoscopic ultrasound examination

43232   with transendoscopic ultrasound-guided intramural or transmural fine needle aspiration/biopsy(s)

(Do not report 76975 in conjunction with 43231, 43232)

(For interpretation of specimen, see 88172-88173)

43234   Upper gastrointestinal endoscopy, simple primary examination (eg, with small diameter flexible endoscope) (separate procedure)

43235   Upper gastrointestinal endoscopy including esophagus, stomach, and either the duodenum and/or jejunum as appropriate; diagnostic, with or without collection of specimen(s) by brushing or washing (separate procedure)

43239   with biopsy, single or multiple

(For upper gastrointestinal endoscopy with suturing of the esophagogastric junction, see Category III code 0008T)

43240   with transmural drainage of pseudocyst

443

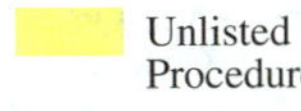

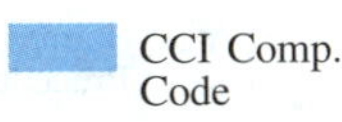

CCI Comp.
Code

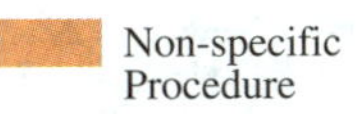

43241   with transendoscopic intraluminal tube or catheter placement

43242   with transendoscopic ultrasound-guided intramural or transmural fine needle aspiration/biopsy(s)

(Do not report 76975 in conjunction with 43242)

(For interpretation of specimen, see 88172-88173)

43243   with injection sclerosis of esophageal and/or gastric varices

43244   with band ligation of esophageal and/or gastric varices

▲ **43245**   with dilation of gastric outlet for obstruction (eg, balloon, guide wire, bougie)

43246   with directed placement of percutaneous gastrostomy tube

(For radiological supervision and interpretation, use 74350)

43247   with removal of foreign body

(For radiological supervision and interpretation, use 74235)

43248   with insertion of guide wire followed by dilation of esophagus over guide wire

43249   with balloon dilation of esophagus (less than 30 mm diameter)

43250   with removal of tumor(s), polyp(s), or other lesion(s) by hot biopsy forceps or bipolar cautery

43251   with removal of tumor(s), polyp(s), or other lesion(s) by snare technique

43255   with control of bleeding, any method

43256   with transendoscopic stent placement (includes predilation)

43258   with ablation of tumor(s), polyp(s), or other lesion(s) not amenable to removal by hot biopsy forceps, bipolar cautery or snare technique

(For injection sclerosis of esophageal varices, use 43204 or 43243)

● New Code   ▲ Revised Code   ✱ Starred Procedure   ✚ Add-On Code   ⊘ Modifier -51 Exempt

43259 with endoscopic ultrasound examination

(For radiological supervision and interpretation, use 76975)

43260 Endoscopic retrograde cholangiopancreatography (ERCP); diagnostic, with or without collection of specimen(s) by brushing or washing (separate procedure)

(For radiological supervision and interpretation, see 74328, 74329, 74330)

43261 with biopsy, single or multiple

43262 with sphincterotomy/papillotomy

(For radiological supervision and interpretation, see 74328, 74329, 74330)

43263 with pressure measurement of sphincter of Oddi (pancreatic duct or common bile duct)

(For radiological supervision and interpretation, see 74328, 74329, 74330)

▲ **43264** with endoscopic retrograde removal of calculus/calculi from biliary and/or pancreatic ducts

(When done with sphincterotomy, also use 43262)

(For radiological supervision and interpretation, see 74328, 74329, 74330)

▲ **43265** with endoscopic retrograde destruction, lithotripsy of calculus/calculi, any method

(When done with sphincterotomy, also use 43262)

(For radiological supervision and interpretation, see 74328, 74329, 74330)

43267 with endoscopic retrograde insertion of nasobiliary or nasopancreatic drainage tube

(When done with sphincterotomy, also use 43262)

(For radiological supervision and interpretation, see 74328, 74329, 74330)

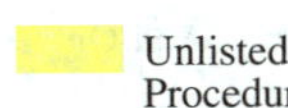

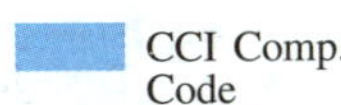

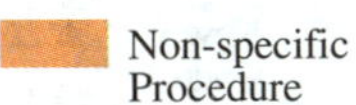

Non-specific
Procedure

43268   with endoscopic retrograde insertion of tube or stent into bile or pancreatic duct

(When done with sphincterotomy, also use 43262)

(For radiological supervision and interpretation, see 74328, 74329, 74330)

43269   with endoscopic retrograde removal of foreign body and/or change of tube or stent

(When done with sphincterotomy, also use 43262)

(For radiological supervision and interpretation, see 74328, 74329, 74330)

43271   with endoscopic retrograde balloon dilation of ampulla, biliary and/or pancreatic duct(s)

(When done with sphincterotomy, also use 43262)

(For radiological supervision and interpretation, see 74328, 74329, 74330)

43272   with ablation of tumor(s), polyp(s), or other lesion(s) not amenable to removal by hot biopsy forceps, bipolar cautery or snare technique

(For radiological supervision and interpretation, see 74328, 74329, 74330)

LAPAROSCOPY

43280   Laparoscopy, surgical, esophagogastric fundoplasty (eg, Nissen, Toupet procedures)

(For open approach, use 43324)

43289   Unlisted laparoscopy procedure, esophagus

REPAIR

43300   Esophagoplasty, (plastic repair or reconstruction), cervical approach; without repair of tracheoesophageal fistula

43305   with repair of tracheoesophageal fistula

43310   Esophagoplasty, (plastic repair or reconstruction), thoracic approach; without repair of tracheoesophageal fistula

---

446 ● New Code ▲ Revised Code ＊ Starred Procedure ＋ Add-On Code ⊘ Modifier -51 Exempt

43312   with repair of tracheoesophageal fistula

● **43313**   Esophagoplasty for congenital defect, (plastic repair or reconstruction), thoracic approach; without repair of congenital tracheoesophageal fistula

● **43314**   with repair of congenital tracheoesophageal fistula

43320   Esophagogastrostomy (cardioplasty), with or without vagotomy and pyloroplasty, transabdominal or transthoracic approach

43324   Esophagogastric fundoplasty (eg, Nissen, Belsey IV, Hill procedures)

(For laparoscopic procedure, use 43280)

43325   Esophagogastric fundoplasty; with fundic patch (Thal-Nissen procedure)

(For cricopharyngeal myotomy, use 43030)

43326   with gastroplasty (eg, Collis)

43330   Esophagomyotomy (Heller type); abdominal approach

43331   thoracic approach

(For thoracoscopic esophagomyotomy, use 32665)

43340   Esophagojejunostomy (without total gastrectomy); abdominal approach

43341   thoracic approach

43350   Esophagostomy, fistulization of esophagus, external; abdominal approach

43351   thoracic approach

43352   cervical approach

43360   Gastrointestinal reconstruction for previous esophagectomy, for obstructing esophageal lesion or fistula, or for previous esophageal exclusion; with stomach, with or without pyloroplasty

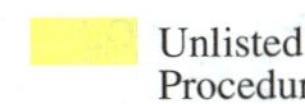
Separate Procedure

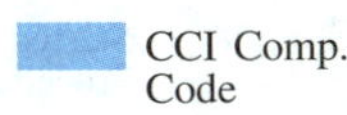
Unlisted Procedure

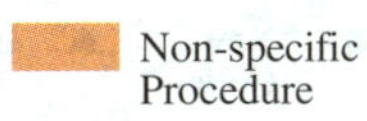
CCI Comp. Code

Non-specific Procedure

▲ **43361**   with colon interposition or small intestine reconstruction, including intestine mobilization, preparation, and anastomosis(es)

43400   Ligation, direct, esophageal varices

43401   Transection of esophagus with repair, for esophageal varices

43405   Ligation or stapling at gastroesophageal junction for pre-existing esophageal perforation

43410   Suture of esophageal wound or injury; cervical approach

43415   transthoracic or transabdominal approach

43420   Closure of esophagostomy or fistula; cervical approach

43425   transthoracic or transabdominal approach

(For repair of esophageal hiatal hernia, see 39520 et seq)

MANIPULATION

(For associated esophagogram, use 74220)

*43450   Dilation of esophagus, by unguided sound or bougie, single or multiple passes

43453   Dilation of esophagus, over guide wire

(For dilation with direct visualization, use 43220)

43456   Dilation of esophagus, by balloon or dilator, retrograde

43458   Dilation of esophagus with balloon (30 mm diameter or larger) for achalasia

(For dilation with balloon less than 30 mm diameter, use 43220)

(For radiological supervision and interpretation, use 74360)

43460   Esophagogastric tamponade, with balloon (Sengstaaken type)

(For removal of esophageal foreign body by balloon catheter, see 43215, 43247, 74235)

---

448   ● New Code   ▲ Revised Code   * Starred Procedure   + Add-On Code   ⊘ Modifier -51 Exempt

OTHER PROCEDURES

43496   Free jejunum transfer with microvascular anastomosis

(Do not report code 69990 in addition to code 43496)

43499   Unlisted procedure, esophagus

STOMACH

INCISION

43500   Gastrotomy; with exploration or foreign body removal

43501   with suture repair of bleeding ulcer

43502   with suture repair of pre-existing esophagogastric laceration (eg, Mallory-Weiss)

43510   with esophageal dilation and insertion of permanent intraluminal tube (eg, Celestin or Mousseaux-Barbin)

43520   Pyloromyotomy, cutting of pyloric muscle (Fredet-Ramstedt type operation)

EXCISION

43600   Biopsy of stomach; by capsule, tube, peroral (one or more specimens)

43605   by laparotomy

43610   Excision, local; ulcer or benign tumor of stomach

43611   malignant tumor of stomach

43620   Gastrectomy, total; with esophagoenterostomy

43621   with Roux-en-Y reconstruction

43622   with formation of intestinal pouch, any type

43631   Gastrectomy, partial, distal; with gastroduodenostomy

43632   with gastrojejunostomy

449

43633   with Roux-en-Y reconstruction

43634   with formation of intestinal pouch

+43635   Vagotomy when performed with partial distal gastrectomy (List separately in addition to code(s) for primary procedure)

(Use 43635 in conjunction with codes 43631, 43632, 43633, 43634)

43638   Gastrectomy, partial, proximal, thoracic or abdominal approach including esophagogastrostomy, with vagotomy;

43639   with pyloroplasty or pyloromyotomy

(For regional thoracic lymphadenectomy, use 38746)

(For regional abdominal lymphadenectomy, use 38747)

43640   Vagotomy including pyloroplasty, with or without gastrostomy; truncal or selective

(For pyloroplasty, use 43800)

(For vagotomy, see 64752-64760)

43641   parietal cell (highly selective)

(For upper gastrointestinal endoscopy, see 43234-43259)

LAPAROSCOPY

43651   Laparoscopy, surgical; transection of vagus nerves, truncal

43652   transection of vagus nerves, selective or highly selective

43653   gastrostomy, without construction of gastric tube (eg, Stamm procedure) (separate procedure)

43659   Unlisted laparoscopy procedure, stomach

INTRODUCTION

43750   Percutaneous placement of gastrostomy tube

(For radiological supervision and interpretation, use 74350)

● New Code   ▲ Revised Code   ✳ Starred Procedure   ✛ Add-On Code   ⊘ Modifier -51 Exempt

43752   Naso- or oro-gastric tube placement, necessitating physician's skill

(If imaging guidance is performed, use 76000)

(For enteric tube placement, see 44500, 74340)

(Do not report 43752 in conjunction with critical care codes 99291-99292, or neonatal intensive care codes, 99295-99298)

∗43760   Change of gastrostomy tube

(For endoscopic placement of gastrostomy tube, use 43246)

(For radiological supervision and interpretation, use 75984)

43761   Repositioning of the gastric feeding tube, any method, through the duodenum for enteric nutrition

(If imaging guidance is performed, use 75984)

OTHER PROCEDURES

43800   Pyloroplasty

(For pyloroplasty and vagotomy, use 43640)

43810   Gastroduodenostomy

43820   Gastrojejunostomy; without vagotomy

43825   with vagotomy, any type

43830   Gastrostomy, open; without construction of gastric tube (eg, Stamm procedure) (separate procedure)

43831   neonatal, for feeding

(For change of gastrostomy tube, use 43760)

43832   with construction of gastric tube (eg, Janeway procedure)

43840   Gastrorrhaphy, suture of perforated duodenal or gastric ulcer, wound, or injury

43842   Gastric restrictive procedure, without gastric bypass, for morbid obesity; vertical-banded gastroplasty

451

| 43843 | other than vertical-banded gastroplasty |

| 43846 | Gastric restrictive procedure, with gastric bypass for morbid obesity; with short limb (less than 100 cm) Roux-en-Y gastroenterostomy |

▲ | 43847 | with small intestine reconstruction to limit absorption |

| 43848 | Revision of gastric restrictive procedure for morbid obesity (separate procedure) |

| 43850 | Revision of gastroduodenal anastomosis (gastroduodenostomy) with reconstruction; without vagotomy |

| 43855 | with vagotomy |

▲ | 43860 | Revision of gastrojejunal anastomosis (gastrojejunostomy) with reconstruction, with or without partial gastrectomy or intestine resection; without vagotomy |

| 43865 | with vagotomy |

| 43870 | Closure of gastrostomy, surgical |

| 43880 | Closure of gastrocolic fistula |

| 43999 | Unlisted procedure, stomach |

INTESTINES (EXCEPT RECTUM)

INCISION

| 44005 | Enterolysis (freeing of intestinal adhesion) (separate procedure) |

(Do not report 44005 in addition to 45136)

(For laparoscopic approach, use 44200)

| 44010 | Duodenotomy, for exploration, biopsy(s), or foreign body removal |

+44015 | Tube or needle catheter jejunostomy for enteral alimentation, intraoperative, any method (List separately in addition to primary procedure)

● New Code   ▲ Revised Code   ✳ Starred Procedure   ✚ Add-On Code   ⊘ Modifier -51 Exempt

▲ **44020** Enterotomy, small intestine, other than duodenum; for exploration, biopsy(s), or foreign body removal

44021 for decompression (eg, Baker tube)

44025 Colotomy, for exploration, biopsy(s), or foreign body removal

44050 Reduction of volvulus, intussusception, internal hernia, by laparotomy

44055 Correction of malrotation by lysis of duodenal bands and/or reduction of midgut volvulus (eg, Ladd procedure)

EXCISION

44100 Biopsy of intestine by capsule, tube, peroral (one or more specimens)

▲ **44110** Excision of one or more lesions of small or large intestine not requiring anastomosis, exteriorization, or fistulization; single enterotomy

44111 multiple enterotomies

44120 Enterectomy, resection of small intestine; single resection and anastomosis

(Do not report 44120 in addition to 45136)

+44121 each additional resection and anastomosis (List separately in addition to code for primary procedure)

(Use 44121 in conjunction with code 44120)

44125 with enterostomy

● **44126** Enterectomy, resection of small intestine for congenital atresia, single resection and anastomosis of proximal segment of intestine; without tapering

● **44127** with tapering

●**+44128** each additional resection and anastomosis (List separately in addition to code for primary procedure)

(Use 44128 in conjunction with codes 44126, 44127)

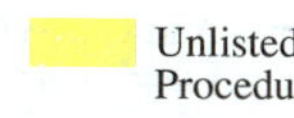

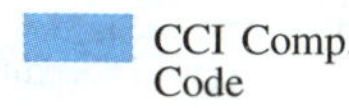

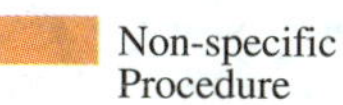

44130   Enteroenterostomy, anastomosis of intestine, with or without cutaneous enterostomy (separate procedure)

44132   Donor enterectomy, open, with preparation and maintenance of allograft; from cadaver donor

44133   partial, from living donor

44135   Intestinal allotransplantation; from cadaver donor

44136   from living donor

+44139   Mobilization (take-down) of splenic flexure performed in conjunction with partial colectomy (List separately in addition to primary procedure)

(Use 44139 in conjunction with codes 44140-44147)

44140   Colectomy, partial; with anastomosis

(For laparoscopic procedure, use 44204)

44141   with skin level cecostomy or colostomy

44143   with end colostomy and closure of distal segment (Hartmann type procedure)

44144   with resection, with colostomy or ileostomy and creation of mucofistula

44145   with coloproctostomy (low pelvic anastomosis)

44146   with coloproctostomy (low pelvic anastomosis), with colostomy

44147   abdominal and transanal approach

44150   Colectomy, total, abdominal, without proctectomy; with ileostomy or ileoproctostomy

44151   with continent ileostomy

44152   with rectal mucosectomy, ileoanal anastomosis, with or without loop ileostomy

● New Code   ▲ Revised Code   * Starred Procedure   + Add-On Code   ⊘ Modifier -51 Exempt

44153   with rectal mucosectomy, ileoanal anastomosis, creation of ileal reservoir (S or J), with or without loop ileostomy

44155   Colectomy, total, abdominal, with proctectomy; with ileostomy

44156   with continent ileostomy

▲ **44160**   Colectomy, partial, with removal of terminal ileum and ileocolostomy

(For laparoscopic procedure, use 44205)

LAPAROSCOPY

44200   Laparoscopy, surgical; enterolysis (freeing of intestinal adhesion) (separate procedure)

(For laparoscopy with salpingolysis, ovariolysis, use 58660)

44201   jejunostomy (eg, for decompression or feeding)

▲ **44202**   enterectomy, resection of small intestine, single resection and anastomosis

●+**44203**   each additional small intestine resection and anastomosis (List separately in addition to code for primary procedure)

(Use 44203 in conjunction with code 44202)

(For open procedure, see 44120, 44121)

● **44204**   colectomy, partial, with anastomosis

(For open procedure, use 44140)

● **44205**   colectomy, partial, with removal of terminal ileum with ileocolostomy

(For open procedure, use 44160)

44209   Unlisted laparoscopy procedure, intestine (except rectum)

ENTEROSTOMY-EXTERNAL FISTULIZATION OF INTESTINES

44300   Enterostomy or cecostomy, tube (eg, for decompression or feeding) (separate procedure)

44310   Ileostomy or jejunostomy, non-tube (separate procedure)

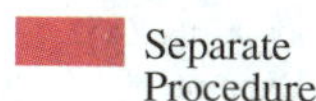

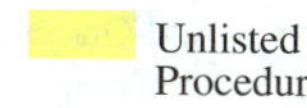

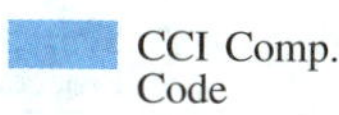

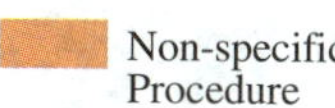

(Do not report 44310 in addition to 45136)

44312 Revision of ileostomy; simple (release of superficial scar) (separate procedure)

44314 complicated (reconstruction in-depth) (separate procedure)

44316 Continent ileostomy (Kock procedure) (separate procedure)

(For fiberoptic evaluation, use 44385)

44320 Colostomy or skin level cecostomy; (separate procedure)

▲ **44322** with multiple biopsies (eg, for congenital megacolon) (separate procedure)

44340 Revision of colostomy; simple (release of superficial scar) (separate procedure)

44345 complicated (reconstruction in-depth) (separate procedure)

44346 with repair of paracolostomy hernia (separate procedure)

ENDOSCOPY, SMALL INTESTINE AND STOMAL

(For upper gastrointestinal endoscopy, see 43234-43258)

44360 Small intestinal endoscopy, enteroscopy beyond second portion of duodenum, not including ileum; diagnostic, with or without collection of specimen(s) by brushing or washing (separate procedure)

44361 with biopsy, single or multiple

44363 with removal of foreign body

44364 with removal of tumor(s), polyp(s), or other lesion(s) by snare technique

44365 with removal of tumor(s), polyp(s), or other lesion(s) by hot biopsy forceps or bipolar cautery

▲ **44366** with control of bleeding (eg, injection, bipolar cautery, unipolar cautery, laser, heater probe, stapler, plasma coagulator)

● New Code   ▲ Revised Code   ✱ Starred Procedure   ✚ Add-On Code   ⊘ Modifier -51 Exempt

44369   with ablation of tumor(s), polyp(s), or other lesion(s) not amenable to removal by hot biopsy forceps, bipolar cautery or snare technique

44370   with transendoscopic stent placement (includes predilation)

44372   with placement of percutaneous jejunostomy tube

44373   with conversion of percutaneous gastrostomy tube to percutaneous jejunostomy tube

44376   Small intestinal endoscopy, enteroscopy beyond second portion of duodenum, including ileum; diagnostic, with or without collection of specimen(s) by brushing or washing (separate procedure)

44377   with biopsy, single or multiple

▲ **44378**   with control of bleeding (eg, injection, bipolar cautery, unipolar cautery, laser, heater probe, stapler, plasma coagulator)

44379   with transendoscopic stent placement (includes predilation)

44380   Ileoscopy, through stoma; diagnostic, with or without collection of specimen(s) by brushing or washing (separate procedure)

44382   with biopsy, single or multiple

44383   with transendoscopic stent placement (includes predilation)

44385   Endoscopic evaluation of small intestinal (abdominal or pelvic) pouch; diagnostic, with or without collection of specimen(s) by brushing or washing (separate procedure)

44386   with biopsy, single or multiple

44388   Colonoscopy through stoma; diagnostic, with or without collection of specimen(s) by brushing or washing (separate procedure)

44389   with biopsy, single or multiple

44390   with removal of foreign body

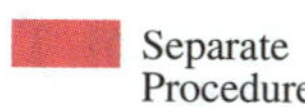 Separate Procedure

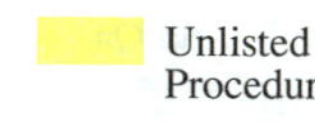 Unlisted Procedure

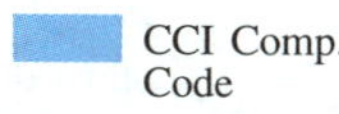 CCI Comp. Code

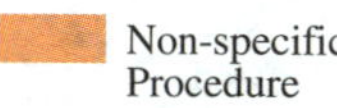 Non-specific Procedure

▲ **44391**   with control of bleeding (eg, injection, bipolar cautery, unipolar cautery, laser, heater probe, stapler, plasma coagulator)

44392   with removal of tumor(s), polyp(s), or other lesion(s) by hot biopsy forceps or bipolar cautery

44393   with ablation of tumor(s), polyp(s), or other lesion(s) not amenable to removal by hot biopsy forceps, bipolar cautery or snare technique

44394   with removal of tumor(s), polyp(s), or other lesion(s) by snare technique

(For colonoscopy per rectum, see 45330-45385)

44397   with transendoscopic stent placement (includes predilation)

INTRODUCTION

⊘ **44500**   Introduction of long gastrointestinal tube (eg, Miller-Abbott) (separate procedure)

(For radiological supervision and interpretation, use 74340)

(For naso- or oro-gastric tube placement, use 43752)

REPAIR

44602   Suture of small intestine (enterorrhaphy) for perforated ulcer, diverticulum, wound, injury or rupture; single perforation

44603   multiple perforations

44604   Suture of large intestine (colorrhaphy) for perforated ulcer, diverticulum, wound, injury, or rupture (single or multiple perforations); without colostomy

44605   with colostomy

44615   Intestinal stricturoplasty (enterotomy and enterorrhaphy) with or without dilation, for intestinal obstruction

44620   Closure of enterostomy, large or small intestine;

44625   with resection and anastomosis other than colorectal

● New Code   ▲ Revised Code   * Starred Procedure   + Add-On Code   ⊘ Modifier -51 Exempt

44626   with resection and colorectal anastomosis (eg, closure of Hartmann type procedure)

44640   Closure of intestinal cutaneous fistula

44650   Closure of enteroenteric or enterocolic fistula

44660   Closure of enterovesical fistula; without intestinal or bladder resection

▲ **44661**   with intestine and/or bladder resection

(For closure of renocolic fistula, see 50525, 50526)

(For closure of gastrocolic fistula, use 43880)

(For closure of rectovesical fistula, see 45800, 45805)

44680   Intestinal plication (separate procedure)

OTHER PROCEDURES

▲ **44700**   Exclusion of small intestine from pelvis by mesh or other prosthesis, or native tissue (eg, bladder or omentum)

(For therapeutic radiation clinical treatment, see Radiation Oncology section)

44799   Unlisted procedure, intestine

MECKEL'S DIVERTICULUM AND THE MESENTERY

EXCISION

44800   Excision of Meckel's diverticulum (diverticulectomy) or omphalomesenteric duct

44820   Excision of lesion of mesentery (separate procedure)

(With intestine resection, see 44120 or 44140 et seq)

SUTURE

44850   Suture of mesentery (separate procedure)

(For reduction and repair of internal hernia, use 44050)

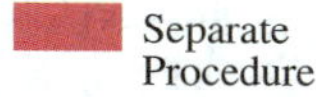 Separate Procedure   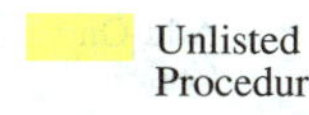 Unlisted Procedure   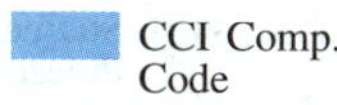 CCI Comp. Code   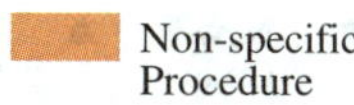 Non-specific Procedure

OTHER PROCEDURES

44899 Unlisted procedure, Meckel's diverticulum and the mesentery

APPENDIX

INCISION

44900 Incision and drainage of appendiceal abscess; open

44901 percutaneous

(For radiological supervision and interpretation, use 75989)

EXCISION

44950 Appendectomy;

(Incidental appendectomy during intra-abdominal surgery does not usually warrant a separate identification. If necessary to report, add modifier -52)

+44955 when done for indicated purpose at time of other major procedure (not as separate procedure) (List separately in addition to code for primary procedure)

44960 for ruptured appendix with abscess or generalized peritonitis

LAPAROSCOPY

44970 Laparoscopy, surgical, appendectomy

44979 Unlisted laparoscopy procedure, appendix

RECTUM

INCISION

45000 Transrectal drainage of pelvic abscess

45005 Incision and drainage of submucosal abscess, rectum

45020 Incision and drainage of deep supralevator, pelvirectal, or retrorectal abscess

(See also 46050, 46060)

● New Code	▲ Revised Code	✳ Starred Procedure	✛ Add-On Code	⊘ Modifier -51 Exempt

EXCISION

45100   Biopsy of anorectal wall, anal approach (eg, congenital megacolon)

(For endoscopic biopsy, use 45305)

45108   Anorectal myomectomy

45110   Proctectomy; complete, combined abdominoperineal, with colostomy

45111   partial resection of rectum, transabdominal approach

45112   Proctectomy, combined abdominoperineal, pull-through procedure (eg, colo-anal anastomosis)

(For colo-anal anastomosis with colonic reservoir or pouch, use 45119)

45113   Proctectomy, partial, with rectal mucosectomy, ileoanal anastomosis, creation of ileal reservoir (S or J), with or without loop ileostomy

45114   Proctectomy, partial, with anastomosis; abdominal and transsacral approach

45116   transsacral approach only (Kraske type)

45119   Proctectomy, combined abdominoperineal pull-through procedure (eg, colo-anal anastomosis), with creation of colonic reservoir (eg, J-pouch), with or without proximal diverting ostomy

45120   Proctectomy, complete (for congenital megacolon), abdominal and perineal approach; with pull-through procedure and anastomosis (eg, Swenson, Duhamel, or Soave type operation)

45121   with subtotal or total colectomy, with multiple biopsies

45123   Proctectomy, partial, without anastomosis, perineal approach

45126   Pelvic exenteration for colorectal malignancy, with proctectomy (with or without colostomy), with removal of bladder and ureteral transplantations, and/or hysterectomy, or cervicectomy, with or without removal of tube(s), with or without removal of ovary(s), or any combination thereof

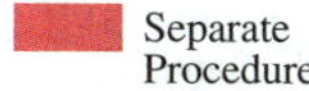 Separate Procedure

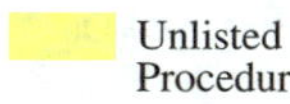 Unlisted Procedure

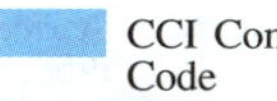 CCI Comp. Code

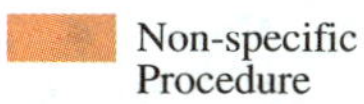 Non-specific Procedure

461

45130 Excision of rectal procidentia, with anastomosis; perineal approach

45135 abdominal and perineal approach

● **45136** Excision of ileoanal reservoir with ileostomy

(Do not report 45136 in addition to 44005, 44120, 44310)

45150 Division of stricture of rectum

45160 Excision of rectal tumor by proctotomy, transsacral or transcoccygeal approach

45170 Excision of rectal tumor, transanal approach

DESTRUCTION

▲ **45190** Destruction of rectal tumor (eg, electrodessiccation, electrosurgery, laser ablation, laser resection, cryosurgery) transanal approach

ENDOSCOPY

45300 Proctosigmoidoscopy, rigid; diagnostic, with or without collection of specimen(s) by brushing or washing (separate procedure)

▲ **45303** with dilation (eg, balloon, guide wire, bougie)

(For radiological supervision and interpretation, use 74360)

45305 with biopsy, single or multiple

45307 with removal of foreign body

45308 with removal of single tumor, polyp, or other lesion by hot biopsy forceps or bipolar cautery

45309 with removal of single tumor, polyp, or other lesion by snare technique

45315 with removal of multiple tumors, polyps, or other lesions by hot biopsy forceps, bipolar cautery or snare technique

---

   ● New Code   ▲ Revised Code   ✳ Starred Procedure   ✚ Add-On Code   ⊘ Modifier -51 Exempt

▲ **45317**   with control of bleeding (eg, injection, bipolar cutery, unipolar cautery, laser, heater probe, stapler, plasma coagulator)

45320   with ablation of tumor(s), polyp(s), or other lesion(s) not amenable to removal by hot biopsy forceps, bipolar cautery or snare technique (eg, laser)

45321   with decompression of volvulus

(45325 colonoscopy has been renumbered 45355 without change in terminology)

45327   with transendoscopic stent placement (includes predilation)

45330   Sigmoidoscopy, flexible; diagnostic, with or without collection of specimen(s) by brushing or washing (separate procedure)

45331   with biopsy, single or multiple

45332   with removal of foreign body

45333   with removal of tumor(s), polyp(s), or other lesion(s) by hot biopsy forceps or bipolar cautery

▲ **45334**   with control of bleeding (eg, injection, bipolar cutery, unipolar cautery, laser, heater probe, stapler, plasma coagulator)

45337   with decompression of volvulus, any method

45338   with removal of tumor(s), polyp(s), or other lesion(s) by snare technique

45339   with ablation of tumor(s), polyp(s), or other lesion(s) not amenable to removal by hot biopsy forceps, bipolar cautery or snare technique

45341   with endoscopic ultrasound examination

45342   with transendoscopic ultrasound guided intramural or transmural fine needle aspiration/biopsy(s)

(Do not report 76975 in conjunction with codes 45341, 45342)

(For interpretation of specimen, see 88172-88173)

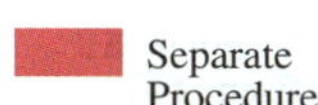 Separate Procedure

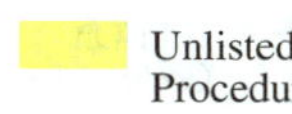 Unlisted Procedure

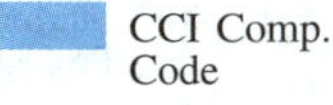 CCI Comp. Code

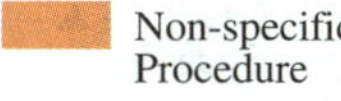 Non-specific Procedure

(For transrectal ultrasound utilizing rigid probe device, use 76872)

45345 with transendoscopic stent placement (includes predilation)

45355 Colonoscopy, rigid or flexible, transabdominal via colotomy, single or multiple

45378 Colonoscopy, flexible, proximal to splenic flexure; diagnostic, with or without collection of specimen(s) by brushing or washing, with or without colon decompression (separate procedure)

45379 with removal of foreign body

45380 with biopsy, single or multiple

▲ **45382** with control of bleeding (eg, injection, bipolar cautery, unipolar cautery, laser, heater probe, stapler, plasma coagulator)

45383 with ablation of tumor(s), polyp(s), or other lesion(s) not amenable to removal by hot biopsy forceps, bipolar cautery or snare technique

45384 with removal of tumor(s), polyp(s), or other lesion(s) by hot biopsy forceps or bipolar cautery

45385 with removal of tumor(s), polyp(s), or other lesion(s) by snare technique

(For small intestine and stomal endoscopy, see 44360-44393)

45387 with transendoscopic stent placement (includes predilation)

REPAIR

45500 Proctoplasty; for stenosis

45505 for prolapse of mucous membrane

45520 Perirectal injection of sclerosing solution for prolapse

45540 Proctopexy for prolapse; abdominal approach

45541 perineal approach

● New Code   ▲ Revised Code   ✳ Starred Procedure   ✛ Add-On Code   ⃠ Modifier -51 Exempt

45550 Proctopexy combined with sigmoid resection, abdominal approach

45560 Repair of rectocele (separate procedure)

(For repair of rectocele with posterior colporrhaphy, use 57250)

45562 Exploration, repair, and presacral drainage for rectal injury;

45563   with colostomy

45800 Closure of rectovesical fistula;

45805   with colostomy

45820 Closure of rectourethral fistula;

45825   with colostomy

(For rectovaginal fistula closure, see 57300-57308)

MANIPULATION

***45900** Reduction of procidentia (separate procedure) under anesthesia

***45905** Dilation of anal sphincter (separate procedure) under anesthesia other than local

45910 Dilation of rectal stricture (separate procedure) under anesthesia other than local

***45915** Removal of fecal impaction or foreign body (separate procedure) under anesthesia

OTHER PROCEDURES

45999 Unlisted procedure, rectum

● **46020** Placement of seton

(Do not report 46020 in addition to 46060, 46280, 46600)

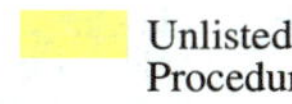
Separate
Procedure

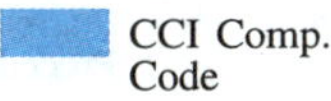
Unlisted
Procedure

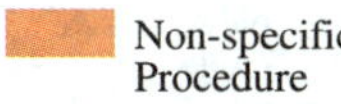
CCI Comp.
Code

Non-specific
Procedure

ANUS

INCISION

***46030**   Removal of anal seton, other marker

46040   Incision and drainage of ischiorectal and/or perirectal abscess (separate procedure)

46045   Incision and drainage of intramural, intramuscular, or submucosal abscess, transanal, under anesthesia

***46050**   Incision and drainage, perianal abscess, superficial

(See also 45020, 46060)

46060   Incision and drainage of ischiorectal or intramural abscess, with fistulectomy or fistulotomy, submuscular, with or without placement of seton

(Do not report 46060 in addition to 46020)

(See also 45020)

46070   Incision, anal septum (infant)

(For anoplasty, see 46700-46705)

***46080**   Sphincterotomy, anal, division of sphincter (separate procedure)

46083   Incision of thrombosed hemorrhoid, external

EXCISION

46200   Fissurectomy, with or without sphincterotomy

46210   Cryptectomy; single

46211   multiple (separate procedure)

46220   Papillectomy or excision of single tag, anus (separate procedure)

46221   Hemorrhoidectomy, by simple ligature (eg, rubber band)

46230   Excision of external hemorrhoid tags and/or multiple papillae

● New Code   ▲ Revised Code   * Starred Procedure   + Add-On Code   ⊘ Modifier -51 Exempt

46250   Hemorrhoidectomy, external, complete

46255   Hemorrhoidectomy, internal and external, simple;

46257   with fissurectomy

46258   with fistulectomy, with or without fissurectomy

46260   Hemorrhoidectomy, internal and external, complex or extensive;

46261   with fissurectomy

46262   with fistulectomy, with or without fissurectomy

46270   Surgical treatment of anal fistula (fistulectomy/fistulotomy); subcutaneous

46275   submuscular

46280   complex or multiple, with or without placement of seton

(Do not report 46280 in addition to 46020)

(46281 has been renumbered to 46288 without change in terminology)

46285   second stage

46288   Closure of anal fistula with rectal advancement flap

***46320**   Enucleation or excision of external thrombotic hemorrhoid

INTRODUCTION

***46500**   Injection of sclerosing solution, hemorrhoids

ENDOSCOPY

46600   Anoscopy; diagnostic, with or without collection of specimen(s) by brushing or washing (separate procedure)

(Do not report 46600 in addition to 46020)

▲ **46604**   with dilation (eg, balloon, guide wire, bougie)

46606   with biopsy, single or multiple

| Separate Procedure | Unlisted Procedure | CCI Comp. Code | Non-specific Procedure |

467

46608	with removal of foreign body
46610	with removal of single tumor, polyp, or other lesion by hot biopsy forceps or bipolar cautery
46611	with removal of single tumor, polyp, or other lesion by snare technique
46612	with removal of multiple tumors, polyps, or other lesions by hot biopsy forceps, bipolar cautery or snare technique
▲ **46614**	with control of bleeding (eg, injection, bipolar cautery, unipolar cautery, laser, heater probe, stapler, plasma coagulator)
46615	with ablation of tumor(s), polyp(s), or other lesion(s) not amenable to removal by hot biopsy forceps, bipolar cautery or snare technique

REPAIR

46700	Anoplasty, plastic operation for stricture; adult
46705	infant

(For simple incision of anal septum, use 46070)

46715	Repair of low imperforate anus; with anoperineal fistula (cut-back procedure)
46716	with transposition of anoperineal or anovestibular fistula
46730	Repair of high imperforate anus without fistula; perineal or sacroperineal approach
46735	combined transabdominal and sacroperineal approaches
46740	Repair of high imperforate anus with rectourethral or rectovaginal fistula; perineal or sacroperineal approach
46742	combined transabdominal and sacroperineal approaches
46744	Repair of cloacal anomaly by anorectovaginoplasty and urethroplasty, sacroperineal approach
46746	Repair of cloacal anomaly by anorectovaginoplasty and urethroplasty, combined abdominal and sacroperineal approach;

● New Code   ▲ Revised Code   * Starred Procedure   + Add-On Code   ⊘ Modifier -51 Exempt

46748	with vaginal lengthening by intestinal graft or pedicle flaps
46750	Sphincteroplasty, anal, for incontinence or prolapse; adult
46751	child
46753	Graft (Thiersch operation) for rectal incontinence and/or prolapse
46754	Removal of Thiersch wire or suture, anal canal
46760	Sphincteroplasty, anal, for incontinence, adult; muscle transplant
46761	levator muscle imbrication (Park posterior anal repair)
46762	implantation artificial sphincter

DESTRUCTION

***46900**	Destruction of lesion(s), anus (eg, condyloma, papilloma, molluscum contagiosum, herpetic vesicle), simple; chemical
***46910**	electrodesiccation
46916	cryosurgery
46917	laser surgery
46922	surgical excision
▲ **46924**	Destruction of lesion(s), anus (eg, condyloma, papilloma, molluscum contagiosum, herpetic vesicle), extensive (eg, laser surgery, electrosurgery, cryosurgery, chemosurgery)
46934	Destruction of hemorrhoids, any method; internal
46935	external
46936	internal and external
46937	Cryosurgery of rectal tumor; benign
46938	malignant
▲ **46940**	Curettage or cautery of anal fissure, including dilation of anal sphincter (separate procedure); initial

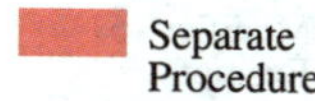
Separate Procedure

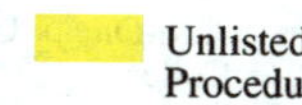
Unlisted Procedure

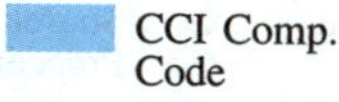
CCI Comp. Code

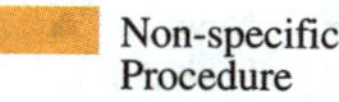
Non-specific Procedure

46942	subsequent

SUTURE

46945	Ligation of internal hemorrhoids; single procedure
46946	multiple procedures

OTHER PROCEDURES

46999	Unlisted procedure, anus

LIVER

INCISION

***47000** Biopsy of liver, needle; percutaneous

(If imaging guidance is performed, see 76003, 76360, 76393, 76942)

+47001 when done for indicated purpose at time of other major procedure (List separately in addition to code for primary procedure)

(If imaging guidance is performed, see 76003, 76942)

(For fine needle aspiration in conjunction with 47000, 47001, see 10021, 10022)

(For evaluation of fine needle aspirate in conjunction with 47000, 47001, see 88172, 88173)

47010 Hepatotomy; for open drainage of abscess or cyst, one or two stages

47011 for percutaneous drainage of abscess or cyst, one or two stages

(For radiological supervision and interpretation, use 75989)

47015 Laparotomy, with aspiration and/or injection of hepatic parasitic (eg, amoebic or echinococcal) cyst(s) or abscess(es)

EXCISION

47100 Biopsy of liver, wedge

● New Code	▲ Revised Code	* Starred Procedure	+ Add-On Code	⊘ Modifier -51 Exempt

47120 Hepatectomy, resection of liver; partial lobectomy

47122 trisegmentectomy

47125 total left lobectomy

47130 total right lobectomy

47133 Donor hepatectomy, with preparation and maintenance of allograft; from cadaver donor

47134 partial, from living donor

47135 Liver allotransplantation; orthotopic, partial or whole, from cadaver or living donor, any age

47136 heterotopic, partial or whole, from cadaver or living donor, any age

REPAIR

47300 Marsupialization of cyst or abscess of liver

47350 Management of liver hemorrhage; simple suture of liver wound or injury

47360 complex suture of liver wound or injury, with or without hepatic artery ligation

47361 exploration of hepatic wound, extensive debridement, coagulation and/or suture, with or without packing of liver

47362 re-exploration of hepatic wound for removal of packing

LAPAROSCOPY

● **47370** Laparoscopy, surgical, ablation of one or more liver tumor(s); radiofrequency

(For imaging guidance, use 76490)

● **47371** cryosurgical

(For imaging guidance, use 76490)

47379 Unlisted laparoscopic procedure, liver

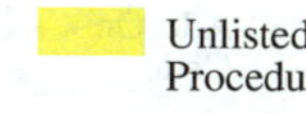

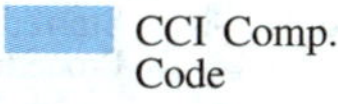

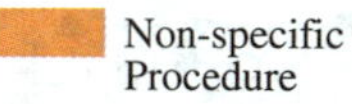

Non-specific
Procedure

OTHER PROCEDURES

● **47380** Ablation, open, of one or more liver tumor(s); radiofrequency

(For imaging guidance, use 76490)

● **47381** cryosurgical

(For imaging guidance, use 76490)

● **47382** Ablation, one or more liver tumor(s), percutaneous, radiofrequency

(For imaging guidance and monitoring, see code 76362, 76394, or 76490)

47399 Unlisted procedure, liver

BILIARY TRACT

INCISION

47400 Hepaticotomy or hepaticostomy with exploration, drainage, or removal of calculus

47420 Choledochotomy or choledochostomy with exploration, drainage, or removal of calculus, with or without cholecystotomy; without transduodenal sphincterotomy or sphincteroplasty

47425 with transduodenal sphincterotomy or sphincteroplasty

47460 Transduodenal sphincterotomy or sphincteroplasty, with or without transduodenal extraction of calculus (separate procedure)

47480 Cholecystotomy or cholecystostomy with exploration, drainage, or removal of calculus (separate procedure)

47490 Percutaneous cholecystostomy

(For radiological supervision and interpretation, use 75989)

INTRODUCTION

47500 Injection procedure for percutaneous transhepatic cholangiography

---

● New Code ▲ Revised Code * Starred Procedure + Add-On Code ⃠ Modifier -51 Exempt

(For radiological supervision and interpretation, use 74320)

47505   Injection procedure for cholangiography through an existing catheter (eg, percutaneous transhepatic or T-tube)

(For radiological supervision and interpretation, use 74305)

47510   Introduction of percutaneous transhepatic catheter for biliary drainage

(For radiological supervision and interpretation, use 75980)

47511   Introduction of percutaneous transhepatic stent for internal and external biliary drainage

(For radiological supervision and interpretation, use 75982)

47525   Change of percutaneous biliary drainage catheter

(For radiological supervision and interpretation, use 75984)

47530   Revision and/or reinsertion of transhepatic tube

(For radiological supervision and interpretation, use 75984)

ENDOSCOPY

+47550   Biliary endoscopy, intraoperative (choledochoscopy) (List separately in addition to code for primary procedure)

47552   Biliary endoscopy, percutaneous via T-tube or other tract; diagnostic, with or without collection of specimen(s) by brushing and/or washing (separate procedure)

47553   with biopsy, single or multiple

▲ **47554**   with removal of calculus/calculi

47555   with dilation of biliary duct stricture(s) without stent

(For ERCP, see 43260-43272, 74363)

(If imaging guidance is performed, see 74363, 75982)

47556   with dilation of biliary duct stricture(s) with stent

(If imaging guidance is performed, see 74363, 75982)

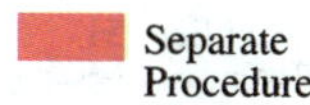 Separate Procedure

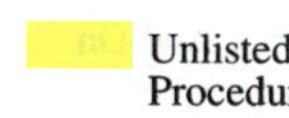 Unlisted Procedure

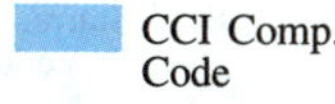 CCI Comp. Code

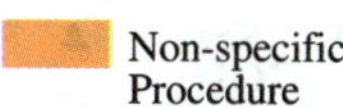 Non-specific Procedure

473

LAPAROSCOPY

47560 Laparoscopy, surgical; with guided transhepatic cholangiography, without biopsy

47561 with guided transhepatic cholangiography with biopsy

47562 cholecystectomy

47563 cholecystectomy with cholangiography

47564 cholecystectomy with exploration of common duct

47570 cholecystoenterostomy

47579 Unlisted laparoscopy procedure, biliary tract

EXCISION

47600 Cholecystectomy;

47605 with cholangiography

(For laparoscopic approach, see 47562-47564)

47610 Cholecystectomy with exploration of common duct;

47612 with choledochoenterostomy

47620 with transduodenal sphincterotomy or sphincteroplasty, with or without cholangiography

47630 Biliary duct stone extraction, percutaneous via T-tube tract, basket, or snare (eg, Burhenne technique)

(For radiological supervision and interpretation, use 74327)

47700 Exploration for congenital atresia of bile ducts, without repair, with or without liver biopsy, with or without cholangiography

47701 Portoenterostomy (eg, Kasai procedure)

47711 Excision of bile duct tumor, with or without primary repair of bile duct; extrahepatic

47712 intrahepatic

(For anastomosis, see 47760-47800)

47715 Excision of choledochal cyst

47716 Anastomosis, choledochal cyst, without excision

REPAIR

47720 Cholecystoenterostomy; direct

(For laparoscopic approach, use 47570)

47721 with gastroenterostomy

47740 Roux-en-Y

47741 Roux-en-Y with gastroenterostomy

47760 Anastomosis, of extrahepatic biliary ducts and gastrointestinal tract

47765 Anastomosis, of intrahepatic ducts and gastrointestinal tract

47780 Anastomosis, Roux-en-Y, of extrahepatic biliary ducts and gastrointestinal tract

47785 Anastomosis, Roux-en-Y, of intrahepatic biliary ducts and gastrointestinal tract

47800 Reconstruction, plastic, of extrahepatic biliary ducts with end-to-end anastomosis

47801 Placement of choledochal stent

47802 U-tube hepaticoenterostomy

47900 Suture of extrahepatic biliary duct for pre-existing injury (separate procedure)

OTHER PROCEDURES

47999 Unlisted procedure, biliary tract

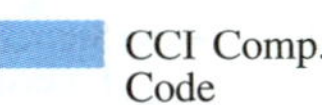
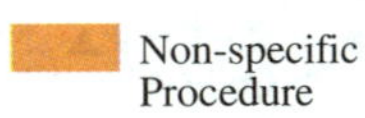

	Separate Procedure		Unlisted Procedure		CCI Comp. Code		Non-specific Procedure

475

PANCREAS

(For peroral pancreatic endoscopic procedures, see 43260-43272)

INCISION

48000 Placement of drains, peripancreatic, for acute pancreatitis;

48001 with cholecystostomy, gastrostomy, and jejunostomy

48005 Resection or debridement of pancreas and peripancreatic tissue for acute necrotizing pancreatitis

48020 Removal of pancreatic calculus

EXCISION

▲ **48100** Biopsy of pancreas, open (eg, fine needle aspiration, needle core biopsy, wedge biopsy)

***48102** Biopsy of pancreas, percutaneous needle

(For radiological supervision and interpretation, see 76003, 76360, 76393, 76942)

(For fine needle aspiration, use 10022)

(For evaluation of fine needle aspirate, see 88172, 88173)

48120 Excision of lesion of pancreas (eg, cyst, adenoma)

48140 Pancreatectomy, distal subtotal, with or without splenectomy; without pancreaticojejunostomy

48145 with pancreaticojejunostomy

48146 Pancreatectomy, distal, near-total with preservation of duodenum (Child-type procedure)

48148 Excision of ampulla of Vater

48150 Pancreatectomy, proximal subtotal with total duodenectomy, partial gastrectomy, choledochoenterostomy and gastrojejunostomy (Whipple-type procedure); with pancreatojejunostomy

48152 without pancreatojejunostomy

● New Code   ▲ Revised Code   * Starred Procedure   + Add-On Code   ⊘ Modifier -51 Exempt

48153 Pancreatectomy, proximal subtotal with near-total duodenectomy, choledochoenterostomy, and duodenojejunostomy (pylorus-sparing, whipple-type procedure); with pancreatojejunostomy

48154 without pancreatojejunostomy

48155 Pancreatectomy, total

▲ **48160** Pancreatectomy, total or subtotal, with autologous transplantation of pancreas or pancreatic islet cells

48180 Pancreaticojejunostomy, side-to-side anastomosis (Puestow-type operation)

INTRODUCTION

+48400 Injection procedure for intraoperative pancreatography (List separately in addition to code for primary procedure)

(For radiological supervision and interpretation, see 74300-74305)

REPAIR

▲ **48500** Marsupialization of pancreatic cyst

48510 External drainage, pseudocyst of pancreas; open

48511 percutaneous

(For radiological supervision and interpretation, use 75989)

48520 Internal anastomosis of pancreatic cyst to gastrointestinal tract; direct

48540 Roux-en-Y

▲ **48545** Pancreatorrhaphy for injury

▲ **48547** Duodenal exclusion with gastrojejunostomy for pancreatic injury

PANCREAS TRANSPLANTATION

48550 Donor pancreatectomy, with preparation and maintenance of allograft from cadaver donor, with or without duodenal segment for transplantation

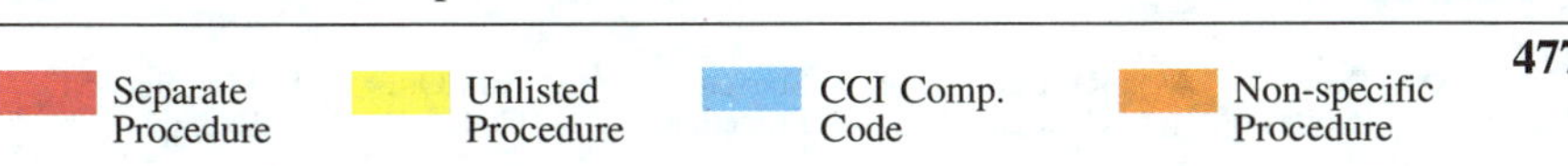

477

48554 Transplantation of pancreatic allograft

48556 Removal of transplanted pancreatic allograft

OTHER PROCEDURES

48999 Unlisted procedure, pancreas

ABDOMEN, PERITONEUM, AND OMENTUM

INCISION

49000 Exploratory laparotomy, exploratory celiotomy with or without biopsy(s) (separate procedure)

(To report wound exploration due to penetrating trauma without laparatomy, use 20102)

49002 Reopening of recent laparotomy

(To report re-exploration of hepatic wound for removal of packing, use 47362)

49010 Exploration, retroperitoneal area with or without biopsy(s) (separate procedure)

(To report wound exploration due to penetrating trauma without laparotomy, use 20102)

49020 Drainage of peritoneal abscess or localized peritonitis, exclusive of appendiceal abscess; open

(For appendiceal abscess, use 44900)

49021 percutaneous

(For radiological supervision and interpretation, use 75989)

49040 Drainage of subdiaphragmatic or subphrenic abscess; open

49041 percutaneous

(For radiological supervision and interpretation, use 75989)

49060 Drainage of retroperitoneal abscess; open

49061 percutaneous

478

● New Code ▲ Revised Code ✳ Starred Procedure ✚ Add-On Code ⊘ Modifier -51 Exempt

(For laparoscopic drainage, use 49323)

(For radiological supervision and interpretation, use 75989)

49062 Drainage of extraperitoneal lymphocele to peritoneal cavity, open

***49080** Peritoneocentesis, abdominal paracentesis, or peritoneal lavage (diagnostic or therapeutic); initial

***49081** subsequent

(If imaging guidance is performed, see 76360, 76942)

49085 Removal of peritoneal foreign body from peritoneal cavity

(For lysis of intestinal adhesions, use 44005)

EXCISION, DESTRUCTION

***49180** Biopsy, abdominal or retroperitoneal mass, percutaneous needle

(If imaging guidance is performed, see 76003, 76360, 76393, 76942)

(For fine needle aspiration, use 10021 or 10022)

(For evaluation of fine needle aspirate, see 88172, 88173)

49200 Excision or destruction by any method of intra-abdominal or retroperitoneal tumors or cysts or endometriomas;

49201 extensive

49215 Excision of presacral or sacrococcygeal tumor

▲ **49220** Staging laparotomy for Hodgkins disease or lymphoma (includes splenectomy, needle or open biopsies of both liver lobes, possibly also removal of abdominal nodes, abdominal node and/or bone marrow biopsies, ovarian repositioning)

49250 Umbilectomy, omphalectomy, excision of umbilicus (separate procedure)

49255 Omentectomy, epiploectomy, resection of omentum (separate procedure)

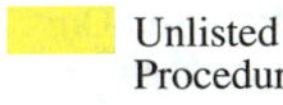

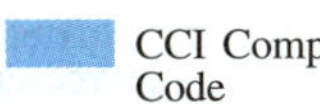

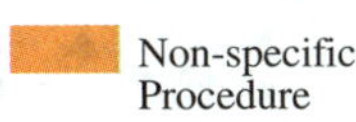

Non-specific
Procedure

LAPAROSCOPY

49320 Laparoscopy, abdomen, peritoneum, and omentum; diagnostic, with or without collection of specimen(s) by brushing or washing (separate procedure)

49321 Laparoscopy, surgical; with biopsy (single or multiple)

49322 with aspiration of cavity or cyst (eg, ovarian cyst) (single or multiple)

49323 with drainage of lymphocele to peritoneal cavity

(For percutaneous or open drainage, see 49060, 49061)

49329 Unlisted laparoscopy procedure, abdomen, peritoneum and omentum

INTRODUCTION, REVISION, AND/OR REMOVAL

*49400** Injection of air or contrast into peritoneal cavity (separate procedure)

(For radiological supervision and interpretation, use 74190)

*49420** Insertion of intraperitoneal cannula or catheter for drainage or dialysis; temporary

49421 permanent

49422 Removal of permanent intraperitoneal cannula or catheter

(For removal of a temporary catheter/cannula, use appropriate E/M code)

49423 Exchange of previously placed abscess or cyst drainage catheter under radiological guidance (separate procedure)

(For radiological supervision and interpretation, use 75984)

▲ **49424** Contrast injection for assessment of abscess or cyst via previously placed drainage catheter or tube (separate procedure)

(For radiological supervision and interpretation, use 76080)

49425 Insertion of peritoneal-venous shunt

● New Code   ▲ Revised Code   * Starred Procedure   + Add-On Code   ⊘ Modifier -51 Exempt

49426   Revision of peritoneal-venous shunt

(For shunt patency test, use 78291)

49427   Injection procedure (eg, contrast media) for evaluation of previously placed peritoneal-venous shunt

(For radiological supervision and interpretation, see 75809, 78291)

49428   Ligation of peritoneal-venous shunt

49429   Removal of peritoneal-venous shunt

REPAIR

Hernioplasty, Herniorrhaphy, Herniotomy

(For reduction and repair of intra-abdominal hernia, use 44050)

(For debridement of abdominal wall, see 11042, 11043)

● **49491**   Repair, initial inguinal hernia, preterm infant (less than 37 weeks gestation at birth), performed from birth up to 50 weeks post-conceptual age, with or without hydrocelectomy; reducible

● **49492**   incarcerated or strangulated

(Post-conceptual age equals gestational age at birth plus age of infant in weeks at the time of the hernia repair. Initial inguinal hernia repairs that are performed on preterm infants who are over 50 weeks postconceptual age and under age 6 months at the time of surgery, should be reported using codes 49495, 49496)

▲ **49495**   Repair, initial inguinal hernia, full term infant under age 6 months, or preterm infant over 50 weeks postconceptual age and under age 6 months at the time of surgery, with or without hydrocelectomy; reducible

49496   incarcerated or strangulated

(Post-conceptual age equals gestational age at birth plus age in weeks at the time of the hernia repair. Initial inguinal hernia repairs that are performed on preterm infants who are under or up to 50 weeks postconceptual age but under 6 months of age since birth, should be reported using codes 49491, 49492. Inguinal hernia repairs on infants age 6 months to under 5 years should be reported using codes 49500-49501)

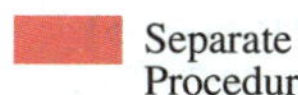 Separate Procedure

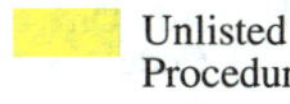 Unlisted Procedure

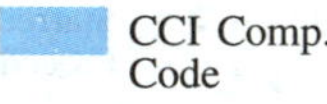 CCI Comp. Code

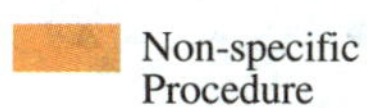 Non-specific Procedure

49500	Repair initial inguinal hernia, age 6 months to under 5 years, with or without hydrocelectomy; reducible
49501	incarcerated or strangulated
49505	Repair initial inguinal hernia, age 5 years or over; reducible
49507	incarcerated or strangulated
49520	Repair recurrent inguinal hernia, any age; reducible
49521	incarcerated or strangulated
49525	Repair inguinal hernia, sliding, any age
49540	Repair lumbar hernia
49550	Repair initial femoral hernia, any age; reducible
49553	incarcerated or strangulated
49555	Repair recurrent femoral hernia; reducible
49557	incarcerated or strangulated
49560	Repair initial incisional or ventral hernia; reducible
49561	incarcerated or strangulated
49565	Repair recurrent incisional or ventral hernia; reducible
49566	incarcerated or strangulated
+49568	Implantation of mesh or other prosthesis for incisional or ventral hernia repair (List separately in addition to code for the incisional or ventral hernia repair)
49570	Repair epigastric hernia (eg, preperitoneal fat); reducible (separate procedure)
49572	incarcerated or strangulated
49580	Repair umbilical hernia, under age 5 years; reducible
49582	incarcerated or strangulated

● New Code	▲ Revised Code	✳ Starred Procedure	✚ Add-On Code	⊘ Modifier -51 Exempt

49585	Repair umbilical hernia, age 5 years or over; reducible
49587	incarcerated or strangulated
49590	Repair spigelian hernia
49600	Repair of small omphalocele, with primary closure
49605	Repair of large omphalocele or gastroschisis; with or without prosthesis
49606	with removal of prosthesis, final reduction and closure, in operating room
49610	Repair of omphalocele (Gross type operation); first stage
49611	second stage

(For diaphragmatic or hiatal hernia repair, see 39502-39541)

LAPAROSCOPY

49650	Laparoscopy, surgical; repair initial inguinal hernia
49651	repair recurrent inguinal hernia
49659	Unlisted laparoscopy procedure, hernioplasty, herniorrhaphy, herniotomy

SUTURE

49900	Suture, secondary, of abdominal wall for evisceration or dehiscence

(For suture of ruptured diaphragm, see 39540, 39541)

(For debridement of abdominal wall, see 11042, 11043)

OTHER PROCEDURES

+49905	Omental flap (eg, for reconstruction of sternal and chest wall defects) (List separately in addition to code for primary procedure)
49906	Free omental flap with microvascular anastomosis

(Do not report code 69990 in addition to code 49906)

49999   Unlisted procedure, abdomen, peritoneum and omentum

● New Code   ▲ Revised Code   ✻ Starred Procedure   ✚ Add-On Code   ⊘ Modifier -51 Exempt

URINARY SYSTEM

(For provision of chemotherapeutic agents, use 96545 in
addition to code for primary procedure)

CPT codes from this section of CPT are used to report invasive and surgical
procedures performed on the kidney; ureter; bladder; prostate (resection); and
urethra.

There are numerous starred (*) procedures in this section of CPT indicating
the possibility of reporting an appropriate visit code in addition to the
surgical procedure.

URODYNAMICS

CPT codes in this section may be used separately or in various
combinations. When multiple procedures are performed in the same session,
modifier -51 should be added to the second and all subsequent CPT codes.
Procedures in this section are performed by, or under the direct supervision
of, a physician.

In addition, all materials and supplies, used in the provision of these
services, such as instruments, equipment, fluids, gases, probes, catheters,
technician's fees, medications, gloves, trays, tubing and other sterile supplies
are considered to be included in the base code. Use modifier -26 to code
and report interpretation of results or operation of equipment only.

CYSTOSCOPY, URETHROSCOPY, and CYSTOURETHROSCOPY

The descriptions of CPT codes in this section are listed so that the main
procedure can be identified without having to list all of the minor related
procedures performed at the same time. For example:

52601   Transurethral electrosurgical resection of prostate, including
control of postoperative bleeding, complete (vasectomy,
meatotomy, cystourethroscopy, urethral calibration and/or
dilation, and internal urethrotomy are included)

All of the secondary procedures are included in the single code 52601. If
any of the secondary procedures requires significant additional time and
effort, to the point of making the procedure "unusual", modifier -22 should
be added with an appropriate increase in fee and a report explaining what
made the procedure unusual.

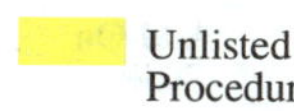 Separate
Procedure

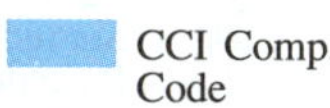 Unlisted
Procedure

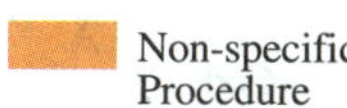 CCI Comp.
Code

Non-specific
Procedure

KIDNEY

INCISION

(For retroperitoneal expoloration, abscess, tumor, or cyst, see 49010, 49060, 49200, 49201)

50010 Renal exploration, not necessitating other specific procedures

50020 Drainage of perirenal or renal abscess; open

50021 percutaneous

(For radiological supervision and interpretation, use 75989)

50040 Nephrostomy, nephrotomy with drainage

50045 Nephrotomy, with exploration

(For renal endoscopy performed in conjunction with this procedure, see 50570-50580)

50060 Nephrolithotomy; removal of calculus

50065 secondary surgical operation for calculus

50070 complicated by congenital kidney abnormality

50075 removal of large staghorn calculus filling renal pelvis and calyces (including anatrophic pyelolithotomy)

50080 Percutaneous nephrostolithotomy or pyelostolithotomy, with or without dilation, endoscopy, lithotripsy, stenting, or basket extraction; up to 2 cm

50081 over 2cm

(For establishment of nephrostomy without nephrostolithotomy, see 50040, 50395, 52334)

(For fluoroscopic guidance, see 76000, 76001)

50100 Transection or repositioning of aberrant renal vessels (separate procedure)

50120 Pyelotomy; with exploration

486

● New Code	▲ Revised Code	✱ Starred Procedure	✚ Add-On Code	⊘ Modifier -51 Exempt

(For renal endoscopy performed in conjunction with this procedure, see 50570-50580)

50125 with drainage, pyelostomy

50130 with removal of calculus (pyelolithotomy, pelviolithotomy, including coagulum pyelolithotomy)

50135 complicated (eg, secondary operation, congenital kidney abnormality)

(For supply of anticarcinogenic agents, use 99070 in addition to code for primary procedure)

EXCISION

(For excision of retroperitoneal tumor or cyst, see 49200, 49201)

∗50200 Renal biopsy; percutaneous, by trocar or needle

(For radiological supervision and interpretation, see 76003, 76360, 76393, 76942)

(For fine needle aspiration, use 10022)

(For evaluation of fine needle aspirate, see 88172, 88173)

50205 by surgical exposure of kidney

▲ **50220** Nephrectomy, including partial ureterectomy, any open approach including rib resection;

50225 complicated because of previous surgery on same kidney

50230 radical, with regional lymphadenectomy and/or vena caval thrombectomy

(When vena caval resection with reconstruction is necessary, use 37799)

50234 Nephrectomy with total ureterectomy and bladder cuff; through same incision

50236 through separate incision

50240 Nephrectomy, partial

50280 Excision or unroofing of cyst(s) of kidney

 Separate Procedure 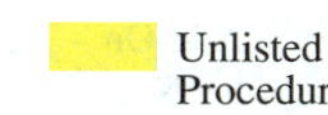 Unlisted Procedure 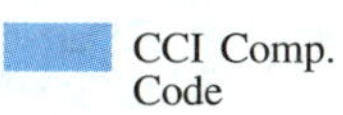 CCI Comp. Code 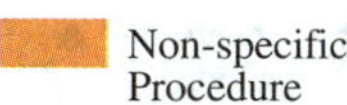 Non-specific Procedure

(For laparoscopic ablation of renal cysts, use 50541)

50290   Excision of perinephric cyst

RENAL TRANSPLANTATION

(For dialysis, see 90935-90999)

(For laparoscopic donor nephrectomy, use 50547)

(For laparoscopic drainage of lymphocele to peritoneal cavity, use 49323)

50300   Donor nephrectomy, with preparation and maintenance of allograft, from cadaver donor, unilateral or bilateral

50320   Donor nephrectomy, open from living donor (excluding preparation and maintenance of allograft)

50340   Recipient nephrectomy (separate procedure)

50360   Renal allotransplantation, implantation of graft; excluding donor and recipient nephrectomy

50365   with recipient nephrectomy

50370   Removal of transplanted renal allograft

50380   Renal autotransplantation, reimplantation of kidney

(For extra-corporeal "bench" surgery, use autotransplantation as the primary procedure and add the secondary procedure (eg, partial nephrectomy, nephrolithotomy), and use the modifier -51)

INTRODUCTION

∗50390   Aspiration and/or injection of renal cyst or pelvis by needle, percutaneous

(For radiological supervision and interpretation, see 74425, 74470, 76003, 76360, 76393, 76942)

(For evaluation of fine needle aspirate, see 88172, 88173)

50392   Introduction of intracatheter or catheter into renal pelvis for drainage and/or injection, percutaneous

(For radiological supervision and interpretation, see 74475, 76360, 76942)

● New Code   ▲ Revised Code   ∗ Starred Procedure   + Add-On Code   ⊘ Modifier -51 Exempt

50393 Introduction of ureteral catheter or stent into ureter through renal pelvis for drainage and/or injection, percutaneous

(For radiological supervision and interpretation, see 74480, 76003, 76360, 76942)

50394 Injection procedure for pyelography (as nephrostogram, pyelostogram, antegrade pyeloureterograms) through nephrostomy or pyelostomy tube, or indwelling ureteral catheter

(For radiological supervision and interpretation, use 74425)

50395 Introduction of guide into renal pelvis and/or ureter with dilation to establish nephrostomy tract, percutaneous

(For radiological supervision and interpretation, see 74475, 74480, 74485)

(For nephrostolithotomy, see 50080, 50081)

(For retrograde percutaneous nephrostomy, use 52334)

(For endoscopic surgery, see 50551-50561)

50396 Manometric studies through nephrostomy or pyelostomy tube, or indwelling ureteral catheter

(For radiological supervision and interpretation, see 74425, 74475, 74480)

***50398** Change of nephrostomy or pyelostomy tube

(For radiological supervision and interpretation, use 75984)

REPAIR

50400 Pyeloplasty (Foley Y-pyeloplasty), plastic operation on renal pelvis, with or without plastic operation on ureter, nephropexy, nephrostomy, pyelostomy, or ureteral splinting; simple

50405 complicated (congenital kidney abnormality, secondary pyeloplasty, solitary kidney, calycoplasty)

(For laparoscopic approach, use 50544)

50500 Nephrorrhaphy, suture of kidney wound or injury

50520 Closure of nephrocutaneous or pyelocutaneous fistula

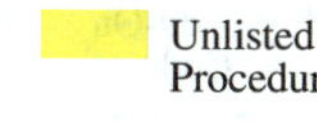

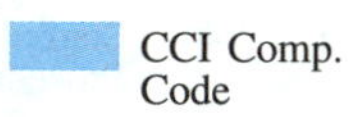

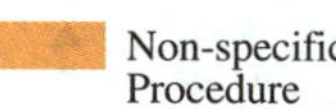

50525 Closure of nephrovisceral fistula (eg, renocolic), including visceral repair; abdominal approach

50526 thoracic approach

50540 Symphysiotomy for horseshoe kidney with or without pyeloplasty and/or other plastic procedure, unilateral or bilateral (one operation)

LAPAROSCOPY

50541 Laparoscopy, surgical; ablation of renal cysts

50544 pyeloplasty

50545 radical nephrectomy (includes removal of Gerota's fascia and surrounding fatty tissue, removal of regional lymph nodes, and adrenalectomy)

(For open procedure, use 50230)

50546 nephrectomy including partial ureterectomy

50547 donor nephrectomy from living donor (excluding preparation and maintenance of allograft)

(For open procedure, use 50320)

50548 nephrectomy with total ureterectomy

(For open procedure, see 50234, 50236)

50549 Unlisted laparoscopy procedure, renal

(For laparoscopic drainage of lymphocele to peritoneal cavity, use 49323)

ENDOSCOPY

(For supplies and materials, use 99070)

(References to office and hospital have been deleted)

50551 Renal endoscopy through established nephrostomy or pyelostomy, with or without irrigation, instillation, or ureteropyelography, exclusive of radiologic service;

  ● New Code ▲ Revised Code ✳ Starred Procedure + Add-On Code ⊘ Modifier -51 Exempt

50553   with ureteral catheterization, with or without dilation of ureter

50555   with biopsy

50557   with fulguration and/or incision, with or without biopsy

50559   with insertion of radioactive substance with or without biopsy and/or fulguration

50561   with removal of foreign body or calculus

(When procedures 50570-50580 provide a significant identifiable service, they may be added to 50045 and 50120)

50570   Renal endoscopy through nephrotomy or pyelotomy, with or without irrigation, instillation, or ureteropyelography, exclusive of radiologic service;

(For nephrotomy, use 50045)

(For pyelotomy, use 50120)

50572   with ureteral catheterization, with or without dilation of ureter

50574   with biopsy

50575   with endopyelotomy (includes cystoscopy, ureteroscopy, dilation of ureter and ureteral pelvic junction, incision of ureteral pelvic junction and insertion of endopyelotomy stent)

50576   with fulguration and/or incision, with or without biopsy

50578   with insertion of radioactive substance, with or without biopsy and/or fulguration

50580   with removal of foreign body or calculus

OTHER PROCEDURES

50590   Lithotripsy, extracorporeal shock wave

URETER

INCISION

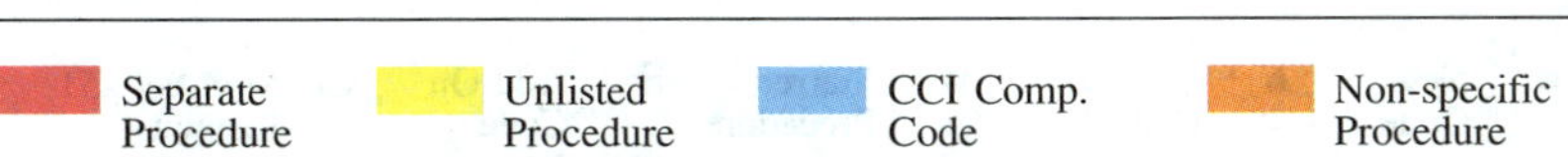

50600 Ureterotomy with exploration or drainage (separate procedure)

(For ureteral endoscopy performed in conjunction with this procedure, see 50970-50980)

50605 Ureterotomy for insertion of indwelling stent, all types

50610 Ureterolithotomy; upper one-third of ureter

50620   middle one-third of ureter

50630   lower one-third of ureter

(For laparoscopic approach, use 50945)

(For transvesical ureterolithotomy, use 51060)

(For cystotomy with stone basket extraction of ureteral calculus, use 51065)

(For endoscopic extraction or manipulation of ureteral calculus, see 50080, 50081, 50561, 50980, 52320-52330, 52352, 52353)

EXCISION

(For ureterocele, see 51535, 52300)

50650 Ureterectomy, with bladder cuff (separate procedure)

50660 Ureterectomy, total, ectopic ureter, combination abdominal, vaginal and/or perineal approach

INTRODUCTION

50684 Injection procedure for ureterography or ureteropyelography through ureterostomy or indwelling ureteral catheter

(For radiological supervision and interpretation, use 74425)

50686 Manometric studies through ureterostomy or indwelling ureteral catheter

***50688** Change of ureterostomy tube

(If imaging guidance is performed, use 75984)

50690 Injection procedure for visualization of ileal conduit and/or ureteropyelography, exclusive of radiologic service

---

● New Code	▲ Revised Code	* Starred Procedure	✛ Add-On Code	⊘ Modifier -51 Exempt

(For radiological supervision and interpretation, use 74425)

REPAIR

50700 Ureteroplasty, plastic operation on ureter (eg, stricture)

50715 Ureterolysis, with or without repositioning of ureter for retroperitoneal fibrosis

50722 Ureterolysis for ovarian vein syndrome

50725 Ureterolysis for retrocaval ureter, with reanastomosis of upper urinary tract or vena cava

50727 Revision of urinary-cutaneous anastomosis (any type urostomy);

50728 with repair of fascial defect and hernia

50740 Ureteropyelostomy, anastomosis of ureter and renal pelvis

50750 Ureterocalycostomy, anastomosis of ureter to renal calyx

50760 Ureteroureterostomy

50770 Transureteroureterostomy, anastomosis of ureter to contralateral ureter

(Codes 50780-50785 include minor procedures to prevent vesicoureteral reflux)

50780 Ureteroneocystostomy; anastomosis of single ureter to bladder

(When combined with cystourethroplasty or vesical neck revision, use 51820)

50782 anastomosis of duplicated ureter to bladder

50783 with extensive ureteral tailoring

50785 with vesico-psoas hitch or bladder flap

50800 Ureteroenterostomy, direct anastomosis of ureter to intestine

▲ **50810** Ureterosigmoidostomy, with creation of sigmoid bladder and establishment of abdominal or perineal colostomy, including intestine anastomosis

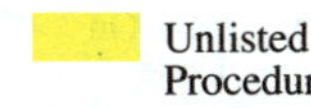
Separate
Procedure

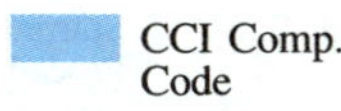
Unlisted
Procedure

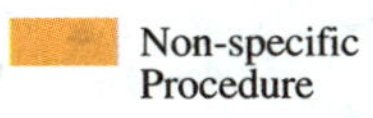
CCI Comp.
Code

Non-specific
Procedure

▲ **50815** Ureterocolon conduit, including intestine anastomosis

▲ **50820** Ureteroileal conduit (ileal bladder), including intestine anastomosis (Bricker operation)

(For combination of 50800-50820 with cystectomy, see 51580-51595)

▲ **50825** Continent diversion, including intestine anastomosis using any segment of small and/or large intestine (Kock pouch or Camey enterocystoplasty)

50830 Urinary undiversion (eg, taking down of ureteroileal conduit, ureterosigmoidostomy or ureteroenterostomy with ureteroureterostomy or ureteroneocystostomy)

▲ **50840** Replacement of all or part of ureter by intestine segment, including intestine anastomosis

50845 Cutaneous appendico-vesicostomy

50860 Ureterostomy, transplantation of ureter to skin

50900 Ureterorrhaphy, suture of ureter (separate procedure)

50920 Closure of ureterocutaneous fistula

50930 Closure of ureterovisceral fistula (including visceral repair)

50940 Deligation of ureter

(For ureteroplasty, ureterolysis, see 50700-50860)

LAPAROSCOPY

50945 Laparoscopy, surgical; ureterolithotomy

50947 ureteroneocystostomy with cystoscopy and ureteral stent placement

50948 ureteroneocystostomy without cystoscopy and ureteral stent placement

(For open ureteroneocystostomy, see 50780-50785)

50949 Unlisted laparoscopy procedure, ureter

● New Code   ▲ Revised Code   ∗ Starred Procedure   + Add-On Code   ⊘ Modifier -51 Exempt

ENDOSCOPY

(References to office and hospital have been deleted)

50951 Ureteral endoscopy through established ureterostomy, with or without irrigation, instillation, or ureteropyelography, exclusive of radiologic service;

50953 with ureteral catheterization, with or without dilation of ureter

50955 with biopsy

50957 with fulguration and/or incision, with or without biopsy

50959 with insertion of radioactive substance, with or without biopsy and/or fulguration (not including provision of material)

50961 with removal of foreign body or calculus

(When procedures 50970-50980 provide a significant identifiable service, they may be added to 50600)

50970 Ureteral endoscopy through ureterotomy, with or without irrigation, instillation, or ureteropyelography, exclusive of radiologic service;

(For ureterotomy, use 50600)

50972 with ureteral catheterization, with or without dilation of ureter

50974 with biopsy

50976 with fulguration and/or incision, with or without biopsy

50978 with insertion of radioactive substance, with or without biopsy and/or fulguration (not including provision of material)

50980 with removal of foreign body or calculus

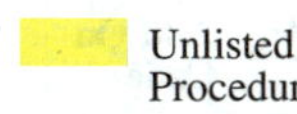 Separate Procedure   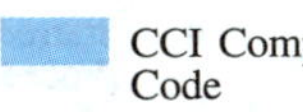 Unlisted Procedure   CCI Comp. Code   Non-specific Procedure

BLADDER

INCISION

***51000** Aspiration of bladder by needle

***51005** Aspiration of bladder; by trocar or intracatheter

51010 with insertion of suprapubic catheter

(If imaging guidance is performed, see 76003, 76360, 76942)

51020 Cystotomy or cystostomy; with fulguration and/or insertion of radioactive material

51030 with cryosurgical destruction of intravesical lesion

51040 Cystostomy, cystotomy with drainage

51045 Cystotomy, with insertion of ureteral catheter or stent (separate procedure)

51050 Cystolithotomy, cystotomy with removal of calculus, without vesical neck resection

51060 Transvesical ureterolithotomy

▲ **51065** Cystotomy, with calculus basket extraction and/or ultrasonic or electrohydraulic fragmentation of ureteral calculus

51080 Drainage of perivesical or prevesical space abscess

EXCISION

51500 Excision of urachal cyst or sinus, with or without umbilical hernia repair

51520 Cystotomy; for simple excision of vesical neck (separate procedure)

51525 for excision of bladder diverticulum, single or multiple (separate procedure)

51530 for excision of bladder tumor

(For transurethral resection, see 52234-52240, 52305)

● New Code	▲ Revised Code	* Starred Procedure	+ Add-On Code	⊘ Modifier -51 Exempt

51535   Cystotomy for excision, incision, or repair of ureterocele

(For transurethral excision, use 52300)

51550   Cystectomy, partial; simple

51555   complicated (eg, postradiation, previous surgery, difficult location)

51565   Cystectomy, partial, with reimplantation of ureter(s) into bladder (ureteroneocystostomy)

51570   Cystectomy, complete; (separate procedure)

51575   with bilateral pelvic lymphadenectomy, including external iliac, hypogastric, and obturator nodes

51580   Cystectomy, complete, with ureterosigmoidostomy or ureterocutaneous transplantations;

51585   with bilateral pelvic lymphadenectomy, including external iliac, hypogastric, and obturator nodes

▲ **51590**   Cystectomy, complete, with ureteroileal conduit or sigmoid bladder, including intestine anastomosis;

51595   with bilateral pelvic lymphadenectomy, including external iliac, hypogastric, and obturator nodes

▲ **51596**   Cystectomy, complete, with continent diversion, any open technique, using any segment of small and/or large intestine to construct neobladder

51597   Pelvic exenteration, complete, for vesical, prostatic or urethral malignancy, with removal of bladder and ureteral transplantations, with or without hysterectomy and/or abdominoperineal resection of rectum and colon and colostomy, or any combination thereof

(For pelvic exenteration for gynecologic malignancy, use 58240)

INTRODUCTION

(For bladder catheterization, see 53670, 53675)

***51600**   Injection procedure for cystography or voiding urethrocystography

	Separate Procedure		Unlisted Procedure		CCI Comp. Code		Non-specific Procedure

(For radiological supervision and interpretation, see 74430, 74455)

51605 Injection procedure and placement of chain for contrast and/or chain urethrocystography

(For radiological supervision and interpretation, use 74430)

51610 Injection procedure for retrograde urethrocystography

(For radiological supervision and interpretation, use 74450)

***51700** Bladder irrigation, simple, lavage and/or instillation

***51705** Change of cystostomy tube; simple

***51710**   complicated

(If imaging guidance is performed, use 75984)

51715 Endoscopic injection of implant material into the submucosal tissues of the urethra and/or bladder neck

51720 Bladder instillation of anticarcinogenic agent (including detention time)

URODYNAMICS

51725 Simple cystometrogram (CMG) (eg, spinal manometer)

51726 Complex cystometrogram (eg, calibrated electronic equipment)

51736 Simple uroflowmetry (UFR) (eg, stop-watch flow rate, mechanical uroflowmeter)

51741 Complex uroflowmetry (eg, calibrated electronic equipment)

51772 Urethral pressure profile studies (UPP) (urethral closure pressure profile), any technique

51784 Electromyography studies (EMG) of anal or urethral sphincter, other than needle, any technique

51785 Needle electromyography studies (EMG) of anal or urethral sphincter, any technique

---

498

● New Code   ▲ Revised Code   ✳ Starred Procedure   ✛ Add-On Code   ⊘ Modifier -51 Exempt

51792 Stimulus evoked response (eg, measurement of bulbocavernosus reflex latency time)

51795 Voiding pressure studies (VP); bladder voiding pressure, any technique

51797 intra-abdominal voiding pressure (AP) (rectal, gastric, intraperitoneal)

REPAIR

51800 Cystoplasty or cystourethroplasty, plastic operation on bladder and/or vesical neck (anterior Y-plasty, vesical fundus resection), any procedure, with or without wedge resection of posterior vesical neck

51820 Cystourethroplasty with unilateral or bilateral ureteroneocystostomy

51840 Anterior vesicourethropexy, or urethropexy (eg, Marshall-Marchetti-Krantz, Burch); simple

51841 complicated (eg, secondary repair)

(For urethropexy (Pereyra type), use 57289)

51845 Abdomino-vaginal vesical neck suspension, with or without endoscopic control (eg, Stamey, Raz, modified Pereyra)

51860 Cystorrhaphy, suture of bladder wound, injury or rupture; simple

51865 complicated

51880 Closure of cystostomy (separate procedure)

51900 Closure of vesicovaginal fistula, abdominal approach

(For vaginal approach, see 57320-57330)

51920 Closure of vesicouterine fistula;

51925 with hysterectomy

(For closure of vesicoenteric fistula, see 44660, 44661)

(For closure of rectovesical fistula, see 45800-45805)

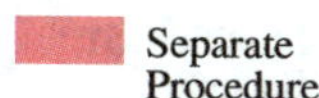
Separate Procedure

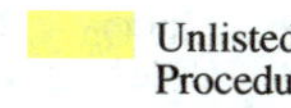
Unlisted Procedure

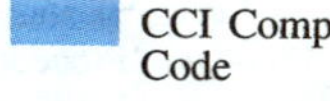
CCI Comp. Code

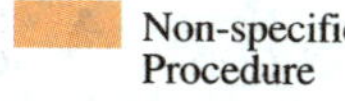
Non-specific Procedure

▲ **51940** Closure, exstrophy of bladder

(See also 54390)

▲ **51960** Enterocystoplasty, including intestinal anastomosis

51980 Cutaneous vesicostomy

LAPAROSCOPY

51990 Laparoscopy, surgical; urethral suspension for stress incontinence

51992 sling operation for stress incontinence (eg, fascia or synthetic)

(For open sling operation for stress incontinence, use 57288)

(For reversal or removal of sling operation for stress incontinence, use 57287)

ENDOSCOPY—CYSTOSCOPY, URETHROSCOPY, CYSTOURETHROSCOPY

(References to office and hospital have been deleted)

52000 Cystourethroscopy (separate procedure)

● **52201** Cystourethroscopy with irrigation and evacuation of clots

(Do not report 52001 in addition to 52000)

52005 Cystourethroscopy, with ureteral catheterization, with or without irrigation, instillation, or ureteropyelography, exclusive of radiologic service;

52007 with brush biopsy of ureter and/or renal pelvis

52010 Cystourethroscopy, with ejaculatory duct catheterization, with or without irrigation, instillation, or duct radiography, exclusive of radiologic service

(For radiological supervision and interpretation, use 74440)

● New Code ▲ Revised Code * Starred Procedure + Add-On Code ⊘ Modifier -51 Exempt

TRANSURETHRAL SURGERY

Urethra and Bladder

(References to office and hospital have been deleted)

52204 Cystourethroscopy, with biopsy

52214 Cystourethroscopy, with fulguration (including cryosurgery or laser surgery) of trigone, bladder neck, prostatic fossa, urethra, or periurethral glands

52224 Cystourethroscopy, with fulguration (including cryosurgery or laser surgery) or treatment of MINOR (less than 0.5 cm) lesion(s) with or without biopsy

52234 Cystourethroscopy, with fulguration (including cryosurgery or laser surgery) and/or resection of; SMALL bladder tumor(s) (0.5 to 2.0 cm)

52235 MEDIUM bladder tumor(s) (2.0 to 5.0 cm)

52240 LARGE bladder tumor(s)

52250 Cystourethroscopy with insertion of radioactive substance, with or without biopsy or fulguration

52260 Cystourethroscopy, with dilation of bladder for interstitial cystitis; general or conduction (spinal) anesthesia

52265 local anesthesia

52270 Cystourethroscopy, with internal urethrotomy; female

52275 male

52276 Cystourethroscopy with direct vision internal urethrotomy

52277 Cystourethroscopy, with resection of external sphincter (sphincterotomy)

52281 Cystourethroscopy, with calibration and/or dilation of urethral stricture or stenosis, with or without meatotomy, with or without injection procedure for cystography, male or female

52282 Cystourethroscopy, with insertion of urethral stent

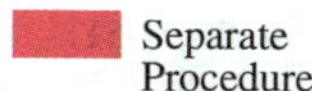

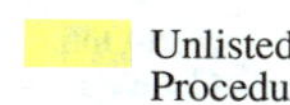

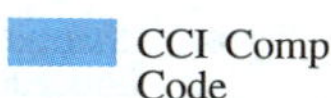

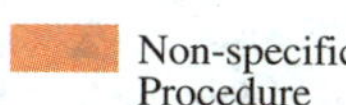

52283   Cystourethroscopy, with steroid injection into stricture

52285   Cystourethroscopy for treatment of the female urethral syndrome with any or all of the following: urethral meatotomy, urethral dilation, internal urethrotomy, lysis of urethrovaginal septal fibrosis, lateral incisions of the bladder neck, and fulguration of polyp(s) of urethra, bladder neck, and/or trigone

52290   Cystourethroscopy; with ureteral meatotomy, unilateral or bilateral

52300   with resection or fulguration of orthotopic ureterocele(s), unilateral or bilateral

52301   with resection or fulguration of ectopic ureterocele(s), unilateral or bilateral

52305   with incision or resection of orifice of bladder diverticulum, single or multiple

52310   Cystourethroscopy, with removal of foreign body, calculus, or ureteral stent from urethra or bladder (separate procedure); simple

52315   complicated

52317   Litholapaxy: crushing or fragmentation of calculus by any means in bladder and removal of fragments; simple or small (less than 2.5 cm)

52318   complicated or large (over 2.5 cm)

URETER AND PELVIS

52320   Cystourethroscopy (including ureteral catheterization); with removal of ureteral calculus

52325   with fragmentation of ureteral calculus (eg, ultrasonic or electro-hydraulic technique)

52327   with subureteric injection of implant material

52330   with manipulation, without removal of ureteral calculus

52332   Cystourethroscopy, with insertion of indwelling ureteral stent (eg, Gibbons or double-J type)

● New Code   ▲ Revised Code   ✳ Starred Procedure   ✛ Add-On Code   ⊘ Modifier -51 Exempt

52334   Cystourethroscopy with insertion of ureteral guide wire through kidney to establish a percutaneous nephrostomy, retrograde

(For percutaneous nephrostolithotomy, see 50080, 50081; for establishment of nephrostomy tract only, use 50395)

(52335   deleted 2001 edition. To report, use 52351)

(52336   deleted 2001 edition. To report, use 52352)

(52337   deleted 2001 edition. To report, use 52353)

(52338   deleted 2001 edition. To report, use 52354)

(52339   deleted 2001 edition. To report, use 52355)

(52340   deleted 2001 edition. To report, use 52400)

52341   Cystourethroscopy; with treatment of ureteral stricture (eg, balloon dilation, laser, electrocautery, and incision)

52342   with treatment of ureteropelvic junction stricture (eg, balloon dilation, laser, electrocautery, and incision)

52343   with treatment of intra-renal stricture (eg, balloon dilation, laser, electrocautery, and incision)

52344   Cystourethroscopy with ureteroscopy; with treatment of ureteral stricture (eg, balloon dilation, laser, electrocautery, and incision)

52345   with treatment of ureteropelvic junction stricture (eg, balloon dilation, laser, electrocautery, and incision)

52346   with treatment of intra-renal stricture (eg, balloon dilation, laser, electrocautery, and incision)

● **52347**   Cystourethroscopy with transurethral resection or incision of ejaculatory ducts

52351   Cystourethroscopy, with ureteroscopy and/or pyeloscopy; diagnostic

(For radiological supervision and interpretation, use 74485)

(Do not report 52351 in conjunction with 52341-52346, 52352-52355)

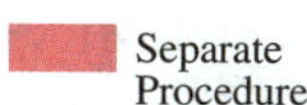 Separate Procedure

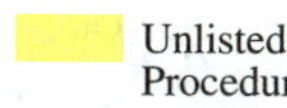 Unlisted Procedure

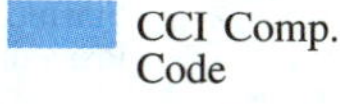 CCI Comp. Code

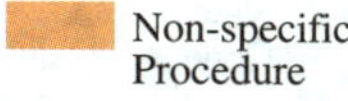 Non-specific Procedure

503

52352   with removal or manipulation of calculus (ureteral catheterization is included)

52353   with lithotripsy (ureteral catheterization is included)

52354   with biopsy and/or fulguration of lesion

52355   with resection of tumor

VESICAL NECK AND PROSTATE

52400   Cystourethroscopy with incision, fulguration, or resection of congenital posterior urethral valves, or congenital obstructive hypertrophic mucosal folds

52450   Transurethral incision of prostate

52500   Transurethral resection of bladder neck (separate procedure)

▲ **52510**   Transurethral balloon dilation of the prostatic urethra

52601   Transurethral electrosurgical resection of prostate, including control of postoperative bleeding, complete (vasectomy, meatotomy, cystourethroscopy, urethral calibration and/or dilation, and internal urethrotomy are included)

(For other approaches, see 55801-55845)

52606   Transurethral fulguration for postoperative bleeding occurring after the usual follow-up time

52612   Transurethral resection of prostate; first stage of two-stage resection (partial resection)

52614   second stage of two-stage resection (resection completed)

52620   Transurethral resection; of residual obstructive tissue after 90 days postoperative

52630   of regrowth of obstructive tissue longer than one year postoperative

52640   of postoperative bladder neck contracture

52647   Non-contact laser coagulation of prostate, including control of postoperative bleeding, complete (vasectomy, meatotomy, cystourethroscopy, urethral calibration and/or dilation, and internal urethrotomy are included)

52648 Contact laser vaporization with or without transurethral resection of prostate, including control of postoperative bleeding, complete (vasectomy, meatotomy, cystourethroscopy, urethral calibration and/or dilation, and internal urethrotomy are included)

52700 Transurethral drainage of prostatic abscess

URETHRA

(For endoscopy, see cystoscopy, urethroscopy, cystourethroscopy, 52000-52700)

(For injection procedure for urethrocystography, see 51600-51610)

INCISION

53000 Urethrotomy or urethrostomy, external (separate procedure); pendulous urethra

53010 perineal urethra, external

53020 Meatotomy, cutting of meatus (separate procedure); except infant

53025 infant

53040 Drainage of deep periurethral abscess

(For subcutaneous abscess, see 10060, 10061)

53060 Drainage of Skene's gland abscess or cyst

53080 Drainage of perineal urinary extravasation; uncomplicated (separate procedure)

53085 complicated

EXCISION

53200 Biopsy of urethra

53210 Urethrectomy, total, including cystostomy; female

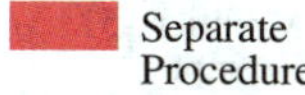 Separate Procedure
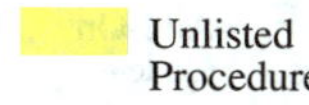 Unlisted Procedure
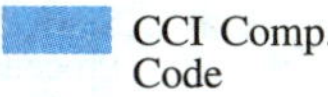 CCI Comp. Code
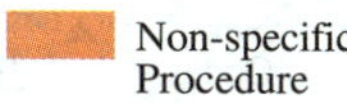 Non-specific Procedure

505

53215   male

53220   Excision or fulguration of carcinoma of urethra

53230   Excision of urethral diverticulum (separate procedure); female

53235   male

53240   Marsupialization of urethral diverticulum, male or female

53250   Excision of bulbourethral gland (Cowper's gland)

53260   Excision or fulguration; urethral polyp(s), distal urethra

     (For endoscopic approach, see 52214, 52224)

53265   urethral caruncle

53270   Skene's glands

53275   urethral prolapse

REPAIR

     (For hypospadias, see 54300-54352)

53400   Urethroplasty; first stage, for fistula, diverticulum, or stricture (eg, Johannsen type)

53405   second stage (formation of urethra), including urinary diversion

53410   Urethroplasty, one-stage reconstruction of male anterior urethra

53415   Urethroplasty, transpubic or perineal, one stage, for reconstruction or repair of prostatic or membranous urethra

53420   Urethroplasty, two-stage reconstruction or repair of prostatic or membranous urethra; first stage

53425   second stage

53430   Urethroplasty, reconstruction of female urethra

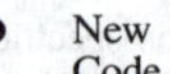 New Code   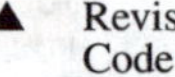 Revised Code   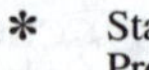 Starred Procedure    Add-On Code   ⊘ Modifier -51 Exempt

● **53431** Urethroplasty with tubularization of posterior urethra and/or lower bladder for incontinence (eg, Tenago, Leadbetter procedure)

53440 Operation for correction of male urinary incontinence, with or without introduction of prosthesis

53442 Removal of perineal prosthesis introduced for continence

(53443 deleted 2002 edition. To report, use 53431)

● **53444** Insertion of tandem cuff (dual cuff)

▲ **53445** Insertion of inflatable urethral/bladder neck sphincter, including placement of pump, reservoir, and cuff

● **53446** Removal of inflatable urethral/bladder neck sphincter, including pump, reservoir, and cuff

▲ **53447** Removal and replacement of inflatable urethral/bladder neck sphincter including pump, reservoir, and cuff at the same operative session

● **53448** Removal and replacement of inflatable urethral/bladder neck sphincter including pump, reservoir, and cuff through an infected field at the same operative session including irrigation and debridement of infected tissue

(Do not report 11040-11043 in addition to 53448)

▲ **53449** Repair of inflatable urethral/bladder neck sphincter, including pump, reservoir, and cuff

53450 Urethromeatoplasty, with mucosal advancement

(For meatotomy, see 53020, 53025)

53460 Urethromeatoplasty, with partial excision of distal urethral segment (Richardson type procedure)

53502 Urethrorrhaphy, suture of urethral wound or injury; female

53505 penile

53510 perineal

| 53515 | prostatomembranous |

| 53520 | Closure of urethrostomy or urethrocutaneous fistula, male (separate procedure) |

(For closure of urethrovaginal fistula, use 57310)

(For closure of urethrorectal fistula, see 45820, 45825)

MANIPULATION

(For radiological supervision and interpretation, use 74485)

| *53600 | Dilation of urethral stricture by passage of sound or urethral dilator, male; initial |

| *53601 | subsequent |

| 53605 | Dilation of urethral stricture or vesical neck by passage of sound or urethral dilator, male, general or conduction (spinal) anesthesia |

| *53620 | Dilation of urethral stricture by passage of filiform and follower, male; initial |

| *53621 | subsequent |

| *53660 | Dilation of female urethra including suppository and/or instillation; initial |

| *53661 | subsequent |

| 53665 | Dilation of female urethra, general or conduction (spinal) anesthesia |

| *53670 | Catheterization, urethra; simple |

| *53675 | complicated (may include difficult removal of balloon catheter) |

OTHER PROCEDURES

| 53850 | Transurethral destruction of prostate tissue; by microwave thermotherapy |

| 53852 | by radiofrequency thermotherapy |

● New Code   ▲ Revised Code   * Starred Procedure   + Add-On Code   ⊘ Modifier -51 Exempt

● **53853**   by water-induced thermotherapy

53899 Unlisted procedure, urinary system

| Separate Procedure | Unlisted Procedure | CCI Comp. Code | Non-specific Procedure |

MALE GENITAL SYSTEM

CPT codes from this section of CPT are used to report invasive and surgical procedures performed on the penis; testis; epididymis; scrotum; spermatic cord and prostate. There are several starred procedures in this section.

PENIS

INCISION

54000 Slitting of prepuce, dorsal or lateral (separate procedure); newborn

54001 except newborn

54015 Incision and drainage of penis, deep

(For skin and subcutaneous abscess, see 10060-10160)

DESTRUCTION

***54050** Destruction of lesion(s), penis (eg, condyloma, papilloma, molluscum contagiosum, herpetic vesicle), simple; chemical

***54055** electrodesiccation

54056 cryosurgery

54057 laser surgery

54060 surgical excision

▲ **54065** Destruction of lesion(s), penis (eg, condyloma, papilloma, molluscum contagiosum, herpetic vesicle), extensive (eg, laser surgery, electosurgery, cryosurgery, chemosurgery)

(For destruction or excision of other lesions, see Integumentary System)

EXCISION

54100 Biopsy of penis; (separate procedure)

54105 deep structures

54110 Excision of penile plaque (Peyronie disease);

● New Code   ▲ Revised Code   * Starred Procedure   + Add-On Code   ⊘ Modifier -51 Exempt

54111   with graft to 5 cm in length

54112   with graft greater than 5 cm in length

54115   Removal foreign body from deep penile tissue (eg, plastic implant)

54120   Amputation of penis; partial

54125   complete

54130   Amputation of penis, radical; with bilateral inguinofemoral lymphadenectomy

54135   in continuity with bilateral pelvic lymphadenectomy, including external iliac, hypogastric and obturator nodes

(for lymphadenectomy (separate procedure) see 38760-38770)

54150   Circumcision, using clamp or other device; newborn

54152   except newborn

54160   Circumcision, surgical excision other than clamp, device or dorsal slit; newborn

54161   except newborn

● **54162**   Lysis or excision of penile post-circumcision adhesions

● **54163**   Repair incomplete circumcision

● **54164**   Frenulotomy of penis

(Do not report with circumcision codes 54150-54161, 54162, 54163)

INTRODUCTION

***54200**   Injection procedure for Peyronie disease;

54205   with surgical exposure of plaque

54220   Irrigation of corpora cavernosa for priapism

54230   Injection procedure for corpora cavernosography

	Separate Procedure		Unlisted Procedure		CCI Comp. Code		Non-specific Procedure

511

(For radiological supervision and interpretation, use 74445)

54231 Dynamic cavernosometry, including intracavernosal injection of vasoactive drugs (eg, papaverine, phentolamine)

54235 Injection of corpora cavernosa with pharmacologic agent(s) (eg, papaverine, phentolamine)

54240 Penile plethysmography

54250 Nocturnal penile tumescence and/or rigidity test

REPAIR

(For other urethroplasties, see 53400-53430)

(For penile revascularization, use 37788)

54300 Plastic operation of penis for straightening of chordee (eg, hypospadias), with or without mobilization of urethra

54304 Plastic operation on penis for correction of chordee or for first stage hypospadias repair with or without transplantation of prepuce and/or skin flaps

54308 Urethroplasty for second stage hypospadias repair (including urinary diversion); less than 3 cm

54312 greater than 3 cm

54316 Urethroplasty for second stage hypospadias repair (including urinary diversion) with free skin graft obtained from site other than genitalia

54318 Urethroplasty for third stage hypospadias repair to release penis from scrotum (eg, third stage Cecil repair)

54322 One stage distal hypospadias repair (with or without chordee or circumcision); with simple meatal advancement (eg, Magpi, V-flap)

54324 with urethroplasty by local skin flaps (eg, flip-flap, prepucial flap)

54326 with urethroplasty by local skin flaps and mobilization of urethra

● New Code   ▲ Revised Code   ✱ Starred Procedure   ✚ Add-On Code   ⊘ Modifier -51 Exempt

54328   with extensive dissection to correct chordee and urethroplasty with local skin flaps, skin graft patch, and/or island flap

54332 One stage proximal penile or penoscrotal hypospadias repair requiring extensive dissection to correct chordee and urethroplasty by use of skin graft tube and/or island flap

54336 One stage perineal hypospadias repair requiring extensive dissection to correct chordee and urethroplasty by use of skin graft tube and/or island flap

54340 Repair of hypospadias complications (ie, fistula, stricture, diverticula); by closure, incision, or excision, simple

54344   requiring mobilization of skin flaps and urethroplasty with flap or patch graft

54348   requiring extensive dissection and urethroplasty with flap, patch or tubed graft (includes urinary diversion)

54352 Repair of hypospadias cripple requiring extensive dissection and excision of previously constructed structures including re-release of chordee and reconstruction of urethra and penis by use of local skin as grafts and island flaps and skin brought in as flaps or grafts

54360 Plastic operation on penis to correct angulation

54380 Plastic operation on penis for epispadias distal to external sphincter;

54385   with incontinence

54390   with exstrophy of bladder

54400 Insertion of penile prosthesis; non-inflatable (semi-rigid)

54401   inflatable (self-contained)

(54402   deleted 2002 edition. To report, see 54415, 54416)

▲ **54405** Insertion of multi-component inflatable penile prosthesis, including placement of pump, cylinders, and reservoir

(For reduced services, report 54405 with modifier -52)

513

● **54406** Removal of all components of a multi-component inflatable penile prosthesis without replacement of prosthesis

(For reduced services, report 54406 with modifier -52)

(54407 deleted 2002 edition. To report, see 54406, 54408, 54410)

● **54408** Repair of component(s) of a multi-component, inflatable penile prosthesis

(54409 deleted 2002 edition. To report, use 54408)

● **54410** Removal and replacement of all component(s) of a multi-component inflatable penile prosthesis at the same operative session

● **54411** Removal and replacement of all components of a multi-component inflatable penile prosthesis through an infected field at the same operative session, including irrigation and debridement of infected tissue

(For reduced services, report 54411 with modifier -52)

(Do not report 11040-11043 in addition to 54411)

● **54415** Removal of non-inflatable (semi-rigid) or inflatable (self-contained) penile prosthesis, without replacement of prosthesis

● **54416** Removal and replacement of non-inflatable (semi-rigid) or inflatable (self-contained) penile prosthesis at the same operative session

● **54417** Removal and replacement of non-inflatable (semi-rigid) or inflatable (self-contained) penile prosthesis through an infected field at the same operative session, including irrigation and debridement of infected tissue

(Do not report 11040-11043 in addition to 54417)

54420 Corpora cavernosa-saphenous vein shunt (priapism operation), unilateral or bilateral

54430 Corpora cavernosa-corpus spongiosum shunt (priapism operation), unilateral or bilateral

---

514 ● New Code ▲ Revised Code * Starred Procedure + Add-On Code ⊘ Modifier -51 Exempt

54435 Corpora cavernosa-glans penis fistulization (eg, biopsy needle, Winter procedure, rongeur, or punch) for priapism

54440 Plastic operation of penis for injury

MANIPULATION

54450 Foreskin manipulation including lysis of preputial adhesions and stretching

TESTIS

EXCISION

54500 Biopsy of testis, needle (separate procedure)

(For fine needle aspiration, see 10021, 10022)

(For evaluation of fine needle aspirate, see 88172, 88173)

54505 Biopsy of testis, incisional (separate procedure)

(When combined with vasogram, seminal vesiculogram, or epididymogram, use 55300)

(54510 deleted 2002 edition. To report, use 54512)

54512 Excision of extraparenchymal lesion of testis

54520 Orchiectomy, simple (including subcapsular), with or without testicular prosthesis, scrotal or inguinal approach

54522 Orchiectomy, partial

54530 Orchiectomy, radical, for tumor; inguinal approach

54535 with abdominal exploration

(For orchiectomy with repair of hernia, see 49505 or 49507 and 54520)

(For radical retroperitoneal lymphadenectomy, use 38780)

54550 Exploration for undescended testis (inguinal or scrotal area)

54560 Exploration for undescended testis with abdominal exploration

---

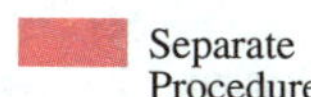 Separate Procedure

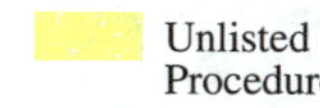 Unlisted Procedure

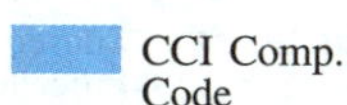 CCI Comp. Code

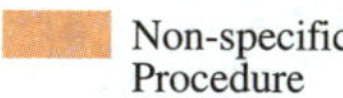 Non-specific Procedure

REPAIR

54600 Reduction of torsion of testis, surgical, with or without fixation of contralateral testis

54620 Fixation of contralateral testis (separate procedure)

54640 Orchiopexy, inguinal approach, with or without hernia repair

(For inguinal hernia repair performed in conjunction with inguinal orchiopexy, see 49495-49525)

54650 Orchiopexy, abdominal approach, for intra-abdominal testis (eg, Fowler-Stephens)

(For laparoscopic approach, use 54692)

54660 Insertion of testicular prosthesis (separate procedure)

54670 Suture or repair of testicular injury

54680 Transplantation of testis(es) to thigh (because of scrotal destruction)

LAPAROSCOPY

54690 Laparoscopy, surgical; orchiectomy

54692   orchiopexy for intra-abdominal testis

54699 Unlisted laparoscopy procedure, testis

EPIDIDYMIS

INCISION

54700 Incision and drainage of epididymis, testis and/or scrotal space (eg, abscess or hematoma)

EXCISION

54800 Biopsy of epididymis, needle

(For fine needle aspiration, see 10021, 10022)

(For evaluation of fine needle aspirate, see 88172, 88173)

---

516 ● New Code ▲ Revised Code * Starred Procedure + Add-On Code ⊘ Modifier -51 Exempt

54820 Exploration of epididymis, with or without biopsy

54830 Excision of local lesion of epididymis

54840 Excision of spermatocele, with or without epididymectomy

54860 Epididymectomy; unilateral

54861   bilateral

REPAIR

54900 Epididymovasostomy, anastomosis of epididymis to vas deferens; unilateral

54901   bilateral

(For operating microscope, use 69990)

TUNICA VAGINALIS

INCISION

***55000** Puncture aspiration of hydrocele, tunica vaginalis, with or without injection of medication

EXCISION

55040 Excision of hydrocele; unilateral

55041   bilateral

(With hernia repair, see 49495-49501)

REPAIR

55060 Repair of tunica vaginalis hydrocele (Bottle type)

SCROTUM

INCISION

***55100** Drainage of scrotal wall abscess

(See also 54700)

55110 Scrotal exploration

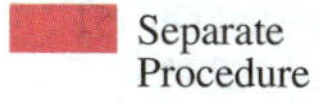 Separate Procedure

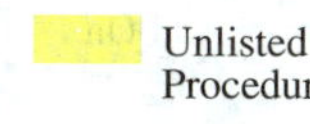 Unlisted Procedure

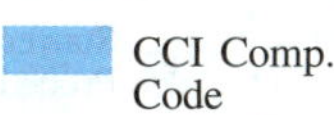 CCI Comp. Code

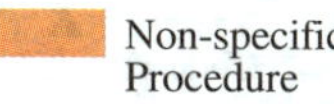 Non-specific Procedure

517

55120   Removal of foreign body in scrotum

EXCISION

(For excision of local lesion of skin of scrotum, see Integumentary System)

55150   Resection of scrotum

REPAIR

55175   Scrotoplasty; simple

55180   complicated

VAS DEFERENS

INCISION

55200   Vasotomy, cannulization with or without incision of vas, unilateral or bilateral (separate procedure)

EXCISION

55250   Vasectomy, unilateral or bilateral (separate procedure), including postoperative semen examination(s)

INTRODUCTION

55300   Vasotomy for vasograms, seminal vesiculograms, or epididymograms, unilateral or bilateral

(For radiological supervision and interpretation, use 74440)

(When combined with biopsy of testis, see 54505 and use modifier -51)

REPAIR

55400   Vasovasostomy, vasovasorrhaphy

(For operating microscope, use 69990)

SUTURE

55450   Ligation (percutaneous) of vas deferens, unilateral or bilateral (separate procedure)

---

518   ● New Code   ▲ Revised Code   ✳ Starred Procedure   ✛ Add-On Code   ⊘ Modifier -51 Exempt

SPERMATIC CORD

EXCISION

55500   Excision of hydrocele of spermatic cord, unilateral (separate procedure)

55520   Excision of lesion of spermatic cord (separate procedure)

55530   Excision of varicocele or ligation of spermatic veins for varicocele; (separate procedure)

55535   abdominal approach

55540   with hernia repair

LAPAROSCOPY

55550   Laparoscopy, surgical, with ligation of spermatic veins for varicocele

55559   Unlisted laparoscopy procedure, spermatic cord

SEMINAL VESICLES

INCISION

55600   Vesiculotomy;

55605   complicated

EXCISION

55650   Vesiculectomy, any approach

55680   Excision of Mullerian duct cyst

     (For injection procedure, see 52010, 55300)

PROSTATE

INCISION

55700   Biopsy, prostate; needle or punch, single or multiple, any approach

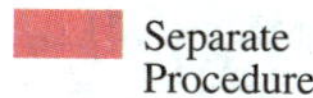
Separate Procedure

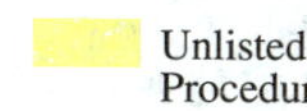
Unlisted Procedure

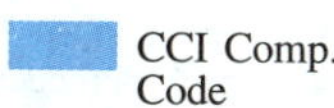
CCI Comp. Code

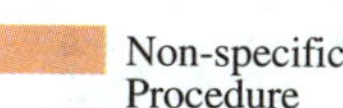
Non-specific Procedure

(If imaging guidance is performed, use 76942)

(For fine needle aspiration, see 10021, 10022)

(For evaluation of fine needle aspirate, see 88172, 88173)

55705   incisional, any approach

55720   Prostatotomy, external drainage of prostatic abscess, any approach; simple

55725   complicated

(For transurethral drainage, use 52700)

EXCISION

(For transurethral removal of prostate, see 52601-52640)

(For transurethral destruction of prostate, see 53850-53852)

(For limited pelvic lymphadenectomy for staging (separate procedure), use 38562)

(For independent node dissection, see 38770-38780)

55801   Prostatectomy, perineal, subtotal (including control of postoperative bleeding, vasectomy, meatotomy, urethral calibration and/or dilation, and internal urethrotomy)

55810   Prostatectomy, perineal radical;

55812   with lymph node biopsy(s) (limited pelvic lymphadenectomy)

55815   with bilateral pelvic lymphadenectomy, including external iliac, hypogastric and obturator nodes

(If 55815 is carried out on separate days, use 38770 with modifier -50 and 55810)

55821   Prostatectomy (including control of postoperative bleeding, vasectomy, meatotomy, urethral calibration and/or dilation, and internal urethrotomy); suprapubic, subtotal, one or two stages

55831   retropubic, subtotal

55840   Prostatectomy, retropubic radical, with or without nerve sparing;

   ● New Code   ▲ Revised Code   ✳ Starred Procedure   ✛ Add-On Code   ⊘ Modifier -51 Exempt

55842   with lymph node biopsy(s) (limited pelvic lymphadenectomy)

55845   with bilateral pelvic lymphadenectomy, including external iliac, hypogastric, and obturator nodes

(If 55845 is carried out on separate days, use 38770 with modifier -50 and 55840)

55859   Transperineal placement of needles or catheters into prostate for interstitial radioelement application, with or without cystoscopy

(For interstitial radioelement application, see 77776-77778)

(For ultrasonic guidance for interstitial radioelement application, use 76965)

55860   Exposure of prostate, any approach, for insertion of radioactive substance;

(For application of interstitial radioelement, see 77776-77778)

55862   with lymph node biopsy(s) (limited pelvic lymphadenectomy)

55865   with bilateral pelvic lymphadenectomy, including external iliac, hypogastric and obturator nodes

OTHER PROCEDURES

(For artificial insemination, see 58321, 58322)

55870   Electroejaculation

55873   Cryosurgical ablation of the prostate (includes ultrasonic guidance for interstitial cryosurgical probe placement)

55899   Unlisted procedure, male genital system

INTERSEX SURGERY

55970   Intersex surgery; male to female

55980   female to male

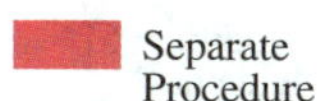 Separate Procedure

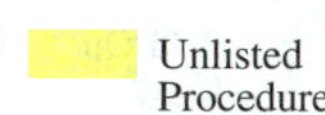 Unlisted Procedure

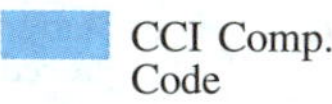 CCI Comp. Code

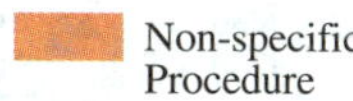 Non-specific Procedure

521

FEMALE GENITAL SYSTEM

CPT codes from this section of the CPT coding system are used to report invasive and surgical procedures performed on the perineum; vulva and introitus; vagina; cervix uteri; corpus uteri; oviduct and ovarium. In vitro fertilization is also coded using CPT codes 58970-58976 from this section.

When coding the removal of multiple vulva or perineal lesions, multiple lesions are coded with multiple codes.

When coding for the insertion of vaginal pessaries, code for the pessary itself (A4560) if purchased by the physician's office.

Select the code describing the excision procedure performed on the specific anatomic site to report LEEP (Loop Electrosurgical Excision Procedure) performed on an anatomic site other than the cervix (57460 and 57522).

Do not code pelvic examination under anesthesia (57410) when D & C or cervical circumferential biopsies with D & Cs are performed. In fact, pelvic examinations under anesthesia (57410) should not be coded separately when any other procedures are performed.

> (For pelvic laparotomy, use 49000)
>
> (For excision or destruction of endometriomas, open method, see 49200, 49201)
>
> (For paracentesis, see 49080, 49081)
>
> (For secondary closure of abdominal wall evisceration or disruption, use 49900)
>
> (For fulguration or excision of lesions, laparoscopic approach, use 58662)
>
> (For chemotherapy, see 96400-96549)

VULVA, PERINEUM AND INTROITUS

INCISION

> (For incision and drainage of sebaceous cyst, furuncle, or abscess, see 10040, 10060, 10061)

***56405** Incision and drainage of vulva or perineal abscess

***56420** Incision and drainage of Bartholin's gland abscess

> (For incision and drainage of Skene's gland abscess or cyst, use 53060)

● New Code	▲ Revised Code	* Starred Procedure	+ Add-On Code	⊘ Modifier -51 Exempt

56440 Marsupialization of Bartholin's gland cyst

56441 Lysis of labial adhesions

DESTRUCTION

▲ **56501** Destruction of lesion(s), vulva; simple (eg, laser surgery, electrosurgery, cryosurgery, chemosurgery)

▲ **56515** extensive (eg, laser surgery, electrosurgery, cryosurgery, chemosurgery)

(For destruction of Skene's gland cyst or abscess, use 53270)

(For cautery destruction of urethral caruncle, use 53265)

EXCISION

***56605** Biopsy of vulva or perineum (separate procedure); one lesion

+ ***56606** each separate additional lesion (List separately in addition to code for primary procedure)

(Use 56606 in conjunction with code 56605)

(For excision of local lesion, see 11420-11426, 11620-11626)

56620 Vulvectomy simple; partial

56625 complete

(For skin graft, see 15000 et seq)

56630 Vulvectomy, radical, partial;

(For skin graft, if used, see 15000, 15120, 15121, 15240, 15241)

56631 with unilateral inguinofemoral lymphadenectomy

56632 with bilateral inguinofemoral lymphadenectomy

56633 Vulvectomy, radical, complete;

56634 with unilateral inguinofemoral lymphadenectomy

56637 with bilateral inguinofemoral lymphadenectomy

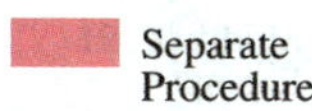 Separate Procedure

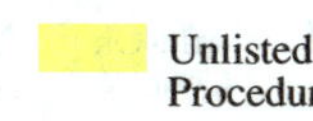 Unlisted Procedure

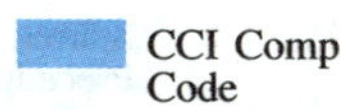 CCI Comp. Code

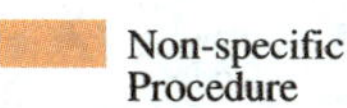 Non-specific Procedure

523

56640 Vulvectomy, radical, complete, with inguinofemoral, iliac, and pelvic lymphadenectomy

(For lymphadenectomy, see 38760-38780)

56700 Partial hymenectomy or revision of hymenal ring

***56720** Hymenotomy, simple incision

56740 Excision of Bartholin's gland or cyst

(For excision of Skene's gland, use 53270)

(For excision of urethral caruncle, use 53265)

(For excision or fulguration of urethral carcinoma, use 53220)

(For excision or marsupialization of urethral diverticulum, see 53230, 53240)

REPAIR

(For repair of urethra for mucosal prolapse, use 53275)

56800 Plastic repair of introitus

56805 Clitoroplasty for intersex state

56810 Perineoplasty, repair of perineum, nonobstetrical (separate procedure)

(See also 56800)

(For repair of wounds to genitalia, see 12001-12007, 12041-12047, 13131-13133)

(For repair of recent injury of vagina and perineum, nonobstetrical, use 57210)

(For anal sphincteroplasty, see 46750, 46751)

(For episiorrhaphy, episioperineorrhaphy for recent injury of vulva and/or perineum, nonobstetrical, use 57210)

VAGINA

INCISION

57000 Colpotomy; with exploration

● New Code ▲ Revised Code ✱ Starred Procedure ✛ Add-On Code ⊘ Modifier -51 Exempt

| 57010 | with drainage of pelvic abscess |

*57020 Colpocentesis (separate procedure)

▲ 57022 Incision and drainage of vaginal hematoma; obstetrical/postpartum

57023 non-obstetrical (eg, post-trauma, spontaneous bleeding)

DESTRUCTION

▲ 57061 Destruction of vaginal lesion(s); simple (eg, laser surgery, electrosurgery, cryosurgery, chemosurgery)

▲ 57065 extensive (eg, laser surgery, electrosurgery, cryosurgery, chemosurgery)

EXCISION

*57100 Biopsy of vaginal mucosa; simple (separate procedure)

57105 extensive, requiring suture (including cysts)

57106 Vaginectomy, partial removal of vaginal wall;

57107 with removal of paravaginal tissue (radical vaginectomy)

57109 with removal of paravaginal tissue (radical vaginectomy) with bilateral total pelvic lymphadenectomy and para-aortic lymph node sampling (biopsy)

57110 Vaginectomy, complete removal of vaginal wall;

57111 with removal of paravaginal tissue (radical vaginectomy)

57112 with removal of paravaginal tissue (radical vaginectomy) with bilateral total pelvic lymphadenectomy and para-aortic lymph node sampling (biopsy)

57120 Colpocleisis (Le Fort type)

57130 Excision of vaginal septum

57135 Excision of vaginal cyst or tumor

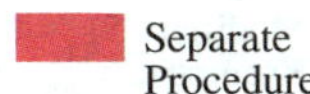

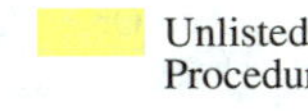

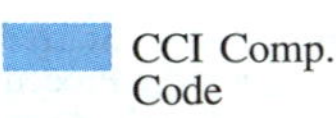

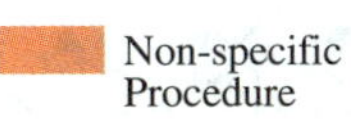

525

INTRODUCTION

***57150** Irrigation of vagina and/or application of medicament for treatment of bacterial, parasitic, or fungoid disease

● **57155** Insertion of uterine tandems and/or vaginal ovoids for clinical brachytherapy

(For insertion of radioelement sources or ribbons, see 77761-77763, 77781-77784)

***57160** Fitting and insertion of pessary or other intravaginal support device

57170 Diaphragm or cervical cap fitting with instructions

57180 Introduction of any hemostatic agent or pack for spontaneous or traumatic nonobstetrical vaginal hemorrhage (separate procedure)

REPAIR

(For urethral suspension, Marshall-Marchetti-Krantz type, abdominal approach, see 51840, 51841)

(For laparoscopic suspension, use 51990)

57200 Colporrhaphy, suture of injury of vagina (nonobstetrical)

57210 Colpoperineorrhaphy, suture of injury of vagina and/or perineum (nonobstetrical)

57220 Plastic operation on urethral sphincter, vaginal approach (eg, Kelly urethral plication)

57230 Plastic repair of urethrocele

57240 Anterior colporrhaphy, repair of cystocele with or without repair of urethrocele

57250 Posterior colporrhaphy, repair of rectocele with or without perineorrhaphy

(For repair of rectocele (separate procedure) without posterior colporrhaphy, use 45560)

57260 Combined anteroposterior colporrhaphy;

526

● New Code   ▲ Revised Code   * Starred Procedure   ✚ Add-On Code   ⊘ Modifier -51 Exempt

57265   with enterocele repair

57268   Repair of enterocele, vaginal approach (separate procedure)

57270   Repair of enterocele, abdominal approach (separate procedure)

57280   Colpopexy, abdominal approach

57282   Sacrospinous ligament fixation for prolapse of vagina

57284   Paravaginal defect repair (including repair of cystocele, stress urinary incontinence, and/or incomplete vaginal prolapse)

57287   Removal or revision of sling for stress incontinence (eg, fascia or synthetic)

57288   Sling operation for stress incontinence (eg, fascia or synthetic)

(For laparoscopic approach, use 51992)

57289   Pereyra procedure, including anterior colporrhaphy

57291   Construction of artificial vagina; without graft

57292   with graft

57300   Closure of rectovaginal fistula; vaginal or transanal approach

57305   abdominal approach

57307   abdominal approach, with concomitant colostomy

57308   transperineal approach, with perineal body reconstruction, with or without levator plication

57310   Closure of urethrovaginal fistula;

57311   with bulbocavernosus transplant

57320   Closure of vesicovaginal fistula; vaginal approach

(For concomitant cystostomy, see 51005-51040)

57330   transvesical and vaginal approach

 Separate Procedure   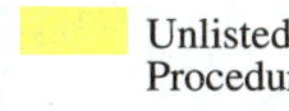 Unlisted Procedure   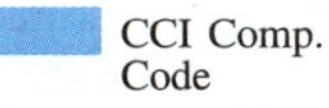 CCI Comp. Code   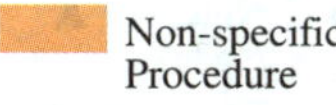 Non-specific Procedure

(For abdominal approach, use 51900)

57335 Vaginoplasty for intersex state

MANIPULATION

***57400** Dilation of vagina under anesthesia

***57410** Pelvic examination under anesthesia

57415 Removal of impacted vaginal foreign body (separate procedure) under anesthesia

(For removal without anesthesia of an impacted vaginal foreign body, use the appropriate E/M code)

ENDOSCOPY

***57452** Colposcopy (vaginoscopy); (separate procedure)

***57454** with biopsy(s) of the cervix and/or endocervical curettage

57460 with loop electrode excision procedure of the cervix

CERVIX UTERI

EXCISION

(For radical surgical procedures, see 58200-58240)

***57500** Biopsy, single or multiple, or local excision of lesion, with or without fulguration (separate procedure)

57505 Endocervical curettage (not done as part of a dilation and curettage)

▲ **57510** Cautery of cervix; electro or thermal

***57511** cryocautery, initial or repeat

57513 laser ablation

57520 Conization of cervix, with or without fulguration, with or without dilation and curettage, with or without repair; cold knife or laser

(See also 58120)

● New Code ▲ Revised Code * Starred Procedure ✛ Add-On Code ⊘ Modifier -51 Exempt

57522   loop electrode excision

57530   Trachelectomy (cervicectomy), amputation of cervix (separate procedure)

57531   Radical trachelectomy, with bilateral total pelvic lymphadenectomy and para-aortic lymph node sampling biopsy, with or without removal of tube(s), with or without removal of ovary(s)

(For radical abdominal hysterectomy, use 58210)

57540   Excision of cervical stump, abdominal approach;

57545   with pelvic floor repair

57550   Excision of cervical stump, vaginal approach;

57555   with anterior and/or posterior repair

57556   with repair of enterocele

(For insertion of intrauterine device, use 58300)

REPAIR

57700   Cerclage of uterine cervix, nonobstetrical

57720   Trachelorrhaphy, plastic repair of uterine cervix, vaginal approach

MANIPULATION

*__57800__   Dilation of cervical canal, instrumental (separate procedure)

57820   Dilation and curettage of cervical stump

CORPUS UTERI

EXCISION

*__58100__   Endometrial sampling (biopsy) with or without endocervical sampling (biopsy), without cervical dilation, any method (separate procedure)

(For endocervical curettage only, use 57505)

529

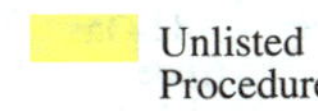

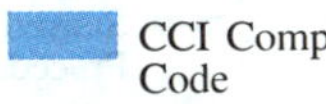

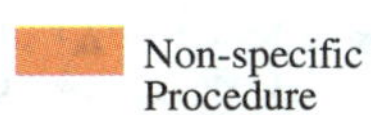

58120 Dilation and curettage, diagnostic and/or therapeutic (nonobstetrical)

(For postpartum hemorrhage, use 59160)

▲ **58140** Myomectomy, excision of leiomyomata of uterus, single or multiple (separate procedure); abdominal approach

58145 vaginal approach

58150 Total abdominal hysterectomy (corpus and cervix), with or without removal of tube(s), with or without removal of ovary(s);

58152 with colpo-urethrocystopexy (eg, Marshall-Marchetti-Krantz, Burch)

(For urethrocystopexy without hysterectomy, see 51840, 51841)

58180 Supracervical abdominal hysterectomy (subtotal hysterectomy), with or without removal of tube(s), with or without removal of ovary(s)

58200 Total abdominal hysterectomy, including partial vaginectomy, with para-aortic and pelvic lymph node sampling, with or without removal of tube(s), with or without removal of ovary(s)

58210 Radical abdominal hysterectomy, with bilateral total pelvic lymphadenectomy and para-aortic lymph node sampling (biopsy), with or without removal of tube(s), with or without removal of ovary(s)

(For radical hysterectomy with ovarian transposition, use also 58825)

58240 Pelvic exenteration for gynecologic malignancy, with total abdominal hysterectomy or cervicectomy, with or without removal of tube(s), with or without removal of ovary(s), with removal of bladder and ureteral transplantations, and/or abdominoperineal resection of rectum and colon and colostomy, or any combination thereof

(For pelvic exenteration for lower urinary tract or male genital malignancy, use 51597)

58260 Vaginal hysterectomy;

58262 with removal of tube(s), and/or ovary(s)

● New Code ▲ Revised Code ✳ Starred Procedure ✛ Add-On Code ⃠ Modifier -51 Exempt

58263   with removal of tube(s), and/or ovary(s), with repair of enterocele

58267   with colpo-urethrocystopexy (Marshall-Marchetti-Krantz type, Pereyra type, with or without endoscopic control)

58270   with repair of enterocele

(For repair of enterocele with removal of tubes and/or ovaries, use 58263)

▲ **58275**   Vaginal hysterectomy, with total or partial vaginectomy;

58280   with repair of enterocele

58285   Vaginal hysterectomy, radical (Schauta type operation)

INTRODUCTION

(For insertion/removal of implantable contraceptive capsules, see 11975, 11976, 11977)

***58300**   Insertion of intrauterine device (IUD)

58301   Removal of intrauterine device (IUD)

58321   Artificial insemination; intra-cervical

58322   intra-uterine

58323   Sperm washing for artificial insemination

***58340**   Catheterization and introduction of saline or contrast material for hysterosonography or hysterosalpingography

(For radiological supervision and interpretation of hysterosonography, use 76831)

(For radiological supervision and interpretation of hysterosalpingography, use 74740)

(For endometrial cryoablation with ultrasonic guidance, use Category III code 0009T)

58345   Transcervical introduction of fallopian tube catheter for diagnosis and/or re-establishing patency (any method), with or without hysterosalpingography

 Separate Procedure   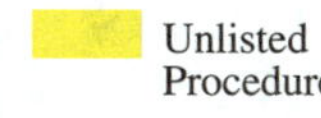 Unlisted Procedure   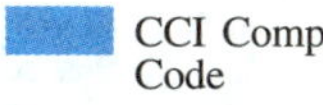 CCI Comp. Code   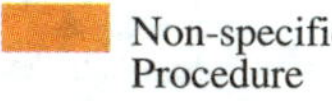 Non-specific Procedure

(For radiological supervision and interpretation, use 74742)

● **58346**   Insertion of Heyman capsules for clinical brachytherapy

(For insertion of radioelement sources or ribbons, see 77761-77763, 77781-77784)

***58350**   Chromotubation of oviduct, including materials

(For materials supplied by physician, use 99070)

58353   Endometrial ablation, thermal, without hysteroscopic guidance

(For hysteroscopic procedure, use 58563)

REPAIR

58400   Uterine suspension, with or without shortening of round ligaments, with or without shortening of sacrouterine ligaments; (separate procedure)

58410   with presacral sympathectomy

58520   Hysterorrhaphy, repair of ruptured uterus (nonobstetrical)

58540   Hysteroplasty, repair of uterine anomaly (Strassman type)

(For closure of vesicouterine fistula, use 51920)

LAPAROSCOPY-HYSTEROSCOPY

The descriptions of CPT codes in this section are listed so that the main procedure can be identified without having to list all of the minor related procedures performed at the same time. For example:

58558   Hysterscopy, surgical; with sampling (biopsy) of endometrium and/or polypectomy, with or without D & C

The secondary procedure(s) is/are included in the single code 58558. If any of the secondary procedures require significant additional time and effort, to the point of making the procedure "unusual", modifier -22 should be added with an appropriate increase in fee and a report explaining why the procedure was unusual.

58550   Laparoscopy, surgical; with vaginal hysterectomy with or without removal of tube(s), with or without removal of ovary(s) (laparoscopic assisted vaginal hysterectomy)

● New Code   ▲ Revised Code   * Starred Procedure   + Add-On Code   ⊘ Modifier -51 Exempt

58551   with removal of leiomyomata (single or multiple)

58555   Hysteroscopy, diagnostic (separate procedure)

58558   Hysteroscopy, surgical; with sampling (biopsy) of endometrium and/or polypectomy, with or without D & C

58559   with lysis of intrauterine adhesions (any method)

58560   with division or resection of intrauterine septum (any method)

58561   with removal of leiomyomata

58562   with removal of impacted foreign body

▲ **58563**   with endometrial ablation (eg, endometrial resection, electrosurgical ablation, thermoablation)

58578   Unlisted laparoscopy procedure, uterus

58579   Unlisted hysteroscopy procedure, uterus

OVIDUCT/OVARY

INCISION

58600   Ligation or transection of fallopian tube(s), abdominal or vaginal approach, unilateral or bilateral

58605   Ligation or transection of fallopian tube(s), abdominal or vaginal approach, postpartum, unilateral or bilateral, during same hospitalization (separate procedure)

(For laparoscopic procedures, use 58670, 58671)

▲ **+58611**   Ligation or transection of fallopian tube(s) when done at the time of cesarean delivery or intra-abdominal surgery (not a separate procedure) (List separately in addition to code for primary procedure)

58615   Occlusion of fallopian tube(s) by device (eg, band, clip, Falope ring) vaginal or suprapubic approach

(For laparoscopic approach, use 58671)

Separate Procedure

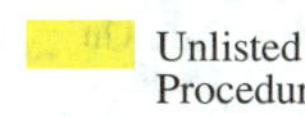
Unlisted Procedure

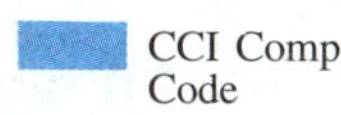
CCI Comp. Code

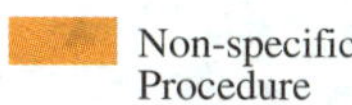
Non-specific Procedure

533

LAPAROSCOPY

(For laparoscopic biopsy of the ovary or fallopian tube, use 49321)

58660 Laparoscopy, surgical; with lysis of adhesions (salpingolysis, ovariolysis) (separate procedure)

58661 with removal of adnexal structures (partial or total oophorectomy and/or salpingectomy)

58662 with fulguration or excision of lesions of the ovary, pelvic viscera, or peritoneal surface by any method

58670 with fulguration of oviducts (with or without transection)

58671 with occlusion of oviducts by device (eg, band, clip, or Falope ring)

58672 with fimbrioplasty

58673 with salpingostomy (salpingoneostomy)

(Codes 58672 and 58673 are used to report unilateral procedures. For bilateral procedure, use modifier -50)

58679 Unlisted laparoscopy procedure, oviduct, ovary

EXCISION

58700 Salpingectomy, complete or partial, unilateral or bilateral (separate procedure)

58720 Salpingo-oophorectomy, complete or partial, unilateral or bilateral (separate procedure)

REPAIR

58740 Lysis of adhesions (salpingolysis, ovariolysis)

(For laparoscopic approach, use 58660)

(For excision or destruction of endometriomas, open method, see 49200, 49201)

(For fulguration or excision of lesions, laparscopic approach, use 58662)

● New Code ▲ Revised Code ∗ Starred Procedure ✛ Add-On Code ⊘ Modifier -51 Exempt

58750   Tubotubal anastomosis

58752   Tubouterine implantation

58760   Fimbrioplasty

(For laparoscopic approach, use 58672)

58770   Salpingostomy (salpingoneostomy)

(For laparscopic approach, use 58673)

OVARY

INCISION

58800   Drainage of ovarian cyst(s), unilateral or bilateral, (separate procedure); vaginal approach

58805   abdominal approach

58820   Drainage of ovarian abscess; vaginal approach, open

58822   abdominal approach

58823   Drainage of pelvic abscess, transvaginal or transrectal approach, percutaneous (eg, ovarian, pericolic)

(For radiological supervision and interpretation, use 75989)

58825   Transposition, ovary(s)

EXCISION

58900   Biopsy of ovary, unilateral or bilateral (separate procedure)

(For laparoscopic biopsy of the ovary or fallopian tube, use 49321)

58920   Wedge resection or bisection of ovary, unilateral or bilateral

58925   Ovarian cystectomy, unilateral or bilateral

58940   Oophorectomy, partial or total, unilateral or bilateral;

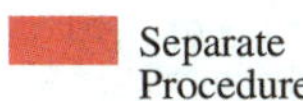

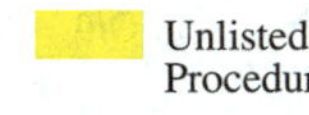

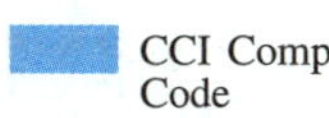

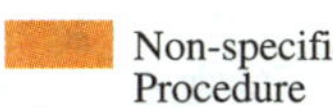

58943   for ovarian, tubal or primary peritoneal malignancy, with para-aortic and pelvic lymph node biopsies, peritoneal washings, peritoneal biopsies, diaphragmatic assessments, with or without salpingectomy(s), with or without omentectomy

58950   Resection of ovarian, tubal or primary peritoneal malignancy with bilateral salpingo-oophorectomy and omentectomy;

58951   with total abdominal hysterectomy, pelvic and limited para-aortic lymphadenectomy

58952   with radical dissection for debulking (ie, radical excision or destruction, intra-abdominal or retroperitoneal tumors)

● **58953**   Bilateral salpingo-oophorectomy with omentectomy, total abdominal hysterectomy and radical dissection for debulking;

● **58954**   with pelvic lymphadenectomy and limited para-aortic lymphadenectomy

58960   Laparotomy, for staging or restaging of ovarian, tubal or primary peritoneal malignancy (second look), with or without omentectomy, peritoneal washing, biopsy of abdominal and pelvic peritoneum, diaphragmatic assessment with pelvic and limited para-aortic lymphadenectomy

IN VITRO FERTILIZATION

58970   Follicle puncture for oocyte retrieval, any method

(For radiological supervision and interpretation, use 76948)

58974   Embryo transfer, intrauterine

58976   Gamete, zygote, or embryo intrafallopian transfer, any method

OTHER PROCEDURES

58999   Unlisted procedure, female genital system (nonobstetrical)

| ● New Code | ▲ Revised Code | ✱ Starred Procedure | + Add-On Code | ⊘ Modifier -51 Exempt |

MATERNITY CARE AND DELIVERY

CPT codes from this section are used to report routine maternity care and invasive and surgical procedures performed as part of prenatal, delivery and post-partum care. The services normally provided in uncomplicated maternity cases include antepartum care, delivery, and postpartum care.

ANTEPARTUM CARE

The definition of antepartum care for coding purposes includes the initial and subsequent history, physical examinations, recording of weight, blood pressures, fetal heart tones, routine chemical urinalysis, and routine visits. Routine antepartum visits are defined as:

- Monthly visits up to 28 weeks gestation

- Biweekly visits up to 36 weeks gestation, and

- Weekly visits until delivery

Any other visits or services provided within this time period should be coded separately. Using 6 to 8 weeks gestation as the typical starting point, the above definition translates into between 9 and 11 routine visits per patient.

DELIVERY

Delivery services are defined as including hospital admission, the admission history and physical examination, management of uncomplicated labor, and vaginal or cesarean delivery.

- The definition of delivery services includes the hospital admission, and admission history and physical.

- Resuscitation of newborn infants when necessary, defined in previous editions, is not included in the delivery services. If the delivering physician has to resuscitate the newborn infant, he/she may code this service as a separate procedure.

- Medical problems "complicating labor and delivery management" may require additional resources and should be reported using or evaluation and management service codes.

POSTPARTUM CARE

Postpartum care is defined as hospital and office visits following vaginal or cesarean delivery. No number of visits is defined by CPT; however, the typical fee for total obstetrical care includes a single office follow-up visit six weeks postpartum.

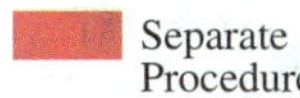 Separate Procedure

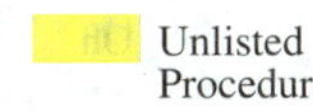 Unlisted Procedure

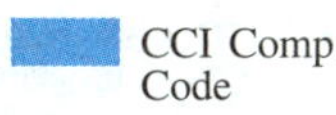 CCI Comp. Code

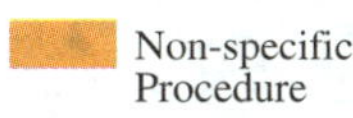 Non-specific Procedure

COMPLICATIONS OF PREGNANCY

The services defined previously are for normal, uncomplicated maternity care. For medical complications of pregnancy, for example, cardiac problems, neurological problems, diabetes, hypertension, toxemia, hyperemesis, pre-term labor and premature rupture of membranes, use evaluation and management service codes.

For surgical complications of pregnancy, such as appendectomy, hernia, ovarian cyst, Bartholin cysts, etc., use CPT codes from the SURGERY section of CPT. Note that in either case, complications are not considered to be part of routine maternity care and should be coded and reported in addition to maternity CPT codes.

PARTIAL MATERNITY SERVICES

Occasionally a physician may provide all or part of the antepartum and/or postpartum care but does not perform the actual delivery due to termination of the pregnancy by abortion, or referral to another physician for delivery. In this circumstance, the physician has the option of using the inclusive CPT codes 59420 or 59430 from the Maternity Care and Delivery section reporting each visit using evaluation and management service codes 99201-99215.

MISCELLANEOUS CODING RULES

Obstetric care can be coded as a global package or can be broken down when necessary into antepartum, delivery and postpartum care.

Complicated pregnancies and deliveries need to be coded appropriately to indicate the increased work on the physician's part during the patient's care. There are several options for recording these circumstances.

(For circumcision of newborn, see 54150, 54160)

ANTEPARTUM SERVICES

(For insertion of transcervical or transvaginal fetal oximetry sensor, use Category III code 0021T)

▲ ***59000**   Amniocentesis, diagnostic

(For radiological supervision and interpretation, use 76946)

● **59001**   therapeutic amniotic fluid reduction (includes ultrasound guidance)

59012   Cordocentesis (intrauterine), any method

(For radiological supervision and interpretation, use 76941)

59015   Chorionic villus sampling, any method

● New Code   ▲ Revised Code   * Starred Procedure   ✛ Add-On Code   ⊘ Modifier -51 Exempt

(For radiological supervision and interpretation, use 76945)

***59020** Fetal contraction stress test

59025 Fetal non-stress test

***59030** Fetal scalp blood sampling

59050 Fetal monitoring during labor by consulting physician (ie, non-attending physician) with written report; supervision and interpretation

59051 interpretation only

EXCISION

59100 Hysterotomy, abdominal (eg, for hydatidiform mole, abortion)

(When tubal ligation is performed at the same time as hysterotomy, use 58611 in addition to 59100)

59120 Surgical treatment of ectopic pregnancy; tubal or ovarian, requiring salpingectomy and/or oophorectomy, abdominal or vaginal approach

59121 tubal or ovarian, without salpingectomy and/or oophorectomy

59130 abdominal pregnancy

59135 interstitial, uterine pregnancy requiring total hysterectomy

59136 interstitial, uterine pregnancy with partial resection of uterus

59140 cervical, with evacuation

59150 Laparoscopic treatment of ectopic pregnancy; without salpingectomy and/or oophorectomy

59151 with salpingectomy and/or oophorectomy

59160 Curettage, postpartum

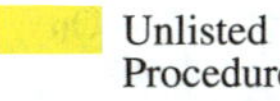

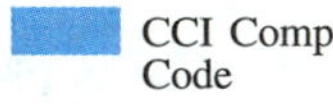

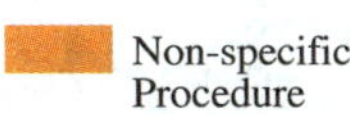

Non-specific
Procedure

INTRODUCTION

(For intrauterine fetal transfusion, use 36460)

(For introduction of hypertonic solution and/or prostaglandins to initiate labor, see 59850-59857)

59200 Insertion of cervical dilator (eg, laminaria, prostaglandin) (separate procedure)

REPAIR

(For tracheoplasty, use 57700)

59300 Episiotomy or vaginal repair, by other than attending physician

59320 Cerclage of cervix, during pregnancy; vaginal

59325 abdominal

59350 Hysterorrhaphy of ruptured uterus

VAGINAL DELIVERY, ANTEPARTUM AND POSTPARTUM CARE

(For insertion of transcervical or transvaginal fetal oximetry sensor, use Category III code 0021T)

59400 Routine obstetric care including antepartum care, vaginal delivery (with or without episiotomy, and/or forceps) and postpartum care

59409 Vaginal delivery only (with or without episiotomy and/or forceps);

59410 including postpartum care

59412 External cephalic version, with or without tocolysis

(Use 59412 in addition to code(s) for delivery)

59414 Delivery of placenta (separate procedure)

(For 1-3 antepartum care visits, see appropriate E/M code(s))

59425 Antepartum care only; 4-6 visits

59426 7 or more visits

59430 Postpartum care only (separate procedure)

● New Code ▲ Revised Code ✳ Starred Procedure ✛ Add-On Code ⊘ Modifier -51 Exempt

CESAREAN DELIVERY

(For standby attendance for infant, use 99360)

(For insertion of transcervical or transvaginal fetal oximetry sensor, use Category III code 0021T)

59510 Routine obstetric care including antepartum care, cesarean delivery, and postpartum care

59514 Cesarean delivery only;

59515 including postpartum care

+59525 Subtotal or total hysterectomy after cesarean delivery (List separately in addition to code for primary procedure)

(Use 59525 in conjunction with codes 59510, 59514, 59515, 59618, 59620, 59622)

DELIVERY AFTER PREVIOUS CESAREAN DELIVERY

(For insertion of transcervical or transvaginal fetal oximetry sensor, use Category III code 0021T)

59610 Routine obstetric care including antepartum care, vaginal delivery (with or without episiotomy, and/or forceps) and postpartum care, after previous cesarean delivery

59612 Vaginal delivery only, after previous cesarean delivery (with or without episiotomy and/or forceps);

59614 including postpartum care

59618 Routine obstetric care including antepartum care, cesarean delivery, and postpartum care, following attempted vaginal delivery after previous cesarean delivery

59620 Cesarean delivery only, following attempted vaginal delivery after previous cesarean delivery;

59622 including postpartum care

Separate Procedure	Unlisted Procedure	CCI Comp. Code	Non-specific Procedure

ABORTION

(For medical treatment of spontaneous complete abortion, any trimester, use E/M codes 99201-99233)

59812 Treatment of incomplete abortion, any trimester, completed surgically

59820 Treatment of missed abortion, completed surgically; first trimester

59821 second trimester

59830 Treatment of septic abortion, completed surgically

59840 Induced abortion, by dilation and curettage

59841 Induced abortion, by dilation and evacuation

59850 Induced abortion, by one or more intra-amniotic injections (amniocentesis-injections), including hospital admission and visits, delivery of fetus and secundines;

59851 with dilation and curettage and/or evacuation

59852 with hysterotomy (failed intra-amniotic injection)

(For insertion of cervical dilator, use 59200)

59855 Induced abortion, by one or more vaginal suppositories (eg, prostaglandin) with or without cervical dilation (eg, laminaria), including hospital admission and visits, delivery of fetus and secundines;

59856 with dilation and curettage and/or evacuation

59857 with hysterotomy (failed medical evacuation)

OTHER PROCEDURES

59866 Multifetal pregnancy reduction(s) (MPR)

59870 Uterine evacuation and curettage for hydatidiform mole

59871 Removal of cerclage suture under anesthesia (other than local)

● New Code   ▲ Revised Code   * Starred Procedure   + Add-On Code   ⊘ Modifier -51 Exempt

59898 Unlisted laparoscopy procedure, maternity care and delivery

59899 Unlisted procedure, maternity care and delivery

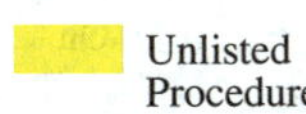

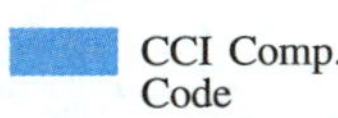

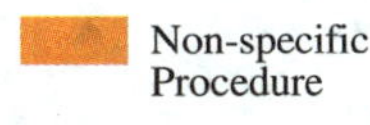

Non-specific
Procedure

ENDOCRINE SYSTEM

CPT codes from this section of CPT are used to report invasive and surgical procedures performed on the thyroid gland, parathyroid, thymus, adrenal glands and carotid body.

(For pituitary and pineal surgery, see Nervous System)

THYROID GLAND

INCISION

▲ *60000   Incision and drainage of thyroglossal duct cyst, infected

EXCISION

60001   Aspiration and/or injection, thyroid cyst

(For fine needle aspiration, see 10021, 10022)

(If imaging guidance is performed, see 76360, 76942)

*60100   Biopsy thyroid, percutaneous core needle

(If imaging guidance is performed, see 76003, 76360, 76393, 76942)

(For fine needle aspiration, use 10021 or 10022)

(For evaluation of fine needle aspirate, see 88172, 88173)

60200   Excision of cyst or adenoma of thyroid, or transection of isthmus

60210   Partial thyroid lobectomy, unilateral; with or without isthmusectomy

60212   with contralateral subtotal lobectomy, including isthmusectomy

60220   Total thyroid lobectomy, unilateral; with or without isthmusectomy

60225   with contralateral subtotal lobectomy, including isthmusectomy

60240   Thyroidectomy, total or complete

● New Code   ▲ Revised Code   * Starred Procedure   + Add-On Code   ⊘ Modifier -51 Exempt

60252 Thyroidectomy, total or subtotal for malignancy; with limited neck dissection

60254   with radical neck dissection

60260 Thyroidectomy, removal of all remaining thyroid tissue following previous removal of a portion of thyroid

▲ **60270** Thyroidectomy, including substernal thyroid; sternal split or transthoracic approach

60271   cervical approach

60280 Excision of thyroglossal duct cyst or sinus;

60281   recurrent

(For thyroid ultrasonography, use 76536)

PARATHYROID, THYMUS, ADRENAL GLANDS, AND CAROTID BODY

EXCISION

(For pituitary and pineal surgery, see Nervous System)

60500 Parathyroidectomy or exploration of parathyroid(s);

60502   re-exploration

60505   with mediastinal exploration, sternal split or transthoracic approach

+60512 Parathyroid autotransplantation (List separately in addition to code for primary procedure)

(Use 60512 in conjunction with codes 60500, 60502, 60505, 60212, 60225, 60240, 60252, 60254, 60260, 60270, 60271)

60520 Thymectomy, partial or total; transcervical approach (separate procedure)

60521   sternal split or transthoracic approach, without radical mediastinal dissection (separate procedure)

60522   sternal split or transthoracic approach, with radical mediastinal dissection (separate procedure)

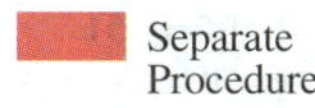

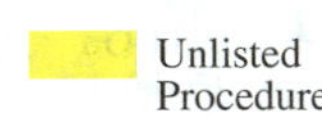

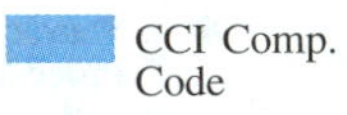

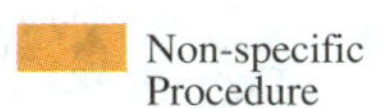

545

60540 Adrenalectomy, partial or complete, or exploration of adrenal gland with or without biopsy, transabdominal, lumbar or dorsal (separate procedure);

60545 with excision of adjacent retroperitoneal tumor

(For excision of remote or disseminated pheochromocytoma, see 49200, 49201)

(For laparoscopic approach, use 56321)

60600 Excision of carotid body tumor; without excision of carotid artery

60605 with excision of carotid artery

LAPAROSCOPY

60650 Laparoscopy, surgical, with adrenalectomy, partial or complete, or exploration of adrenal gland with or without biopsy, transabdominal, lumbar or dorsal

60659 Unlisted laparoscopy procedure, endocrine system

OTHER PROCEDURES

60699 Unlisted procedure, endocrine system

● New Code   ▲ Revised Code   ✳ Starred Procedure   + Add-On Code   ⊘ Modifier -51 Exempt

NERVOUS SYSTEM

CPT codes from this section of the CPT coding system are used to report invasive and surgical procedures on the skull; meninges and brain; spine and spinal cord; and the extracranial nerves, peripheral nerves and autonomic nervous system.

There are numerous codes for spinal injections found in this section. Review documentation for whether the injection is a single one, differential one or continuous. Also determine the number of levels involved when a regional block is administered.

SKULL, MENINGES, AND BRAIN

(For injection procedure for cerebral angiography, see 36100-36218)

(For injection procedure for ventriculography, see 61026, 61120, 61130)

(For injection procedure for pneumoencephalography, use 61055)

INJECTION, DRAINAGE OR ASPIRATION

***61000** Subdural tap through fontanelle, or suture, infant, unilateral or bilateral; initial

***61001** subsequent taps

***61020** Ventricular puncture through previous burr hole, fontanelle, suture, or implanted ventricular catheter/reservoir; without injection

▲***61026** with injection of medication or other substance for diagnosis or treatment

***61050** Cisternal or lateral cervical (C1-C2) puncture; without injection (separate procedure)

▲***61055** with injection of medication or other substance for diagnosis or treatment (eg, C1-C2)

(For radiological supervision and interpretation, see Radiology)

***61070** Puncture of shunt tubing or reservoir for aspiration or injection procedure

(For radiological supervision and interpretation, see 75809)

547

Separate Procedure

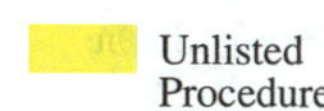
Unlisted Procedure

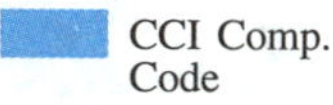
CCI Comp. Code

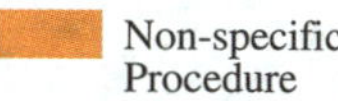
Non-specific Procedure

TWIST DRILL, BURR HOLE(S), OR TREPHINE

***61105** Twist drill hole for subdural or ventricular puncture;

⊘***61107** for implanting ventricular catheter or pressure recording device

61108 for evacuation and/or drainage of subdural hematoma

61120 Burr hole(s) for ventricular puncture (including injection of gas, contrast media, dye, or radioactive material)

61140 Burr hole(s) or trephine; with biopsy of brain or intracranial lesion

61150 with drainage of brain abscess or cyst

61151 with subsequent tapping (aspiration) of intracranial abscess or cyst

61154 Burr hole(s) with evacuation and/or drainage of hematoma, extradural or subdural

61156 Burr hole(s); with aspiration of hematoma or cyst, intracerebral

⊘***61210** for implanting ventricular catheter, reservoir, EEG electrode(s) or pressure recording device (separate procedure)

61215 Insertion of subcutaneous reservoir, pump or continuous infusion system for connection to ventricular catheter

(For chemotherapy, use 96450)

61250 Burr hole(s) or trephine, supratentorial, exploratory, not followed by other surgery

61253 Burr hole(s) or trephine, infratentorial, unilateral or bilateral

(If burr hole(s) or trephine are followed by craniotomy at same operative session, use 61304-61321; do not use 61250 or 61253)

CRANIECTOMY OR CRANIOTOMY

61304 Craniectomy or craniotomy, exploratory; supratentorial

61305 infratentorial (posterior fossa)

● New Code   ▲ Revised Code   * Starred Procedure   + Add-On Code   ⊘ Modifier -51 Exempt

61312 Craniectomy or craniotomy for evacuation of hematoma, supratentorial; extradural or subdural

61313 intracerebral

61314 Craniectomy or craniotomy for evacuation of hematoma, infratentorial; extradural or subdural

61315 intracerebellar

61320 Craniectomy or craniotomy, drainage of intracranial abscess; supratentorial

61321 infratentorial

61330 Decompression of orbit only, transcranial approach

61332 Exploration of orbit (transcranial approach); with biopsy

61333 with removal of lesion

61334 with removal of foreign body

61340 Other cranial decompression (eg, subtemporal), supratentorial

61343 Craniectomy, suboccipital with cervical laminectomy for decompression of medulla and spinal cord, with or without dural graft (eg, Arnold-Chiari malformation)

61345 Other cranial decompression, posterior fossa

(For orbital decompression by lateral wall approach, Kroenlein type, use 67445)

61440 Craniotomy for section of tentorium cerebelli (separate procedure)

61450 Craniectomy, subtemporal, for section, compression, or decompression of sensory root of gasserian ganglion

61458 Craniectomy, suboccipital; for exploration or decompression of cranial nerves

61460 for section of one or more cranial nerves

61470 for medullary tractotomy

Separate Procedure	Unlisted Procedure	CCI Comp. Code	Non-specific Procedure

549

61480	for mesencephalic tractotomy or pedunculotomy
61490	Craniotomy for lobotomy, including cingulotomy
61500	Craniectomy; with excision of tumor or other bone lesion of skull
61501	for osteomyelitis
61510	Craniectomy, trephination, bone flap craniotomy; for excision of brain tumor, supratentorial, except meningioma
61512	for excision of meningioma, supratentorial
61514	for excision of brain abscess, supratentorial
61516	for excision or fenestration of cyst, supratentorial

(For excision of pituitary tumor or craniopharyngioma, see 61545, 61546, 61548)

61518	Craniectomy for excision of brain tumor, infratentorial or posterior fossa; except meningioma, cerebellopontine angle tumor, or midline tumor at base of skull
61519	meningioma
61520	cerebellopontine angle tumor
61521	midline tumor at base of skull
61522	Craniectomy, infratentorial or posterior fossa; for excision of brain abscess
61524	for excision or fenestration of cyst
61526	Craniectomy, bone flap craniotomy, transtemporal (mastoid) for excision of cerebellopontine angle tumor;
61530	combined with middle/posterior fossa craniotomy/craniectomy
61531	Subdural implantation of strip electrodes through one or more burr or trephine hole(s) for long term seizure monitoring

(For stereotactic implantation of electrodes, use 61760)

● New Code	▲ Revised Code	∗ Starred Procedure	**+** Add-On Code	⊘ Modifier -51 Exempt

61533 Craniotomy with elevation of bone flap; for subdural implantation of an electrode array, for long term seizure monitoring

(For continuous EEG monitoring, see 95950-95954)

61534 for excision of epileptogenic focus without electrocorticography during surgery

61535 for removal of epidural or subdural electrode array, without excision of cerebral tissue (separate procedure)

61536 for excision of cerebral epileptogenic focus, with electrocorticography during surgery (includes removal of electrode array)

61538 for lobectomy with electrocorticography during surgery, temporal lobe

61539 for lobectomy with electrocorticography during surgery, other than temporal lobe, partial or total

61541 for transection of corpus callosum

61542 for total hemispherectomy

61543 for partial or subtotal hemispherectomy

61544 for excision or coagulation of choroid plexus

61545 for excision of craniopharyngioma

61546 Craniotomy for hypophysectomy or excision of pituitary tumor, intracranial approach

61548 Hypophysectomy or excision of pituitary tumor, transnasal or transseptal approach, nonstereotactic

(Do not report code 69990 in addition to code 61548)

61550 Craniectomy for craniosynostosis; single cranial suture

61552 multiple cranial sutures

(For cranial reconstruction for orbital hypertelorism, see 21260-21263)

 Separate Procedure

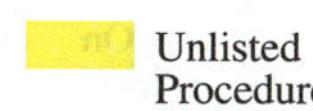 Unlisted Procedure

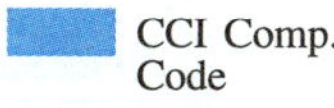 CCI Comp. Code

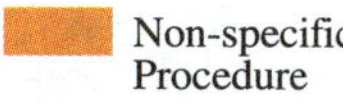 Non-specific Procedure

61556 Craniotomy for craniosynostosis; frontal or parietal bone flap

61557 bifrontal bone flap

61558 Extensive craniectomy for multiple cranial suture craniosynostosis (eg, cloverleaf skull); not requiring bone grafts

61559 recontouring with multiple osteotomies and bone autografts (eg, barrel-stave procedure) (includes obtaining grafts)

61563 Excision, intra and extracranial, benign tumor of cranial bone (eg, fibrous dysplasia); without optic nerve decompression

61564 with optic nerve decompression

(For reconstruction, see 21181-21183)

61570 Craniectomy or craniotomy; with excision of foreign body from brain

61571 with treatment of penetrating wound of brain

(For sequestrectomy for osteomyelitis, use 61501)

61575 Transoral approach to skull base, brain stem or upper spinal cord for biopsy, decompression or excision of lesion;

61576 requiring splitting of tongue and/or mandible (including tracheostomy)

(For arthrodesis, use 22548)

APPROACH PROCEDURES

Anterior Cranial Fossa

61580 Craniofacial approach to anterior cranial fossa; extradural, including lateral rhinotomy, ethmoidectomy, sphenoidectomy, without maxillectomy or orbital exenteration

61581 extradural, including lateral rhinotomy, orbital exenteration, ethmoidectomy, sphenoidectomy and/or maxillectomy

61582 extradural, including unilateral or bifrontal craniotomy, elevation of frontal lobe(s), osteotomy of base of anterior cranial fossa

---

● New Code   ▲ Revised Code   * Starred Procedure   + Add-On Code   ⊘ Modifier -51 Exempt

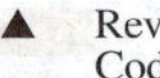

61583   intradural, including unilateral or bifrontal craniotomy, elevation or resection of frontal lobe, osteotomy of base of anterior cranial fossa

61584   Orbitocranial approach to anterior cranial fossa, extradural, including supraorbital ridge osteotomy and elevation of frontal and/or temporal lobe(s); without orbital exenteration

61585   with orbital exenteration

61586   Bicoronal, transzygomatic and/or LeFort I osteotomy approach to anteriorcranial fossa with or without internal fixation, without bone graft

Middle Cranial Fossa

61590   Infratemporal pre-auricular approach to middle cranial fossa (parapharyngeal space, infratemporal and midline skull base, nasopharynx), with or without disarticulation of the mandible, including parotidectomy, craniotomy, decompression and/or mobilization of the facial nerve and/or petrous carotid artery

61591   Infratemporal post-auricular approach to middle cranial fossa (internal auditory meatus, petrous apex, tentorium, cavernous sinus, parasellar area, infratemporal fossa) including mastoidectomy, resection of sigmoid sinus, with or without decompression and/or mobilization of contents of auditory canal or petrous carotid artery

61592   Orbitocranial zygomatic approach to middle cranial fossa (cavernous sinus and carotid artery, clivus, basilar artery or petrous apex) including osteotomy of zygoma, craniotomy, extra- or intradural elevation of temporal lobe

Posterior Cranial Fossa

61595   Transtemporal approach to posterior cranial fossa, jugular foramen or midline skull base, including mastoidectomy, decompression of sigmoid sinus and/or facial nerve, with or without mobilization

61596   Transcochlear approach to posterior cranial fossa, jugular foramen or midline skull base, including labyrinthectomy, decompression, with or without mobilization of facial nerve and/or petrous carotid artery

61597   Transcondylar (far lateral) approach to posterior cranial fossa, jugular foramen or midline skull base, including occipital

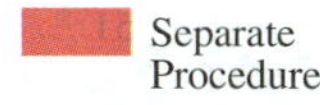

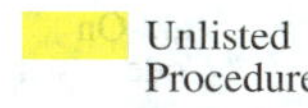

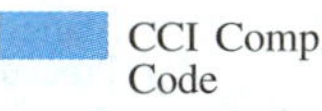

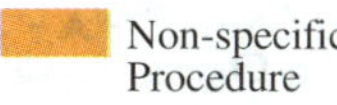

553

condylectomy, mastoidectomy, resection of C1-C3 vertebral body(s), decompression of vertebral artery, with or without mobilization

61598 Transpetrosal approach to posterior cranial fossa, clivus or foramen magnum, including ligation of superior petrosal sinus and/or sigmoid sinus

DEFINITIVE PROCEDURES

Base of Anterior Cranial Fossa

61600 Resection or excision of neoplastic, vascular or infectious lesion of base of anterior cranial fossa; extradural

61601 intradural, including dural repair, with or without graft

Base of Middle Cranial Fossa

61605 Resection or excision of neoplastic, vascular or infectious lesion of infratemporal fossa, parapharyngeal space, petrous apex; extradural

61606 intradural, including dural repair, with or without graft

61607 Resection or excision of neoplastic, vascular or infectious lesion of parasellar area, cavernous sinus, clivus or midline skull base; extradural

61608 intradural, including dural repair, with or without graft

+61609 Transection or ligation, carotid artery in cavernous sinus; without repair (List separately in addition to code for primary procedure)

+61610 with repair by anastomosis or graft (List separately in addition to code for primary procedure)

+61611 Transection or ligation, carotid artery in petrous canal; without repair (List separately in addition to code for primary procedure)

+61612 with repair by anastomosis or graft (List separately in addition to code for primary procedure)

61613 Obliteration of carotid aneurysm, arteriovenous malformation, or carotid-cavernous fistula by dissection within cavernous sinus

●	New Code	▲	Revised Code	*	Starred Procedure	+	Add-On Code	⊘	Modifier -51 Exempt

Base of Posterior Cranial Fossa

61615   Resection or excision of neoplastic, vascular or infectious lesion of base of posterior cranial fossa, jugular foramen, foramen magnum, or C1-C3 vertebral bodies; extradural

61616   intradural, including dural repair, with or without graft

REPAIR AND/OR RECONSTRUCTION OF SURGICAL DEFECTS OF SKULL BASE

▲ **61618**   Secondary repair of dura for cerebrospinal fluid leak, anterior, middle or posterior cranial fossa following surgery of the skull base; by free tissue graft (eg, pericranium, fascia, tensor fascia lata, adipose tissue, homologous or synthetic grafts)

61619   by local or regionalized vascularized pedicle flap or myocutaneous flap (including galea, temporalis, frontalis or occipitalis muscle)

ENDOVASCULAR THERAPY

61624   Transcatheter occlusion or embolization (eg, for tumor destruction, to achieve hemostasis, to occlude a vascular malformation), percutaneous, any method; central nervous system (intracranial, spinal cord)

(See also 37204)

(For radiological supervision and interpretation, use 75894)

61626   non-central nervous system, head or neck (extracranial, brachiocephalic branch)

(See also 37204)

(For radiological supervision and interpretation, use 75894)

SURGERY FOR ANEURYSM, ARTERIOVENOUS MALFORMATION OR VASCULAR DISEASE

61680   Surgery of intracranial arteriovenous malformation; supratentorial, simple

61682   supratentorial, complex

61684   infratentorial, simple

61686   infratentorial, complex

 Separate Procedure

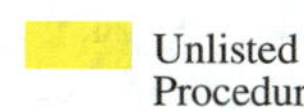 Unlisted Procedure

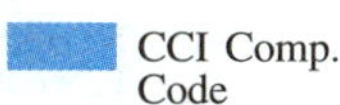 CCI Comp. Code

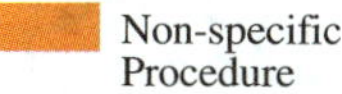 Non-specific Procedure

555

61690   dural, simple

61692   dural, complex

61697   Surgery of complex intracranial aneurysm, intracranial
approach; carotid circulation

61698   vertebrobasilar circulation

(61697, 61698 involve aneurysms that are larger than 15 mm or
with calcification of the aneurysm neck, or with incorporation
of normal vessels into the aneurysm neck, or a procedure
requiring temporary vessel occlusion, trapping or
cardiopulmonary bypass to successfully treat the aneurysm)

61700   Surgery of simple intracranial aneurysm, intracranial approach;
carotid circulation

61702   vertebralbasilar circulation

61703   Surgery of intracranial aneurysm, cervical approach by
application of occluding clamp to cervical carotid artery
(Selverstone-Crutchfield type)

(For cervical approach for direct ligation of carotid artery, see
37600-37606)

61705   Surgery of aneurysm, vascular malformation or
carotid-cavernous fistula; by intracranial and cervical occlusion
of carotid artery

61708   by intracranial electrothrombosis

(For ligation or gradual occlusion of internal/common carotid
artery, see 37605, 37606)

61710   by intra-arterial embolization, injection procedure, or
balloon catheter

61711   Anastomosis, arterial, extracranial-intracranial (eg, middle
cerebral/cortical) arteries

(For carotid or vertebral thromboendarterectomy, use 35301)

● New
Code   ▲ Revised
Code   * Starred
Procedure   + Add-On
Code   ⊘ Modifier -51
Exempt

STEREOTAXIS

61720 Creation of lesion by stereotactic method, including burr hole(s) and localizing and recording techniques, single or multiple stages; globus pallidus or thalamus

61735 subcortical structure(s) other than globus pallidus or thalamus

61750 Stereotactic biopsy, aspiration, or excision, including burr hole(s), for intracranial lesion;

61751 with computerized axial tomography and/or magnetic resonance guidance

(For radiological supervision and interpretation of computerized tomography, see 70450, 70460, or 70470 as appropriate)

(For radiological supervision and interpretation of magnetic resonance imaging, see 70551, 70552, or 70553 as appropriate)

61760 Stereotactic implantation of depth electrodes into the cerebrum for long term seizure monitoring

61770 Stereotactic localization, including burr hole(s), with insertion of catheter(s) or probe(s) for placement of radiation source

61790 Creation of lesion by stereotactic method, percutaneous, by neurolytic agent (eg, alcohol, thermal, electrical, radiofrequency); gasserian ganglion

61791 trigeminal medullary tract

61793 Stereotactic radiosurgery (particle beam, gamma ray or linear accelerator), one or more sessions

(For intensity modulated beam delivery plan and treatment, see 77301, 77418)

+61795 Stereotactic computer assisted volumetric (navigational) procedure, intracranial, extracranial, or spinal (List separately in addition to code for primary procedure)

NEUROSTIMULATORS (INTRACRANIAL)

61850 Twist drill or burr hole(s) for implantation of neurostimulator electrodes, cortical

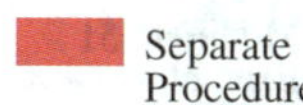
Separate Procedure

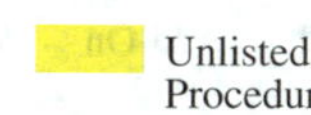
Unlisted Procedure

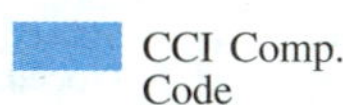
CCI Comp. Code

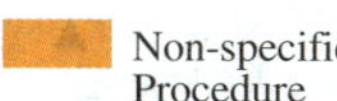
Non-specific Procedure

557

61860 Craniectomy or craniotomy for implantation of neurostimulator electrodes, cerebral, cortical

61862 Twist drill, burr hole, craniotomy, or craniectomy for stereotactic implantation of one neurostimulator array in subcortical site (eg, thalamus, globus pallidus, subthalamic nucleus, periventricular, periaqueductal gray)

61870 Craniectomy for implantation of neurostimulator electrodes, cerebellar; cortical

61875   subcortical

61880 Revision or removal of intracranial neurostimulator electrodes

61885 Incision and subcutaneous placement of cranial neurostimulator pulse generator or receiver, direct or inductive coupling; with connection to a single electrode array

61886   with connection to two or more electrode arrays

(For open placement of cranial nerve (eg, vagal, trigeminal) neurostimulator electrode(s), use 64573)

(For percutaneous placement of cranial nerve (eg, vagal, trigeminal) neurostimulator electrode(s), use 64553)

(For revision or removal of cranial nerve (eg, vagal, trigeminal) neurostimulator electrode(s), use 64585)

61888 Revision or removal of cranial neurostimulator pulse generator or receiver

REPAIR

62000 Elevation of depressed skull fracture; simple, extradural

62005   compound or comminuted, extradural

62010   with repair of dura and/or debridement of brain

▲ **62100** Craniotomy for repair of dural/cerebrospinal fluid leak, including surgery for rhinorrhea/otorrhea

(For repair of spinal dural/CSF leak, see 63707, 63709)

● New Code　　▲ Revised Code　　✱ Starred Procedure　　✚ Add-On Code　　⃠ Modifier -51 Exempt

62115   Reduction of craniomegalic skull (eg, treated hydrocephalus); not requiring bone grafts or cranioplasty

62116   with simple cranioplasty

62117   requiring craniotomy and reconstruction with or without bone graft (includes obtaining grafts)

62120   Repair of encephalocele, skull vault, including cranioplasty

62121   Craniotomy for repair of encephalocele, skull base

62140   Cranioplasty for skull defect; up to 5 cm diameter

62141   larger than 5 cm diameter

62142   Removal of bone flap or prosthetic plate of skull

62143   Replacement of bone flap or prosthetic plate of skull

62145   Cranioplasty for skull defect with reparative brain surgery

62146   Cranioplasty with autograft (includes obtaining bone grafts); up to 5 cm diameter

62147   larger than 5 cm diameter

CEREBROSPINAL FLUID (CSF) SHUNT

62180   Ventriculocisternostomy (Torkildsen type operation)

62190   Creation of shunt; subarachnoid/subdural-atrial, -jugular, -auricular

62192   subarachnoid/subdural-peritoneal, -pleural, other terminus

62194   Replacement or irrigation, subarachnoid/subdural catheter

62200   Ventriculocisternostomy, third ventricle;

62201   stereotactic method

62220   Creation of shunt; ventriculo-atrial, -jugular, -auricular

62223   ventriculo-peritoneal, -pleural, other terminus

Separate Procedure	Unlisted Procedure	CCI Comp. Code	Non-specific Procedure

559

| | 62225 | Replacement or irrigation, ventricular catheter |

▲ 62230   Replacement or revision of cerebrospinal fluid shunt, obstructed valve, or distal catheter in shunt system

▲ 62252   Reprogramming of programmable cerebrospinal shunt

▲ 62256   Removal of complete cerebrospinal fluid shunt system; without replacement

62258   with replacement by similar or other shunt at same operation

(For percutaneous irrigation or aspiration of shunt reservoir, use 61070)

(For reprogramming of programmable CSF shunt, use 62252)

SPINE AND SPINAL CORD

(For application of caliper or tongs, use 20660)

(For treatment of fracture or dislocation of spine, see 22305-22327)

INJECTION, DRAINAGE, OR ASPIRATION

62263   Percutaneous lysis of epidural adhesions using solution injection (eg, hypertonic saline, enzyme) or mechanical means (eg, spring-wound catheter) including radiologic localization (includes contrast when administered)

*62268   Percutaneous aspiration, spinal cord cyst or syrinx

(For radiological supervision and interpretation, see 76003, 76360, 76942)

*62269   Biopsy of spinal cord, percutaneous needle

(For radiological supervision and interpretation, see 76003, 76360, 76942)

*62270   Spinal puncture, lumbar, diagnostic

▲*62272   Spinal puncture, therapeutic, for drainage of cerebrospinal fluid (by needle or catheter)

*62273   Injection, epidural, of blood or clot patch

● New Code   ▲ Revised Code   * Starred Procedure   + Add-On Code   ⊘ Modifier -51 Exempt

***62280**   Injection/infusion of neurolytic substance (eg, alcohol, phenol, iced saline solutions), with or without other therapeutic substance; subarachnoid

***62281**   epidural, cervical or thoracic

***62282**   epidural, lumbar, sacral (caudal)

⊘***62284**   Injection procedure for myelography and/or computerized axial tomography, spinal (other than C1-C2 and posterior fossa)

       (For injection procedure at C1-C2, use 61055)

       (For radiological supervision and interpretation, see Radiology)

62287   Aspiration or decompression procedure, percutaneous, of nucleus pulposus of intervertebral disk, any method, single or multiple levels, lumbar (eg, manual or automated percutaneous diskectomy, percutaneous laser diskectomy)

       (For fluoroscopic guidance, use 76003)

***62290**   Injection procedure for diskography, each level; lumbar

***62291**   cervical or thoracic

       (For radiological supervision or interpretation, see 72285, 72295)

62292   Injection procedure for chemonucleolysis, including diskography, intervertebral disk, single or multiple levels, lumbar

62294   Injection procedure, arterial, for occlusion of arteriovenous malformation, spinal

62310   Injection, single (not via indwelling catheter), not including neurolytic substances, with or without contrast (for either localization or epidurography), of diagnostic or therapeutic substance(s) (including anesthetic, antispasmodic, opioid, steroid, other solution), epidural or subarachnoid; cervical or thoracic

62311   lumbar, sacral (caudal)

62318   Injection, including catheter placement, continuous infusion with intermittent bolus not including neurolytic substances, with or without contrast (for either localization or epidurography), of diagnostic or therapeutic substances (including anesthetic, antispasmodic, opioid, steroid, other solution), epidural or subarachnoid; cervical or thoracic

62319   lumbar, sacral (caudal)

(For transforaminal epidural injection, see 64479-64484)

CATHETER IMPLANTATION

(For percutaneous placement of intrathecal or epidural catheter, see codes 62270-62273, 62280-62284, 62310-62319)

62350 Implantation, revision or repositioning of tunneled intrathecal or epidural catheter, for long-term medication administration via an external pump or implantable reservoir/infusion pump; without laminectomy

62351   with laminectomy

(For refilling and maintenance of an implantable reservoir or infusion pump, use 96530)

62355 Removal of previously implanted intrathecal or epidural catheter

RESERVOIR/PUMP IMPLANTATION

62360 Implantation or replacement of device for intrathecal or epidural drug infusion; subcutaneous reservoir

62361   non-programmable pump

62362   programmable pump, including preparation of pump, with or without programming

62365 Removal of subcutaneous reservoir or pump, previously implanted for intrathecal or epidural infusion

62367 Electronic analysis of programmable, implanted pump for intrathecal or epidural drug infusion (includes evaluation of reservoir status, alarm status, drug prescription status); without reprogramming

62368   with reprogramming

(To report implantable pump or reservoir refill, use 96530)

● New Code   ▲ Revised Code   ＊ Starred Procedure   ＋ Add-On Code   ⊘ Modifier -51 Exempt

POSTERIOR EXTRADURAL LAMINOTOMY OR LAMINECTOMY FOR EXPLORATION/DECOMPRESSION OF NEURAL ELEMENTS OR EXCISION OF HERNIATED INTERVERTEBRAL DISKS

(When 63001-63048 are followed by arthrodesis, see 22590-22614)

63001 Laminectomy with exploration and/or decompression of spinal cord and/or cauda equina, without facetectomy, foraminotomy or diskectomy, (eg, spinal stenosis), one or two vertebral segments; cervical

63003 thoracic

63005 lumbar, except for spondylolisthesis

63011 sacral

63012 Laminectomy with removal of abnormal facets and/or pars inter-articularis with decompression of cauda equina and nerve roots for spondylolisthesis, lumbar (Gill type procedure)

63015 Laminectomy with exploration and/or decompression of spinal cord and/or cauda equina, without facetectomy, foraminotomy or diskectomy, (eg, spinal stenosis), more than 2 vertebral segments; cervical

63016 thoracic

63017 lumbar

63020 Laminotomy (hemilaminectomy), with decompression of nerve root(s), including partial facetectomy, foraminotomy and/or excision of herniated intervertebral disk; one interspace, cervical

63030 one interspace, lumbar (including open or endoscopically assisted approach)

+63035 each additional interspace, cervical or lumbar (List separately in addition to code for primary procedure)

(Use 63035 in conjunction with codes 63020-63030)

63040 Laminotomy (hemilaminectomy), with decompression of nerve root(s), including partial facetectomy, foraminotomy and/or excision of herniated intervertebral disk, reexploration, single interspace; cervical

---

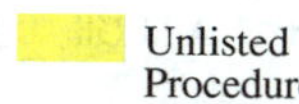 Separate Procedure

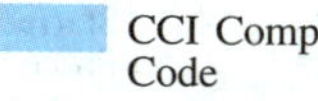 Unlisted Procedure

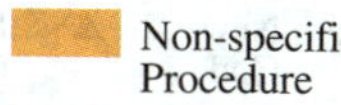 CCI Comp. Code

Non-specific Procedure

563

63042	lumbar

(Codes 63040-63044 are unilateral procedures. For bilateral procedures, use modifier -50)

+63043   each additional cervical interspace (List separately in addition to code for primary procedure)

(Use 63043 in conjunction with code 63040)

+63044   each additional lumbar interspace (List separately in addition to code for primary procedure)

Use 63044 in conjunction with code 63042)

63045   Laminectomy, facetectomy and foraminotomy (unilateral or bilateral with decompression of spinal cord, cauda equina and/or nerve root(s), (eg, spinal or lateral recess stenosis)), single vertebral segment; cervical

63046   thoracic

63047   lumbar

+63048   each additional segment, cervical, thoracic, or lumbar (List separately in addition to code for primary procedure)

(Use 63048 in conjunction with codes 63045-63047)

TRANSPEDICULAR OR COSTOVERTEBRAL APPROACH FOR POSTEROLATERAL EXTRADURAL EXPLORATION/ DECOMPRESSION

63055   Transpedicular approach with decompression of spinal cord, equina and/or nerve root(s) (eg, herniated intervertebral disk), single segment; thoracic

63056   lumbar (including transfacet, or lateral extraforaminal approach) (eg, far lateral herniated intervertebral disk)

+63057   each additional segment, thoracic or lumbar (List separately in addition to code for primary procedure)

(Use 63057 in conjunction with codes 63055, 63056)

63064   Costovertebral approach with decompression of spinal cord or nerve root(s), (eg, herniated intervertebral disk), thoracic; single segment

---

● New Code   ▲ Revised Code   ✱ Starred Procedure   + Add-On Code   ⊘ Modifier -51 Exempt

+63066   each additional segment (List separately in addition to code for primary procedure)

(Use 63066 in conjunction with code 63064)

(For excision of thoracic intraspinal lesions by laminectomy, see 63266, 63271, 63276, 63281, 63286)

ANTERIOR OR ANTEROLATERAL APPROACH FOR EXTRADURAL EXPLORATION/DECOMPRESSION

63075   Diskectomy, anterior, with decompression of spinal cord and/or nerve root(s), including osteophytectomy; cervical, single interspace

+63076   cervical, each additional interspace (List separately in addition to code for primary procedure)

(Use 63076 in conjunction with code 63075)

63077   thoracic, single interspace

+63078   thoracic, each additional interspace (List separately in addition to code for primary procedure)

(Use 63078 in conjunction with code 63077)

(Do not report code 69990 in addition to codes 63075-63078)

63081   Vertebral corpectomy (vertebral body resection), partial or complete, anterior approach with decompression of spinal cord and/or nerve root(s); cervical, single segment

+63082   cervical, each additional segment (List separately in addition to code for primary procedure)

(Use 63082 in conjunction with code 63081)

(For transoral approach, see 61575, 61576)

63085   Vertebral corpectomy (vertebral body resection), partial or complete, transthoracic approach with decompression of spinal cord and/or nerve root(s); thoracic, single segment

+63086   thoracic, each additional segment (List separately in addition to code for primary procedure)

(Use 63086 in conjunction with code 63085)

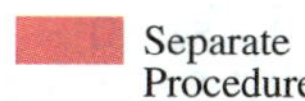 Separate Procedure

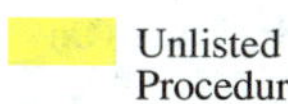 Unlisted Procedure

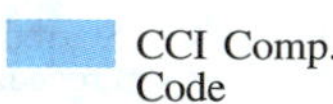 CCI Comp. Code

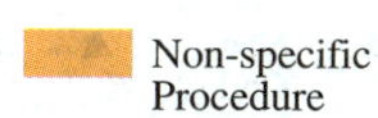 Non-specific Procedure

565

63087 Vertebral corpectomy (vertebral body resection), partial or complete, combined thoracolumbar approach with decompression of spinal cord, cauda equina or nerve root(s), lower thoracic or lumbar; single segment

+63088 each additional segment (List separately in addition to code for primary procedure)

(Use 63088 in conjunction with code 63087)

63090 Vertebral corpectomy (vertebral body resection), partial or complete, transperitoneal or retroperitoneal approach with decompression of spinal cord, cauda equina or nerve root(s), lower thoracic, lumbar, or sacral; single segment

+63091 each additional segment (List separately in addition to code for primary procedure)

(Use 63091 in conjunction with code 63090)

(Procedures 63081-63091 include diskectomy above and/or below vertebral segment)

(If followed by arthrodesis, see 22548-22812)

(For reconstruction of spine, use appropriate vertebral corpectomy codes 63081-63091, bone graft codes 20930-20938, arthrodesis codes 22548-22812, and spinal instrumentation codes 22840-22855)

INCISION

63170 Laminectomy with myelotomy (eg, Bischof or DREZ type), cervical, thoracic, or thoracolumbar

63172 Laminectomy with drainage of intramedullary cyst/syrinx; to subarachnoid space

63173 to peritoneal space

63180 Laminectomy and section of dentate ligaments, with or without dural graft, cervical; one or two segments

63182 more than two segments

63185 Laminectomy with rhizotomy; one or two segments

63190 more than two segments

● New Code   ▲ Revised Code   ✳ Starred Procedure   + Add-On Code   ⊘ Modifier -51 Exempt

63191 Laminectomy with section of spinal accessory nerve

(For resection of sternocleidomastoid muscle, use 21720)

63194 Laminectomy with cordotomy, with section of one spinothalamic tract, one stage; cervical

63195 thoracic

63196 Laminectomy with cordotomy, with section of both spinothalamic tracts, one stage; cervical

63197 thoracic

63198 Laminectomy with cordotomy with section of both spinothalamic tracts, two stages within 14 days; cervical

63199 thoracic

63200 Laminectomy, with release of tethered spinal cord, lumbar

EXCISION BY LAMINECTOMY OF LESION OTHER THAN HERNIATED DISK

63250 Laminectomy for excision or occlusion of arteriovenous malformation of spinal cord; cervical

63251 thoracic

63252 thoracolumbar

63265 Laminectomy for excision or evacuation of intraspinal lesion other than neoplasm, extradural; cervical

63266 thoracic

63267 lumbar

63268 sacral

63270 Laminectomy for excision of intraspinal lesion other than neoplasm, intradural; cervical

63271 thoracic

63272 lumbar

Separate Procedure | Unlisted Procedure | CCI Comp. Code | Non-specific Procedure

63273		sacral
63275		Laminectomy for biopsy/excision of intraspinal neoplasm; extradural, cervical
63276		extradural, thoracic
63277		extradural, lumbar
63278		extradural, sacral
63280		intradural, extramedullary, cervical
63281		intradural, extramedullary, thoracic
63282		intradural, extramedullary, lumbar
63283		intradural, sacral
63285		intradural, intramedullary, cervical
63286		intradural, intramedullary, thoracic
63287		intradural, intramedullary, thoracolumbar
63290		combined extradural-intradural lesion, any level

(For drainage of intramedullary cyst/syrinx, use 63172, 63173)

EXCISION, ANTERIOR OR ANTEROLATERAL APPROACH, INTRASPINAL LESION

(For arthrodesis, see 22548-22585)

(For reconstruction of spine, see 20930-20938)

63300		Vertebral corpectomy (vertebral body resection), partial or complete, for excision of intraspinal lesion, single segment; extradural, cervical
63301		extradural, thoracic by transthoracic approach
63302		extradural, thoracic by thoracolumbar approach
63303		extradural, lumbar or sacral by transperitoneal or retroperitoneal approach

● New Code ▲ Revised Code ✱ Starred Procedure ✛ Add-On Code ⊘ Modifier -51 Exempt

63304 intradural, cervical

63305 intradural, thoracic by transthoracic approach

63306 intradural, thoracic by thoracolumbar approach

63307 intradural, lumbar or sacral by transperitoneal or retroperitoneal approach

+63308 each additional segment (List separately in addition to codes for single segment)

(Use 63308 in conjunction with codes 63300-63307)

STEREOTAXIS

63600 Creation of lesion of spinal cord by stereotactic method, percutaneous, any modality (including stimulation and/or recording)

63610 Stereotactic stimulation of spinal cord, percutaneous, separate procedure not followed by other surgery

63615 Stereotactic biopsy, aspiration, or excision of lesion, spinal cord

NEUROSTIMULATORS (SPINAL)

63650 Percutaneous implantation of neurostimulator electrode array, epidural

63655 Laminectomy for implantation of neurostimulator electrodes, plate/paddle, epidural

63660 Revision or removal of spinal neurostimulator electrode percutaneous array(s) or plate/paddle(s)

63685 Incision and subcutaneous placement of spinal neurostimulator pulse generator or receiver, direct or inductive coupling

63688 Revision or removal of implanted spinal neurostimulator pulse generator or receiver

REPAIR

63700 Repair of meningocele; less than 5 cm diameter

63702 larger than 5 cm diameter

Separate Procedure	Unlisted Procedure	CCI Comp. Code	Non-specific Procedure

569

63704   Repair of myelomeningocele; less than 5 cm diameter

63706   larger than 5 cm diameter

(For complex skin closure, see Integumentary System)

▲ **63707**   Repair of dural/cerebrospinal fluid leak, not requiring laminectomy

▲ **63709**   Repair of dural/cerebrospinal fluid leak or pseudomeningocele, with laminectomy

63710   Dural graft, spinal

(For laminectomy and section of dentate ligaments, with or without dural graft, cervical, see 63180, 63182)

SHUNT, SPINAL CSF

63740   Creation of shunt, lumbar, subarachnoid-peritoneal, -pleural, or other; including laminectomy

63741   percutaneous, not requiring laminectomy

63744   Replacement, irrigation or revision of lumbosubarachnoid shunt

63746   Removal of entire lumbosubarachnoid shunt system without replacement

EXTRACRANIAL NERVES, PERIPHERAL NERVES, AND AUTONOMIC NERVOUS SYSTEM

(For intracranial surgery on cranial nerves, see 61450, 61460, 61790)

INTRODUCTION/INJECTION OF ANESTHETIC AGENT (NERVE BLOCK), DIAGNOSTIC OR THERAPEUTIC

Somatic Nerves

*✱**64400**   Injection, anesthetic agent; trigeminal nerve, any division or branch

✱**64402**   facial nerve

✱**64405**   greater occipital nerve

| ● New Code | ▲ Revised Code | ✱ Starred Procedure | ✛ Add-On Code | ⊘ Modifier -51 Exempt |

***64408**   vagus nerve

***64410**   phrenic nerve

***64412**   spinal accessory nerve

***64413**   cervical plexus

***64415**   brachial plexus

***64417**   axillary nerve

***64418**   suprascapular nerve

***64420**   intercostal nerve, single

***64421**   intercostal nerves, multiple, regional block

***64425**   ilioinguinal, iliohypogastric nerves

***64430**   pudendal nerve

***64435**   paracervical (uterine) nerve

***64445**   sciatic nerve

***64450**   other peripheral nerve or branch

(For phenol destruction, see 64622-64627)

(For subarachnoid or subdural injection, see 62280, 62310-62319)

(For epidural or caudal injection, see 62273, 62281-62282, 62310-62319)

(Codes 64470-64484 are unilateral procedures. For bilateral procedures, use modifier -50)

(For fluoroscopic guidance and localization for needle placement and injection in conjunction with codes 64470-64484, use code 76005)

64470   Injection, anesthetic agent and/or steroid, paravertebral facet joint or facet joint nerve; cervical or thoracic, single level

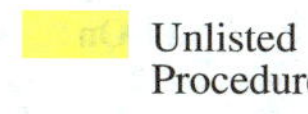

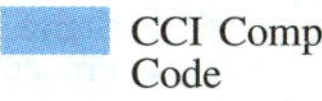

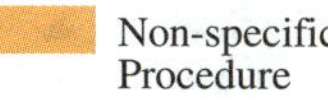

Non-specific
Procedure

+64472   cervical or thoracic, each additional level (List separately in addition to code for primary procedure)

(Use code 64472 in conjunction with code 64470)

64475   lumbar or sacral, single level

+64476   lumbar or sacral, each additional level (List separately in addition to code for primary procedure)

(Use code 64476 in conjunction with code 64475)

64479   Injection, anesthetic agent and/or steroid, transforaminal epidural; cervical or thoracic, single level

+64480   cervical or thoracic, each additional level (List separately in addition to code for primary procedure)

(Use code 64480 in conjunction with code 64479)

64483   lumbar or sacral, single level

+64484   lumbar or sacral, each additional level (List separately in addition to code for primary procedure)

(Use code 64484 in conjunction with code 64483)

Sympathetic Nerves

***64505**   Injection, anesthetic agent; sphenopalatine ganglion

***64508**   carotid sinus (separate procedure)

***64510**   stellate ganglion (cervical sympathetic)

***64520**   lumbar or thoracic (paravertebral sympathetic)

***64530**   celiac plexus, with or without radiologic monitoring

NEUROSTIMULATORS (PERIPHERAL NERVE)

64550   Application of surface (transcutaneous) neurostimulator

64553   Percutaneous implantation of neurostimulator electrodes; cranial nerve

▲ 64555   peripheral nerve (excludes sacral nerve)

| ● New Code | ▲ Revised Code | * Starred Procedure | + Add-On Code | ⊘ Modifier -51 Exempt |

| 64560 | autonomic nerve |

● **64561**   sacral nerve (transforaminal placement)

| 64565 | neuromuscular |

| 64573 | Incision for implantation of neurostimulator electrodes; cranial nerve |

(For open placement of cranial nerve (eg, vagal, trigeminal) neurostimulator pulse generator or receiver, see 61885, 61886, as appropriate)

(For revision or removal of cranial nerve (eg, vagal trigeminal) neurostimulator pulse generator or receiver, use 61888)

▲ **64575**   peripheral nerve (excludes sacral nerve)

| 64577 | autonomic nerve |

| 64580 | neuromuscular |

● **64581**   sacral nerve (transforaminal placement)

| 64585 | Revision or removal of peripheral neurostimulator electrodes |

| 64590 | Incision and subcutaneous placement of peripheral neurostimulator pulse generator or receiver, direct or inductive coupling |

| 64595 | Revision or removal of peripheral neurostimulator pulse generator or receiver |

DESTRUCTION BY NEUROLYTIC AGENT (eg, CHEMICAL, THERMAL, ELECTRICAL, RADIOFREQUENCY, OR CHEMODENERVATION)

Somatic Nerves

| 64600 | Destruction by neurolytic agent, trigeminal nerve; supraorbital, infraorbital, mental, or inferior alveolar branch |

| 64605 | second and third division branches at foramen ovale |

| 64610 | second and third division branches at foramen ovale under radiologic monitoring |

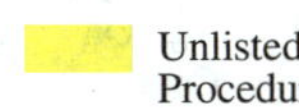

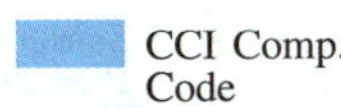

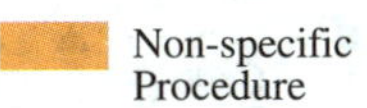

64612 Chemodenervation of muscle(s); muscles innervated by facial nerve (eg, for blepharospasm, hemifacial spasm)

64613 cervical spinal muscles (eg, for spasmodic torticollis)

64614 extremity(s) and/or trunk muscle(s) (eg, for dystonia, cerebral palsy, multiple sclerosis)

(For chemodenervation for strabismus involving the extraocular muscles, use 67345)

64620 Destruction by neurolytic agent, intercostal nerve

(Codes 64622-64627 are unilateral procedures. For bilateral procedures, use modifier -50)

(For fluoroscopic guidance and localization for needle placement and neurolysis in conjunction with codes 64622-64627, use 76005)

64622 Destruction by neurolytic agent, paravertebral facet joint nerve; lumbar or sacral, single level

+64623 lumbar or sacral, each additional level (List separately in addition to code for primary procedure)

(Use 64623 in conjunction with code 64622)

64626 cervical or thoracic, single level

+64627 cervical or thoracic, each additional level (List separately in addition to code for primary procedure)

(Use 64627 in conjunction with code 64626)

64630 Destruction by neurolytic agent; pudendal nerve

64640 other peripheral nerve or branch

Sympathetic Nerves

64680 Destruction by neurolytic agent, celiac plexus, with or without radiologic monitoring

---

● New Code   ▲ Revised Code   ✱ Starred Procedure   ✛ Add-On Code   ⊘ Modifier -51 Exempt

NEUROPLASTY (EXPLORATION, NEUROLYSIS OR NERVE DECOMPRESSION)

(For internal neurolysis requiring use of operating microscope, use 64727)

(For facial nerve decompression, use 69720)

64702 Neuroplasty; digital, one or both, same digit

64704 nerve of hand or foot

64708 Neuroplasty, major peripheral nerve, arm or leg; other than specified

64712 sciatic nerve

64713 brachial plexus

64714 lumbar plexus

64716 Neuroplasty and/or transposition; cranial nerve (specify)

64718 ulnar nerve at elbow

64719 ulnar nerve at wrist

64721 median nerve at carpal tunnel

(For arthroscopic procedure, use 29848)

64722 Decompression; unspecified nerve(s) (specify)

64726 plantar digital nerve

+64727 Internal neurolysis, requiring use of operating microscope (List separately in addition to code for neuroplasty) (Neuroplasty includes external neurolysis)

(Do not report code 69990 in addition to code 64727)

TRANSECTION OR AVULSION

(For stereotactic lesion of gasserian ganglion, use 61790)

64732 Transection or avulsion of; supraorbital nerve

64734 infraorbital nerve

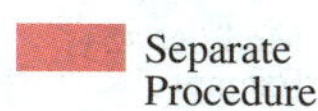

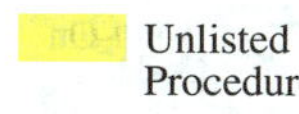

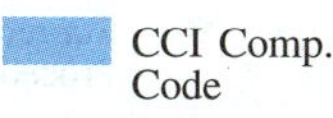

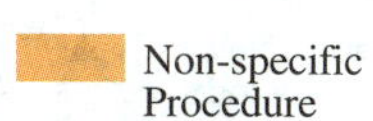

64736	mental nerve
64738	inferior alveolar nerve by osteotomy
64740	lingual nerve
64742	facial nerve, differential or complete
64744	greater occipital nerve
64746	phrenic nerve

(For section of recurrent laryngeal nerve, use 31595)

64752	vagus nerve (vagotomy), transthoracic
▲ **64755**	vagus nerves limited to proximal stomach (selective proximal vagotomy, proximal gastric vagotomy, parietal cell vagotomy, supra- or highly selective vagotomy)

(For laparoscopic approach, use 43652)

64760	vagus nerve (vagotomy), abdominal

(For laparoscopic approach, use 43651)

64761	pudendal nerve
64763	Transection or avulsion of obturator nerve, extrapelvic, with or without adductor tenotomy
64766	Transection or avulsion of obturator nerve, intrapelvic, with or without adductor tenotomy
64771	Transection or avulsion of other cranial nerve, extradural
64772	Transection or avulsion of other spinal nerve, extradural

(For excision of tender scar, skin and subcutaneous tissue, with or without tiny neuroma, see 11400-11446, 13100-13153)

EXCISION

Somatic Nerves

(For Morton neurectomy, use 28080)

64774	Excision of neuroma; cutaneous nerve, surgically identifiable

● New Code	▲ Revised Code	✱ Starred Procedure	✚ Add-On Code	⊘ Modifier -51 Exempt

64776   digital nerve, one or both, same digit

+64778   digital nerve, each additional digit (List separately in addition to code for primary procedure)

(Use 64778 in conjunction with code 64776)

64782   hand or foot, except digital nerve

+64783   hand or foot, each additional nerve, except same digit (List separately in addition to code for primary procedure)

(Use 64783 in conjunction with code 64782)

64784   major peripheral nerve, except sciatic

64786   sciatic nerve

+64787 Implantation of nerve end into bone or muscle (List separately in addition to neuroma excision)

(Use 64787 in conjunction with codes 64774-64786)

64788 Excision of neurofibroma or neurolemmoma; cutaneous nerve

64790   major peripheral nerve

64792   extensive (including malignant type)

64795 Biopsy of nerve

Sympathetic Nerves

64802 Sympathectomy, cervical

64804 Sympathectomy, cervicothoracic

64809 Sympathectomy, thoracolumbar

64818 Sympathectomy, lumbar

▲ **64820** Sympathectomy; digital arteries, each digit

(Do not report 69990 in addition to code 64820)

● **64821**   radial artery

Separate Procedure	Unlisted Procedure	CCI Comp. Code	Non-specific Procedure

(Do not report 69990 in addition to code 64821)

● **64822**   ulnar artery

(Do not report 69990 in addition to code 64822)

● **64823**   superficial palmar arch

(Do not report 69990 in addition to code 64823)

NEURORRPHAPHY

64831   Suture of digital nerve, hand or foot; one nerve

+64832   each additional digital nerve (List separately in addition to code for primary procedure)

(Use 64832 in conjunction with code 64831)

64834   Suture of one nerve, hand or foot; common sensory nerve

64835   median motor thenar

64836   ulnar motor

+64837   Suture of each additional nerve, hand or foot (List separately in addition to code for primary procedure)

(Use 64837 in conjunction with codes 64834-64836)

64840   Suture of posterior tibial nerve

64856   Suture of major peripheral nerve, arm or leg, except sciatic; including transposition

64857   without transposition

64858   Suture of sciatic nerve

+64859   Suture of each additional major peripheral nerve (List separately in addition to code for primary procedure)

(Use 64859 in conjunction with codes 64856, 64857)

64861   Suture of; brachial plexus

64862   lumbar plexus

● New Code   ▲ Revised Code   ✳ Starred Procedure   ✛ Add-On Code   ⊘ Modifier -51 Exempt

64864 Suture of facial nerve; extracranial

64865 infratemporal, with or without grafting

64866 Anastomosis; facial-spinal accessory

64868 facial-hypoglossal

64870 facial-phrenic

+64872 Suture of nerve; requiring secondary or delayed suture (List separately in addition to code for primary neurorrhaphy)

(Use 64872 in conjunction with codes 64831-64865)

+64874 requiring extensive mobilization, or transposition of nerve (List separately in addition to code for nerve suture)

(Use 64874 in conjunction with codes 64831-64865)

+64876 requiring shortening of bone of extremity (List separately in addition to code for nerve suture)

(Use 64876 in conjunction with codes 64831-64865)

NEURORRHAPHY WITH NERVE GRAFT

64885 Nerve graft (includes obtaining graft), head or neck; up to 4 cm in length

64886 more than 4 cm length

64890 Nerve graft (includes obtaining graft), single strand, hand or foot; up to 4 cm length

64891 more than 4 cm length

64892 Nerve graft (includes obtaining graft), single strand, arm or leg; up to 4 cm length

64893 more than 4 cm length

64895 Nerve graft (includes obtaining graft), multiple strands (cable), hand or foot; up to 4 cm length

64896 more than 4 cm length

Separate Procedure	Unlisted Procedure	CCI Comp. Code	Non-specific Procedure

579

64897   Nerve graft (includes obtaining graft), multiple strands (cable), arm or leg; up to 4 cm length

64898   more than 4 cm length

+64901   Nerve graft, each additional nerve; single strand (List separately in addition to code for primary procedure)

(Use 64901 in conjunction with codes 64885-64893)

+64902   multiple strands (cable) (List separately in addition to code for primary procedure)

(Use 64902 in conjunction with codes 64885, 64886, 64895-64898)

64905   Nerve pedicle transfer; first stage

64907   second stage

OTHER PROCEDURES

64999   Unlisted procedure, nervous system

● New Code   ▲ Revised Code   ✳ Starred Procedure   ✛ Add-On Code   ⃠ Modifier -51 Exempt

EYE AND OCULAR ADNEXA

CPT codes from this section of the CPT coding system are used to report surgical procedures on the eye and ocular adnexa. Diagnostic services and medical treatment of the eye are defined in the Medicine Section of the CPT manual.

If surgical procedures are performed only on the eyelid, code from the Integumentary System subsection of the CPT coding system. Cataract codes are selected on the type of procedure performed. Whenever injections are performed during cataract surgery, do not report them separately.

> (For diagnostic and treatment ophthalmological services, see Medicine, Ophthalmology, and 92002 et seq)

> (Do not report code 69990 in addition to codes 65091-68850)

EYEBALL

REMOVAL OF EYE

65091 Evisceration of ocular contents; without implant

65093 with implant

65101 Enucleation of eye; without implant

65103 with implant, muscles not attached to implant

65105 with implant, muscles attached to implant

> (For conjunctivoplasty after enucleation, see 68320 et seq)

65110 Exenteration of orbit (does not include skin graft), removal of orbital contents; only

65112 with therapeutic removal of bone

65114 with muscle or myocutaneous flap

> (For skin graft to orbit (split skin), see 15120, 15121; free, full thickness, see 15260, 15261)

> (For eyelid repair involving more than skin, see 67930 et seq)

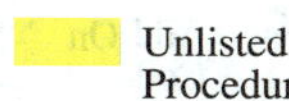 Separate Procedure

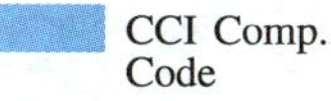 Unlisted Procedure

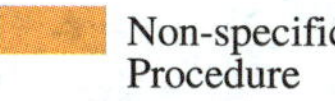 CCI Comp. Code

Non-specific Procedure

SECONDARY IMPLANT(S) PROCEDURES

65125 Modification of ocular implant with placement or replacement of pegs (eg, drilling receptacle for prosthesis appendage) (separate procedure)

65130 Insertion of ocular implant secondary; after evisceration, in scleral shell

65135 after enucleation, muscles not attached to implant

65140 after enucleation, muscles attached to implant

65150 Reinsertion of ocular implant; with or without conjunctival graft

65155 with use of foreign material for reinforcement and/or attachment of muscles to implant

65175 Removal of ocular implant

(For orbital implant (implant outside muscle cone) insertion, use 67550; removal, use 67560)

REMOVAL OF FOREIGN BODY

(For removal of implanted material: ocular implant, use 65175; anterior segment implant, use 65920; posterior segment implant, use 67120; orbital implant, use 67560)

(For diagnostic x-ray for foreign body, use 70030)

(For diagnostic echography for foreign body, use 76529)

(For removal of foreign body from orbit: frontal approach, use 67413; lateral approach, use 67430; transcranial approach, use 61334)

(For removal of foreign body from eyelid, embedded, use 67938)

(For removal of foreign body from lacrimal system, use 68530)

***65205** Removal of foreign body, external eye; conjunctival superficial

***65210** conjunctival embedded (includes concretions), subconjunctival, or scleral nonperforating

***65220** corneal, without slit lamp

● New Code	▲ Revised Code	* Starred Procedure	+ Add-On Code	⃠ Modifier -51 Exempt

***65222**   corneal, with slit lamp

(For repair of corneal laceration with foreign body, use 65275)

▲ **65235**   Removal of foreign body, intraocular; from anterior chamber of eye or lens

(For removal of implanted material from anterior segment, use 65920)

65260   from posterior segment, magnetic extraction, anterior or posterior route

65265   from posterior segment, nonmagnetic extraction

(For removal of implanted material from posterior segment, use 67120)

REPAIR OF LACERATION

(For fracture of orbit, see 21385 et seq)

(For repair of wound of eyelid, skin, linear, simple, see 12011-12018; intermediate, layered closure, see 12051-12057; linear, complex, see 13150-13160; other, see 67930, 67935)

(For repair of wound of lacrimal system, use 68700)

(For repair of operative wound, use 66250)

***65270**   Repair of laceration; conjunctiva, with or without nonperforating laceration sclera, direct closure

65272   conjunctiva, by mobilization and rearrangement, without hospitalization

65273   conjunctiva, by mobilization and rearrangement, with hospitalization

65275   cornea, nonperforating, with or without removal foreign body

65280   cornea and/or sclera, perforating, not involving uveal tissue

65285   cornea and/or sclera, perforating, with reposition or resection of uveal tissue

65286   application of tissue glue, wounds of cornea and/or sclera

 Separate Procedure

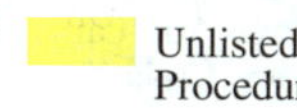 Unlisted Procedure

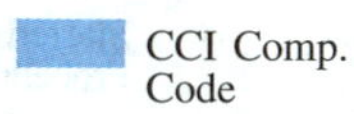 CCI Comp. Code

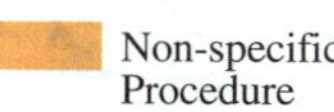 Non-specific Procedure

583

(Repair of laceration includes use of conjunctival flap and restoration of anterior chamber, by air or saline injection when indicated)

(For repair of iris or ciliary body, use 66680)

65290 Repair of wound, extraocular muscle, tendon and/or Tenon's capsule

ANTERIOR SEGMENT

CORNEA

Excision

65400 Excision of lesion, cornea (keratectomy, lamellar, partial), except pterygium

***65410** Biopsy of cornea

65420 Excision or transposition of pterygium; without graft

65426 with graft

Removal or Destruction

***65430** Scraping of cornea, diagnostic, for smear and/or culture

***65435** Removal of corneal epithelium; with or without chemocauterization (abrasion, curettage)

65436 with application of chelating agent (eg, EDTA)

65450 Destruction of lesion of cornea by cryotherapy, photocoagulation or thermocauterization

65600 Multiple punctures of anterior cornea (eg, for corneal erosion, tattoo)

Keratoplasty

(Keratoplasty excludes refractive keratoplasty procedures, 65760, 65765, and 65767)

65710 Keratoplasty (corneal transplant); lamellar

65730 penetrating (except in aphakia)

● New Code   ▲ Revised Code   * Starred Procedure   + Add-On Code   ⊘ Modifier -51 Exempt

65750   penetrating (in aphakia)

65755   penetrating (in pseudophakia)

Other Procedures

65760   Keratomileusis

65765   Keratophakia

65767   Epikeratoplasty

65770   Keratoprosthesis

65771   Radial keratotomy

65772   Corneal relaxing incision for correction of surgically induced astigmatism

65775   Corneal wedge resection for correction of surgically induced astigmatism

(For fitting of contact lens for treatment of disease, use 92070)

(For unlisted procedures on cornea, use 66999)

ANTERIOR CHAMBER

Incision

***65800**   Paracentesis of anterior chamber of eye (separate procedure); with diagnostic aspiration of aqueous

***65805**   with therapeutic release of aqueous

65810   with removal of vitreous and/or discission of anterior hyaloid membrane, with or without air injection

65815   with removal of blood, with or without irrigation and/or air injection

(For injection, see 66020-66030)

(For removal of blood clot, use 65930)

65820   Goniotomy

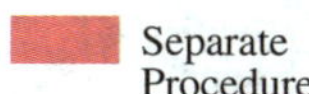

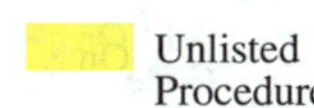

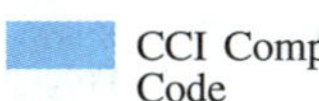

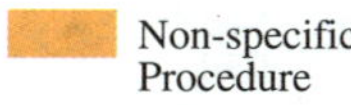

65850　Trabeculotomy ab externo

65855　Trabeculoplasty by laser surgery, one or more sessions (defined treatment series)

(If re-treatment is necessary after several months because of disease progression, a new treatment or treatment series should be reported with a modifier, if necessary, to indicate lesser or greater complexity)

(For trabeculectomy, use 66170)

65860　Severing adhesions of anterior segment, laser technique (separate procedure)

Other Procedures

65865　Severing adhesions of anterior segment of eye, incisional technique (with or without injection of air or liquid) (separate procedure); goniosynechiae

(For trabeculoplasty by laser surgery, use 65855)

65870　　anterior synechiae, except goniosynechiae

65875　　posterior synechiae

65880　　corneovitreal adhesions

(For laser surgery, use 66821)

▲ **65900**　Removal of epithelial downgrowth, anterior chamber of eye

▲ **65920**　Removal of implanted material, anterior segment of eye

▲ **65930**　Removal of blood clot, anterior segment of eye

▲ **66020**　Injection, anterior chamber of eye (separate procedure); air or liquid

***66030**　　medication

(For unlisted procedures on anterior segment, use 66999)

ANTERIOR SCLERA

Excision

(For removal of intraocular foreign body, use 65235)

(For operations on posterior sclera, use 67250, 67255)

66130 Excision of lesion, sclera

66150 Fistulization of sclera for glaucoma; trephination with iridectomy

66155 thermocauterization with iridectomy

66160 sclerectomy with punch or scissors, with iridectomy

66165 iridencleisis or iridotasis

66170 trabeculectomy ab externo in absence of previous surgery

(For trabeculotomy ab externo, use 65850)

(For repair of operative wound, use 66250)

66172 trabeculectomy ab externo with scarring from previous ocular surgery or trauma (includes injection of antifibrotic agents)

66180 Aqueous shunt to extraocular reservoir (eg, Molteno, Schocket, Denver-Krupin)

66185 Revision of aqueous shunt to extraocular reservoir

(For removal of implanted shunt, use 67120)

Repair or Revision

(For scleral procedures in retinal surgery, see 67101 et seq)

66220 Repair of scleral staphyloma; without graft

66225 with graft

(For scleral reinforcement, see 67250, 67255)

66250 Revision or repair of operative wound of anterior segment, any type, early or late, major or minor procedure

(For unlisted procedures on anterior sclera, use 66999)

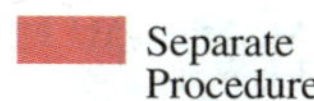

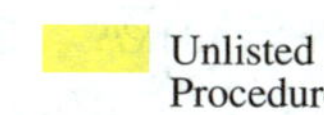

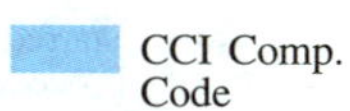

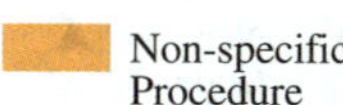

IRIS, CILIARY BODY

Incision

66500   Iridotomy by stab incision (separate procedure); except transfixion

66505   with transfixion as for iris bombe

(For iridotomy by photocoagulation, use 66761)

Excision

66600   Iridectomy, with corneoscleral or corneal section; for removal of lesion

66605   with cyclectomy

66625   peripheral for glaucoma (separate procedure)

66630   sector for glaucoma (separate procedure)

66635   optical (separate procedure)

(For coreoplasty by photocoagulation, use 66762)

Repair

66680   Repair of iris, ciliary body (as for iridodialysis)

(For reposition or resection of uveal tissue with perforating wound of cornea or sclera, use 65285)

66682   Suture of iris, ciliary body (separate procedure) with retrieval of suture through small incision (eg, McCannel suture)

Destruction

66700   Ciliary body destruction; diathermy

66710   cyclophotocoagulation

66720   cryotherapy

66740   cyclodialysis

---

588   ● New Code   ▲ Revised Code   ∗ Starred Procedure   ＋ Add-On Code   ⊘ Modifier -51 Exempt

66761   Iridotomy/iridectomy by laser surgery (eg, for glaucoma) (one or more sessions)

66762   Iridoplasty by photocoagulation (one or more sessions) (eg, for improvement of vision, for widening of anterior chamber angle)

66770   Destruction of cyst or lesion iris or ciliary body (nonexcisional procedure)

     (For excision lesion iris, ciliary body, see 66600, 66605; for removal of epithelial downgrowth, use 65900)

     (For unlisted procedures on iris, ciliary body, use 66999)

LENS

Incision

66820   Discission of secondary membranous cataract (opacified posterior lens capsule and/or anterior hyaloid); stab incision technique (Ziegler or Wheeler knife)

66821   laser surgery (eg, YAG laser) (one or more stages)

66825   Repositioning of intraocular lens prosthesis, requiring an incision (separate procedure)

Removal Cataract

66830   Removal of secondary membranous cataract (opacified posterior lens capsule and/or anterior hyaloid) with corneo-scleral section, with or without iridectomy (iridocapsulotomy, iridocapsulectomy)

66840   Removal of lens material; aspiration technique, one or more stages

66850   phacofragmentation technique (mechanical or ultrasonic) (eg, phacoemulsification), with aspiration

66852   pars plana approach, with or without vitrectomy

66920   intracapsular

66930   intracapsular, for dislocated lens

66940   extracapsular (other than 66840, 66850, 66852)

589

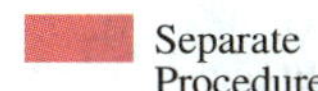 Separate Procedure
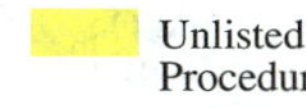 Unlisted Procedure
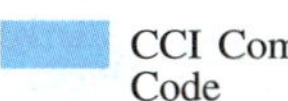 CCI Comp. Code
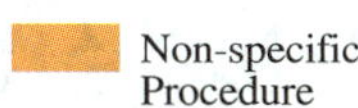 Non-specific Procedure

(For removal of intralenticular foreign body without lens extraction, use 65235)

(For repair of operative wound, use 66250)

▲ **66982** Extracapsular cataract removal with insertion of intraocular lens prosthesis (one stage procedure), manual or mechanical technique (eg, irrigation and aspiration or phacoemulsification), complex, requiring devices or techniques not generally used in routine cataract surgery (eg, iris expansion device, suture support for intraocular lens, or primary posterior capsulorrhexis) or performed on patients in the amblyogenic developmental stage

66983 Intracapsular cataract extraction with insertion of intraocular lens prosthesis (one stage procedure)

66984 Extracapsular cataract removal with insertion of intraocular lens prosthesis (one stage procedure), manual or mechanical technique (eg, irrigation and aspiration or phacoemulsification)

(For complex extracapsular cataract removal, use 66982)

66985 Insertion of intraocular lens prosthesis (secondary implant), not associated with concurrent cataract removal

(To code implant at time of concurrent cataract surgery, see 66982, 66983, 66984)

(For intraocular lens prosthesis supplied by physician, use 99070)

(For ultrasonic determination of intraocular lens power, use 76519)

(For removal of implanted material from anterior segment, use 65920)

(For secondary fixation (separate procedure), use 66682)

66986 Exchange of intraocular lens

OTHER PROCEDURES

66999 Unlisted procedure, anterior segment of eye

● New Code   ▲ Revised Code   ✳ Starred Procedure   ✚ Add-On Code   ⊘ Modifier -51 Exempt

POSTERIOR SEGMENT

VITREOUS

67005 Removal of vitreous, anterior approach (open sky technique or limbal incision); partial removal

67010 subtotal removal with mechanical vitrectomy

(For removal of vitreous by paracentesis of anterior chamber, use 65810)

(For removal of corneovitreal adhesions, use 65880)

67015 Aspiration or release of vitreous, subretinal or choroidal fluid, pars plana approach (posterior sclerotomy)

67025 Injection of vitreous substitute, pars plana or limbal approach, (fluid-gas exchange), with or without aspiration (separate procedure)

67027 Implantation of intravitreal drug delivery system (eg, ganciclovir implant), includes concomitant removal of vitreous

(For removal, use 67121)

67028 Intravitreal injection of a pharmacologic agent (separate procedure)

67030 Discission of vitreous strands (without removal), pars plana approach

67031 Severing of vitreous strands, vitreous face adhesions, sheets, membranes or opacities, laser surgery (one or more stages)

67036 Vitrectomy, mechanical, pars plana approach;

67038 with epiretinal membrane stripping

67039 with focal endolaser photocoagulation

67040 with endolaser panretinal photocoagulation

(For associated lensectomy, use 66850)

(For use of vitrectomy in retinal detachment surgery, use 67108)

(For associated removal of foreign body, see 65260, 65265)

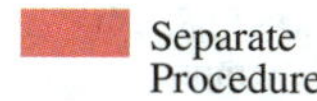

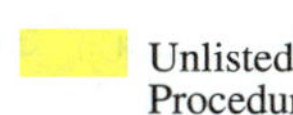

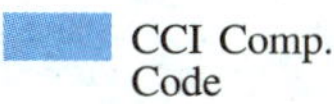

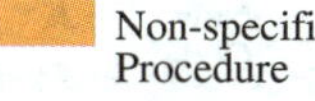

(For unlisted procedures on vitreous, use 67299)

RETINA OR CHOROID

Repair

(If diathermy, cryotherapy and/or photocoagulation are combined, report under principal modality used)

67101   Repair of retinal detachment, one or more sessions; cryotherapy or diathermy, with or without drainage of subretinal fluid

67105   photocoagulation, with or without drainage of subretinal fluid

67107   Repair of retinal detachment; scleral buckling (such as lamellar scleral dissection, imbrication or encircling procedure), with or without implant, with or without cryotherapy, photocoagulation, and drainage of subretinal fluid

67108   with vitrectomy, any method, with or without air or gas tamponade, focal endolaser photocoagulation, cryotherapy, drainage of subretinal fluid, scleral buckling, and/or removal of lens by same technique

67110   by injection of air or other gas (eg, pneumatic retinopexy)

67112   by scleral buckling or vitrectomy, on patient having previous ipsilateral retinal detachment repair(s) using scleral buckling or vitrectomy techniques

(For aspiration of drainage of subretinal or subchoroidal fluid, use 67015)

67115   Release of encircling material (posterior segment)

67120   Removal of implanted material, posterior segment; extraocular

67121   intraocular

(For removal from anterior segment, use 65920)

(For removal of foreign body, see 65260, 65265)

Prophylaxis

67141   Prophylaxis of retinal detachment (eg, retinal break, lattice degeneration) without drainage, one or more sessions; cryotherapy, diathermy

● New Code   ▲ Revised Code   ✱ Starred Procedure   ✛ Add-On Code   ⊘ Modifier -51 Exempt

67145   photocoagulation (laser or xenon arc)

Destruction

67208 Destruction of localized lesion of retina (eg, macular edema, tumors), one or more sessions; cryotherapy, diathermy

67210   photocoagulation

67218   radiation by implantation of source (includes removal of source)

67220 Destruction of localized lesion of choroid (eg, choroidal neovascularization); photocoagulation (eg, laser), one or more sessions

(For destruction of macular drusen, photocoagulation, use Category III code 0017T)

(For destruction of localized lesion of choroid by transpupillary thermotherapy, use Category III code 0016T)

67221   photodynamic therapy (includes intravenous infusion)

●+**67225**   photodynamic therapy, second eye, at single session (List separately in addition to code for primary eye treatment)

(Use 67225 in conjunction with code 67221)

67227 Destruction of extensive or progressive retinopathy (eg, diabetic retinopathy), one or more sessions; cryotherapy, diathermy

67228   photocoagulation (laser or xenon arc)

(For unlisted procedures on retina, use 67299)

SCLERA

Repair Sclera

(For excision lesion sclera, use 66130)

67250 Scleral reinforcement (separate procedure); without graft

67255   with graft

(For repair scleral staphyloma, see 66220, 66225)

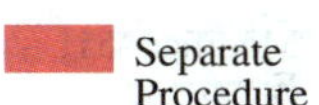
Separate Procedure

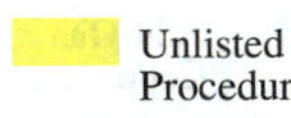
Unlisted Procedure

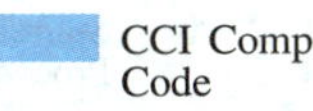
CCI Comp. Code

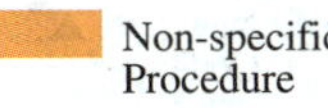
Non-specific Procedure

OTHER PROCEDURES

67299   Unlisted procedure, posterior segment

OCULAR ADNEXA

EXTRAOCULAR MUSCLES

67311   Strabismus surgery, recession or resection procedure; one horizontal muscle

67312   two horizontal muscles

67314   one vertical muscle (excluding superior oblique)

67316   two or more vertical muscles (excluding superior oblique)

(For adjustable sutures, use 67335 in addition to codes 67311-67334 for primary procedure reflecting number of muscles operated on)

67318   Strabismus surgery, any procedure, superior oblique muscle

+67320   Transposition procedure (eg, for paretic extraocular muscle), any extraocular muscle (specify) (List separately in addition to code for primary procedure)

(Use 67320 in conjunction with codes 67311-67318)

+67331   Strabismus surgery on patient with previous eye surgery or injury that did not involve the extraocular muscles (List separately in addition to code for primary procedure)

(Use 67331 in conjunction with codes 67311-67318)

+67332   Strabismus surgery on patient with scarring of extraocular muscles (eg, prior ocular injury, strabismus or retinal detachment surgery) or restrictive myopathy (eg, dysthyroid ophthalmopathy) (List separately in addition to code for primary procedure)

(Use 67332 in conjunction with codes 67311-67318)

+67334   Strabismus surgery by posterior fixation suture technique, with or without muscle recession (List separately in addition to code for primary procedure)

● New Code   ▲ Revised Code   ✳ Starred Procedure   ✚ Add-On Code   ⊘ Modifier -51 Exempt

(Use 67334 in conjunction with codes 67311-67318)

+67335 Placement of adjustable suture(s) during strabismus surgery, including postoperative adjustment(s) of suture(s) (List separately in addition to code for specific strabismus surgery)

(Use 67335 in conjunction with codes 67311-67334)

+67340 Strabismus surgery involving exploration and/or repair of detached extraocular muscle(s) (List separately in addition to code for primary procedure)

(Use 67340 in conjunction with codes 67311-67334)

67343 Release of extensive scar tissue without detaching extraocular muscle (separate procedure)

(Use 67343 in conjunction with codes 67311-67340 when such procedures are performed other than on the affected muscle)

67345 Chemodenervation of extraocular muscle

(For chemodenervation for blepharospasm and other neurological disorders, see 64612 and 64613)

Other Procedures

67350 Biopsy of extraocular muscle

(For repair of wound, extraocular muscle, tendon or Tenon's capsule, use 65290)

67399 Unlisted procedure, ocular muscle

ORBIT

Exploration, Excision, Decompression

67400 Orbitotomy without bone flap (frontal or transconjunctival approach); for exploration, with or without biopsy

67405   with drainage only

67412   with removal of lesion

67413   with removal of foreign body

67414   with removal of bone for decompression

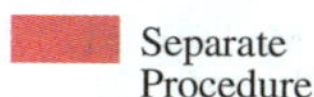

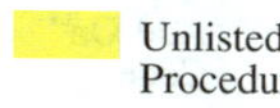

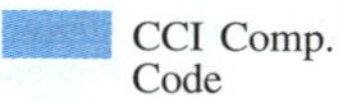

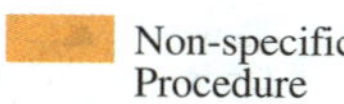

67415   Fine needle aspiration of orbital contents

(For exenteration, enucleation, and repair, see 65101 et seq; for optic nerve decompression, use 67570)

67420   Orbitotomy with bone flap or window, lateral approach (eg, Kroenlein); with removal of lesion

67430   with removal of foreign body

67440   with drainage

67445   with removal of bone for decompression

(For optic nerve sheath decompression, use 67570)

67450   for exploration, with or without biopsy

(For orbitotomy, transcranial approach, see 61330-61334)

(For orbital implant, see 67550, 67560)

(For removal of eyeball or for repair after removal, see 65091-65175)

Other Procedures

***67500**   Retrobulbar injection; medication (separate procedure, does not include supply of medication)

67505   alcohol

▲***67515**   Injection of medication or other substance into Tenon's capsule

(For subconjunctival injection, use 68200)

67550   Orbital implant (implant outside muscle cone); insertion

67560   removal or revision

(For ocular implant (implant inside muscle cone), see 65093-65105, 65130-65175)

(For treatment of fractures of malar area, orbit, see 21355 et seq)

67570   Optic nerve decompression (eg, incision or fenestration of optic nerve sheath)

● New Code   ▲ Revised Code   * Starred Procedure   + Add-On Code   ⊘ Modifier -51 Exempt

67599   Unlisted procedure, orbit

EYELIDS

Incision

***67700**   Blepharotomy, drainage of abscess, eyelid

***67710**   Severing of tarsorrhaphy

***67715**   Canthotomy (separate procedure)

(For canthoplasty, use 67950)

(For division of symblepharon, use 68340)

Excision

(For removal of lesion, involving mainly skin of eyelid, see 11310-11313; 11440-11446, 11640-11646; 17000-17004)

(For repair of wounds, blepharoplasty, grafts, reconstructive surgery, see 67930-67975)

67800   Excision of chalazion; single

67801   multiple, same lid

67805   multiple, different lids

67808   under general anesthesia and/or requiring hospitalization, single or multiple

***67810**   Biopsy of eyelid

***67820**   Correction of trichiasis; epilation, by forceps only

***67825**   epilation by other than forceps (eg, by electrosurgery, cryotherapy, laser surgery)

67830   incision of lid margin

67835   incision of lid margin, with free mucous membrane graft

***67840**   Excision of lesion of eyelid (except chalazion) without closure or with simple direct closure

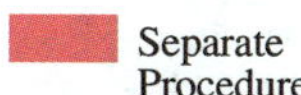
Separate Procedure

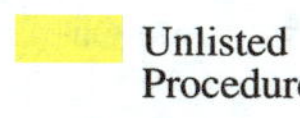
Unlisted Procedure

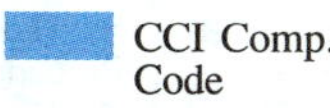
CCI Comp. Code

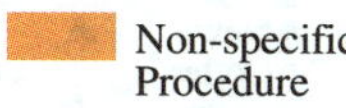
Non-specific Procedure

(For excision and repair of eyelid by reconstructive surgery, see 67961, 67966)

***67850** Destruction of lesion of lid margin (up to 1 cm)

(For Mohs micrographic surgery, see 17304-17310)

(For initiation or follow-up care of topical chemotherapy (eg, 5-FU or similar agents), see appropriate office visits)

Tarsorrhaphy

67875 Temporary closure of eyelids by suture (eg, Frost suture)

67880 Construction of intermarginal adhesions, median tarsorrhaphy, or canthorrhaphy;

67882 with transposition of tarsal plate

(For severing of tarsorrhaphy, use 67710)

(For canthoplasty, reconstruction canthus, use 67950)

(For canthotomy, use 67715)

Repair (Brow Ptosis, Blepharoptosis, Lid Retraction, Ectropion, Entropion)

67900 Repair of brow ptosis (supraciliary, mid-forehead or coronal approach)

(For forehead rhytidectomy, use 15824)

67901 Repair of blepharoptosis; frontalis muscle technique with suture or other material

67902 frontalis muscle technique with fascial sling (includes obtaining fascia)

67903 (tarso)levator resection or advancement, internal approach

67904 (tarso)levator resection or advancement, external approach

67906 superior rectus technique with fascial sling (includes obtaining fascia)

67908 conjunctivo-tarso-Muller's muscle-levator resection (eg, Fasanella-Servat type)

● New Code   ▲ Revised Code   * Starred Procedure   + Add-On Code   ⊘ Modifier -51 Exempt

67909 Reduction of overcorrection of ptosis

67911 Correction of lid retraction

(For obtaining autogenous graft materials, see 20920, 20922, or 20926)

(For correction of trichiasis by mucous membrane graft, use 67835)

67914 Repair of ectropion; suture

67915 thermocauterization

67916 blepharoplasty, excision tarsal wedge

67917 blepharoplasty, extensive (eg, Kuhnt-Szymanowski or tarsal strip operations)

(For correction of everted punctum, use 68705)

67921 Repair of entropion; suture

67922 thermocauterization

67923 blepharoplasty, excision tarsal wedge

67924 blepharoplasty, extensive (eg, Wheeler operation)

(For repair of cicatricial ectropion or entropion requiring scar excision or skin graft, see also 67961 et seq)

Reconstruction

67930 Suture of recent wound, eyelid, involving lid margin, tarsus, and/or palpebral conjunctiva direct closure; partial thickness

67935 full thickness

67938 Removal of embedded foreign body, eyelid

(For repair of skin of eyelid, see 12011-12018; 12051-12057; 13150-13153)

(For tarsorrhaphy, canthorrhaphy, see 67880, 67882)

(For repair of blepharoptosis and lid retraction, see 67901, 67911)

 Separate Procedure

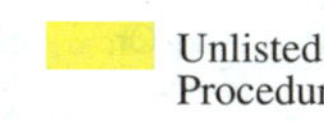 Unlisted Procedure

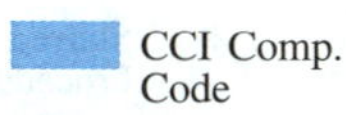 CCI Comp. Code

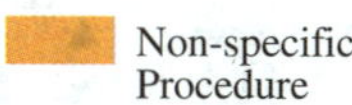 Non-specific Procedure

599

(For blepharoplasty for entropion, ectropion, see 67916, 67917, 67923, 67924)

(For correction of blepharochalasis (blepharorhytidectomy), see 15820-15823)

(For repair of skin of eyelid, adjacent tissue transfer, see 14060, 14061; preparation for graft, use 15000; free graft, see 15120, 15121, 15260, 15261)

(For excision of lesion of eyelid, use 67800 et seq)

(For repair of lacrimal canaliculi, use 68700)

67950 Canthoplasty (reconstruction of canthus)

67961 Excision and repair of eyelid, involving lid margin, tarsus, conjunctiva, canthus, or full thickness, may include preparation for skin graft or pedicle flap with adjacent tissue transfer or rearrangement; up to one-fourth of lid margin

67966 over one-fourth of lid margin

(For canthoplasty, use 67950)

(For free skin grafts, see 15120, 15121, 15260, 15261)

(For tubed pedicle flap preparation, use 15576; for delay, use 15630; for attachment, use 15650)

67971 Reconstruction of eyelid, full thickness by transfer of tarsoconjunctival flap from opposing eyelid; up to two-thirds of eyelid, one stage or first stage

67973 total eyelid, lower, one stage or first stage

67974 total eyelid, upper, one stage or first stage

67975 second stage

Other Procedures

67999 Unlisted procedure, eyelids

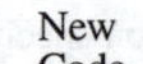

● New Code   ▲ Revised Code   ✽ Starred Procedure   ✚ Add-On Code   ⃠ Modifier -51 Exempt

CONJUNCTIVA

(For removal of foreign body, see 65205 et seq)

INCISION AND DRAINAGE

68020 Incision of conjunctiva, drainage of cyst

68040 Expression of conjunctival follicles (eg, for trachoma)

EXCISION AND/OR DESTRUCTION

68100 Biopsy of conjunctiva

68110 Excision of lesion, conjunctiva; up to 1 cm

68115 over 1 cm

68130 with adjacent sclera

***68135** Destruction of lesion, conjunctiva

INJECTION

(For injection into Tenon's capsule or retrobulbar injection, see 67500-67515)

***68200** Subconjunctival injection

CONJUNCTIVOPLASTY

(For wound repair, see 65270-65273)

68320 Conjunctivoplasty; with conjunctival graft or extensive rearrangement

68325 with buccal mucous membrane graft (includes obtaining graft)

68326 Conjunctivoplasty, reconstruction cul-de-sac; with conjunctival graft or extensive rearrangement

68328 with buccal mucous membrane graft (includes obtaining graft)

68330 Repair of symblepharon; conjunctivoplasty, without graft

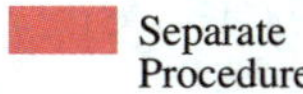
Separate Procedure

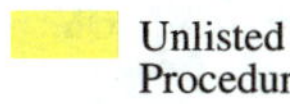
Unlisted Procedure

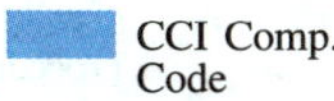
CCI Comp. Code

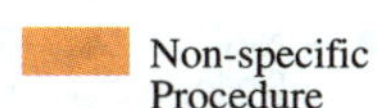
Non-specific Procedure

68335	with free graft conjunctiva or buccal mucous membrane (includes obtaining graft)
68340	division of symblepharon, with or without insertion of conformer or contact lens

OTHER PROCEDURES

68360	Conjunctival flap; bridge or partial (separate procedure)
68362	total (such as Gunderson thin flap or purse string flap)

(For conjunctival flap for perforating injury, see 65280, 65285)

(For repair of operative wound, use 66250)

(For removal of conjunctival foreign body, see 65205, 65210)

68399	Unlisted procedure, conjunctiva

LACRIMAL SYSTEM

Incision

68400	Incision, drainage of lacrimal gland
68420	Incision, drainage of lacrimal sac (dacryocystotomy or dacryocystostomy)
***68440**	Snip incision of lacrimal punctum

Excision

68500	Excision of lacrimal gland (dacryoadenectomy), except for tumor; total
68505	partial
68510	Biopsy of lacrimal gland
68520	Excision of lacrimal sac (dacryocystectomy)
68525	Biopsy of lacrimal sac
68530	Removal of foreign body or dacryolith, lacrimal passages
68540	Excision of lacrimal gland tumor; frontal approach

● New Code　　▲ Revised Code　　* Starred Procedure　　+ Add-On Code　　⊘ Modifier -51 Exempt

| **68550** | involving osteotomy |

Repair

| **68700** | Plastic repair of canaliculi |

| **68705** | Correction of everted punctum, cautery |

| **68720** | Dacryocystorhinostomy (fistulization of lacrimal sac to nasal cavity) |

| **68745** | Conjunctivorhinostomy (fistulization of conjunctiva to nasal cavity); without tube |

| **68750** | with insertion of tube or stent |

| **68760** | Closure of the lacrimal punctum; by thermocauterization, ligation, or laser surgery |

| **68761** | by plug, each |

| **68770** | Closure of lacrimal fistula (separate procedure) |

Probing and/or Related Procedures

| ***68801** | Dilation of lacrimal punctum, with or without irrigation |

(To report a bilateral procedure, use 68801 with modifier -50)

| ***68810** | Probing of nasolacrimal duct, with or without irrigation; |

| **68811** | requiring general anesthesia |

| **68815** | with insertion of tube or stent |

(See also 92018)

(To report a bilateral procedure, use 68810, 68811, or 68815 with modifier -50)

| ***68840** | Probing of lacrimal canaliculi, with or without irrigation |

| ***68850** | Injection of contrast medium for dacryocystography |

(For radiological supervision and interpretation, see 70170, 78660)

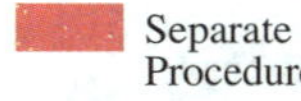 Separate Procedure

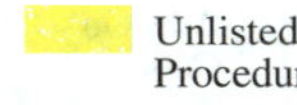 Unlisted Procedure

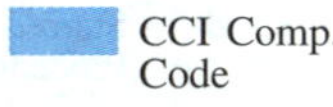 CCI Comp. Code

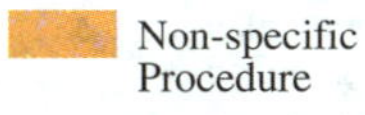 Non-specific Procedure

Other Procedures

68899 Unlisted procedure, lacrimal system

● New Code   ▲ Revised Code   ✳ Starred Procedure   ✛ Add-On Code   ⊘ Modifier -51 Exempt

AUDITORY SYSTEM

CPT codes from this subsection of the CPT coding system are used to report invasive and surgical procedures performed on the external ear; middle ear; inner ear and temporal bone. Includes procedures performed on the inner, outer and middle ear and to the temporal bone.

Diagnostic services, such as otoscopy under general anesthesia, audiometry and vestibular tests, are defined in the Medicine Section of the CPT manual.

Wound repairs to the external ear are located in the Integumentary Subsection of the CPT coding system.

(For diagnostic services (eg, audiometry, vestibular tests), see 92502 et seq)

EXTERNAL EAR

INCISION

***69000**   Drainage external ear, abscess or hematoma; simple

69005   complicated

***69020**   Drainage external auditory canal, abscess

69090   Ear piercing

EXCISION

69100   Biopsy external ear

69105   Biopsy external auditory canal

69110   Excision external ear; partial, simple repair

69120   complete amputation

(For reconstruction of ear, see 15120 et seq)

69140   Excision exostosis(es), external auditory canal

69145   Excision soft tissue lesion, external auditory canal

69150   Radical excision external auditory canal lesion; without neck dissection

---

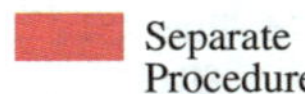

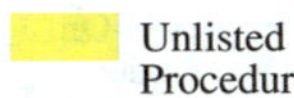

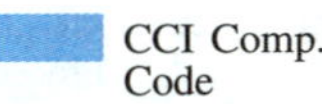

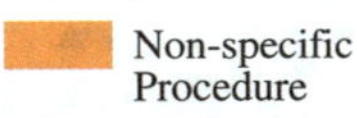

69155   with neck dissection

(For resection of temporal bone, use 69535)

(For skin grafting, see 15000-15261)

REMOVAL OF FOREIGN BODY

69200   Removal foreign body from external auditory canal; without general anesthesia

69205   with general anesthesia

69210   Removal impacted cerumen (separate procedure), one or both ears

69220   Debridement, mastoidectomy cavity, simple (eg, routine cleaning)

69222   Debridement, mastoidectomy cavity, complex (eg, with anesthesia or more than routine cleaning)

REPAIR

(For suture of wound or injury of external ear, see 12011-14300)

69300   Otoplasty, protruding ear, with or without size reduction

▲ **69310**   Reconstruction of external auditory canal (meatoplasty) (eg, for stenosis due to injury, infection) (separate procedure)

69320   Reconstruction external auditory canal for congenital atresia, single stage

(For combination with middle ear reconstruction, see 69631, 69641)

(For other reconstructive procedures with grafts (eg, skin, cartilage, bone), see 13150-15760, 21230-21235)

OTHER PROCEDURES

(For otoscopy under general anesthesia, use 92502)

69399   Unlisted procedure, external ear

● New Code   ▲ Revised Code   ✳ Starred Procedure   ✛ Add-On Code   ⊘ Modifier -51 Exempt

MIDDLE EAR

INTRODUCTION

69400 Eustachian tube inflation, transnasal; with catheterization

69401 without catheterization

69405 Eustachian tube catheterization, transtympanic

69410 Focal application of phase control substance, middle ear (baffle technique)

INCISION

***69420** Myringotomy including aspiration and/or eustachian tube inflation

***69421** Myringotomy including aspiration and/or eustachian tube inflation requiring general anesthesia

69424 Ventilating tube removal when originally inserted by another physician

***69433** Tympanostomy (requiring insertion of ventilating tube), local or topical anesthesia

69436 Tympanostomy (requiring insertion of ventilating tube), general anesthesia

69440 Middle ear exploration through postauricular or ear canal incision

(For atticotomy, see 69601 et seq)

69450 Tympanolysis, transcanal

EXCISION

69501 Transmastoid antrotomy (simple mastoidectomy)

69502 Mastoidectomy; complete

69505 modified radical

69511 radical

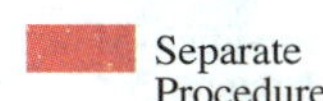 Separate Procedure

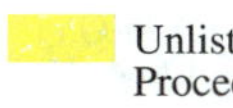 Unlisted Procedure

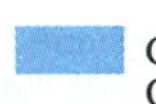 CCI Comp. Code

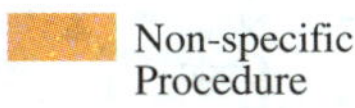 Non-specific Procedure

607

(For skin graft, see 15000 et seq)

(For mastoidectomy cavity debridement, see 69220, 69222)

69530 Petrous apicectomy including radical mastoidectomy

69535 Resection temporal bone, external approach

(For middle fossa approach, see 69950-69970)

69540 Excision aural polyp

69550 Excision aural glomus tumor; transcanal

69552 transmastoid

69554 extended (extratemporal)

REPAIR

69601 Revision mastoidectomy; resulting in complete mastoidectomy

69602 resulting in modified radical mastoidectomy

69603 resulting in radical mastoidectomy

69604 resulting in tympanoplasty

(For planned secondary tympanoplasty after mastoidectomy, see 69631, 69632)

69605 with apicectomy

(For skin graft, see 15120, 15121, 15260, 15261)

69610 Tympanic membrane repair, with or without site preparation or perforation for closure, with or without patch

69620 Myringoplasty (surgery confined to drumhead and donor area)

69631 Tympanoplasty without mastoidectomy (including canalplasty, atticotomy and/or middle ear surgery), initial or revision; without ossicular chain reconstruction

69632 with ossicular chain reconstruction (eg, postfenestration)

● New Code   ▲ Revised Code   * Starred Procedure   ✛ Add-On Code   ⊘ Modifier -51 Exempt

69633   with ossicular chain reconstruction and synthetic prosthesis (eg, partial ossicular replacement prosthesis (PORP), total ossicular replacement prosthesis (TORP))

69635   Tympanoplasty with antrotomy or mastoidotomy (including canalplasty, atticotomy, middle ear surgery, and/or tympanic membrane repair); without ossicular chain reconstruction

69636   with ossicular chain reconstruction

69637   with ossicular chain reconstruction and synthetic prosthesis (eg, partial ossicular replacement prosthesis (PORP), total ossicular replacement prosthesis (TORP))

69641   Tympanoplasty with mastoidectomy (including canalplasty, middle ear surgery, tympanic membrane repair); without ossicular chain reconstruction

69642   with ossicular chain reconstruction

69643   with intact or reconstructed wall, without ossicular chain reconstruction

69644   with intact or reconstructed canal wall, with ossicular chain reconstruction

69645   radical or complete, without ossicular chain reconstruction

69646   radical or complete, with ossicular chain reconstruction

69650   Stapes mobilization

69660   Stapedectomy or stapedotomy with reestablishment of ossicular continuity, with or without use of foreign material;

69661   with footplate drill out

69662   Revision of stapedectomy or stapedotomy

69666   Repair oval window fistula

69667   Repair round window fistula

69670   Mastoid obliteration (separate procedure)

69676   Tympanic neurectomy

	Separate Procedure		Unlisted Procedure		CCI Comp. Code		Non-specific Procedure

OTHER PROCEDURES

69700 Closure postauricular fistula, mastoid (separate procedure)

69710 Implantation or replacement of electromagnetic bone conduction hearing device in temporal bone

(Replacement procedure includes removal of old device)

69711 Removal or repair of electromagnetic bone conduction hearing device in temporal bone

69714 Implantation, osseointegrated implant, temporal bone, with percutaneous attachment to external speech processor/cochlear stimulator; without mastoidectomy

69715 with mastoidectomy

69717 Replacement (including removal of existing device), osseointegrated implant, temporal bone, with percutaneous attachment to external speech processor/cochlear stimulator; without mastoidectomy

69718 with mastoidectomy

69720 Decompression facial nerve, intratemporal; lateral to geniculate ganglion

69725 including medial to geniculate ganglion

69740 Suture facial nerve, intratemporal, with or without graft or decompression; lateral to geniculate ganglion

69745 including medial to geniculate ganglion

(For extracranial suture of facial nerve, use 64864)

69799 Unlisted procedure, middle ear

INNER EAR

INCISION AND/OR DESTRUCTION

69801 Labyrinthotomy, with or without cryosurgery including other nonexcisional destructive procedures or perfusion of vestibuloactive drugs (single or multiple perfusions); transcanal

---

● New Code ▲ Revised Code ✱ Starred Procedure ✚ Add-On Code ⊘ Modifier -51 Exempt

(69801 includes all required infusions performed on initial and subsequent days of treatment)

69802 with mastoidectomy

69805 Endolymphatic sac operation; without shunt

69806 with shunt

69820 Fenestration semicircular canal

69840 Revision fenestration operation

EXCISION

69905 Labyrinthectomy; transcanal

69910 with mastoidectomy

69915 Vestibular nerve section, translabyrinthine approach

(For transcranial approach, use 69950)

INTRODUCTION

69930 Cochlear device implantation, with or without mastoidectomy

OTHER PROCEDURES

69949 Unlisted procedure, inner ear

TEMPORAL BONE, MIDDLE FOSSA APPROACH

(For external approach, use 69535)

69950 Vestibular nerve section, transcranial approach

69955 Total facial nerve decompression and/or repair (may include graft)

69960 Decompression internal auditory canal

69970 Removal of tumor, temporal bone

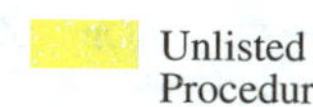

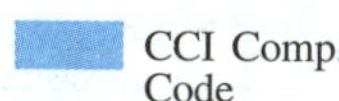

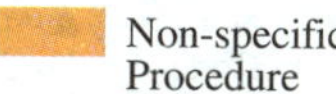

Non-specific
Procedure

OTHER PROCEDURES

69979   Unlisted procedure, temporal bone, middle fossa approach

OPERATING MICROSCOPE

▲ **+69990**   Microsurgical techniques, requiring use of operating microscope
(List separately in addition to code for primary procedure)

● New
Code   ▲ Revised
Code   * Starred
Procedure   + Add-On
Code   ⊘ Modifier -51
Exempt

RADIOLOGY SECTION OVERVIEW

The fourth section of the CPT coding system is the radiology section, which includes diagnostic and therapeutic radiology, nuclear medicine and diagnostic ultrasound services. Within each subsection, the CPT codes are arranged by anatomical site.

Diagnostic radiology uses all modalities of radiant energy in medical diagnosis and therapeutic procedures requiring radiologic guidance. This includes imaging techniques and methodologies using radiation emitted by x-ray tubes, radionuclides, ultrasonographic devices, and radiofrequency electromagnetic radiation.

RADIOLOGY SUBSECTIONS

The RADIOLOGY section of the CPT coding system is divided into 4 subsections; namely:

Diagnostic Radiology (Diagnostic Imaging)	70000-76499
Diagnostic Ultrasound	76500-76999
Radiation Oncology	77261-77999
Nuclear Medicine	78000-79999

COMPLETE PROCEDURES

Interventional radiologic procedures or diagnostic studies involving injection of contrast media include all usual preinjection and postinjection services, for example, necessary local anesthesia, placement of needle or catheter, injection of contrast media, supervision of the study, and interpretation of results. When one of these procedures is performed in full by a single physician, it is designated as a "complete procedure."

SUPERVISION AND INTERPRETATION ONLY

When a procedure is performed by a radiologist-clinician team, it is designated as "supervision and interpretation only" and the separate injection procedure is listed in the appropriate section of the SURGERY section of the CPT coding system. These CPT codes are used only when a procedure is performed by more than one physician, for example, a radiologist-clinician team.

613

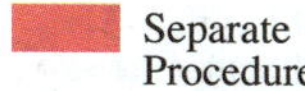

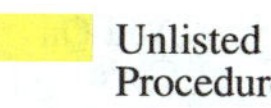

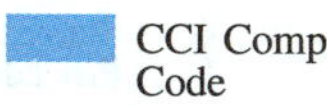

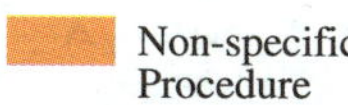

RADIOLOGY SERVICE MODIFIERS

Listed surgical services and procedures may be modified under certain circumstances. When applicable, the modifying circumstance is identified by adding the appropriate two digit modifier to the base procedure code(s). Modifiers commonly used to report RADIOLOGY services include:

-22	Unusual services
-26	Professional component
-32	Mandated services
-51	Multiple procedures
-52	Reduced services
-62	Two surgeons
-66	Surgical team
-76	Repeat procedure by same physician
-77	Repeat procedure by another physician
-78	Return to the operating room for a related procedure during the postoperative period
-79	Unrelated procedure or service by the same physician during the postoperative period
-80	Assistant surgeon
-90	Reference (outside) laboratory
-99	Multiple modifiers
-LT	Left side of body
-RT	Right side of body

BILATERAL PROCEDURE CODES

The RADIOLOGY section includes some CPT codes which include the term "bilateral" in the definition. When reporting these services, do not add the modifier -50, because the procedure is already defined as "bilateral."

● New Code   ▲ Revised Code   ✱ Starred Procedure   ✚ Add-On Code   ⊘ Modifier -51 Exempt

RADIOLOGY SERVICES MEDICARE CONSIDERATIONS

Most of the CPT codes in this section are subject to Medicare Purchased Diagnostic Services guidelines. Coding and reporting should be as instructed by your local Medicare carrier.

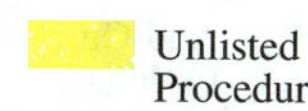 Separate Procedure

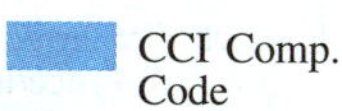 Unlisted Procedure

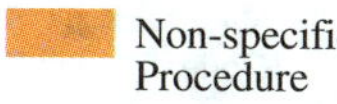 CCI Comp. Code

Non-specific Procedure

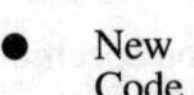

● New Code	▲ Revised Code	✳ Starred Procedure	✚ Add-On Code	⊘ Modifier -51 Exempt

RADIOLOGY CODES

DIAGNOSTIC RADIOLOGY (DIAGNOSTIC IMAGING)

HEAD AND NECK

70010 Myelography, posterior fossa, radiological supervision and interpretation

70015 Cisternography, positive contrast, radiological supervision and interpretation

70030 Radiologic examination, eye, for detection of foreign body

70100 Radiologic examination, mandible; partial, less than four views

70110 complete, minimum of four views

70120 Radiologic examination, mastoids; less than three views per side

70130 complete, minimum of three views per side

70134 Radiologic examination, internal auditory meati, complete

70140 Radiologic examination, facial bones; less than three views

70150 complete, minimum of three views

70160 Radiologic examination, nasal bones, complete, minimum of three views

70170 Dacryocystography, nasolacrimal duct, radiological supervision and interpretation

70190 Radiologic examination; optic foramina

70200 orbits, complete, minimum of four views

70210 Radiologic examination, sinuses, paranasal, less than three views

70220 Radiologic examination, sinuses, paranasal, complete, minimum of three views

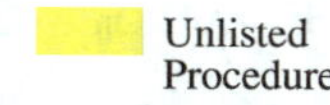 Separate Procedure

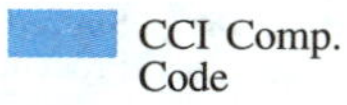 Unlisted Procedure

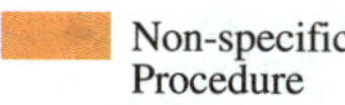 CCI Comp. Code

Non-specific Procedure

70240	Radiologic examination, sella turcica
70250	Radiologic examination, skull; less than four views, with or without stereo
70260	complete, minimum of four views, with or without stereo
70300	Radiologic examination, teeth; single view
70310	partial examination, less than full mouth
70320	complete, full mouth
70328	Radiologic examination, temporomandibular joint, open and closed mouth; unilateral
70330	bilateral
70332	Temporomandibular joint arthrography, radiological supervision and interpretation

(Do not report 76003 in addition to 70332)

70336	Magnetic resonance (eg, proton) imaging, temporomandibular joint(s)
70350	Cephalogram, orthodontic
70355	Orthopantogram
70360	Radiologic examination; neck, soft tissue
70370	pharynx or larynx, including fluoroscopy and/or magnification technique
70371	Complex dynamic pharyngeal and speech evaluation by cine or video recording
70373	Laryngography, contrast, radiological supervision and interpretation
70380	Radiologic examination, salivary gland for calculus
70390	Sialography, radiological supervision and interpretation

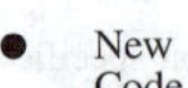 New Code   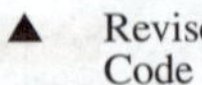 Revised Code   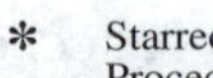 Starred Procedure   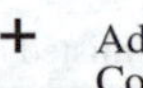 Add-On Code   ⊘ Modifier -51 Exempt

70450 Computerized axial tomography, head or brain; without contrast material

70460 with contrast material(s)

70470 without contrast material, followed by contrast material(s) and further sections

(For coronal, sagittal, and/or oblique sections, use 76375)

70480 Computerized axial tomography, orbit, sella, or posterior fossa or outer, middle, or inner ear; without contrast material

70481 with contrast material(s)

70482 without contrast material, followed by contrast material(s) and further sections

(For coronal, sagittal, and/or oblique sections, use 76375)

70486 Computerized axial tomography, maxillofacial area; without contrast material

70487 with contrast material(s)

70488 without contrast material, followed by contrast material(s) and further sections

(For coronal, sagittal, and/or oblique sections, use 76375)

70490 Computerized axial tomography, soft tissue neck; without contrast material

70491 with contrast material(s)

70492 without contrast material followed by contrast material(s) and further sections

(For coronal, sagittal, and/or oblique sections, use 76375)

(For cervical spine, see 72125, 72126)

70496 Computed tomographic angiography, head, without contrast material(s), followed by contrast material(s) and further sections, including image post-processing

Separate Procedure

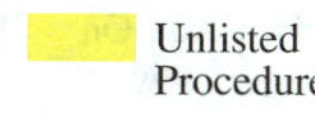
Unlisted Procedure

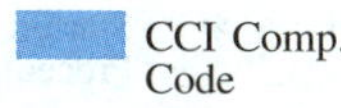
CCI Comp. Code

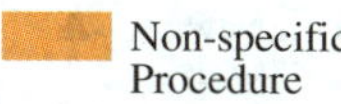
Non-specific Procedure

70498 Computed tomographic angiography, neck, without contrast material(s), followed by contrast material(s) and further sections, including image post-processing

70540 Magnetic resonance (eg, proton) imaging, orbit, face, and neck; without contrast material(s)

(70541 deleted 2001 edition. To report head or neck magnetic resonance angiography studies, see 70544-70546, 70547-70549)

70542 with contrast material(s)

70543 without contrast material(s), followed by contrast material(s) and further sequences

70544 Magnetic resonance angiography, head; without contrast materials

70545 with contrast materials

70546 without contrast material(s), followed by contrast material(s) and further sequences

70547 Magnetic resonance angiography, neck; without contrast materials

70548 with contrast materials

70549 without contrast material(s), followed by contrast material(s) and further sequences

70551 Magnetic resonance (eg, proton) imaging, brain (including brain stem); without contrast material

70552 with contrast material(s)

70553 without contrast material, followed by contrast material(s) and further sequences

  (For magnetic spectroscopy, use 76390)

CHEST

71010 Radiologic examination, chest; single view, frontal

71015 stereo, frontal

 ● New Code ▲ Revised Code ✶ Starred Procedure ✛ Add-On Code ⊘ Modifier -51 Exempt

71020 Radiologic examination, chest, two views, frontal and lateral;

71021 with apical lordotic procedure

71022 with oblique projections

71023 with fluoroscopy

71030 Radiologic examination, chest, complete, minimum of four views;

71034 with fluoroscopy

(For separate chest fluoroscopy, use 76000)

71035 Radiologic examination, chest, special views (eg, lateral decubitus, Bucky studies)

(71036 deleted 2001 edition. To report, use 76003)

71040 Bronchography, unilateral, radiological supervision and interpretation

71060 Bronchography, bilateral, radiological supervision and interpretation

71090 Insertion pacemaker, fluoroscopy and radiography, radiological supervision and interpretation

(For procedure, see appropriate organ or site)

71100 Radiologic examination, ribs, unilateral; two views

71101 including posteroanterior chest, minimum of three views

71110 Radiologic examination, ribs, bilateral; three views

71111 including posteroanterior chest, minimum of four views

71120 Radiologic examination; sternum, minimum of two views

71130 sternoclavicular joint or joints, minimum of three views

71250 Computerized axial tomography, thorax; without contrast material

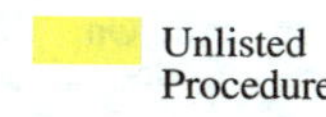

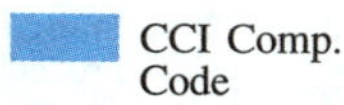

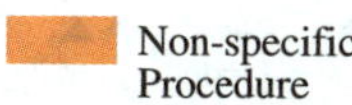

71260   with contrast material(s)

71270   without contrast material, followed by contrast material(s) and further sections

(For coronal, sagittal, and/or oblique sections, use 76375)

71275   Computed tomographic angiography, chest, without contrast material(s), followed by contrast material(s) and further sections, including image post-processing

71550   Magnetic resonance (eg, proton) imaging, chest (eg, for evaluation of hilar and mediastinal lymphadenopathy); without contrast material(s)

71551   with contrast material(s)

71552   without contrast material(s), followed by contrast material(s) and further sequences

(For breast MRI, see 76093 and 76094)

71555   Magnetic resonance angiography, chest (excluding myocardium), with or without contrast material(s)

SPINE AND PELVIS

72010   Radiologic examination, spine, entire, survey study, anteroposterior and lateral

72020   Radiologic examination, spine, single view, specify level

72040   Radiologic examination, spine, cervical; two or three views

72050   minimum of four views

72052   complete, including oblique and flexion and/or extension studies

72069   Radiologic examination, spine, thoracolumbar, standing (scoliosis)

72070   Radiologic examination, spine; thoracic, two views

72072   thoracic, three views

● New Code   ▲ Revised Code   ✱ Starred Procedure   ✚ Add-On Code   ⊘ Modifier -51 Exempt

72074   thoracic, minimum of four views

72080   thoracolumbar, two views

72090   scoliosis study, including supine and erect studies

72100   Radiologic examination, spine, lumbosacral; two or three views

72110   minimum of four views

72114   complete, including bending views

72120   Radiologic examination, spine, lumbosacral, bending views only, minimum of four views

(Contrast material in CT of spine is either by intrathecal or intravenous injection. For intrathecal injection, use also 61055 or 62284. IV injection of contrast material is part of the CT procedure)

72125   Computerized axial tomography, cervical spine; without contrast material

72126   with contrast material

72127   without contrast material, followed by contrast material(s) and further sections

(For intrathecal injection procedure, see 61055, 62284)

72128   Computerized axial tomography, thoracic spine; without contrast material

72129   with contrast material

(For intrathecal injection procedure, see 61055, 62284)

72130   without contrast material, followed by contrast material(s) and further sections

(For intrathecal injection procedure, see 61055, 62284)

72131   Computerized axial tomography, lumbar spine; without contrast material

72132   with contrast material

72133   without contrast material, followed by contrast material(s) and further sections

(For intrathecal injection procedure, see 61055, 62284)

(For coronal, sagittal, and/or oblique sections, use 76375)

72141   Magnetic resonance (eg, proton) imaging, spinal canal and contents, cervical; without contrast material

72142   with contrast material(s)

(For cervical spinal canal imaging without contrast material followed by contrast material, use 72156)

72146   Magnetic resonance (eg, proton) imaging, spinal canal and contents, thoracic; without contrast material

72147   with contrast material(s)

(For thoracic spinal canal imaging without contrast material followed by contrast material, use 72157)

72148   Magnetic resonance (eg, proton) imaging, spinal canal and contents, lumbar; without contrast material

72149   with contrast material(s)

(For lumbar spinal canal imaging without contrast material followed by contrast material, use 72158)

72156   Magnetic resonance (eg, proton) imaging, spinal canal and contents, without contrast material, followed by contrast material(s) and further sequences; cervical

72157   thoracic

72158   lumbar

72159   Magnetic resonance angiography, spinal canal and contents, with or without contrast material(s)

72170   Radiologic examination, pelvis; one or two views

72190   complete, minimum of three views

(For pelvimetry, use 74710)

| ● New Code | ▲ Revised Code | ✱ Starred Procedure | ✛ Add-On Code | ⊘ Modifier -51 Exempt |

72191   Computed tomographic angiography, pelvis; without contrast material(s), followed by contrast material(s) and further sections, including image post-processing

(For CTA aorto-iliofemoral runoff, use 75635)

72192   Computerized axial tomography, pelvis; without contrast material

72193   with contrast material(s)

72194   without contrast material, followed by contrast material(s) and further sections

(For coronal, sagittal, and/or oblique sections, use 76375)

72195   Magnetic resonance (eg, proton) imaging, pelvis; without contrast material(s)

72196   with contrast material(s)

72197   without contrast material(s), followed by contrast material(s) and further sequences

72198   Magnetic resonance angiography, pelvis, with or without contrast material(s)

72200   Radiologic examination, sacroiliac joints; less than three views

72202   three or more views

72220   Radiologic examination, sacrum and coccyx, minimum of two views

72240   Myelography, cervical, radiological supervision and interpretation

72255   Myelography, thoracic, radiological supervision and interpretation

72265   Myelography, lumbosacral, radiological supervision and interpretation

72270   Myelography, entire spinal canal, radiological supervision and interpretation

72275   Epidurography, radiological supervision and interpretation

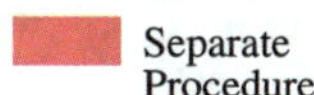 Separate Procedure   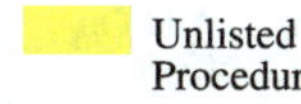 Unlisted Procedure   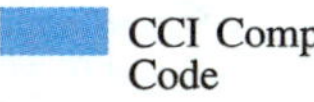 CCI Comp. Code   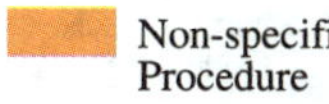 Non-specific Procedure

(For injection procedure, see 62280-62282, 62310-62319, 64479-64484)

72285 Diskography, cervical or thoracic, radiological supervision and interpretation

72295 Diskography, lumbar, radiological supervision and interpretation

UPPER EXTREMITIES

(For stress views, any joint, use 76006)

73000 Radiologic examination; clavicle, complete

73010   scapula, complete

73020 Radiologic examination, shoulder; one view

73030   complete, minimum of two views

73040 Radiologic examination, shoulder, arthrography, radiological supervision and interpretation

(Do not report 76003 in addition to 73040)

73050 Radiologic examination; acromioclavicular joints, bilateral, with or without weighted distraction

73060   humerus, minimum of two views

73070 Radiologic examination, elbow; two views

73080   complete, minimum of three views

73085 Radiologic examination, elbow, arthrography, radiological supervision and interpretation

(Do not report 76003 in addition to 73085)

73090 Radiologic examination; forearm, two views

73092   upper extremity, infant, minimum of two views

73100 Radiologic examination, wrist; two views

73110   complete, minimum of three views

● New Code   ▲ Revised Code   ✳ Starred Procedure   ✛ Add-On Code   ⊘ Modifier -51 Exempt

73115 Radiologic examination, wrist, arthrography, radiological supervision and interpretation

(Do not report 76003 in addition to 73115)

73120 Radiologic examination, hand; two views

73130 minimum of three views

73140 Radiologic examination, finger(s), minimum of two views

73200 Computerized axial tomography, upper extremity; without contrast material

73201 with contrast material(s)

73202 without contrast material, followed by contrast material(s) and further sections

(For coronal, sagittal, and/or oblique sections, use 76375)

73206 Computed tomographic angiography, upper extremity, without contrast material(s), followed by contrast material(s) and further sections, including image post-processing

73218 Magnetic resonance (eg, proton) imaging, upper extremity, other than joint; without contrast material(s)

73219 with contrast material(s)

73220 without contrast material(s), followed by contrast material(s) and further sequences

73221 Magnetic resonance (eg, proton) imaging, any joint of upper extremity; without contrast material(s)

73222 with contrast material(s)

73223 without contrast material(s), followed by contrast material(s) and further sequences

73225 Magnetic resonance angiography, upper extremity, with or without contrast material(s)

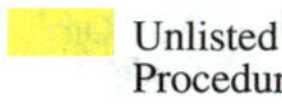
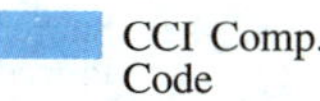
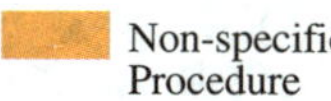

Separate Procedure   Unlisted Procedure   CCI Comp. Code   Non-specific Procedure

LOWER EXTREMITIES

(For stress views, any joint, use 76006)

73500 Radiologic examination, hip, unilateral; one view

73510 complete, minimum of two views

73520 Radiologic examination, hips, bilateral, minimum of two views of each hip, including anteroposterior view of pelvis

73525 Radiologic examination, hip, arthrography, radiological supervision and interpretation

(Do not report 76003 in addition to 73525)

73530 Radiologic examination, hip, during operative procedure

73540 Radiologic examination, pelvis and hips, infant or child, minimum of two views

73542 Radiological examination, sacroiliac joint arthrography, radiological supervision and interpretation

(Do not report 76003 in addition to 73542)

(For procedure, use 27096. If formal arthrography is not performed, recorded, and a formal radiologic report is not issued, use 76005 for fluoroscopic guidance for sacroiliac joint injections)

73550 Radiologic examination, femur, two views

73560 Radiologic examination, knee; one or two views

73562 three views

73564 complete, four or more views

73565 both knees, standing, anteroposterior

73580 Radiologic examination, knee, arthrography, radiological supervision and interpretation

(Do not report 76003 in addition to 73580)

73590 Radiologic examination; tibia and fibula, two views

73592   lower extremity, infant, minimum of two views

73600   Radiologic examination, ankle; two views

73610   complete, minimum of three views

73615   Radiologic examination, ankle, arthrography, radiological supervision and interpretation

(Do not report 76003 in addition to 73615)

73620   Radiologic examination, foot; two views

73630   complete, minimum of three views

73650   Radiologic examination; calcaneus, minimum of two views

73660   toe(s), minimum of two views

73700   Computerized axial tomography, lower extremity; without contrast material

73701   with contrast material(s)

73702   without contrast material, followed by contrast material(s) and further sections

(For coronal, sagittal, and/or oblique sections, use 76375)

73706   Computed tomographic angiography, lower extremity, without contrast material(s), followed by contrast material(s) and further sections, including image post-processing

(For CTA aorto-iliofemoral runoff, use 75635)

73718   Magnetic resonance (eg, proton) imaging, lower extremity, other than joint; without contrast material(s)

73719   with contrast material(s)

73720   without contrast material(s), followed by contrast material(s) and further sequences

73721   Magnetic resonance (eg, proton) imaging, any joint of lower extremity; without contrast material

Separate
Procedure

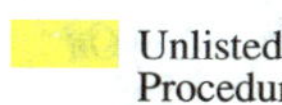
Unlisted
Procedure

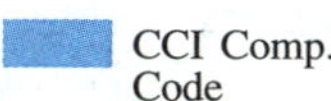
CCI Comp.
Code

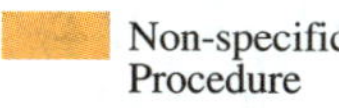
Non-specific
Procedure

73722   with contrast material

73723   without contrast material followed by contrast material(s) and further sequences

73725   Magnetic resonance angiography, lower extremity, with or without contrast material(s)

ABDOMEN

74000   Radiologic examination, abdomen; single anteroposterior view

74010   anteroposterior and additional oblique and cone views

74020   complete, including decubitus and/or erect views

74022   complete acute abdomen series, including supine, erect, and/or decubitus views, upright PA chest

74150   Computerized axial tomography, abdomen; without contrast material

74160   with contrast material(s)

74170   without contrast material, followed by contrast material(s) and further sections

(For coronal, sagittal, and/or oblique sections, use 76375)

74175   Computed tomographic angiography, abdomen, without contrast material(s), followed by contrast material(s) and further sections, including image post-processing

(For CTA aorto-iliofemoral runoff, use 75635)

74181   Magnetic resonance (eg, proton) imaging, abdomen; without contrast material(s)

74182   with contrast material(s)

74183   without contrast material, followed by contrast material(s) and further sequences

74185   Magnetic resonance angiography, abdomen, with or without contrast material(s)

● New Code   ▲ Revised Code   * Starred Procedure   + Add-On Code   ⊘ Modifier -51 Exempt

74190   Peritoneogram (eg, after injection of air or contrast), radiological supervision and interpretation

(For procedure, use 49400)

(For computerized axial tomography, see 72192 or 74150)

GASTROINTESTINAL TRACT

(For percutaneous placement of gastrostomy tube, use 43750)

74210   Radiologic examination; pharynx and/or cervical esophagus

74220   esophagus

▲ **74230**   Swallowing function, with cineradiography/videoradiography

74235   Removal of foreign body(s), esophageal, with use of balloon catheter, radiological supervision and interpretation

(For procedure, see 43215, 43247)

74240   Radiologic examination, gastrointestinal tract, upper; with or without delayed films, without KUB

74241   with or without delayed films, with KUB

▲ **74245**   with small intestine, includes multiple serial films

74246   Radiological examination, gastrointestinal tract, upper, air contrast, with specific high density barium, effervescent agent, with or without glucagon; with or without delayed films, without KUB

74247   with or without delayed films, with KUB

▲ **74249**   with small intestine follow-through

▲ **74250**   Radiologic examination, small intestine, includes multiple serial films;

74251   via enteroclysis tube

74260   Duodenography, hypotonic

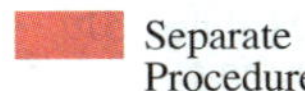

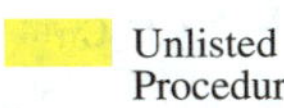

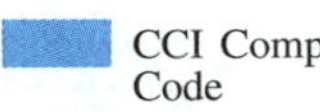

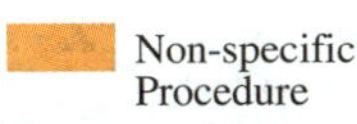

74270 Radiologic examination, colon; barium enema, with or without KUB

74280 air contrast with specific high density barium, with or without glucagon

74283 Therapeutic enema, contrast or air, for reduction of intussusception or other intraluminal obstruction (eg, meconium ileus)

74290 Cholecystography, oral contrast;

74291 additional or repeat examination or multiple day examination

74300 Cholangiography and/or pancreatography; intraoperative, radiological supervision and interpretation

+74301 additional set intraoperative, radiological supervision and interpretation (List separately in addition to code for primary procedure)

(Use 74301 in conjunction with code 74300)

▲ **74305** through existing catheter, radiological supervision and interpretation

(For procedure, see 47505, 48400, 47560-47561, 47563)

(For biliary duct stone extraction, percutaneous, see 47630, 74327)

74320 Cholangiography, percutaneous, transhepatic, radiological supervision and interpretation

▲ **74327** Postoperative biliary duct calculus removal, percutaneous via T-tube tract, basket, or snare (eg, Burhenne technique), radiological supervision and interpretation

(For procedure, use 47630)

74328 Endoscopic catheterization of the biliary ductal system, radiological supervision and interpretation

(For procedure, see 43260-43272 as appropriate)

74329 Endoscopic catheterization of the pancreatic ductal system, radiological supervision and interpretation

● New Code   ▲ Revised Code   * Starred Procedure   + Add-On Code   ⊘ Modifier -51 Exempt

(For procedure, see 43260-43272 as appropriate)

74330 Combined endoscopic catheterization of the biliary and pancreatic ductal systems, radiological supervision and interpretation

(For procedure, see 43260-43272 as appropriate)

74340 Introduction of long gastrointestinal tube (eg, Miller-Abbott), including multiple fluoroscopies and films, radiological supervision and interpretation

(For tube placement, use 44500)

74350 Percutaneous placement of gastrostomy tube, radiological supervision and interpretation

74355 Percutaneous placement of enteroclysis tube, radiological supervision and interpretation

74360 Intraluminal dilation of strictures and/or obstructions (eg, esophagus), radiological supervision and interpretation

▲ **74363** Percutaneous transhepatic dilation of biliary duct stricture with or without placement of stent, radiological supervision and interpretation

(For procedure, see 47510, 47511, 47555, 47556)

URINARY TRACT

74400 Urography (pyelography), intravenous, with or without KUB, with or without tomography

74410 Urography, infusion, drip technique and/or bolus technique;

74415   with nephrotomography

74420 Urography, retrograde, with or without KUB

74425 Urography, antegrade, (pyelostogram, nephrostogram, loopogram), radiological supervision and interpretation

74430 Cystography, minimum of three views, radiological supervision and interpretation

---

633

74440 Vasography, vesiculography, or epididymography, radiological supervision and interpretation

74445 Corpora cavernosography, radiological supervision and interpretation

74450 Urethrocystography, retrograde, radiological supervision and interpretation

74455 Urethrocystography, voiding, radiological supervision and interpretation

74470 Radiologic examination, renal cyst study, translumbar, contrast visualization, radiological supervision and interpretation

74475 Introduction of intracatheter or catheter into renal pelvis for drainage and/or injection, percutaneous, radiological supervision and interpretation

74480 Introduction of ureteral catheter or stent into ureter through renal pelvis for drainage and/or injection, percutaneous, radiological supervision and interpretation

(For transurethral surgery (ureter and pelvis), see 52320-52355)

74485 Dilation of nephrostomy, ureters, or urethra, radiological supervision and interpretation

(For dilation of ureter without radiologic guidance, use 52341, 52344)

(For change of nephrostomy or pyelostomy tube, use 50398)

GYNECOLOGICAL AND OBSTETRICAL

(For abdomen and pelvis, see 72170-72190, 74000-74170)

74710 Pelvimetry, with or without placental localization

74740 Hysterosalpingography, radiological supervision and interpretation

(For introduction of saline or contrast for hysterosalpingography, see 58340)

74742 Transcervical catheterization of fallopian tube, radiological supervision and interpretation

---

634   ● New Code   ▲ Revised Code   * Starred Procedure   + Add-On Code   ⊘ Modifier -51 Exempt

(For procedure, use 58345)

74775 Perineogram (eg, vaginogram, for sex determination or extent of anomalies)

HEART

(For separate injection procedures for vascular radiology, see Surgery section, 36000-36299)

(For cardiac catheterization procedures, see 93501-93556)

75552 Cardiac magnetic resonance imaging for morphology; without contrast material

75553 with contrast material

75554 Cardiac magnetic resonance imaging for function, with or without morphology; complete study

75555 limited study

75556 Cardiac magnetic resonance imaging for velocity flow mapping

AORTA AND ARTERIES

(For intravenous procedure, see 36000-36013, 36400-36425 and 36100-36248 for intra-arterial procedure)

(For radiological supervision and interpretation, see 75600-75978)

75600 Aortography, thoracic, without serialography, radiological supervision and interpretation

(For injection procedure, use 93544)

75605 Aortography, thoracic, by serialography, radiological supervision and interpretation

(For injection procedure, use 93544)

75625 Aortography, abdominal, by serialography, radiological supervision and interpretation

(For injection procedure, use 93544)

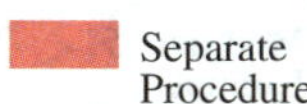

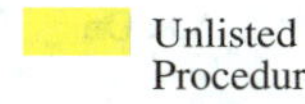

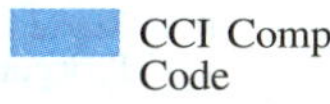

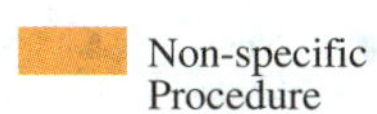

75630   Aortography, abdominal plus bilateral iliofemoral lower extremity, catheter, by serialography, radiological supervision and interpretation

75635   Computed tomographic angiography, abdominal aorta and bilateral iliofemoral lower extremity runoff, radiological supervision and interpretation, without contrast material(s), followed by contrast material(s) and further sections, including image post-processing

75650   Angiography, cervicocerebral, catheter, including vessel origin, radiological supervision and interpretation

75658   Angiography, brachial, retrograde, radiological supervision and interpretation

75660   Angiography, external carotid, unilateral, selective, radiological supervision and interpretation

75662   Angiography, external carotid, bilateral, selective, radiological supervision and interpretation

75665   Angiography, carotid, cerebral, unilateral, radiological supervision and interpretation

75671   Angiography, carotid, cerebral, bilateral, radiological supervision and interpretation

75676   Angiography, carotid, cervical, unilateral, radiological supervision and interpretation

75680   Angiography, carotid, cervical, bilateral, radiological supervision and interpretation

75685   Angiography, vertebral, cervical, and/or intracranial, radiological supervision and interpretation

75705   Angiography, spinal, selective, radiological supervision and interpretation

75710   Angiography, extremity, unilateral, radiological supervision and interpretation

75716   Angiography, extremity, bilateral, radiological supervision and interpretation

---

● New Code   ▲ Revised Code   ✳ Starred Procedure   ✚ Add-On Code   ⊘ Modifier -51 Exempt

75722 Angiography, renal, unilateral, selective (including flush aortogram), radiological supervision and interpretation

75724 Angiography, renal, bilateral, selective (including flush aortogram), radiological supervision and interpretation

75726 Angiography, visceral, selective or supraselective, (with or without flush aortogram), radiological supervision and interpretation

(For selective angiography, each additional visceral vessel studied after basic examination, use 75774)

75731 Angiography, adrenal, unilateral, selective, radiological supervision and interpretation

75733 Angiography, adrenal, bilateral, selective, radiological supervision and interpretation

75736 Angiography, pelvic, selective or supraselective, radiological supervision and interpretation

75741 Angiography, pulmonary, unilateral, selective, radiological supervision and interpretation

(For injection procedure, use 93541)

75743 Angiography, pulmonary, bilateral, selective, radiological supervision and interpretation

(For injection procedure, use 93541)

75746 Angiography, pulmonary, by nonselective catheter or venous injection, radiological supervision and interpretation

75756 Angiography, internal mammary, radiological supervision and interpretation

(For introduction of catheter, injection procedure, see 93501-93533, 93545, 93556)

+75774 Angiography, selective, each additional vessel studied after basic examination, radiological supervision and interpretation (List separately in addition to code for primary procedure)

(Use 75774 in addition to code for specific initial vessel studied)

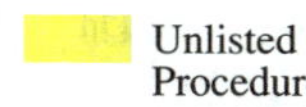
Separate
Procedure

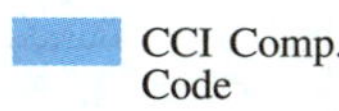
Unlisted
Procedure

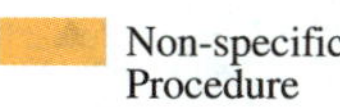
CCI Comp.
Code

Non-specific
Procedure

637

(For angiography, see codes 75600-75790)

(For catheterizations, see codes 36215-36248)

(For introduction of catheter, injection procedure, see 93501-93533, 93545, 93555, 93556)

75790 Angiography, arteriovenous shunt (eg, dialysis patient), radiological supervision and interpretation

For introduction of catheter, use 36140, 36145, 36215-36217, 36245-36247)

VEINS AND LYMPHATICS

(For injection procedure for venous system, see 36000-36015, 36400-36510)

(For injection procedure for lymphatic system, use 38790)

75801 Lymphangiography, extremity only, unilateral, radiological supervision and interpretation

75803 Lymphangiography, extremity only, bilateral, radiological supervision and interpretation

75805 Lymphangiography, pelvic/abdominal, unilateral, radiological supervision and interpretation

75807 Lymphangiography, pelvic/abdominal, bilateral, radiological supervision and interpretation

75809 Shuntogram for investigation of previously placed indwelling nonvascular shunt (eg, LeVeen shunt, ventriculoperitoneal shunt, indwelling infusion pump), radiological supervision and interpretation

(For procedure, see 49427 or 61070)

75810 Splenoportography, radiological supervision and interpretation

75820 Venography, extremity, unilateral, radiological supervision and interpretation

75822 Venography, extremity, bilateral, radiological supervision and interpretation

● New Code   ▲ Revised Code   ✻ Starred Procedure   ✚ Add-On Code   ⊘ Modifier -51 Exempt

75825 Venography, caval, inferior, with serialography, radiological supervision and interpretation

75827 Venography, caval, superior, with serialography, radiological supervision and interpretation

75831 Venography, renal, unilateral, selective, radiological supervision and interpretation

75833 Venography, renal, bilateral, selective, radiological supervision and interpretation

75840 Venography, adrenal, unilateral, selective, radiological supervision and interpretation

75842 Venography, adrenal, bilateral, selective, radiological supervision and interpretation

75860 Venography, sinus or jugular, catheter, radiological supervision and interpretation

75870 Venography, superior sagittal sinus, radiological supervision and interpretation

75872 Venography, epidural, radiological supervision and interpretation

75880 Venography, orbital, radiological supervision and interpretation

75885 Percutaneous transhepatic portography with hemodynamic evaluation, radiological supervision and interpretation

75887 Percutaneous transhepatic portography without hemodynamic evaluation, radiological supervision and interpretation

75889 Hepatic venography, wedged or free, with hemodynamic evaluation, radiological supervision and interpretation

75891 Hepatic venography, wedged or free, without hemodynamic evaluation, radiological supervision and interpretation

75893 Venous sampling through catheter, with or without angiography (eg, for parathyroid hormone, renin), radiological supervision and interpretation

(For procedure, use 36500)

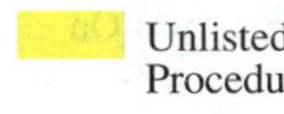
Separate Procedure

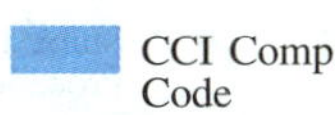
Unlisted Procedure

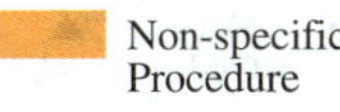
CCI Comp. Code

Non-specific Procedure

TRANSCATHETER PROCEDURES

75894 Transcatheter therapy, embolization, any method, radiological supervision and interpretation

75896 Transcatheter therapy, infusion, any method (eg, thrombolysis other than coronary), radiological supervision and interpretation

(For infusion for coronary disease, see 92975, 92977)

▲ **75898** Angiography through existing catheter for follow-up study for transcatheter therapy, embolization or infusion

75900 Exchange of a previously placed arterial catheter during thrombolytic therapy with contrast monitoring, radiological supervision and interpretation

(For procedure, use 37209)

75940 Percutaneous placement of IVC filter, radiological supervision and interpretation

75945 Intravascular ultrasound (non-coronary vessel), radiological supervision and interpretation; initial vessel

+75946 each additional non-coronary vessel (List separately in addition to code for primary procedure)

(Use 75946 in conjunction with code 75945)

(For catheterizations, see codes 36215-36248)

(For transcatheter therapies, see codes 37200-37208, 61624, 61626)

(For procedure, see 37250, 37251)

75952 Endovascular repair of infrarenal abdominal aortic aneurysm or dissection, radiological supervision and interpretation

(For implantation of endovascular grafts, see 34800-34808)

75953 Placement of proximal or distal extension prosthesis for endovascular repair of infrarenal abdominal aortic aneurysm, radiological supervision and interpretation

(For implantation of endovascular extension prostheses, see 34825, 34826)

● New Code   ▲ Revised Code   * Starred Procedure   + Add-On Code   ⊘ Modifier -51 Exempt

75960 Transcatheter introduction of intravascular stent(s), (non-coronary vessel), percutaneous and/or open, radiological supervision and interpretation, each vessel

(For procedure, see 37205-37208)

(For radiologic supervision and interpretation for transcatheter placement of extracranial cerebrovascular artery stent(s), use Category III code 0007T)

75961 Transcatheter retrieval, percutaneous, of intravascular foreign body (eg, fractured venous or arterial catheter), radiological supervision and interpretation

(For procedure, use 37203)

75962 Transluminal balloon angioplasty, peripheral artery, radiological supervision and interpretation

+75964 Transluminal balloon angioplasty, each additional peripheral artery, radiological supervision and interpretation (List separately in addition to code for primary procedure)

(Use 75964 in conjunction with code 75962)

75966 Transluminal balloon angioplasty, renal or other visceral artery, radiological supervision and interpretation

+75968 Transluminal balloon angioplasty, each additional visceral artery, radiological supervision and interpretation (List separately in addition to code for primary procedure)

(Use 75968 in conjunction with code 75966)

(For percutaneous transluminal coronary angioplasty, see 92982-92984)

75970 Transcatheter biopsy, radiological supervision and interpretation

(For injection procedure only for transcatheter therapy or biopsy, see 36100-36299)

(For transcatheter renal and ureteral biopsy, use 52007)

(For percutaneous needle biopsy of pancreas, use 48102; of retroperitoneal lymph node or mass, use 49180)

75978 Transluminal balloon angioplasty, venous (eg, subclavian stenosis), radiological supervision and interpretation

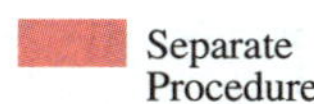
Separate
Procedure

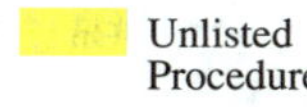
Unlisted
Procedure

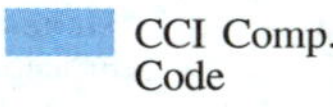
CCI Comp.
Code

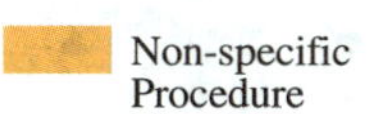
Non-specific
Procedure

75980 Percutaneous transhepatic biliary drainage with contrast monitoring, radiological supervision and interpretation

75982 Percutaneous placement of drainage catheter for combined internal and external biliary drainage or of a drainage stent for internal biliary drainage in patients with an inoperable mechanical biliary obstruction, radiological supervision and interpretation

75984 Change of percutaneous tube or drainage catheter with contrast monitoring (eg, gastrointestinal system, genitourinary system, abscess), radiological supervision and interpretation

(For change of nephrostomy or pyelostomy tube only, use 50398)

(For introduction procedure only for percutaneous biliary drainage, see 47510, 47511)

(For percutaneous choloecystostomy, use 47490)

(For change of percutaneous biliary drainage catheter only, use 47525)

(For percutaneous nephrostolithotomy or pyelostolithotomy, see 50080, 50081)

▲ **75989** Radiological guidance for percutaneous drainage of abscess, or specimen collection (ie, fluoroscopy, ultrasound, or computed axial tomography), with placement of indwelling catheter, radiological supervision and interpretation

TRANSLUMINAL ATHERECTOMY

75992 Transluminal atherectomy, peripheral artery, radiological supervision and interpretation

(For procedure, see 35481-35485, 35491-35495)

+75993 Transluminal atherectomy, each additional peripheral artery, radiological supervision and interpretation (List separately in addition to code for primary procedure)

(Use 75993 in conjunction with code 75992)

(For procedure, see 35481-35485, 35491-35495)

75994 Transluminal atherectomy, renal, radiological supervision and interpretation

● New Code	▲ Revised Code	* Starred Procedure	+ Add-On Code	⊘ Modifier -51 Exempt

(For procedure, see 35480, 35490)

75995   Transluminal atherectomy, visceral, radiological supervision and interpretation

(For procedure, see 35480, 35490)

+75996   Transluminal atherectomy, each additional visceral artery, radiological supervision and interpretation (List separately in addition to code for primary procedure)

(Use 75996 in conjunction with code 75995)

(For procedure, see 35480, 35490)

OTHER PROCEDURES

(For arthrography of shoulder, use 73040; elbow, use 73085; wrist, use 73115; hip, use 73525; knee, use 73580; ankle, use 73615)

76000   Fluoroscopy (separate procedure), up to one hour physician time, other than 71023 or 71034 (eg, cardiac fluoroscopy)

76001   Fluoroscopy, physician time more than one hour, assisting a non-radiologic physician (eg, nephrostolithotomy, ERCP, bronchoscopy, transbronchial biopsy)

76003   Fluoroscopic guidance for needle placement (eg, biopsy, aspiration, injection, localization device)

(See appropriate surgical code for procedure and anatomic location)

(Fluoroscopy 76003 is considered inclusive of all radiographic arthrography with the exception of supervision and interpretation for CT and MR arthrography)

(Do not report 76003 in addition to 70332, 73040, 73085, 73115, 73525, 73580, 73615)

(Fluoroscopy 76003 is considered inclusive of organ/anatomic specific radiological supervision and interpretation procedures 74320, 74350, 74355, 74445, 74470, 74475, 75809, 75810, 75885, 75887, 75980, 75982, 75989)

76005   Fluoroscopic guidance and localization of needle or catheter tip for spine or paraspinous diagnostic or therapeutic injection procedures (epidural, transforaminal epidural, subarachnoid,

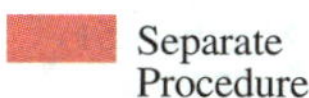

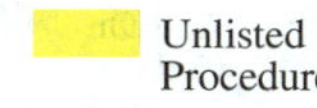

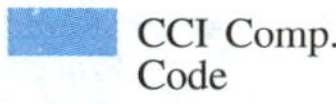

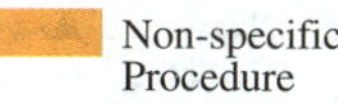

643

paravertebral facet joint, paravertebral facet joint nerve or sacroiliac joint), including neurolytic agent destruction

(Injection of contrast during fluoroscopic guidance and localization is an inclusive component of codes 62270-62273, 62280-62282, 62310-32319)

(Fluoroscopic guidance for subarachnoid puncture for diagnostic radiographic myelography is included in supervision and interpretation codes 72240, 72255, 72265, 72270)

(For epidural or subarachnoid needle or catheter placement and injection, see codes 62270-62273, 62280-62282, 62310-62319)

(For sacroiliac joint arthrography, see 27096, 73542. If formal arthrography is not performed, recorded, and a formal radiographic report is not issued, use 76005 for fluoroscopic guidance for sacroiliac joint injections)

(For paravertebral facet joint injection, see 64470-64476. For transforaminal epidural needle placement and injection, see 64479-64484)

(For destruction by neurolytic agent, see 64600-64680)

76006 Radiologic examination, stress view(s), any joint, stress applied by a physician (includes comparison views)

76010 Radiologic examination from nose to rectum for foreign body, single view, child

76012 Radiological supervision and interpretation, percutaneous vertebroplasty, per vertebral body; under fluoroscopic guidance

76013   under CT guidance

(For procedure, see 22520-22522)

76020 Bone age studies

76040 Bone length studies (orthoroentgenogram, scanogram)

76061 Radiologic examination, osseous survey; limited (eg, for metastases)

76062   complete (axial and appendicular skeleton)

76065 Radiologic examination, osseous survey, infant

▲ **76066**   Joint survey, single view, two or more joints (specify)

▲ **76070**   Computerized axial tomography bone density study, one or more sites

76075   Dual energy x-ray absorptiometry (DEXA), bone density study, one or more sites; axial skeleton (eg, hips, pelvis, spine)

76076   appendicular skeleton (peripheral) (eg, radius, wrist, heel)

▲ **76078**   Radiographic absorptiometry (eg, photodensitometry, radiogrammetry), one or more sites

76080   Radiologic examination, abscess, fistula or sinus tract study, radiological supervision and interpretation

●+**76085**   Digitization of film radiographic images with computer analysis for lesion detection and further physician review for interpretation, screening mammography (List separately in addition to code for primary procedure)

(Use 76085 in conjunction with code 76092)

76086   Mammary ductogram or galactogram, single duct, radiological supervision and interpretation

76088   Mammary ductogram or galactogram, multiple ducts, radiological supervision and interpretation

76090   Mammography; unilateral

76091   bilateral

76092   Screening mammography, bilateral (two view film study of each breast)

(For computer aided detection applied to a screening mammogram, use 76085)

76093   Magnetic resonance imaging, breast, without and/or with contrast material(s); unilateral

76094   bilateral

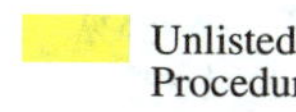

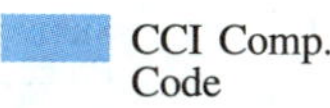

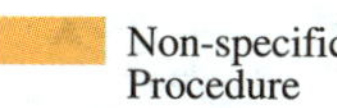

76095   Stereotactic localization for breast biopsy or needle placement (eg, for wire localization or for injection), each lesion, radiological supervision and interpretation

(For procedure, see 10022, 19000, 19001, 19102, 19103, 19290, 19291)

(For injection for sentinel node localization without lymphoscintigraphy, use 38792)

76096   Mammographic guidance for needle placement, breast, (eg, for wire localization or for injection), each lesion, radiological supervision and interpretation

(For procedure, see 10022, 19000, 19102, 19103, 19290, 19291)

(For injection for sentinel node localization without lymphoscintigraphy, use 38792)

76098   Radiological examination, surgical specimen

76100   Radiologic examination, single plane body section (eg, tomography), other than with urography

76101   Radiologic examination, complex motion (ie, hypercycloidal) body section (eg, mastoid polytomography), other than with urography; unilateral

76102   bilateral

(For nephrotomography, use 74415)

▲ **76120**   Cineradiography/videoradiography, except where specifically included

▲ **+76125**   Cineradiography/videoradiography to complement routine examination (List separately in addition to code for primary procedure)

76140   Consultation on x-ray examination made elsewhere, written report

76150   Xeroradiography

(76150 is to be used for non-mammographic studies only)

76350   Subtraction in conjunction with contrast studies

---

646   ● New Code   ▲ Revised Code   * Starred Procedure   + Add-On Code   ⊘ Modifier -51 Exempt

▲ **76355**   Computerized axial tomographic guidance for stereotactic localization

▲ **76360**   Computerized axial tomographic guidance for needle biopsy, radiological supervision and interpretation

● **76362**   Computerized axial tomographic guidance for, and monitoring of, tissue ablation

(For percutaneous radiofrequency ablation, use 47382)

(76365   deleted 2001 edition. For computed tomographic guidance for cyst aspiration, see appropriate organ or site and 76360)

▲ **76370**   Computerized axial tomographic guidance for placement of radiation therapy fields

▲ **76375**   Coronal, sagittal, multiplanar, oblique, 3-dimensional and/or holographic reconstruction of computerized axial tomography, magnetic resonance imaging, or other tomographic modality

(Use 76375 in addition to code for imaging procedure)

▲ **76380**   Computerized axial tomography, limited or localized follow-up study

76390   Magnetic resonance spectroscopy

(For magnetic resonance imaging, use appropriate MRI body site code)

76393   Magnetic resonance guidance for needle placement (eg, for biopsy, needle aspiration, injection, or placement of localization device) radiological supervision and interpretation

(For procedure see appropriate organ or site)

● **76394**   Magnetic resonance guidance for, and monitoring of, tissue ablation

(For percutaneous radiofrequency ablation, use 47382)

76400   Magnetic resonance (eg, proton) imaging, bone marrow blood supply

● **76490**   Ultrasound guidance for, and monitoring of, tissue ablation

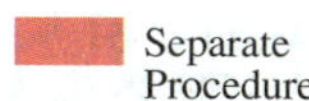
Separate Procedure

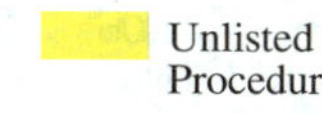
Unlisted Procedure

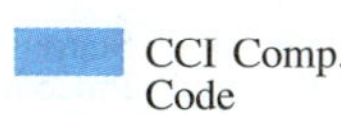
CCI Comp. Code

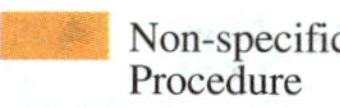
Non-specific Procedure

647

(Do not report 76490 in addition to 76986)

(For ablation, see codes 47370-47382)

76499 Unlisted diagnostic radiologic procedure

● New
Code

▲ Revised
Code

* Starred
Procedure

+ Add-On
Code

⊘ Modifier -51
Exempt

DIAGNOSTIC ULTRASOUND

Diagnostic ultrasound is a non-invasive medical imaging technology that uses high frequency sound waves to form an image of body tissues. Information obtained from these images can be utilized along with other patient data in order to arrive at a medical diagnosis. Ultrasound, when compared to other imaging modalities like MRI (Magnetic Resonance Imaging) and CT (Computed Tomography), is a relatively low cost non-invasive procedure that does not utilize either magnetic fields or ionizing radiation (x-rays).

The following definitions are important when choosing CPT codes for diagnostic ultrasound services and procedures.

A-MODE — Implies a one-dimensional ultrasonic measurement procedure.

M-MODE — Implies a one-dimensional ultrasonic measurement procedure with movement of the trace to record amplitude and velocity of moving echo-producing structures.

B-SCAN — Implies a two-dimensional ultrasonic scanning procedure with a two-dimensional display.

REAL-TIME — Implies a two-dimensional ultrasonic scanning procedure with display of both two-dimensional structure and motion with time.

HEAD AND NECK

(For determination of corneal thickness (eg, pachymetry) with interpretation and report, bilateral, use Category III code 0025T)

76506 Echoencephalography, B-scan and/or real time with image documentation (gray scale) (for determination of ventricular size, delineation of cerebral contents and detection of fluid masses or other intracranial abnormalities), including A-mode encephalography as secondary component where indicated

76511 Ophthalmic ultrasound, echography, diagnostic; A-scan only, with amplitude quantification

76512 contact B-scan (with or without simultaneous A-scan)

76513 anterior segment ultrasound, immersion (water bath) B-scan or high resolution biomicroscopy

76516 Ophthalmic biometry by ultrasound echography, A-scan;

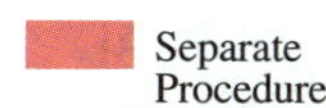

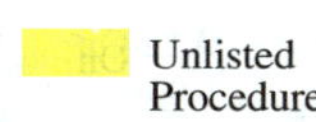

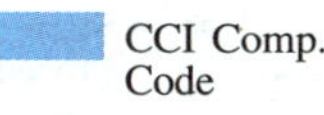

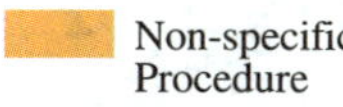

76519 with intraocular lens power calculation

(For partial coherence interferometry, use 92136)

76529 Ophthalmic ultrasonic foreign body localization

▲ **76536** Ultrasound, soft tissues of head and neck (eg, thyroid, parathyroid, parotid), B-scan and/or real time with image documentation

CHEST

▲ **76604** Ultrasound, chest, B-scan (includes mediastinum) and/or real time with image documentation

▲ **76645** Ultrasound, breast(s) (unilateral or bilateral), B-scan and/or real time with image documentation

ABDOMEN AND PERITONEUM

▲ **76700** Ultrasound, abdominal, B-scan and/or real time with image documentation; complete

76705 limited (eg, single organ, quadrant, follow-up)

▲ **76770** Ultrasound, retroperitoneal (eg, renal, aorta, nodes), B-scan and/or real time with image documentation; complete

76775 limited

▲ **76778** Ultrasound, transplanted kidney, B-scan and/or real time with image documentation, with or without duplex Doppler study

SPINAL CANAL

▲ **76800** Ultrasound, spinal canal and contents

PELVIS

▲ **76805** Ultrasound, pregnant uterus, B-scan and/or real time with image documentation; complete (complete fetal and maternal evaluation)

76810 complete (complete fetal and maternal evaluation), multiple gestation, after the first trimester

---

650

● New Code   ▲ Revised Code   ✳ Starred Procedure   ✛ Add-On Code   ⦸ Modifier -51 Exempt

76815   limited (fetal size, heart beat, placental location, fetal position, or emergency in the delivery room)

76816   follow-up or repeat

76818   Fetal biophysical profile; with non-stress testing

▲ **76819**   without non-stress testing

(Fetal biophysical profile assessments for the second and any additional fetuses, should be reported separately by code 76818 or 76819 with the modifier -51 appended)

(For amniotic fluid index without non-stress test, use 76815)

76825   Echocardiography, fetal, cardiovascular system, real time with image documentation (2D), with or without M-mode recording;

76826   follow-up or repeat study

76827   Doppler echocardiography, fetal, cardiovascular system, pulsed wave and/or continuous wave with spectral display; complete

76828   follow-up or repeat study

(To report the use of color mapping, use 93325)

▲ **76830**   Ultrasound, transvaginal

76831   Hysterosonography, with or without color flow Doppler

(For introduction of saline or contrast for hysterosonography, use 58340)

▲ **76856**   Ultrasound, pelvic (nonobstetric), B-scan and/or real time with image documentation; complete

76857   limited or follow-up (eg, for follicles)

GENITALIA

▲ **76870**   Ultrasound, scrotum and contents

76872   Echography, transrectal;

76873   prostate volume study for brachytherapy treatment planning (separate procedure)

EXTREMITIES

▲ **76880**   Ultrasound, extremity, non-vascular, B-scan and/or real time with image documentation

▲ **76885**   Ultrasound of infant hips, real time with imaging documentation; dynamic (requiring physician manipulation)

▲ **76886**   limited, static (not requiring physician manipulation)

VASCULAR STUDIES

ULTRASONIC GUIDANCE PROCEDURES

76930   Ultrasonic guidance for pericardiocentesis, imaging supervision and interpretation

76932   Ultrasonic guidance for endomyocardial biopsy, imaging supervision and interpretation

(76934   deleted 2001 edition. To report, see 32000 and 76942)

76936   Ultrasound guided compression repair of arterial pseudoaneurysm or arteriovenous fistulae (includes diagnostic ultrasound evaluation, compression of lesion and imaging)

(76938   deleted 2001 edition. To report, see appropriate organ or site and 76942)

76941   Ultrasonic guidance for intrauterine fetal transfusion or cordocentesis, imaging supervision and interpretation

(For procedure, see 36460, 59012)

76942   Ultrasonic guidance for needle placement (eg, biopsy, aspiration, injection, localization device) imaging supervision and interpretation

76945   Ultrasonic guidance for chorionic villus sampling, imaging supervision and interpretation

(For procedure, use 59015)

● New Code   ▲ Revised Code   ✱ Starred Procedure   ✚ Add-On Code   ⊘ Modifier -51 Exempt

76946   Ultrasonic guidance for amniocentesis, imaging supervision and interpretation

76948   Ultrasonic guidance for aspiration of ova, imaging supervision and interpretation

76950   Ultrasonic guidance for placement of radiation therapy fields

(**76960**   deleted 2001 edition. To report, use 76950)

76965   Ultrasonic guidance for interstitial radioelement application

OTHER ULTRASOUND PROCEDURES

76970   Ultrasound study follow-up (specify)

76975   Gastrointestinal endoscopic ultrasound, imaging supervision and interpretation

(For procedure, use 43259)

(Do not report 76975 in conjunction with 43231, 43232, 43242, 45341, 45342)

76977   Ultrasound bone density measurement and interpretation, peripheral site(s), any method

76986   Ultrasonic guidance, intraoperative

(Do not report 76986 in addition to 47370-47382)

(For ultrasound guidance for open and laparoscopic radiofrequency tissue ablation, use 76490)

76999   Unlisted ultrasound procedure

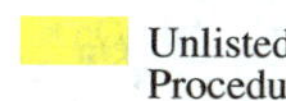
Separate Procedure

Unlisted Procedure

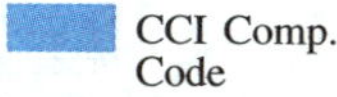
CCI Comp. Code

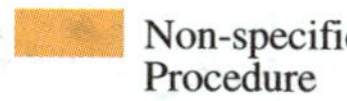
Non-specific Procedure

653

RADIATION ONCOLOGY

Radiation therapy is the use of high level radiation to destroy cancer cells. Both tumor cells and healthy cells may be affected by this radiation. The radiation injures the cancer cells so they can no longer continue to divide or multiply. With each treatment, more of the cells die and the tumor shrinks. The dead cells are broken down, carried away by the blood and excreted by the body. Most of the healthy cells are able to recover from this injury. However, the damage to the healthy cells is the reason for the side effects of radiation therapy.

The dose of radiation is determined by the size, extent, type and grade of tumor along with its response to radiation therapy. Complex calculations are done to determine the dose and timing of radiation in treatment planning. Often, the treatment is given over several different angles in order to deliver the maximum amount of radiation to the tumor and the minimum amount to normal tissues.

Services defined in this section of the CPT book coding system teletherapy and brachytherapy. To report Radiation Oncology services, the following must be performed and documented:

- The initial consultation

- Clinical treatment planning with/without simulation

- Medical radiation physics, dosimetry, treatment devices and special services

- Clinical treatment management procedures

- Normal follow-up care during treatment and for three months following completion of treatment

CONSULTATION OR CLINICAL MANAGEMENT

All consultations, pre-treatment patient evaluations, and/or medical care services are coded using evaluation and management service codes

CLINICAL TREATMENT PLANNING

Clinical treatment planning includes test interpretation, localization of tumor(s), treatment determination, and choice of treatment modality and treatment devices. Clinical treatment planning may be simple, intermediate or complex.

PLANNING

77261	Therapeutic radiology treatment planning; simple
77262	intermediate

● New Code	▲ Revised Code	✳ Starred Procedure	✚ Add-On Code	⊘ Modifier -51 Exempt

| 77263 | complex |

SIMULATION

| 77280 | Therapeutic radiology simulation-aided field setting; simple |

| 77285 | intermediate |

| 77290 | complex |

| 77295 | three-dimensional |

| 77299 | Unlisted procedure, therapeutic radiology clinical treatment planning |

MEDICAL RADIATION PHYSICS, DOSIMETRY, TREATMENT DEVICES, AND SPECIAL SERVICES

▲ **77300** Basic radiation dosimetry calculation, central axis depth dose calculation, TDF, NSD, gap calculation, off axis factor, tissue inhomogeneity factors, calculation of non-ionizing radiation surface and depth dose, as required during course of treatment, only when prescribed by the treating physician

● **77301** Intensity modulated radiotherapy plan, including dose-volume histograms for target and critical structure partial tolerance specifications

(Dose plan is optimized using inverse or forward planning technique for modulated beam delivery (eg, binary, dynamic MLC) to create highly conformal dose distribution. Computer plan distribution must be verified for positional accuracy based on dosimetric verification of the intensity map with verification of treatment set up and interpretation of verification methodology)

| 77305 | Teletherapy, isodose plan (whether hand or computer calculated); simple (one or two parallel opposed unmodified ports directed to a single area of interest) |

| 77310 | intermediate (three or more treatment ports directed to a single area of interest) |

| 77315 | complex (mantle or inverted Y, tangential ports, the use of wedges, compensators, complex blocking, rotational beam, or special beam considerations) |

655

(Only one teletherapy isodose plan may be reported for a given course of therapy to a specific treatment area)

77321 Special teletherapy port plan, particles, hemibody, total body

77326 Brachytherapy isodose calculation; simple (calculation made from single plane, one to four sources/ ribbon application, remote afterloading brachytherapy, 1 to 8 sources)

(For definition of source/ribbon, see Clinical Brachytherapy)

77327 intermediate (multiplane dosage calculations, application involving 5 to 10 sources/ribbons, remote afterloading brachytherapy, 9 to 12 sources)

77328 complex (multiplane isodose plan, volume implant calculations, over 10 sources/ribbons used, special spatial reconstruction, remote afterloading brachytherapy, over 12 sources)

77331 Special dosimetry (eg, TLD, microdosimetry) (specify), only when prescribed by the treating physician

77332 Treatment devices, design and construction; simple (simple block, simple bolus)

77333 intermediate (multiple blocks, stents, bite blocks, special bolus)

77334 complex (irregular blocks, special shields, compensators, wedges, molds or casts)

77336 Continuing medical physics consultation, including assessment of treatment parameters, quality assurance of dose delivery, and review of patient treatment documentation in support of the radiation oncologist, reported per week of therapy

77370 Special medical radiation physics consultation

77399 Unlisted procedure, medical radiation physics, dosimetry and treatment devices, and special services

RADIATION TREATMENT DELIVERY

77401 Radiation treatment delivery, superficial and/or ortho voltage

● New Code ▲ Revised Code ✴ Starred Procedure + Add-On Code ⊘ Modifier -51 Exempt

77402 Radiation treatment delivery, single treatment area, single port or parallel opposed ports, simple blocks or no blocks; up to 5 MeV

77403 6-10 MeV

77404 11-19 MeV

77406 20 MeV or greater

77407 Radiation treatment delivery, two separate treatment areas, three or more ports on a single treatment area, use of multiple blocks; up to 5 MeV

77408 6-10 MeV

77409 11-19 MeV

77411 20 MeV or greater

77412 Radiation treatment delivery, three or more separate treatment areas, custom blocking, tangential ports, wedges, rotational beam, compensators, special particle beam (eg, electron or neutrons); up to 5 MeV

77413 6-10 MeV

77414 11-19 MeV

77416 20 MeV or greater

77417 Therapeutic radiology port film(s)

● **77418** Intensity modulated treatment delivery, single or multiple fields/arcs, via narrow spatially and temporally modulated beams (eg, binary, dynamic MLC), per treatment session

(For intensity modulated treatment planning, use 77301)

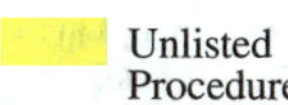
Separate
Procedure

Unlisted
Procedure

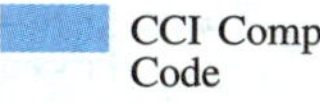
CCI Comp.
Code

Non-specific
Procedure

RADIATION TREATMENT MANAGEMENT

CPT codes in this section presume treatment on a daily basis (4 or 5 fractions per week) with the use of megavoltage photon or high energy particle sources. Daily and weekly clinical treatment management are mutually exclusive for the same dates. CPT defines three distinct levels of clinical treatment management: simple, intermediate and complex. Review this section of CPT for detailed definitions of these levels of service.

77427 Radiation treatment management, five treatments

77431 Radiation therapy management with complete course of therapy consisting of one or two fractions only

(77431 is not to be used to fill in the last week of a long course of therapy)

77432 Stereotactic radiation treatment management of cerebral lesion(s) (complete course of treatment consisting of one session)

77470 Special treatment procedure (eg, total body irradiation, hemibody irradiation, per oral, endocavitary or vaginal cone irradiation)

(77470 assumes that the procedure is performed one or more times during the course of therapy, in addition to daily or weekly patient management)

77499 Unlisted procedure, therapeutic radiology treatment management

PROTON BEAM TREATMENT DELIVERY

77520 Proton treatment delivery; simple, without compensation

77522   simple, with compensation

77523   intermediate

77525   complex

HYPERTHERMIA

77600 Hyperthermia, externally generated; superficial (ie, heating to a depth of 4 cm or less)

● New Code	▲ Revised Code	✳ Starred Procedure	✚ Add-On Code	⊘ Modifier -51 Exempt

77605	deep (ie, heating to depths greater than 4 cm)
77610	Hyperthermia generated by interstitial probe(s); 5 or fewer interstitial applicators
77615	more than 5 interstitial applicators

CLINICAL INTRACAVITARY HYPERTHERMIA

77620	Hyperthermia generated by intracavitary probe(s)

CLINICAL BRACHYTHERAPY

77750	Infusion or instillation of radioelement solution
77761	Intracavitary radiation source application; simple
77762	intermediate
77763	complex
77776	Interstitial radiation source application; simple
77777	intermediate
77778	complex
77781	Remote afterloading high intensity brachytherapy; 1-4 source positions or catheters
77782	5-8 source positions or catheters
77783	9-12 source positions or catheters
77784	over 12 source positions or catheters
77789	Surface application of radiation source
77790	Supervision, handling, loading of radiation source
77799	Unlisted procedure, clinical brachytherapy

	Separate Procedure		Unlisted Procedure		CCI Comp. Code		Non-specific Procedure

NUCLEAR MEDICINE

Nuclear medicine is used in the diagnosis, management, treatment, and prevention of serious disease. Nuclear medicine imaging procedures often identify abnormalities very early in the progression of a disease. This early detection allows a disease to be treated early in its course when there may be a more successful prognosis.

Nuclear medicine uses very small amounts of radioactive materials or radiopharmaceuticals to diagnose and treat disease. Radiopharmaceuticals are substances that are attracted to specific organs, bones, or tissues. The radiopharmaceuticals used in nuclear medicine emit gamma rays that can be detected externally by special types of cameras: gamma or PET cameras. These cameras work in conjunction with computers used to form images that provide data and information about the area of body being imaged. The amount of radiation from a nuclear medicine procedure is comparable to that received during a diagnostic x-ray.

Nuclear medicine procedures may be performed independently or in the course of overall medical care. If the physician providing nuclear medicine services is also responsible for the diagnostic work-up and/or follow-up care of the patient, evaluation and management service codes should be coded in addition to the nuclear medicine procedures.

Radioimmunoassay tests are located in the clinical pathology section, code series 82000-84999. These CPT codes can be used by any specialist performing such tests in a laboratory licensed and/or certified for radioimmunoassays. The reporting of these tests is not confined to clinical pathology laboratories alone.

Note that the services listed in this section do not include the provision of radium or other elements. When those materials are supplied by the physician they should be listed as separate procedures using code 78990 for diagnostic radionuclide(s) and 79900 for therapeutic radionuclide.

DIAGNOSTIC NUCLEAR MEDICINE

ENDOCRINE SYSTEM

78000 Thyroid uptake; single determination

78001 multiple determinations

78003 stimulation, suppression or discharge (not including initial uptake studies)

78006 Thyroid imaging, with uptake; single determination

● New Code ▲ Revised Code * Starred Procedure + Add-On Code ⊘ Modifier -51 Exempt

78007   multiple determinations

78010 Thyroid imaging; only

78011   with vascular flow

78015 Thyroid carcinoma metastases imaging; limited area (eg, neck and chest only)

78016   with additional studies (eg, urinary recovery)

78018   whole body

(For calcitonin, use 82308)

(For triiodothyronin (true TT-3), use 84480)

(For triiodothyronin, free (FT-3), (unbound T-3 only), use 84481)

(For TT-4 thyroxine, use 84436)

(For T-4 thyroxine, neonatal, use 84437)

(For FT-4 thyroxine, free, (unbound T-4 only), use 84439)

+78020 Thyroid carcinoma metastases uptake (List separately in addition to code for primary procedure)

(Use 78020 in conjunction with code 78018 only)

78070 Parathyroid imaging

(For parathormone (parathyroid hormone), use 83970)

78075 Adrenal imaging, cortex and/or medulla

(For cortisol, plasma, use 82533)

(For cortisol, urine, use 82533)

(For aldosterone, double isotope technique, use 82088)

(For aldosterone, blood, use 82088)

(For aldosterone, urine, use 82088)

(For 17-ketosteroids, use 83586)

(For 17-OH ketosteroids, use 83586)

(For 17-hydroxycorticosteroids, use 83491)

Separate
Procedure

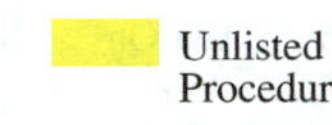
Unlisted
Procedure

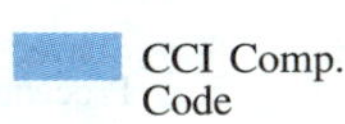
CCI Comp.
Code

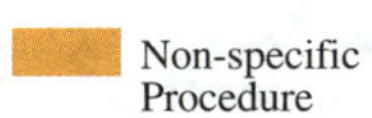
Non-specific
Procedure

(For insulin, use 83525)

(For insulin antibodies, use 86337)

(For proinsulin, use 84206)

(For glucagon, use 82943)

(For adrenocorticotropic hormone (ACTH), use 82024)

(For human growth hormone (HGH), (somatotropin), use 83003)

(For human growth antibody, use 86277)

(For thyroglobulin antibody, use 86800)

(For thyroid microsomal antibody, use 86376)

(For thyroid stimulating hormone (TSH), use 84443)

(For thyrotropin releasing factor, see 80438, 80439)

(For plus long-acting thyroid stimulator (LATS), use 84445)

(For follicle stimulating hormone (FSH component of pituitary gonadotropin), use 83001)

(For luteinizing hormone (LH component of pituitary gonadotropin), (ICSH), use 83002)

(For luteinizing releasing factor (LRH), use 83727)

(For prolactin level (mammotropin), use 84146)

(For vasopressin level (antidiuretic hormone), use 84588)

(For estradiol, use 82670)

(For progesterone, use 84144)

(For testosterone, blood, use 84403)

(For testosterone, urine, use 84403)

(For etiocholanolone, use 82696)

78099   Unlisted endocrine procedure, diagnostic nuclear medicine

(For chemical analysis, see Chemistry section)

HEMATOPOIETIC, RETICULOENDOTHELIAL AND LYMPHATIC SYSTEM

78102   Bone marrow imaging; limited area

● New Code   ▲ Revised Code   ＊ Starred Procedure   ＋ Add-On Code   ⃠ Modifier -51 Exempt

78103	multiple areas
78104	whole body
78110	Plasma volume, radiopharmaceutical volume-dilution technique (separate procedure); single sampling
78111	multiple samplings
78120	Red cell volume determination (separate procedure); single sampling
78121	multiple samplings
78122	Whole blood volume determination, including separate measurement of plasma volume and red cell volume (radiopharmaceutical volume-dilution technique)
78130	Red cell survival study;
78135	differential organ/tissue kinetics, (eg, splenic and/or hepatic sequestration)
78140	Labeled red cell sequestration, differential organ/tissue, (eg, splenic and/or hepatic)
78160	Plasma radioiron disappearance (turnover) rate
78162	Radioiron oral absorption
78170	Radioiron red cell utilization
78172	Chelatable iron for estimation of total body iron

(For hemosiderin, use 83071)

(For intrinsic factor antibodies, use 86340)

(For cyanocobalamin (vitamin B-12), use 82607)

(For folic acid (folate) serum, use 82746)

(For hepatitis B antigen, see 87340, 37350)

(For hepatitis A antibody (HAAb), see 86708, 86709)

(For hepatitis B core antibody (HBcAb), see 86704, 86705)

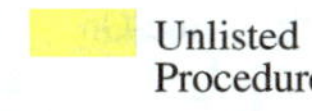 Separate Procedure

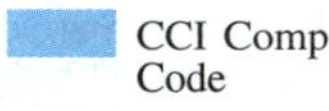 Unlisted Procedure

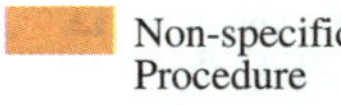 CCI Comp. Code

Non-specific Procedure

(For hepatitis B surface antigen (HBsAb), use 87340)

(For hepatitis B surface antibody (HBsAb), use 86706)

(For hepatitis Be antigen (HBeAg), use 87350)

(For hepatitis Be antibody (HBeAb), use 86707)

78185 Spleen imaging only, with or without vascular flow

(If combined with liver study, use procedures 78215 and 78216)

78190 Kinetics, study of platelet survival, with or without differential organ/tissue localization

78191 Platelet survival study

▲ **78195** Lymphatics and lymph nodes imaging

(For sentinel node identification without scintigraphy imaging, use 38792)

(For sentinal node excision, see 38500-38542)

78199 Unlisted hematopoietic, reticuloendothelial and lymphatic procedure, diagnostic nuclear medicine

(For chemical analysis, see Chemistry section)

GASTROINTESTINAL SYSTEM

78201 Liver imaging; static only

78202 with vascular flow

(For spleen imaging only, use 78185)

78205 Liver imaging (SPECT);

78206 with vascular flow

78215 Liver and spleen imaging; static only

78216 with vascular flow

78220 Liver function study with hepatobiliary agents, with serial images

---

● New Code   ▲ Revised Code   * Starred Procedure   ✛ Add-On Code   ⊘ Modifier -51 Exempt

78223 Hepatobiliary ductal system imaging, including gallbladder, with or without pharmacologic intervention, with or without quantitative measurement of gallbladder function

78230 Salivary gland imaging;

78231   with serial images

78232 Salivary gland function study

78258 Esophageal motility

78261 Gastric mucosa imaging

78262 Gastroesophageal reflux study

78264 Gastric emptying study

78267 Urea breath test, C-14; acquisition for analysis

78268   analysis

78270 Vitamin B-12 absorption study (eg, Schilling test); without intrinsic factor

78271   with intrinsic factor

78272 Vitamin B-12 absorption studies combined, with and without intrinsic factor

78278 Acute gastrointestinal blood loss imaging

78282 Gastrointestinal protein loss

(For gastrin, use 82941)

(For intrinsic factor level, use 83528)

(For carcinoembryonic antigen level (CEA), use 82378)

▲ **78290** Intestine imaging (eg, ectopic gastric mucosa, Meckels localization, volvulus)

78291 Peritoneal-venous shunt patency test (eg, for LeVeen, Denver shunt)

Separate Procedure

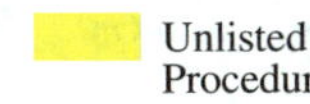
Unlisted Procedure

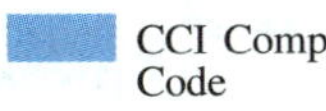
CCI Comp. Code

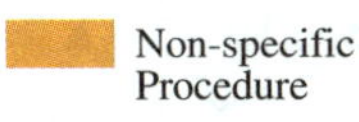
Non-specific Procedure

(For injection procedure, use 49427)

78299 Unlisted gastrointestinal procedure, diagnostic nuclear medicine

(For chemical analysis, see Chemistry section)

MUSCULOSKELETAL SYSTEM

78300 Bone and/or joint imaging; limited area

78305 multiple areas

78306 whole body

78315 three phase study

78320 tomographic (SPECT)

78350 Bone density (bone mineral content) study, one or more sites; single photon absorptiometry

78351 dual photon absorptiometry, one or more sites

(For radiographic bone density (photodensitometry), use 76078)

78399 Unlisted musculoskeletal procedure, diagnostic nuclear medicine

CARDIOVASCULAR SYSTEM

78414 Determination of central c-v hemodynamics (non-imaging) (eg, ejection fraction with probe technique) with or without pharmacologic intervention or exercise, single or multiple determinations

78428 Cardiac shunt detection

78445 Non-cardiac vascular flow imaging (ie, angiography, venography)

78455 Venous thrombosis study (eg, radioactive fibrinogen)

78456 Acute venous thrombosis imaging, peptide

78457 Venous thrombosis imaging, venogram; unilateral

78458 bilateral

● New Code   ▲ Revised Code   * Starred Procedure   + Add-On Code   ⊘ Modifier -51 Exempt

78459 Myocardial imaging, positron emission tomography (PET), metabolic evaluation

(For myocardial perfusion study, see 78491-78492)

78460 Myocardial perfusion imaging; (planar) single study, at rest or stress (exercise and/or pharmacologic), with or without quantification

78461 multiple studies, (planar) at rest and/or stress (exercise and/or pharmacologic), and redistribution and/or rest injection, with or without quantification

78464 tomographic (SPECT), single study at rest or stress (exercise and/or pharmacologic), with or without quantification

78465 tomographic (SPECT), multiple studies, at rest and/or stress (exercise and/or pharmacologic) and redistribution and/or rest injection, with or without quantification

78466 Myocardial imaging, infarct avid, planar; qualitative or quantitative

78468 with ejection fraction by first pass technique

78469 tomographic SPECT with or without quantification

78472 Cardiac blood pool imaging, gated equilibrium; planar, single study at rest or stress (exercise and/or pharmacologic), wall motion study plus ejection fraction, with or without additional quantitative processing

(For assessment of cardiac function by first pass technique, use 78496)

78473 multiple studies, wall motion study plus ejection fraction, at rest and stress (exercise and/or pharmacologic), with or without additional quantification

+78478 Myocardial perfusion study with wall motion, qualitative or quantitative study (List separately in addition to code for primary procedure)

(Use 78478 in conjunction with codes 78460, 78461, 78464, 78465)

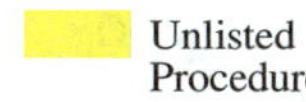
Separate Procedure

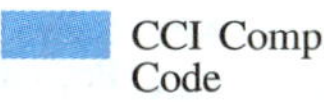
Unlisted Procedure

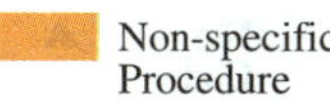
CCI Comp. Code

Non-specific Procedure

+78480   Myocardial perfusion study with ejection fraction (List separately in addition to code for primary procedure)

(Use 78480 in conjunction with codes 78460, 78461, 78464, 78465)

78481   Cardiac blood pool imaging, (planar), first pass technique; single study, at rest or with stress (exercise and/or pharmacologic), wall motion study plus ejection fraction, with or without quantification

78483   multiple studies, at rest and with stress (exercise and/or pharmacologic), wall motion study plus ejection fraction, with or without quantification

(For digoxin, use 80162)

(For cerebral blood flow study, use 78615)

78491   Myocardial imaging, positron emission tomography (PET), perfusion; single study at rest or stress

78492   multiple studies at rest and/or stress

78494   Cardiac blood pool imaging, gated equilibrium, SPECT, at rest, wall motion study plus ejection fraction, with or without quantitative processing

+78496   Cardiac blood pool imaging, gated equilibrium, single study, at rest, with right ventricular ejection fraction by first pass technique (List separately in addition to code for primary procedure)

(Use 78496 in conjunction with code 78472)

78499   Unlisted cardiovascular procedure, diagnostic nuclear medicine

(For chemical analysis, see Chemistry section)

RESPIRATORY SYSTEM

78580   Pulmonary perfusion imaging, particulate

78584   Pulmonary perfusion imaging, particulate, with ventilation; single breath

78585   rebreathing and washout, with or without single breath

---

● New Code   ▲ Revised Code   ✱ Starred Procedure   ✚ Add-On Code   ⊘ Modifier -51 Exempt

78586 Pulmonary ventilation imaging, aerosol; single projection

78587   multiple projections (eg, anterior, posterior, lateral views)

78588 Pulmonary perfusion imaging, particulate, with ventilation imaging, aerosol, one or multiple projections

78591 Pulmonary ventilation imaging, gaseous, single breath, single projection

78593 Pulmonary ventilation imaging, gaseous, with rebreathing and washout with or without single breath; single projection

78594   multiple projections (eg, anterior, posterior, lateral views)

78596 Pulmonary quantitative differential function (ventilation/perfusion) study

78599 Unlisted respiratory procedure, diagnostic nuclear medicine

NERVOUS SYSTEM

78600 Brain imaging, limited procedure; static

78601   with vascular flow

78605 Brain imaging, complete study; static

78606   with vascular flow

78607   tomographic (SPECT)

78608 Brain imaging, positron emission tomography (PET); metabolic evaluation

78609   perfusion evaluation

78610 Brain imaging, vascular flow only

▲ **78615** Cerebral vascular flow

78630 Cerebrospinal fluid flow, imaging (not including introduction of material); cisternography

(For injection procedure, see 61000-61070, 62270-62319)

78635   ventriculography

(For injection procedure, see 61000-61070, 62270-62294)

78645   shunt evaluation

(For injection procedure, see 61000-61070, 62270-62294)

78647   tomographic (SPECT)

▲ **78650** Cerebrospinal fluid leakage detection and localization

(For injection procedure, see 61000-61070, 62270-62294)

(For myelin basic protein, CSF, use 83873)

(78652 has been deleted. To report, use 78647)

78660 Radiopharmaceutical dacryocystography

78699 Unlisted nervous system procedure, diagnostic nuclear medicine

GENITOURINARY SYSTEM

78700 Kidney imaging; static only

78701   with vascular flow

78704   with function study (ie, imaging renogram)

78707 Kidney imaging with vascular flow and function; single study without pharmacological intervention

78708   single study, with pharmacological intervention (eg, angiotensin converting enzyme inhibitor and/or diuretic)

78709   multiple studies, with and without pharmacological intervention (eg, angiotensin converting enzyme inhibitor and/or diuretic)

(For introduction of radioactive substance in association with renal endoscopy, see 50559, 50578)

78710 Kidney imaging, tomographic (SPECT)

78715 Kidney vascular flow only

● New Code ▲ Revised Code * Starred Procedure + Add-On Code ⊘ Modifier -51 Exempt

78725 Kidney function study, non-imaging radioisotopic study

(For renin (angiotensin I), use 84244)

(For angiotensin II, use 82163)

(For beta-2 microglobulin, use 82232)

78730 Urinary bladder residual study

(For introduction of radioactive substance in association with cystotomy or cystostomy, use 51020; in association with cystourethroscopy, use 52250)

78740 Ureteral reflux study (radiopharmaceutical voiding cystogram)

(For catheterization, see 53670, 53675)

(For estradiol, use 82670)

(For estriol, use 82677)

(For progesterone, use 84144)

(For prostatic acid phosphatase, use 84066)

78760 Testicular imaging;

78761   with vascular flow

(For testosterone, blood or urine, use 84403)

(For introduction of radioactive substance in association with ureteral endoscopy, see 50959, 50978)

(For lactogen, human placental (HPL) chorionic somatomammotropin, use 83632)

(For chronic gonadotropin, beta subunit, see 84702, 84703)

(For pregnanediol, use 84135)

(For pregnanetriol, use 84138)

78799 Unlisted genitourinary procedure, diagnostic nuclear medicine

(For chemical analysis, see Chemistry section)

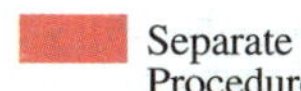
Separate
Procedure

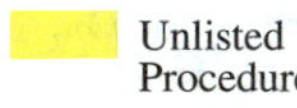
Unlisted
Procedure

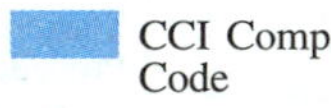
CCI Comp.
Code

Non-specific
Procedure

OTHER PROCEDURES

(For specific organ, see appropriate heading)

(For radiophosphorus tumor identification, ocular, see 78800)

78800 Radiopharmaceutical localization of tumor; limited area

(For specific organ, see appropriate heading)

78801   multiple areas

78802   whole body

78803   tomographic (SPECT)

78805 Radiopharmaceutical localization of inflammatory process; limited area

78806   whole body

78807   tomographic (SPECT)

(For imaging bone infectious or inflammatory disease with a bone imaging radiopharmaceutical, see 78300, 78305, 78306)

(For RAST, see 82785, 83518, 86003, 86005)

(For gamma-E immunoglobulin, use 82785)

(For gamma-G immunoglobulin, use 82784)

(For alpha-1 antitrypsin, see 82103, 82104)

(For alpha-1 fetoprotein, see 82105, 82106)

(For amikacin, use 80150)

(For aminophylline, use 80198)

(For amitriptyline, use 80152)

(For amphetamine, chemical quantitative, use 82145)

(For chlordiazepoxide, see code for specific method)

(For chlorpromazine, see phenothiazine, urine 84022)

(For clonazepam, use 80154)

(For cocaine, quantitative, use 82520)

● New Code   ▲ Revised Code   ✶ Starred Procedure   ✚ Add-On Code   ⊘ Modifier -51 Exempt

(For diazepam, use 80154)

(For dihydromorphinone, quantititave, use 82649)

(For diphenylhydantoin, use 80185)

(For flucytosine, see code for specific method)

(For gentamicin, use 80170)

(For lactic dehydrogenase, use 83615)

(For lysergic acid diethylamide (LSD), see 80100-80103, 80299)

(For morphine (heroin), see 80100-80103, 83925)

(For phencyclidine (PCP), see 80100-80103, 83992)

(For phenobarbital, see barbiturates 80100-80103, 82205)

(For phenytoin (diphenylthydantoin), use 80185)

(For tobramycin, use 80200)

78810 Tumor imaging, positron emission tomography (PET), metabolic evaluation

78890 Generation of automated data: interactive process involving nuclear physician and/or allied health professional personnel; simple manipulations and interpretation, not to exceed 30 minutes

78891 complex manipulations and interpretation, exceeding 30 minutes

(Use 78890 or 78891 in addition to primary procedure)

78990 Provision of diagnostic radiopharmaceutical(s)

78999 Unlisted miscellaneous procedure, diagnostic nuclear medicine

THERAPEUTIC

79000 Radiopharmaceutical therapy, hyper-thyroidism; initial, including evaluation of patient

79001 subsequent, each therapy

(For follow-up visit, see 99211-99215)

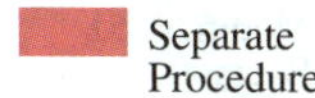 Separate Procedure

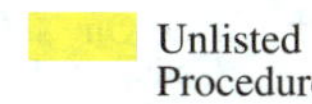 Unlisted Procedure

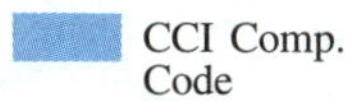 CCI Comp. Code

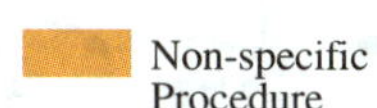 Non-specific Procedure

79020 Radiopharmaceutical therapy, thyroid suppression (euthyroid cardiac disease), including evaluation of patient

79030 Radiopharmaceutical ablation of gland for thyroid carcinoma

79035 Radiopharmaceutical therapy for metastases of thyroid carcinoma

79100 Radiopharmaceutical therapy, polycythemia vera, chronic leukemia, each treatment

79200 Intracavitary radioactive colloid therapy

79300 Interstitial radioactive colloid therapy

79400 Radiopharmaceutical therapy, nonthyroid, nonhematologic

79420 Intravascular radiopharmaceutical therapy, particulate

79440 Intra-articular radiopharmaceutical therapy

79900 Provision of therapeutic radiopharmaceutical(s)

79999 Unlisted radiopharmaceutical therapeutic procedure

● New Code   ▲ Revised Code   ＊ Starred Procedure   ＋ Add-On Code   ⊘ Modifier -51 Exempt

PATHOLOGY/ LABORATORY

LABORATORY SECTION OVERVIEW

The fifth section of the CPT coding system is the laboratory section, which includes codes for pathology and laboratory services. Within each subsection, the CPT codes are arranged by the type of testing or service.

LABORATORY SUBSECTIONS

The PATHOLOGY AND LABORATORY section of CPT is divided into 16 subsections:

Organ or Disease Oriented Panels	80048-80090
Drug Testing	80100-80103
Therapeutic Drug Assays	80150-80299
Evocative/Suppression Testing	80400-80440
Consultations (Clinical Pathology)	80500-80502
Urinalysis	81000-81999
Chemistry	82000-84999
Hematology and Coagulation	85000-85999
Immunology	86000-86849
Transfusion Medicine	86850-86999
Microbiology	87000-87999
Anatomic Pathology	88000-88099
Cytopathology	88100-88199
Cytogenetic Studies	88200-88299
Surgical Pathology	88300-88399
Other Procedures	89000-89399

LABORATORY SERVICES MODIFIERS

Pathology and laboratory services and procedures may be modified under certain circumstances. When applicable, the modifying circumstances should be identified by adding the appropriate modifier to the basic service code. The addition of modifier -22 requires a special report. Modifiers commonly used to report PATHOLOGY and LABORATORY procedures include:

-22   unusual services

-26   professional component

-32   mandated services

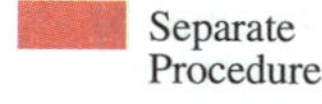

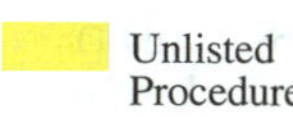

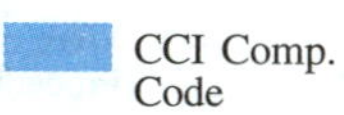

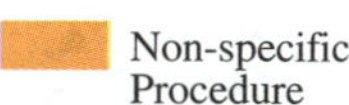

-52   reduced services

-90   reference (outside) laboratory

ANATOMIC/CLINICAL PATHOLOGY

Pathology is that discipline of the practice of medicine that deals with the causes and nature of disease. It contributes to diagnosis, prognosis, and treatment through knowledge gained by the laboratory application of the biologic, chemical, and physical sciences to man, or materials obtained from man. Pathologists diagnose, exclude, and monitor disease by means of information gathered from the microscopic examination of tissue specimens, cells, and body fluids, and from clinical laboratory tests on body fluids and secretions. Pathologists are involved with the management of laboratories and in data processing and with new developments in high technology.

CLINICAL PATHOLOGY

Clinical Pathology focuses on microbiology (including bacteriology, mycology, parasitology, and virology), immunopathology, blood banking/transfusion medicine, chemical pathology, cytogenetics, hematology, coagulation, toxicology, medical microscopy (including urinalysis), molecular biologic techniques, and other advanced diagnostic techniques as they become available.

---

676   ● New Code   ▲ Revised Code   ✻ Starred Procedure   ✚ Add-On Code   ⊘ Modifier -51 Exempt

PATHOLOGY AND LABORATORY

ORGAN OR DISEASE ORIENTED PANELS

CPT codes for organ or disease oriented panels were included in CPT due to the increased use of general screening programs by physicians, clinics, hospitals, and other health care facilities. Other codes in this section define profiles that combine laboratory tests together under a problem oriented classification.

There is a list of specific laboratory tests under each of the panel CPT codes which define the components of each panel. However, each laboratory typically establishes its own profile and provides a listing of the components of that panel performed by the laboratory with test results.

80048   Basic metabolic panel

This panel must include the following:
Calcium (82310)
Carbon dioxide (82374)
Chloride (82435)
Creatinine (82565)
Glucose (82947)
Potassium (84132)
Sodium (84295)
Urea Nitrogen (BUN) (84520)

(Do not use 80048 in addition to 80053)

80050   General health panel

This panel must include the following:
Comprehensive metabolic panel (80054)
Hemogram, automated, and manual differential WBC count
  (CBC) (85022) OR
Hemogram and platelet count, automated, and automated
  complete differential WBC count (CBC) (85025)
Thyroid stimulating hormone (TSH) (84443)

80051   Electrolyte panel

This panel must include the following:
Carbon dioxide (82374)
Chloride (82435)
Potassium (84132)
Sodium (84295)

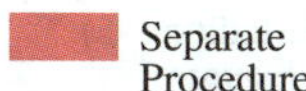

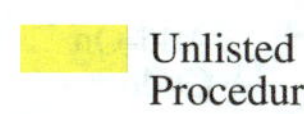

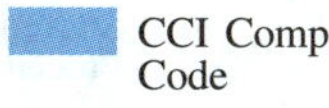

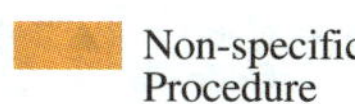

80053   Comprehensive metabolic panel

This panel must include the following:
Albumin (82040)
Bilirubin, total (82247)
Calcium (82310)
Carbon dioxide (bicarbonate) (82374)
Chloride (82435)
Creatinine (82565)
Glucose (82947)
Phosphatase, alkaline (84075)
Potassium (84132)
Protein, total (84155)
Sodium (84295)
Transferase, alanine amino (ALT) (SGPT) (84460)
Transferase, aspartate amino (AST) (SGOT) (84450)
Urea Nitrogen (BUN) (84520)

(Do not use 80053 in addition to 80048, 80076)

80055   Obstetric panel

This panel must include the following:
Hemogram, automated, and manual differential WBC count
   (CBC) (85022) OR
Hemogram and platelet count, automated, and automated
   complete differential WBC count (CBC) (85025)
Hepatitis B surface antigen (HBsAg) (87340)
Antibody, rubella (86762)
Syphilis test, qualitative (eg, VDRL, RPR, ART) (86592)
Antibody screen, RBC, each serum technique (86850)
Blood typing, ABO (86900) AND
Blood typing, Rh (D) (86901)

80061   Lipid panel

This panel must include the following:
Cholesterol, serum, total (82465)
Lipoprotein, direct measurement, high density cholesterol (HDL
   cholesterol) (83718)
Triglycerides (84478)

  ● New Code   ▲ Revised Code   ✳ Starred Procedure   ✚ Add-On Code   ⊘ Modifier -51 Exempt

80069 Renal function panel

This panel must include the following:
Albumin (82040)
Calcium (82310)
Carbon dioxide (bicarbonate) (82374)
Chloride (82435)
Creatinine (82565)
Glucose (82947)
Phosphorus inorganic (phosphate) (84100)
Potassium (84132)
Sodium (84295)
Urea nitrogen (BUN) (84520)

(80072 deleted 2002 edition. To report, see 84550, 85651, 86255, 86430)

80074 Acute hepatitis panel

This panel must include the following:
Hepatitis A antibody (HAAb), IgM antibody (86709)
Hepatitis B core antibody (HbcAb), IgM antibody (86705)
Hepatitis B surface antigen (HbsAg) (87340)
Hepatitis C antibody (86803)

80076 Hepatic function panel

This panel must include the following:
Albumin (82040)
Bilirubin, total (82247)
Bilirubin, direct (82248)
Phosphatase, alkaline (84075)
Protein, total (84155)
Transferase, alanine amino (ALT) (SGPT) (84460)
Transferase, aspartate amino (AST) (SGOT) (84450)

80090 TORCH antibody panel

This panel must include the following tests:
Antibody, cytomegalovirus (CMV) (86644)
Antibody, herpes simplex, non-specific type test (86694)
Antibody, rubella (86762)
Antibody, toxoplasma (86777)

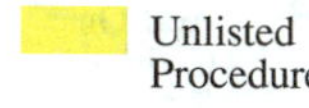

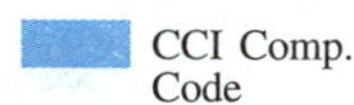

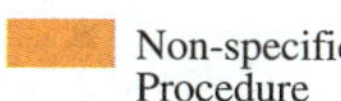

Non-specific
Procedure

679

DRUG TESTING

80100 Drug screen, qualitative; multiple drug classes, chromatographic method, each procedure

80101 single drug class method (eg, immunoassay, enzyme assay), each drug class

80102 Drug, confirmation, each procedure

80103 Tissue preparation for drug analysis

THERAPEUTIC DRUG ASSAYS

80150 Amikacin

80152 Amitriptyline

80154 Benzodiazepines

80156 Carbamazepine; total

80157 free

80158 Cyclosporine

80160 Desipramine

80162 Digoxin

80164 Dipropylacetic acid (valproic acid)

80166 Doxepin

80168 Ethosuximide

80170 Gentamicin

80172 Gold

80173 Haloperidol

80174 Imipramine

---

680   ● New Code   ▲ Revised Code   ✳ Starred Procedure   ✛ Add-On Code   ⊘ Modifier -51 Exempt

80176   Lidocaine

80178   Lithium

80182   Nortriptyline

80184   Phenobarbital

80185   Phenytoin; total

80186   free

80188   Primidone

80190   Procainamide;

80192   with metabolites (eg, n-acetyl procainamide)

80194   Quinidine

80196   Salicylate

80197   Tacrolimus

80198   Theophylline

80200   Tobramycin

80201   Topiramate

80202   Vancomycin

80299   Quantitation of drug, not elsewhere specified

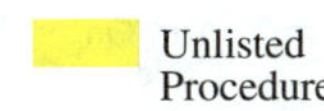 Separate Procedure   Unlisted Procedure   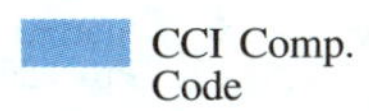 CCI Comp. Code   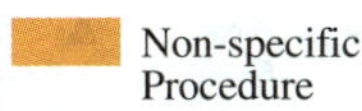 Non-specific Procedure

EVOCATIVE/SUPPRESSION TESTING

80400 ACTH stimulation panel; for adrenal insufficiency

This panel must include the following:
Cortisol (82533 x 2)

80402 for 21 hydroxylase deficiency

This panel must include the following:
Cortisol (82533 x 2)
17 hydroxyprogesterone (83498 x 2)

80406 for 3 beta-hydroxydehydrogenase deficiency

This panel must include the following:
Cortisol (82533 x 2)
17 hydroxypregnenolone (84143 x 2)

80408 Aldosterone suppression evaluation panel (eg, saline infusion)

This panel must include the following:
Aldosterone (82088 x 2)
Renin (84244 x 2)

80410 Calcitonin stimulation panel (eg, calcium, pentagastrin)

This panel must include the following:
Calcitonin (82308 x 3)

80412 Corticotropic releasing hormone (CRH) stimulation panel

This panel must include the following:
Cortisol (82533 x 6)
Adrenocorticotropic hormone (ACTH) (82024 x 6)

80414 Chorionic gonadotropin stimulation panel; testosterone response.

This panel must include the following:
Testosterone (84403 x 2 on three pooled blood samples)

80415 estradiol response.

This panel must include the following:
Estradiol (82670 x 2 on three pooled blood samples)

● New Code   ▲ Revised Code   ✳ Starred Procedure   ✚ Add-On Code   ⊘ Modifier -51 Exempt

80416   Renal vein renin stimulation panel (eg, captopril)

This panel must include the following:
Renin (84244 x 6)

80417   Peripheral vein renin stimulation panel (eg, captopril)

This panel must include the following:
Renin (84244 x 2)

80418   Combined rapid anterior pituitary evaluation panel

This panel must include the following:
Adrenocorticotropic hormone (ACTH) (82024 x 4)
Luteinizing hormone (LH) (83002 x 4)
Follicle stimulating hormone (FSH) (83001 x 4)
Prolactin (84146 x 4)
Human growth hormone (HGH)(83003 x 4)
Cortisol (82533 x 4)
Thyroid stimulating hormone (TSH) (84443 x 4)

80420   Dexamethasone suppression panel, 48 hour

This panel must include the following:
Free cortisol, urine (82530 x 2)
Cortisol (82533 x 2)
Volume measurement for timed collection (81050 x 2)
(For single dose dexamethasone, use 82533)

80422   Glucagon tolerance panel; for insulinoma

This panel must include the following:
Glucose (82947 x 3)
Insulin (83525 x 3)

80424   for pheochromocytoma.

This panel must include the following:
Catecholamines, fractionated (82384 x 2)

80426   Gonadotropin releasing hormone stimulation panel

This panel must include the following:
Follicle stimulating hormone (FSH) (83001 x 4)
Luteinizing hormone (LH)(83002 x 4)

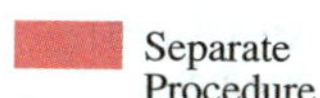 Separate Procedure

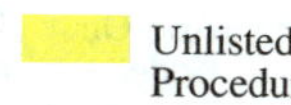 Unlisted Procedure

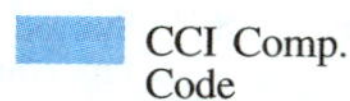 CCI Comp. Code

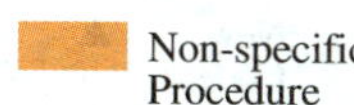 Non-specific Procedure

80428   Growth hormone stimulation panel (eg, arginine infusion, l-dopa administration)

This panel must include the following:
Human growth hormone (HGH)(83003 x 4)

80430   Growth hormone suppression panel (glucose administration)

This panel must include the following:
Glucose (82947 x 3)
Human growth hormone (HGH)(83003 x 4)

80432   Insulin-induced C-peptide suppression panel

This panel must include the following:
Insulin (83525)
C-peptide (84681 x 5)
Glucose (82947 x 5)

80434   Insulin tolerance panel; for ACTH insufficiency

This panel must include the following:
Cortisol (82533 x 5)
Glucose (82947 x 5)

80435   for growth hormone deficiency

This panel must include the following:
Glucose (82947 x 5)
Human growth hormone (HGH) (83003 x 5)

80436   Metyrapone panel

This panel must include the following:
Cortisol (82533 x 2)
11 deoxycortisol (82634 x 2)

80438   Thyrotropin releasing hormone (TRH) stimulation panel; one hour

This panel must include the following:
Thyroid stimulating hormone (TSH) (84443 x 3)

80439   two hour

This panel must include the following:
Thyroid stimulating hormone (TSH) (84443 x 4)

   ● New Code   ▲ Revised Code   * Starred Procedure   + Add-On Code   ⊘ Modifier -51 Exempt

80440   for hyperprolactinemia

This panel must include the following:
Prolactin (84146 x 3)

CONSULTATIONS (CLINICAL PATHOLOGY)

80500   Clinical pathology consultation; limited, without review of patients history and medical records

80502   comprehensive, for a complex diagnostic problem, with review of patients history and medical records

(These codes may also be used for pharmacokinetic consultations)

(For consultations involving the examination and evaluation of the patient, see 99241-99275)

URINALYSIS

81000   Urinalysis, by dip stick or tablet reagent for bilirubin, glucose, hemoglobin, ketones, leukocytes, nitrite, pH, protein, specific gravity,urobilinogen, any number of these constituents; non-automated, with microscopy

81001   automated, with microscopy

81002   non-automated, without microscopy

81003   automated, without microscopy

81005   Urinalysis; qualitative or semiquantitative, except immunoassays

(For non-immunoassay reagent strip urinalysis, see 81000, 81002)

(For immunoassay, qualitative or semiquantitative, use 83518)

(For microalbumin, see 82043, 82044)

81007   bacteriuria screen, except by culture or dipstick

(For culture, see 87086-87088)

(For dipstick, use 81000 or 81002)

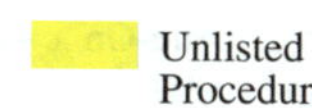

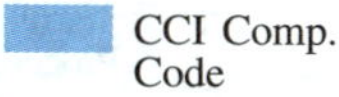

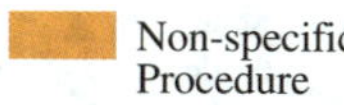

685

81015	microscopic only
81020	two or three glass test
81025	Urine pregnancy test, by visual color comparison methods
81050	Volume measurement for timed collection, each
81099	Unlisted urinalysis procedure

CHEMISTRY

82000	Acetaldehyde, blood
82003	Acetaminophen
82009	Acetone or other ketone bodies, serum; qualitative
82010	quantitative
82013	Acetylcholinesterase

(Acid, gastric, see gastric acid, 82926, 82928)

(Acid phosphatase, see 84060-84066)

82016	Acylcarnitines; qualitative, each specimen
82017	quantitative, each specimen

(For carnitine, use 82379)

82024	Adrenocorticotropic hormone (ACTH)
82030	Adenosine, 5-monophosphate, cyclic (cyclic AMP)
82040	Albumin; serum
82042	urine, quantitative, each specimen
82043	urine, microalbumin, quantitative
82044	urine, microalbumin, semiquantitative (eg, reagent strip assay)

● New Code	▲ Revised Code	✳ Starred Procedure	✚ Add-On Code	⊘ Modifier -51 Exempt

(For prealbumin, use 84134)

82055   Alcohol (ethanol); any specimen except breath

(For other volatiles, alcohol, use 84600)

82075   breath

82085   Aldolase

82088   Aldosterone

(Alkaline phosphatase, see 84075, 84080)

82101   Alkaloids, urine, quantitative

(Alphaketoglutarate, see 82009, 82010)

(Alpha tocopherol (Vitamin E), use 84446)

82103   Alpha-1-antitrypsin; total

82104   phenotype

82105   Alpha-fetoprotein; serum

82106   amniotic fluid

82108   Aluminum

82120   Amines, vaginal fluid, qualitative

(For combined pH and amines test for vaginitis, use 82120 and 83986)

82127   Amino acids; single, qualitative, each specimen

82128   multiple, qualitative, each specimen

82131   single, quantitative, each specimen

82135   Aminolevulinic acid, delta (ALA)

82136   Amino acids, 2 to 5 amino acids, quantitative, each specimen

Separate Procedure	Unlisted Procedure	CCI Comp. Code	Non-specific Procedure

82139 Amino acids, 6 or more amino acids, quantitative, each specimen

82140 Ammonia

82143 Amniotic fluid scan (spectrophotometric)

(For L/S ratio, use 83661)

(Amobarbital, see 80100-80103 for qualitative analysis, 82205 for quantitative analysis)

82145 Amphetamine or methamphetamine

(For qualitative analysis, see 80100-80103)

82150 Amylase

82154 Androstanediol glucuronide

82157 Androstenedione

82160 Androsterone

82163 Angiotensin II

82164 Angiotensin I - converting enzyme (ACE)

(Antidiuretic hormone (ADH), use 84588)

(Antimony, use 83015)

(Antitrypsin, alph-1-, see 82103, 82104)

82172 Apolipoprotein, each

82175 Arsenic

(For heavy metal screening, use 83015)

82180 Ascorbic acid (Vitamin C), blood

(Aspirin, see acetylsalicylic acid, 80196)

(Atherogenic index, blood, ultracentrifugation, quantitative, use 83717)

82190 Atomic absorption spectroscopy, each analyte

● New Code   ▲ Revised Code   ✳ Starred Procedure   ✚ Add-On Code   ⃠ Modifier -51 Exempt

82205   Barbiturates, not elsewhere specified

(For qualitative analysis, see 80100-80103)

82232   Beta-2 microglobulin

(Bicarbonate, use 82374)

82239   Bile acids; total

82240   cholylglycine

(For bile pigments, urine, see 81000-81005)

82247   Bilirubin; total

82248   direct

(82251   deleted 2001 edition. To report, use 82247 and 82248)

82252   feces, qualitative

82261   Biotinidase, each specimen

▲ **82270**   Blood, occult, by peroxidase activity (eg, guaiac), qualitative; feces, 1-3 simultaneous determinations

▲ **82273**   other sources

(Blood urea nitrogen (BUN), see 84520, 84525)

● **82274**   Blood, occult, by fecal hemoglobin determination by immunoassay, qualitative, feces, 1-3 simultaneous determinations

82286   Bradykinin

82300   Cadmium

82306   Calcifediol (25-OH Vitamin D-3)

82307   Calciferol (Vitamin D)

(For 1,25-Dihydroxyvitamin D, use 82652)

82308   Calcitonin

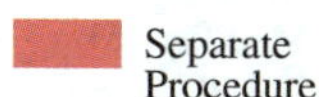

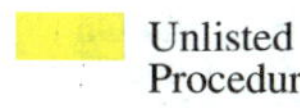

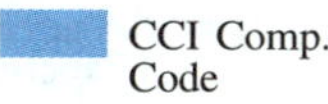

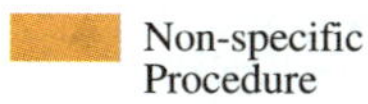

689

82310	Calcium; total	
82330		ionized
82331		after calcium infusion test
82340		urine quantitative, timed specimen

▲ **82355** Calculus; qualitative analysis

82360 quantitative analysis, chemical

82365 infrared spectroscopy

82370 x-ray diffraction

(Carbamates, see individual listings)

82373 Carbohydrate deficient transferrin

82374 Carbon dioxide (bicarbonate)

(See also 82803)

82375 Carbon monoxide, (carboxyhemoglobin); quantitative

82376 qualitative

82378 Carcinoembryonic antigen (CEA)

82379 Carnitine (total and free), quantitative, each specimen

(For acylcarnitine, see 82016, 82017)

82380 Carotene

82382 Catecholamines; total urine

82383 blood

82384 fractionated

(For urine metabolites, see 83835, 84585)

82387 Cathepsin-D

● New Code ▲ Revised Code ✳ Starred Procedure ✦ Add-On Code ⊘ Modifier -51 Exempt

82390   Ceruloplasmin

82397   Chemiluminescent assay

82415   Chloramphenicol

82435   Chloride; blood

82436   urine

82438   other source

(For sweat collection by iontophoresis, use 89360)

82441   Chlorinated hydrocarbons, screen

(Chlorpromazine, use 84022)

(Cholecalciferol (Vitamin D), use 82307)

82465   Cholesterol, serum or whole blood, total

(For high density lipoprotein (HDL), use 83718)

82480   Cholinesterase; serum

82482   RBC

82485   Chondroitin B sulfate, quantitative

(Chorionic gonadotropin, see gonadotropin, 84702, 84703)

82486   Chromatography, qualitative; column (eg, gas liquid or HPLC), analyte not elsewhere specified

82487   paper, 1-dimensional, analyte not elsewhere specified

82488   paper, 2-dimensional, analyte not elsewhere specified

82489   thin layer, analyte not elsewhere specified

82491   Chromatography, quantitative, column (eg, gas liquid or HPLC); single analyte not elsewhere specified, single stationary and mobile phase

82492   multiple analytes, single stationary and mobile phase

691

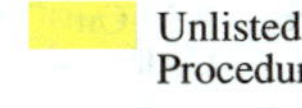
Separate
Procedure

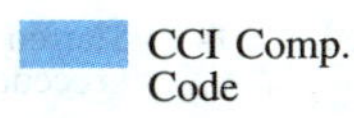
Unlisted
Procedure

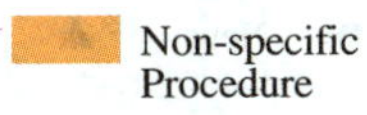
CCI Comp.
Code

Non-specific
Procedure

82495 Chromium

82507 Citrate

82520 Cocaine or metabolite

(Cocaine, qualitative analysis, see 80100-80103)

(Codeine, qualitative analysis, see 80100-80103)

(Codeine, quantitative analysis, see 82101)

(Complement, see 86160-86162)

82523 Collagen cross links, any method

82525 Copper

(Coproporphyrin, see 84119, 84120)

(Corticosteroids, use 83491)

82528 Corticosterone

82530 Cortisol; free

82533 total

(C-peptide, use 84681)

82540 Creatine

82541 Column chromatography/mass spectrometry (eg, GC/MS, or HPLC/MS), analyte not elsewhere specified; qualitative, single stationary and mobile phase

82542 quantitative, single stationary and mobile phase

82543 stable isotope dilution, single analyte, quantitative, single stationary and mobile phase

82544 stable isotope dilution, multiple analytes, quantitative, single stationary and mobile phase

82550 Creatine kinase (CK), (CPK); total

82552 isoenzymes

● New Code ▲ Revised Code ✳ Starred Procedure ✛ Add-On Code ⊘ Modifier -51 Exempt

82553   MB fraction only

82554   isoforms

82565   Creatinine; blood

82570   other source

82575   clearance

82585   Cryofibrinogen

82595   Cryoglobulin, qualitative or semi-quantitative (eg,cryocrit)

(For quantitative, cryoglobulin, see 82784, 82785)

(Crystals, pyrophosphate vs. urate, use 89060)

82600   Cyanide

82607   Cyanocobalamin (Vitamin B-12);

82608   unsaturated binding capacity

(Cyclic AMP, use 82030)

(Cyclic GMP, use 83008)

(Cyclosporine, use 80158)

82615   Cystine and homocystine, urine, qualitative

82626   Dehydroepiandrosterone (DHEA)

82627   Dehydroepiandrosterone-sulfate (DHEA-S)

(Delta-aminolevulinic acid (ALA), use 82135)

82633   Desoxycorticosterone, 11-

82634   Deoxycortisol, 11-

(Dexamethasone suppression test, use 80420)

(Diastase, urine, use 82150)

82638   Dibucaine number

(Dichloroethane, use 84600)

(Dichloromethane, use 84600)

(Diethylether, use 84600)

82646 Dihydrocodeinone

(For qualitative analysis, see 80100-80103)

82649 Dihydromorphinone

(For qualitative analysis, see 80100-80103)

82651 Dihydrotestosterone (DHT)

82652 Dihydroxyvitamin D, 1,25-

82654 Dimethadione

(For qualitative analysis, see 80100-80103)

(Diphenylhydantoin, use 80185)

(Dipropylacetic acid, use 80164)

(Dopamine, see 82382-82384)

(Duodenal contents, see individual enzymes; for intubation and collection, use 89100)

82657 Enzyme activity in blood cells, cultured cells, or tissue, not elsewhere specified; nonradioactive substrate, each specimen

82658   radioactive substrate, each specimen

82664 Electrophoretic technique, not elsewhere specified

(Endocrine receptor assays, see 84233-84235)'

82666 Epiandrosterone

(Epinephrine, see 82382-82384)

82668 Erythropoietin

82670 Estradiol

● New Code   ▲ Revised Code   * Starred Procedure   + Add-On Code   ⊘ Modifier -51 Exempt

82671   Estrogens; fractionated

82672   total

(Estrogen receptor assay, use 84233)

82677   Estriol

82679   Estrone

(Ethanol, see 82055 and 82075)

82690   Ethchlorvynol

(Ethyl alcohol, see 82055 and 82075)

82693   Ethylene glycol

82696   Etiocholanolone

(For fractionation of ketosteroids, use 83593)

82705   Fat or lipids, feces; qualitative

82710   quantitative

82715   Fat differential, feces, quantitative

82725   Fatty acids, nonesterified

82726   Very long chain fatty acids

82728   Ferritin

(Fetal hemoglobin, see hemoglobin 83030, 83033, and 85460)

(Fetoprotein, alpha-1, see 82105, 82106)

82731   Fetal fibronectin, cervicovaginal secretions, semi-quantitative

82735   Fluoride

82742   Flurazepam

(For qualitative analysis, see 80100-80103)

(Foam stability test, use 83662)

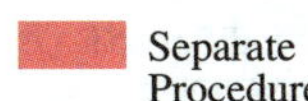
Separate
Procedure

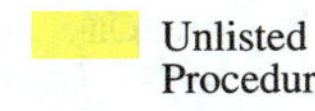
Unlisted
Procedure

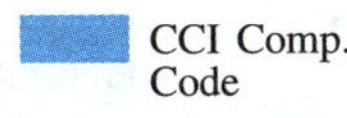
CCI Comp.
Code

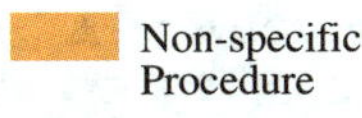
Non-specific
Procedure

82746   Folic acid; serum

82747   RBC

(Follicle stimulating hormone (FSH), use 83001)

82757   Fructose, semen

(Fructosamine, use 82985)

(Fructose, TLC screen, use 84375)

82759   Galactokinase, RBC

82760   Galactose

82775   Galactose-1-phosphate uridyl transferase; quantitative

82776   screen

82784   Gammaglobulin; IgA, IgD, IgG, IgM, each

82785   IgE

(For allergen specific IgE, see 86003, 86005)

82787   immunoglobulin subclasses, (IgG1, 2, 3, or 4), each

(Gamma-glutamyltransferase (GGT), use 82977)

82800   Gases, blood, pH only

82803   Gases, blood, any combination of pH, pCO$_2$, pO$_2$, CO$_2$, HCO3 (including calculated O2 saturation);

(Use 82803 for two or more of the above listed analytes)

82805   with O$_2$ saturation, by direct measurement, except pulse oximetry

82810   Gases, blood, O$_2$ saturation only, by direct measurement, except pulse oximetry

(For pulse oximetry, use 94760)

82820   Hemoglobin-oxygen affinity (pO$_2$ for 50% hemoglobin saturation with oxygen)

● New Code	▲ Revised Code	✳ Starred Procedure	✛ Add-On Code	⃠ Modifier -51 Exempt

82926 Gastric acid, free and total, each specimen

82928 Gastric acid, free or total; each specimen

82938 Gastrin after secretin stimulation

82941 Gastrin

(Gentamicin, use 80170)

(GGT, use 82977)

(GLC, gas liquid chromatography, use 82486)

82943 Glucagon

82945 Glucose, body fluid, other than blood

82946 Glucagon tolerance test

82947 Glucose; quantitative, blood, (except reagent strip)

82948 blood, reagent strip

82950 post glucose dose (includes glucose)

82951 tolerance test (GTT), three specimens (includes glucose)

82952 tolerance test, each additional beyond three specimens

82953 tolbutamide tolerance test

(For insulin tolerance test, see 80434, 80435)

(For leucine tolerance test, use 80428)

(For semiquantitative urine glucose, see 81000, 81002, 81005, 81099)

82955 Glucose-6-phosphate dehydrogenase (G6PD); quantitative

82960 screen

(For glucose tolerance test with medication, use 90784 in addition)

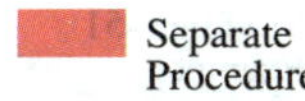 Separate Procedure

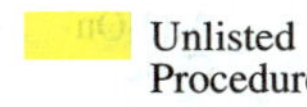 Unlisted Procedure

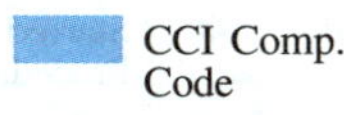 CCI Comp. Code

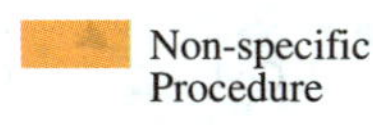 Non-specific Procedure

82962 Glucose, blood by glucose monitoring device(s) cleared by the FDA specifically for home use

82963 Glucosidase, beta

82965 Glutamate dehydrogenase

82975 Glutamine (glutamic acid amide)

82977 Glutamyltransferase, gamma (GGT)

82978 Glutathione

82979 Glutathione reductase, RBC

82980 Glutethimide

(Glycohemoglobin, use 83036)

82985 Glycated protein

(Gonadotropin, chorionic, see 84702, 84703)

83001 Gonadotropin; follicle stimulating hormone (FSH)

83002   luteinizing hormone (LH)

(For luteinizing releasing factor (LRH), use 83727)

83003 Growth hormone, human (HGH) (somatotropin)

(For antibody to human growth hormone, use 86277)

83008 Guanosine monophosphate (GMP), cyclic

83010 Haptoglobin; quantitative

83012   phenotypes

▲ **83013** Helicobacter pylori; analysis for urease activity, non-radioactive isotope

83014   drug administration and sample collection

● New Code ▲ Revised Code ✻ Starred Procedure ✚ Add-On Code ⊘ Modifier -51 Exempt

(For H. pylori, stool, use 87338. For H. pylori, liquid scintillation counter, see 78267, 78268. For H. pylori, enzyme immunoassay, use 87339)

83015 Heavy metal (arsenic, barium, beryllium, bismuth, antimony, mercury); screen

83018 quantitative, each

83020 Hemoglobin fractionation and quantitation; electrophoresis (eg, A2, S, C, and/or F)

83021 chromotography (eg, A2, S, C,and/or F)

83026 Hemoglobin; by copper sulfate method, non-automated

83030 F (fetal), chemical

83033 F (fetal), qualitative

83036 glycated

(For fecal hemoglobin detection by immunoassay, use 82274)

83045 methemoglobin, qualitative

83050 methemoglobin, quantitative

83051 plasma

83055 sulfhemoglobin, qualitative

83060 sulfhemoglobin, quantitative

83065 thermolabile

83068 unstable, screen

83069 urine

83070 Hemosiderin; qualitative

83071 quantitative

(Heroin, see 80100-80103)

(HIAA, use 83497)

(High performance liquid chromatography (HPLC), use 82486)

83080   b-Hexosaminidase, each assay

83088   Histamine

(Hollander test, use 91052)

83090   Homocystine

83150   Homovanillic acid (HVA)

(Hormones, see individual alphabetic listings in Chemistry section)

(Hydrogen breath test, use 91065)

83491   Hydroxycorticosteroids, 17- (17-OHCS)

(For cortisol, see 82530, 82533. For deoxycortisol, use 82634)

83497   Hydroxyindolacetic acid, 5-(HIAA)

(For urine qualitative test, use 81005)

(5-Hydroxytryptamine, use 84260)

83498   Hydroxyprogesterone, 17-d

83499   Hydroxyprogesterone, 20-

83500   Hydroxyproline; free

83505   total

83516   Immunoassay for analyte other than infectious agent antibody or infectious agent antigen, qualitative or semiquantitative; multiple step method

83518   single step method (eg, reagent strip)

83519   Immunoassay, analyte, quantitative; by radiopharmaceutical technique (eg, RIA)

83520   not otherwise specified

● New Code   ▲ Revised Code   * Starred Procedure   + Add-On Code   ⊘ Modifier -51 Exempt

(For immunoassays for antibodies to infectious agent antigens, see analyte and method specific codes in the Immunology section)

(For immunoassay of tumor antigen not elsewhere specified, use 86316)

(Immunoglobulins, see 82784, 82785)

83525   Insulin; total

(For proinsulin, use 84206)

83527   free

83528   Intrinsic factor

(For intrinsic factor antibodies, use 86340)

83540   Iron

83550   Iron binding capacity

83570   Isocitric dehydrogenase (IDH)

(Isonicotinic acid hydrazide, INH, see code for specific method)

(Isopropyl alcohol, use 84600)

83582   Ketogenic steroids, fractionation

(Ketone bodies, for serum, see 82009, 82010; for urine, see 81000-81003)

83586   Ketosteroids, 17- (17-KS); total

83593   fractionation

83605   Lactate (lactic acid)

83615   Lactate dehydrogenase (LD), (LDH);

83625   isoenzymes, separation and quantitation

83632   Lactogen, human placental (HPL) human chorionic somatomammotropin

---

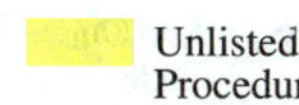
Separate
Procedure

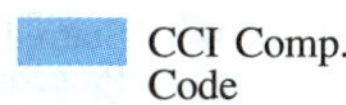
Unlisted
Procedure

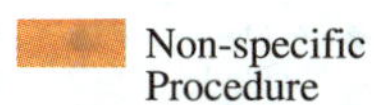
CCI Comp.
Code

Non-specific
Procedure

83633   Lactose, urine; qualitative

83634   quantitative

(For tolerance, see 82951, 82952)

(For breath hydrogen test for lactase deficiency, use 91065)

83655   Lead

83661   Fetal lung maturity assessment; lecithin-sphingomyelin ratio (L/S ratio)

83662   foam stability test

83663   fluorescence polarization

83664   lamellar body density

(For phosphatidylglycerol, use 84081)

83670   Leucine aminopeptidase (LAP)

83690   Lipase

83715   Lipoprotein, blood; electrophoretic separation and quantitation

83716   high resolution fractionation and quantitation of lipoprotein cholesterols (eg, electrophoresis, nuclear magnetic resonance, ultracentrifugation)

83718   Lipoprotein, direct measurement; high density cholesterol (HDL cholesterol)

83719   direct measurement, VLDL cholesterol

83721   direct measurement, LDL cholesterol

(For fractionation by nuclear magnetic resonance or high resolution electrophoresis, use 83716)

(To report direct measurement, intermediate density lipoproteins (remnant lipoproteins), use Category III code 0026T)

(Luteinizing hormone (LH), use 83002)

83727   Luteinizing releasing factor (LRH)

● New Code   ▲ Revised Code   ✱ Starred Procedure   + Add-On Code   ⊘ Modifier -51 Exempt

(For qualitative analysis, see 80100-80103)

(Macroglobulins, alpha-2, use 86329)

83735   Magnesium

83775   Malate dehydrogenase

(Maltose tolerance, see 82951, 82952)

(Mammotropin, use 84146)

83785   Manganese

(Marijuana, see 80100-80103)

83788   Mass spectrometry and tandem mass spectrometry (MS, MS/MS), analyte not elsewhere specified; qualitative, each specimen

83789   quantitative, each specimen

83805   Meprobamate

(For qualitative analysis, see 80100-80103)

83825   Mercury, quantitative

(Mercury screen, use 83015)

83835   Metanephrines

(For catecholamines, see 82382-82384)

83840   Methadone

(For methadone qualitative analysis, see 80100-80103)

(Methamphetamine, see 80100-80103, 82145)

(Methanol, use 84600)

83857   Methemalbumin

(Methemoglobin, see hemoglobin 83045, 83050)

83858   Methsuximide

 Separate Procedure

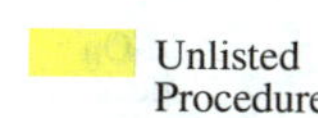 Unlisted Procedure

CCI Comp. Code

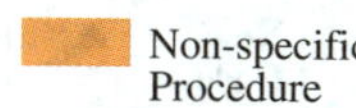 Non-specific Procedure

(Methyl alcohol, use 84600)

(Microalbumin, see 82043 for quantitative, see 82044 for semiquantitative)

(Microglobulin, beta-2, use 82232)

83864 Mucopolysaccharides, acid; quantitative

83866 screen

83872 Mucin, synovial fluid (Ropes test)

▲ **83873** Myelin basic protein, cerebrospinal fluid

(For oligoclonal bands, use 83916)

83874 Myoglobin

83883 Nephelometry, each analyte not elsewhere specified

83885 Nickel

83887 Nicotine

(For microbial identification, see 87797, 87798)

83890 Molecular diagnostics; molecular isolation or extraction

83891 isolation or extraction of highly purified nucleic acid

83892 enzymatic digestion

83893 dot/slot blot production

83894 separation by gel electrophoresis (eg, agarose, polyacrylamide)

83896 nucleic acid probe, each

83897 nucleic acid transfer (eg, Southern, Northern)

83898 amplification of patient nucleic acid (eg, PCR, LCR), single primer pair, each primer pair

83901 amplification of patient nucleic acid, multiplex, each multiplex reaction

● New Code　　▲ Revised Code　　＊ Starred Procedure　　✚ Add-On Code　　⊘ Modifier -51 Exempt

83902   reverse transcription

83903   mutation scanning, by physical properties (eg, single strand conformational polymorphisms (SSCP), heteroduplex, denaturing gradient gel electrophoresis (DGGE), RNA'ase A), single segment, each

83904   mutation identification by sequencing, single segment, each segment

83905   mutation identification by allele specific transcription, single segment, each segment

83906   mutation identification by allele specific translation, single segment, each segment

83912   interpretation and report

83915   Nucleotidase 5-

▲ **83916**   Oligoclonal immune (oligoclonal bands)

83918   Organic acids; total, quantitative, each specimen

83919   qualitative, each specimen

83921   Organic acid, single; quantitative

83925   Opiates, (eg, morphine, meperidine)

83930   Osmolality; blood

83935   urine

83937   Osteocalcin (bone g1a protein)

83945   Oxalate

● **83950**   Oncoprotein, HER-2/neu

(For tissue, see 88342, 88365)

83970   Parathormone (parathyroid hormone)

(Pesticide, quantitative, see code for specific method. For screen for chlorinated hydrocarbons, use 82441)

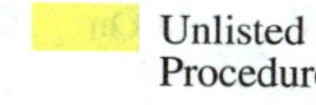
Separate Procedure

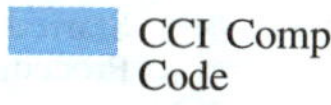
Unlisted Procedure

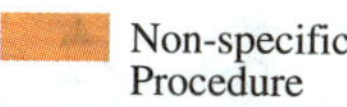
CCI Comp. Code

Non-specific Procedure

705

83986 pH, body fluid, except blood

(For blood pH, see 82800, 82803)

83992 Phencyclidine (PCP)

(For qualitative analysis, see 80100-80103)

(Phenobarbital, use 80184)

84022 Phenothiazine

(For qualitative analysis, see 80100, 80101)

84030 Phenylalanine (PKU), blood

(Phenylalanine-tyrosine ratio, see 84030, 84510)

84035 Phenylketones, qualitative

84060 Phosphatase, acid; total

84061 forensic examination

84066 prostatic

84075 Phosphatase, alkaline;

84078 heat stable (total not included)

84080 isoenzymes

84081 Phosphatidylglycerol

(Phosphates inorganic, use 84100)

(Phosphates, organic, see code for specific method. For cholinesterase, see 82480, 82482)

84085 Phosphogluconate, 6-, dehydrogenase, RBC

84087 Phosphohexose isomerase

84100 Phosphorus inorganic (phosphate);

84105 urine

● New Code   ▲ Revised Code   ✳ Starred Procedure   ✛ Add-On Code   ⊘ Modifier -51 Exempt

(Pituitary gonadotropins, see 83001-83002)

(PKU, see 84030, 84035)

84106 Porphobilinogen, urine; qualitative

84110   quantitative

84119 Porphyrins, urine; qualitative

84120   quantitation and fractionation

84126 Porphyrins, feces; quantitative

84127   qualitative

(Porphyrin precursors, see 82135, 84106, 84110)

(For protoporphyrin, RBC, see 84202, 84203)

84132 Potassium; serum

84133   urine

84134 Prealbumin

(For microalbumin, see 82043, 82044)

84135 Pregnanediol

84138 Pregnanetriol

84140 Pregnenolone

84143 17-hydroxypregnenolone

84144 Progesterone

(Progesterone receptor assay, use 84234)

(For proinsulin, use 84206)

84146 Prolactin

84150 Prostaglandin, each

84152 Prostate specific antigen (PSA); complexed (direct measurement)

Separate Procedure   Unlisted Procedure   CCI Comp. Code   Non-specific Procedure

84153   total

84154   free

84155   Protein; total, except refractometry

84160   refractometric

84165   electrophoretic fractionation and quantitation

84181   Western Blot, with interpretation and report, blood or other body fluid

84182   Western Blot, with interpretation and report, blood or other body fluid, immunological probe for band identification, each

(For Western Blot tissue analysis, use 88371)

84202   Protoporphyrin, RBC; quantitative

84203   screen

84206   Proinsulin

(Pseudocholinesterase, use 82480)

84207   Pyridoxal phosphate (Vitamin B-6)

84210   Pyruvate

84220   Pyruvate kinase

84228   Quinine

84233   Receptor assay; estrogen

84234   progesterone

84235   endocrine, other than estrogen or progesterone (specify hormone)

84238   non-endocrine (eg, acetylcholine) (specify receptor)

84244   Renin

● New Code   ▲ Revised Code   ✳ Starred Procedure   ✚ Add-On Code   ⊘ Modifier -51 Exempt

84252 Riboflavin (Vitamin B-2)

(Salicylates, use 80196)

(Secretin test, see 99070, 89100 and appropriate analyses)

84255 Selenium

84260 Serotonin

(For urine metabolites (HIAA), use 83497)

84270 Sex hormone binding globulin (SHBG)

84275 Sialic acid

(Sickle hemoglobin, use 85660)

84285 Silica

84295 Sodium; serum

84300 urine

(Somatomammotropin, use 83632)

(Somatotropin, use 83003)

84305 Somatomedin

84307 Somatostatin

84311 Spectrophotometry, analyte not elsewhere specified

84315 Specific gravity (except urine)

(For specific gravity, urine, see 81000-81003)

(Stone analysis, see 82355-82370)

84375 Sugars, chromatographic, TLC or paper chromatography

84376 Sugars (mono, di, and oligosaccharides); single qualitative, each specimen

84377 multiple qualitative, each specimen

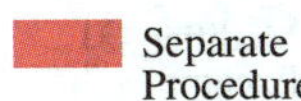 Separate Procedure

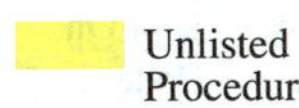 Unlisted Procedure

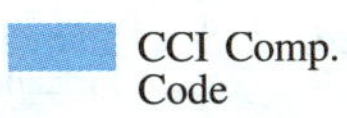 CCI Comp. Code

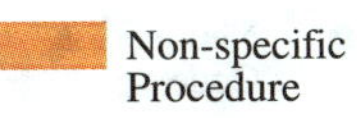 Non-specific Procedure

84378   single quantitative, each specimen

84379   multiple quantitative, each specimen

84392   Sulfate, urine

              (Sulfhemoglobin, see hemoglobin, 83055, 83060)

              (T-3, see 84479-84481)

              (T-4, see 84436-84439)

84402   Testosterone; free

84403   total

84425   Thiamine (Vitamin B-1)

84430   Thiocyanate

84432   Thyroglobulin

              (Thyroglobulin, antibody, use 86800)

              (Thyrotropin releasing hormone (TRH) test, see 80438, 80439)

84436   Thyroxine; total

84437   requiring elution (eg, neonatal)

84439   free

84442   Thyroxine binding globulin (TBG)

84443   Thyroid stimulating hormone (TSH)

▲ **84445**   Thyroid stimulating immune globulins (TSI)

              (Tobramycin, use 80200)

84446   Tocopherol alpha (Vitamin E)

              (Tolbutamide tolerance, use 82953)

84449   Transcortin (cortisol binding globulin)

84450   Transferase; aspartate amino (AST) (SGOT)

710

| ● New Code | ▲ Revised Code | ✱ Starred Procedure | ✛ Add-On Code | ⊘ Modifier -51 Exempt |

84460   alanine amino (ALT) (SGPT)

84466   Transferrin

(Iron binding capacity, use 83550)

84478   Triglycerides

84479   Thyroid hormone (T3 or T4) uptake or thyroid hormone binding ratio (THBR)

84480   Triiodothyronine T3; total (TT-3)

84481   free

84482   reverse

84484   Troponin, quantitative

(For Troponin, qualitative assay, use 84512)

84485   Trypsin; duodenal fluid

84488   feces, qualitative

84490   feces, quantitative, 24-hour collection

84510   Tyrosine

(Urate crystal identification, use 89060)

84512   Troponin, qualitative

(For Troponin, quantitative assay, use 84484)

84520   Urea nitrogen; quantitative

84525   semiquantitative (eg, reagent strip test)

84540   Urea nitrogen, urine

84545   Urea nitrogen, clearance

84550   Uric acid; blood

84560   other source

711

Separate Procedure   Unlisted Procedure   CCI Comp. Code   Non-specific Procedure

84577 Urobilinogen, feces, quantitative

84578 Urobilinogen, urine; qualitative

84580   quantitative, timed specimen

84583   semiquantitative

(Uroporphyrins, use 84120)

(Valproic acid (dipropylacetic acid), ues 80164)

84585 Vanillylmandelic acid (VMA), urine

84586 Vasoactive intestinal peptide (VIP)

84588 Vasopressin (antidiuretic hormone, ADH)

84590 Vitamin A

(Vitamin B-1, use 84425)

(Vitamin B-2, use 84252)

(Vitamin B-6, use 84207)

(Vitamin B-12, use 82607)

(Vitamin B-12, absorption (Schilling), see 78270, 78271)

(Vitamin C, use 82180)

(Vitamin D, see 82306, 82307, 82652)

(Vitamin E, use 84446)

84591 Vitamin, not otherwise specified

84597 Vitamin K

(VMA, use 84585)

84600 Volatiles (eg, acetic anhydride, carbon tetrachloride, dichloroethane, dichloromethane, diethylether, isopropyl alcohol, methanol)

(For acetaldehyde, use 82000)

(Volume, blood, RISA or Cr-51, see 78110, 78111)

● New Code   ▲ Revised Code   * Starred Procedure   + Add-On Code   ⊘ Modifier -51 Exempt

84620   Xylose absorption test, blood and/or urine

(For administration, use 99070)

84630   Zinc

84681   C-peptide

84702   Gonadotropin, chorionic (hCG); quantitative

84703   qualitative

(For urine pregnancy test by visual color comparison, use 81025)

84830   Ovulation tests, by visual color comparison methods for human luteinizing hormone

84999   Unlisted chemistry procedure

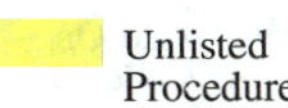 Separate Procedure

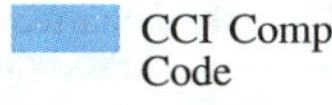 Unlisted Procedure

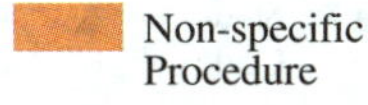 CCI Comp. Code

Non-specific Procedure

HEMATOLOGY AND COAGULATION

(For blood banking procedures, see Transfusion Medicine)

(Agglutinins, see Immunology)

(Antiplasmin, use 85410)

(Antithrombin III, see 85300, 85301)

85002 Bleeding time

85007 Blood count; manual differential WBC count (includes RBC morphology and platelet estimation)

85008 manual blood smear examination without differential parameters

(See also 85585)

(For other fluids (eg, CSF), see 89050, 89051)

85009 differential WBC count, buffy coat

(Eosinophils, nasal smear, use 89190)

85013 spun microhematocrit

85014 other than spun hematocrit

85018 hemoglobin

(For other hemoglobin determination, see 83020-83069)

(For immunoassay, hemoglobin, fecal, use 86683)

85021 hemogram, automated (RBC, WBC, Hgb, Hct and indices only)

85022 hemogram, automated, and manual differential WBC count (CBC)

85023 hemogram and platelet count, automated, and manual differential WBC count (CBC)

85024 hemogram and platelet count, automated, and automated partial differential WBC count (CBC)

● New Code   ▲ Revised Code   ✱ Starred Procedure   ✛ Add-On Code   ⃠ Modifier -51 Exempt

85025   hemogram and platelet count, automated, and automated complete differential WBC count (CBC)

85027   hemogram and platelet count, automated

85031   Blood count; hemogram, manual, complete CBC (RBC, WBC, Hgb, Hct, differential and indices)

85041   red blood cell (RBC) only

(See also 85021-85031, 89050)

85044   reticulocyte count, manual

85045   reticulocyte count, flow cytometry

85046   reticulocytes, hemoglobin concentration

85048   white blood cell (WBC)

(See also 85021-85031)

85060   Blood smear, peripheral, interpretation by physician with written report

(**85095**   deleted 2002 edition. To report, use 38220)

▲ **85097**   Bone marrow, smear interpretation

(For special stains, see 85540, 88312, 88313)

(**85102**   deleted 2002 edition. To report, use 38221)

(For bone biopsy, see 20220, 20225, 20240, 20245, 20250, 20251)

85130   Chromogenic substrate assay

(Circulating anti-coagulant screen (mixing studies), see 85611, 85732)

85170   Clot retraction

85175   Clot lysis time, whole blood dilution

(Clotting factor I (fibrinogen), see 85384, 85385)

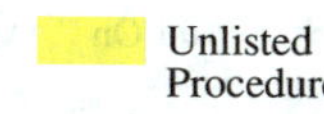
Separate Procedure

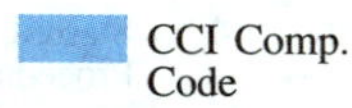
Unlisted Procedure

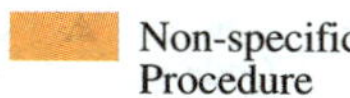
CCI Comp. Code

Non-specific Procedure

715

85210 Clotting; factor II, prothrombin, specific

(See also 85610-85613)

85220 factor V (AcG or proaccelerin), labile factor

85230 factor VII (proconvertin, stable factor)

85240 factor VIII (AHG), one stage

85244 factor VIII related antigen

85245 factor VIII, VW factor, ristocetin cofactor

85246 factor VIII, VW factor antigen

85247 factor VIII, von Willebrands factor, multimetric analysis

85250 factor IX (PTC or Christmas)

85260 factor X (Stuart-Prower)

85270 factor XI (PTA)

85280 factor XII (Hageman)

85290 factor XIII (fibrin stabilizing)

85291 factor XIII (fibrin stabilizing), screen solubility

85292 prekallikrein assay (Fletcher factor assay)

85293 high molecular weight kininogen assay (Fitzgerald factor assay)

85300 Clotting inhibitors or anticoagulants; antithrombin III, activity

85301 antithrombin III, antigen assay

85302 protein C, antigen

85303 protein C, activity

85305 protein S, total

● New Code ▲ Revised Code ✳ Starred Procedure ✚ Add-On Code ⊘ Modifier -51 Exempt

85306   protein S, free

85307 Activated Protein C (APC) resistance assay

85335 Factor inhibitor test

85337 Thrombomodulin

(For mixing studies for inhibitors, use 85732)

85345 Coagulation time; Lee and White

85347   activated

85348   other methods

(Differential count, see 85007 et seq)

(Duke bleeding time, use 85002)

(Eosinophils, nasal smear, use 89190)

85360 Euglobulin lysis

(Fetal hemoglobin, see 83030, 83033, 85460)

85362 Fibrin(ogen) degradation (split) products (FDP)(FSP); agglutination slide, semiquantitative

(Immunoelectrophoresis, use 86320)

85366   paracoagulation

85370   quantitative

85378 Fibrin degradation products, D-dimer; semiquantitative

85379   quantitative

85384 Fibrinogen; activity

85385   antigen

85390 Fibrinolysins or coagulopathy screen, interpretation and report

85400 Fibrinolytic factors and inhibitors; plasmin

Separate Procedure   Unlisted Procedure   CCI Comp. Code   Non-specific Procedure

85410	alpha-2 antiplasmin
85415	plasminogen activator
85420	plasminogen, except antigenic assay
85421	plasminogen, antigenic assay

(Fragility, red blood cell, see 85547, 85555-85557)

85441	Heinz bodies; direct
85445	induced, acetyl phenylhydrazine

(Hematocrit (PCV), see 85014, 85021-85031)

(Hemoglobin, see 83020-83068, 85018-85031)

85460 Hemoglobin or RBCs, fetal, for fetomaternal hemorrhage; differential lysis (Kleihauer-Betke)

(See also 83030, 83033)

(Hemogram, see 85021-85031)

(Hemolysins, see 86940, 86941)

85461	rosette
85475	Hemolysin, acid

(See also 86940, 86941)

85520	Heparin assay
85525	Heparin neutralization
85530	Heparin-protamine tolerance test

(85535   deleted 2002 edition. To report, use 85536)

85536 Iron stain, peripheral blood

(For iron stains on bone marrow or other tissues with physician evaluation, use 88313)

85540 Leukocyte alkaline phosphatase with count

85547   Mechanical fragility, RBC

85549   Muramidase

(Nitroblue tetrazolium dye test, use 86384)

85555   Osmotic fragility, RBC; unincubated

85557   incubated

(Packed cell volume, use 85013)

(Partial thromboplastin time, see 85730, 85732)

(Parasites, blood (eg, malaria smears), use 87207)

(Plasmin, use 85400)

(Plasminogen, use 85420)

(Plasminogen activator, use 85415)

85576   Platelet; aggregation (in vitro), each agent

85585   estimation on smear, only

(See also 85008)

85590   manual count

85595   automated count

85597   Platelet neutralization

85610   Prothrombin time;

85611   substitution, plasma fractions, each

85612   Russell viper venom time (includes venom); undiluted

85613   diluted

(Red blood cell count, see 85021, 85031, 85041)

85635   Reptilase test

(Reticulocyte count, see 85044, 85045)

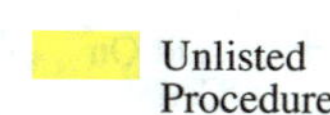

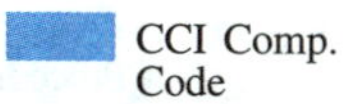

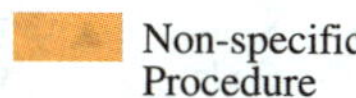

85651   Sedimentation rate, erythrocyte; non-automated

85652   automated

85660   Sickling of RBC, reduction

(Hemoglobin electrophoresis, use 83020)

(Smears (eg, for parasites, malaria), use 87207)

85670   Thrombin time; plasma

85675   titer

85705   Thromboplastin inhibition; tissue

(For individual clotting factors, see 85245-85247)

85730   Thromboplastin time, partial (PTT); plasma or whole blood

85732   substitution, plasma fractions, each

85810   Viscosity

(von Willebrand factor assay, see 85245-85247)

(WBC count, see 85021-85031, 85048, 89050)

85999   Unlisted hematology and coagulation procedure

● New Code   ▲ Revised Code   ✳ Starred Procedure   ✛ Add-On Code   ⊘ Modifier -51 Exempt

IMMUNOLOGY

(Acetylcholine receptor antibody, see 86255, 86256)

(Actinomyces, antibodies to, use 86602)

(Adrenal cortex antibodies, see 86255, 86256)

(For tuberculosis test, cell mediated immunity measurement of gamma interferon antigen response, use Category III code 0010T)

86000   Agglutinins, febrile (eg, Brucella, Francisella, Murine typhus, Q fever,Rocky Mountain spotted fever, scrub typhus), each antigen

(For antibodies to infectious agents, see 86602-86804)

86001   Allergen specific IgG quantitative or semiquantitative, each allergen

(Agglutinins and autohemolysins, see 86940, 86941)

86003   Allergen specific IgE; quantitative or semiquantitative, each allergen

(For total quantitative IgE, use 82785)

86005   qualitative, multiallergen screen (dipstick, paddle or disk)

(For total qualitative IgE, use 83518)

(Alpha-1 antitrypsin, see 82103, 82104)

(Alpha-1 feto-protein, see 82105, 82106)

(Anti-AChR (acetylcholine receptor) antibody titer, see 86255, 86256)

(Anticardiolipin antibody, use 86147)

(Anti-DNA, use 86225)

(Anti-deoxyribonuclease titer, use 86215)

86021   Antibody identification; leukocyte antibodies

86022   platelet antibodies

86023   platelet associated immunoglobulin assay

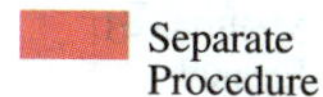

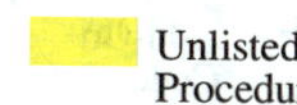

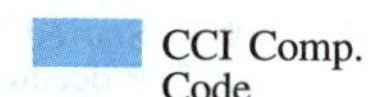

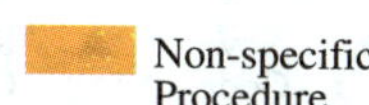

721

86038   Antinuclear antibodies (ANA);

86039   titer

      (Antistreptococcal antibody, ie, anti-DNAse, use 86215)

      (Antistreptokinase titer, use 86590)

86060   Antistreptolysin 0; titer

      (For antibodies to infectious agents, see 86602-86804)

86063   screen

      (For antibodies to infectious agents, see 86602-86804)

      (Blastomyces, antibodies to, use 86612)

86077   Blood bank physician services; difficult cross match and/or evaluation of irregular antibody(s), interpretation and written report

86078   investigation of transfusion reaction including suspicion of transmissible disease, interpretation and written report

86079   authorization for deviation from standard blood banking procedures (eg, use of outdated blood, transfusion of Rh incompatible units), with written report

      (Brucella, antibodies to, use 86622)

      (Candida, antibodies to, use 86628. For skin testing, use 86485)

86140   C-reactive protein;

      (Candidiasis, use 86628)

● **86141**   high sensitivity (hsCRP)

86146   Beta 2 Glycoprotein 1 antibody, each

86147   Cardiolipin (phospholipid) antibody, each lg class

86148   Anti-phosphatidylserine (phospholipid) antibody

86155   Chemotaxis assay, specify method

      (Clostridium difficile toxin, use 87230)

(Coccidioides, antibodies, to, see 86635. For skin testing, use 86490)

86156 Cold agglutinin; screen

86157 titer

86160 Complement; antigen, each component

86161 functional activity, each component

86162 total hemolytic (CH50)

86171 Complement fixation tests, each antigen

(Coombs test, see 86880-86886)

86185 Counterimmunoelectrophoresis, each antigen

(Cryptococcus, antibodies to, use 86641)

86215 Deoxyribonuclease, antibody

86225 Deoxyribonucleic acid (DNA) antibody; native or double stranded

(Echinococcus, antibodies to, see code for specific method)

(For HIV antibody tests, see 86701-86703)

86226 single stranded

(Anti D.S., DNA, IFA, eg, using C.Lucilae, see 86255 and 86256)

86235 Extractable nuclear antigen, antibody to, any method (eg, nRNP, SS-A, SS-B, Sm, RNP, Sc170, J01), each antibody

86243 Fc receptor

(Filaria, antibodies to, see code for specific method)

86255 Fluorescent noninfectious agent antibody; screen, each antibody

86256 titer, each antibody

 Separate Procedure

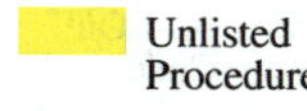 Unlisted Procedure

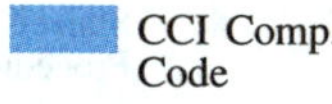 CCI Comp. Code

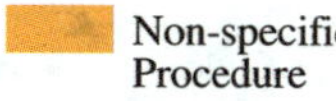 Non-specific Procedure

723

(Fluorescent technique for antigen identification in tissue, use 88346; for indirect fluorescence, use 88347)

(FTA, see 86781)

(Gel (agar) diffusion tests, use 86331)

86277 Growth hormone, human (HGH), antibody

86280 Hemagglutination inhibition test (HAI)

(For rubella, use 86762)

(For antibodies to infectious agents, see 86602-86804)

86294 Immunoassay for tumor antigen, qualitative or semiquantitative (eg, bladder tumor antigen)

86300 Immunoassay for tumor antigen, quantitative; CA 15-3 (27.29)

86301 CA 19-9

86304 CA 125

(For measurement of serum HER-2/neu oncoprotein, see 83950)

(For hepatitis delta agent, antibody, use 86692)

86308 Heterophile antibodies; screening

(For antibodies to infectious agents, see 86602-86804)

86309 titer

(For antibodies to infectious agents, see 86602-86804)

86310 titers after absorption with beef cells and guinea pig kidney

(Histoplasma, antibodies to, use 86698. For skin testing, use 86510)

(For antibodies to infectious agents, see 86602-86804)

(Human growth hormone antibody, use 86277)

86316 Immunoassay for tumor antigen ; other antigen, quantitative (eg, CA 50, 72-4, 549), each

---

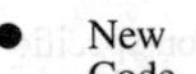

● New Code   ▲ Revised Code   ✳ Starred Procedure   ✛ Add-On Code   ⊘ Modifier -51 Exempt

86317   Immunoassay for infectious agent antibody, quantitative, not otherwise specified

(For immunoassay techniques for antigens, see 83516, 83518, 83519, 83520, 87301-87450, 87810-87899)

(For particle agglutination procedures, use 86403)

86318   Immunoassay for infectious agent antibody, qualitative or semiquantitative, single step method (eg, reagent strip)

86320   Immunoelectrophoresis; serum

▲ **86325**   other fluids (eg, urine, cerebrospinal fluid) with concentration

86327   crossed (2-dimensional assay)

86329   Immunodiffusion; not elsewhere specified

86331   gel diffusion, qualitative (Ouchterlony), each antigen or antibody

86332   Immune complex assay

86334   Immunofixation electrophoresis

● **86336**   Inhibin A

86337   Insulin antibodies

86340   Intrinsic factor antibodies

(Leptospira, antibodies to, use 86720)

(Leukoagglutinins, use 86021)

86341   Islet cell antibody

86343   Leukocyte histamine release test (LHR)

86344   Leukocyte phagocytosis

86353   Lymphocyte transformation, mitogen (phytomitogen) or antigen induced blastogenesis

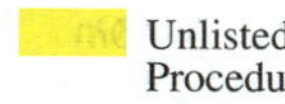 Separate Procedure   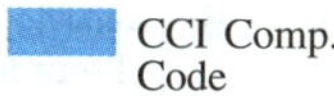 Unlisted Procedure   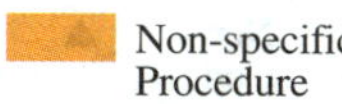 CCI Comp. Code   Non-specific Procedure

(Lymphocytes immunophenotyping, use 88180 for cytometry; see 88342, 88346 for microscopic techniques)

(Malaria antibodies, use 86750)

86359   T cells; total count

86360   absolute CD4 and CD8 count, including ratio

86361   absolute CD4 count

86376   Microsomal antibodies (eg, thyroid or liver-kidney), each

86378   Migration inhibitory factor test (MIF)

(Mitochondrial antibody, liver, see 86255, 86256)

(Mononucleosis, see 86308-86310)

86382   Neutralization test, viral

86384   Nitroblue tetrazolium dye test (NTD)

(Ouchterlony diffusion, use 86331)

(Platelet antibodies, see 86022, 86023)

86403   Particle agglutination; screen, each antibody

86406   titer, each antibody

(Pregnancy test, see 84702, 84703)

(Rapid plasma reagin test (RPR), see 86592, 86593)

86430   Rheumatoid factor; qualitative

86431   quantitative

(Serologic test for syphilis, see 86592, 86593)

86485   Skin test; candida

(For antibody, candida, use 86628)

86490   coccidioidomycosis

86510   histoplasmosis

● New Code   ▲ Revised Code   ∗ Starred Procedure   ✚ Add-On Code   ⊘ Modifier -51 Exempt

(For histoplasma, antibody, use 86698)

86580   tuberculosis, intradermal

86585   tuberculosis, tine test

(For tuberculosis test, cell mediated immunity measurement of gamma interferon antigen response, use Category III code 0010T)

(For skin tests for allergy, see 95010-95199)

(Smooth muscle antibody, see 86255, 86256)

(Sporothrix, antibodies to, see code for specific method)

86586   unlisted antigen, each

86590   Streptokinase, antibody

(For antibodies to infectious agents, see 86602-86804)

(Streptolysin O antibody, see antistreptolysin O, 86060, 86063)

86592   Syphilis test; qualitative (eg, VDRL, RPR, ART)

(For antibodies to infectious agents, see 86602-86804)

86593   quantitative

(For antibodies to infectious agents, see 86602-86804)

(Tetanus antibody, use 86774)

(Thyroglobulin antibody, use 86800)

(Thyroglobulin, use 84432)

(Thyroid microsomal antibody, use 86376)

(For toxoplasma antibody, see 86777-86778)

(For the detection of antibodies other than those to infectious agents, see specific antibody (eg, 86021, 86022, 86023, 86376, 86800, 86850-86870) or specific method (eg, 83516, 86255, 86256))

(For infectious agent/antigen detection, see 87260-87899)

86602   Antibody; actinomyces

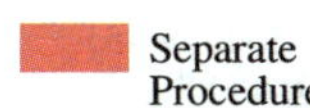

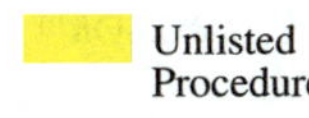

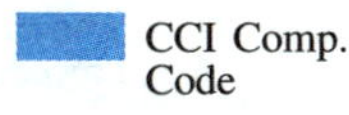

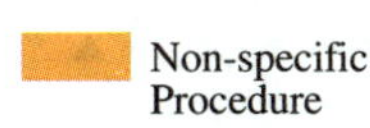

86603	adenovirus
86606	Aspergillus
86609	bacterium, not elsewhere specified
86611	Bartonella
86612	Blastomyces
86615	Bordetella
86617	Borrelia burgdorferi (Lyme disease) confirmatory test (eg, Western blot or immunoblot)
86618	Borrelia burgdorferi (Lyme disease)
86619	Borrelia (relapsing fever)
86622	Brucella
86625	Campylobacter
86628	Candida

(For skin test, candida, use 86485)

86631	Chlamydia
86632	Chlamydia, IgM

(For chlamydia antigen, see 87270, 87320. For fluorescent antibody technique, see 86255, 86256)

86635	Coccidioides
86638	Coxiella Brunetii (Q fever)
86641	Cryptococcus
86644	cytomegalovirus (CMV)

(For TORCH panel, use 80090)

86645	cytomegalovirus (CMV), IgM

● New Code   ▲ Revised Code   ✳ Starred Procedure   + Add-On Code   ⊘ Modifier -51 Exempt

86648	Diphtheria
86651	encephalitis, California (La Crosse)
86652	encephalitis, Eastern equine
86653	encephalitis, St. Louis
86654	encephalitis, Western equine
86658	enterovirus (eg, coxsackie, echo, polio)

(Trichinella, antibodies to, use 86784)

(Trypanosoma, antibodies to, see code for specific method)

(Tuberculosis, use 86580 for skin testing)

(Viral antibodies, see code for specific method)

86663	Epstein-Barr (EB) virus, early antigen (EA)
86664	Epstein-Barr (EB) virus, nuclear antigen (EBNA)
86665	Epstein-Barr (EB) virus, viral capsid (VCA)
86666	Ehrlichia
86668	Francisella Tularensis
86671	fungus, not elsewhere specified
86674	Giardia Lamblia
86677	Helicobacter Pylori
86682	helminth, not elsewhere specified
86683	hemoglobin, fecal
86684	Hemophilus influenza
86687	HTLV-I
86688	HTLV-II
86689	HTLV or HIV antibody, confirmatory test (eg, Western Blot)

729

Separate Procedure   Unlisted Procedure   CCI Comp. Code   Non-specific Procedure

86692   hepatitis, delta agent

(For hepatitis delta agent, antigen, use 87380)

86694   herpes simplex, non-specific type test

(For TORCH panel, use 80090)

86695   herpes simplex, type 1

86696   herpes simplex, type 2

86698   histoplasma

86701   HIV-1

86702   HIV-2

86703   HIV-1 and HIV-2, single assay

(For HIV-1 antigen, use 87390)

(For HIV-2 antigen, use 87391)

(For confirmatory test for HIV antibody (eg, Western Blot), use 86689)

86704 Hepatitis B core antibody (HBcAb); total

86705   IgM antibody

86706 Hepatitis B surface antibody (HBsAb)

86707 Hepatitis Be antibody (HBeAb)

86708 Hepatitis A antibody (HAAb); total

86709   IgM antibody

86710 Antibody; influenza virus

86713   Legionella

86717   Leishmania

86720   Leptospira

86723	Listeria monocytogenes
86727	lymphocytic choriomeningitis
86729	Lymphogranuloma Venereum
86732	mucormycosis
86735	mumps
86738	Mycoplasma
86741	Neisseria meningitidis
86744	Nocardia
86747	parvovirus
86750	Plasmodium (malaria)
86753	protozoa, not elsewhere specified
86756	respiratory syncytial virus
86757	Rickettsia
86759	rotavirus
86762	rubella
86765	rubeola
86768	Salmonella
86771	Shigella
86774	tetanus
86777	Toxoplasma
86778	Toxoplasma, IgM
86781	Treponema Pallidum, confirmatory test (eg, FTA-abs)
86784	trichinella

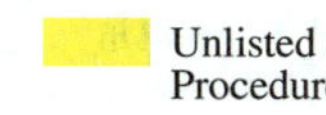 Separate Procedure

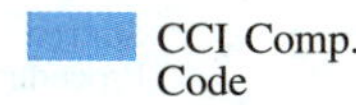 Unlisted Procedure

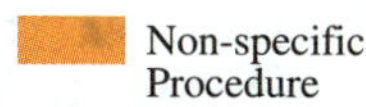 CCI Comp. Code

Non-specific Procedure

86787	varicella-zoster
86790	virus, not elsewhere specified
86793	Yersinia
86800	Thyroglobulin antibody

(For thyroglobulin, use 84432)

86803	Hepatitis C antibody;
86804	confirmatory test (eg, immunoblot)

TISSUE TYPING

(For pretransplant cross-match, see appropriate code or codes)

86805	Lymphocytotoxicity assay, visual crossmatch; with titration
86806	without titration
86807	Serum screening for cytotoxic percent reactive antibody (PRA); standard method
86808	quick method
86812	HLA typing; A, B, or C (eg, A10, B7, B27), single antigen
86813	A, B, or C, multiple antigens
86816	DR/DQ, single antigen
86817	DR/DQ, multiple antigens
86821	lymphocyte culture, mixed (MLC)
86822	lymphocyte culture, primed (PLC)
86849	Unlisted immunology procedure

● New Code   ▲ Revised Code   ✳ Starred Procedure   ✛ Add-On Code   ⊘ Modifier -51 Exempt

TRANSFUSION MEDICINE

(For apheresis, use 36520)

(For therapeutic phlebotomy, use 99195)

86850   Antibody screen, RBC, each serum technique

86860   Antibody elution (RBC), each elution

86870   Antibody identification, RBC antibodies, each panel for each serum technique

86880   Antihuman globulin test (Coombs test); direct, each antiserum

86885   indirect, qualitative, each antiserum

86886   indirect, titer, each antiserum

86890   Autologous blood or component, collection processing and storage; predeposited

86891   intra-or postoperative salvage

(For physician services to autologous donors, see 99201-99204)

86900   Blood typing; ABO

86901   Rh (D)

86903   antigen screening for compatible blood unit using reagent serum, per unit screened

86904   antigen screening for compatible unit using patient serum, per unit screened

86905   RBC antigens, other than ABO or Rh (D), each

86906   Rh phenotyping, complete

86910   Blood typing, for paternity testing, per individual; ABO, Rh and MN

86911   each additional antigen system

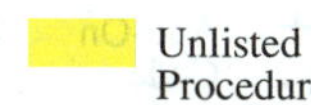

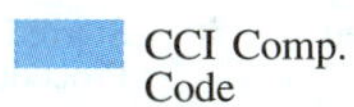

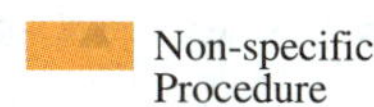

Non-specific
Procedure

86915   Bone marrow or peripheral stem cell harvest, modification or treatment to eliminate cell type(s) (eg, T-cells, metastatic carcinoma)

86920   Compatibility test each unit; immediate spin technique

86921   incubation technique

86922   antiglobulin technique

86927   Fresh frozen plasma, thawing, each unit

86930   Frozen blood, preparation for freezing, each unit;

86931   with thawing

86932   with freezing and thawing

86940   Hemolysins and agglutinins; auto, screen, each

86941   incubated

86945   Irradiation of blood product, each unit

86950   Leukocyte transfusion

          (For leukapheresis, use 36520)

86965   Pooling of platelets or other blood products

86970   Pretreatment of RBCs for use in RBC antibody detection, identification, and/or compatibility testing; incubation with chemical agents or drugs, each

86971   incubation with enzymes, each

86972   by density gradient separation

86975   Pretreatment of serum for use in RBC antibody identification; incubation with drugs, each

86976   by dilution

86977   incubation with inhibitors, each

● New Code   ▲ Revised Code   * Starred Procedure   + Add-On Code   ⊘ Modifier -51 Exempt

86978   by differential red cell absorption using patient RBCs or RBCs of known phenotype, each absorption

86985   Splitting of blood or blood products, each unit

86999   Unlisted transfusion medicine procedure

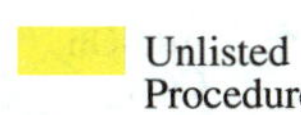

MICROBIOLOGY

87001   Animal inoculation, small animal; with observation

87003   with observation and dissection

87015   Concentration (any type), for infectious agents

    (Do not report 87015 in conjunction with 87177)

87040   Culture, bacterial; blood with isolation and presumptive identification of isolates (includes anaerobic culture, if appropriate)

▲ **87045**   feces, with isolation and preliminary examination (eg, KIA, LIA), Salmonella and Shigella species

87046   stool, additional pathogens, isolation and preliminary examination (eg, Campylobacter, Yersinia, Vibro, E. coli 0157), each plate

87070   any other source except urine, blood or stool, with isolation and presumptive identification of isolates

    (For urine, use 87088)

87071   quantitative, aerobic with isolation and presumptive identification of isolates, any source except urine, blood or stool

    (For urine, use 87088)

87073   quantitative, anaerobic with isolation and presumptive identification of isolates, any source except urine, blood or stool

    (For definitive identification of isolates, use 87076 or 87077. for typing of isolates see 87140-87158)

87075   any source, anaerobic with isolation and presumptive identification of isolates

87076   anaerobic isolate, additional methods required for definitive identification, each isolate

    (For gas liquid chromatography (GLC) or high pressure liquid chromatography (HPLC), use 87143)

● New Code   ▲ Revised Code   ✳ Starred Procedure   ✚ Add-On Code   ⊘ Modifier -51 Exempt

87077   aerobic isolate, additional methods required for definitive identification, each isolate

(For gas liquid chromatography (GLC) or high pressure liquid chromatography (HPLC), use 87143)

87081   Culture, presumptive, pathogenic organisms, screening only;

(**87082**   deleted 2001 edition. To report, use 87081)

(**87083**   deleted 2001 edition. To report, use 87081)

87084   with colony estimation from density chart

(**87085**   deleted 2001 edition. To report, use 87086)

87086   Culture, bacterial; quantitative colony count, urine

87088   with isolation and presumptive identification of isolates, urine

87101   Culture, fungi (mold or yeast) isolation, with presumptive identification of isolates; skin, hair, or nail

87102   other source (except blood)

87103   blood

87106   Culture, fungi, definitive identification, each organism; yeast

(Use 87106 in addition to codes 87101, 87102 or 87103 when appropriate)

87107   mold

87109   Culture, mycoplasma, any source

87110   Culture, chlamydia, any source

(For immunofluorescence staining of shell vials, use 87140)

87116   Culture, tubercle or other acid-fast bacilli (eg, TB, AFB, mycobacteria) any source, with isolation and presumptive identification of isolates

(**87117**   deleted 2001 edition. For concentration, use 87015)

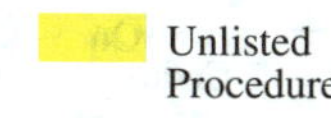 Separate Procedure   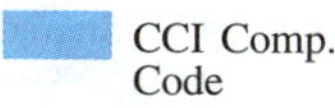 Unlisted Procedure   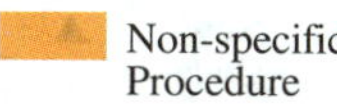 CCI Comp. Code   Non-specific Procedure

87118 Culture, mycobacteria, definitive identification, each isolate

(For nucleic acid probe identification, use 87149)

(For GLC or HPLC identification, use 87143)

87140 Culture, typing; immunofluorescent method, each antiserum

87143 gas liquid chromatography (GLC) or high pressure liquid chromotography (HPLC) method

(87145 deleted 2001 edition. No replacement code identified)

87147 immunologic method, other than immunofluorescence (eg, agglutination grouping), per antiserum

87149 identification by nucleic acid probe

(87151 deleted 2001 edition. To report, use 87147)

87152 identification by pulse field gel typing

(87155 deleted 2001 edition. To report, use 87147)

87158 other methods

(87163 deleted 2001 edition. To report, use 87076 or 87077)

87164 Dark field examination, any source (eg, penile, vaginal, oral, skin); includes specimen collection

87166 without collection

87168 Macroscopic examination; arthropod

87169 parasite

87172 Pinworm exam (eg, cellophane tape prep)

(87174 deleted 2001 edition.)

(87175 deleted 2001 edition.)

87176 Homogenization, tissue, for culture

87177 Ova and parasites, direct smears, concentration and identification

---

● New Code   ▲ Revised Code   ✳ Starred Procedure   + Add-On Code   ⊘ Modifier -51 Exempt

(Do not report 87177 in conjunction with 87015)

(For coccidia or microsporidia exam, use 87207)

(For trichrome, iron hemotoxylin and other special stains, use 88313)

(For nucleic acid probes in cytologic material, use 88365)

(For molecular diagnostics, see 83890-83898, 87470-87799)

87181 Susceptibility studies, antimicrobial agent; agar diffusion method, per agent (eg, antibiotic gradient strip)

87184 disk method, per plate (12 or fewer disks)

87185 enzyme detection (eg, beta lactamase), per enzyme

87186 microdilution or agar dilution (minimum inhibitory concentration (MIC) or breakpoint), each multi-antimicrobial, per plate

+87187 microdilution or agar dilution, minimum lethal concentration (MLC), each plate ((List separately in addition to code for primary procedure)

(Use 87187 in conjunction with 87186 or 87188)

87188 macrobroth dilution method, each agent

87190 mycobacteria, proportion method, each agent

(For other mycobacterial susceptibility studies, see 87181, 87184, 87186, or 87188)

(87192 deleted 2001 edition. For fungal susceptibility studies, see 87181, 87184, 87186, 87187, or 87188)

87197 Serum bactericidal titer (Schlicter test)

● **87198** Cytomegalovirus, direct fluorescent antibody (DFA)

● **87199** Enterovirus, direct fluorescent antibody (DFA)

87205 Smear, primary source with interpretation; Gram or Giemsa stain for bacteria, fungi, or cell types

---

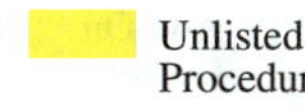

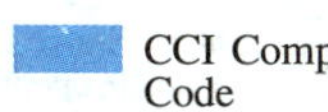

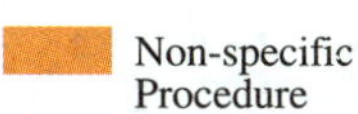

Non-specific
Procedure

87206   fluorescent and/or acid fast stain for bacteria, fungi, or cell types

87207   special stain for inclusion bodies or intracellular parasites (eg, malaria, coccidia, microsporidia, cytomegalovirus, herpes viruses)

(For thick smear preparation, use 87015)

(For complex special stains, see 88312, 88313)

(For fat, meat, fibers, nasal eosinophils, and starch, see miscellaneous section)

(87208   deleted 2001 edition.)

87210   wet mount for infectious agents (eg, saline, India ink, KOH preps)

(For KOH examination of skin, hair or nails, see 87220)

(87211   deleted 2001 edition. To report, use 87177)

87220   Tissue examination by KOH slide of samples from skin, hair, or nails for fungi or ectoparasite ova or mites (eg, scabies)

87230   Toxin or antitoxin assay, tissue culture (eg, Clostridium difficile toxin)

87250   Virus isolation; inoculation of embryonated eggs, or small animal, includes observation and dissection

87252   tissue culture inoculation, observation, and presumptive identification by cytopathic effect

87253   tissue culture, additional studies or definitive identification (eg, hemabsorption, neutralization, immunofluorescence stain) each isolate

(Electron microscopy, use 88348)

(Inclusion bodies in tissue sections, see 88304-88309; in smears, see 87207-87210; in fluids, use 88106)

87254   shell vial, includes identification with immunofluorescence stain, each virus

(Report 87254 in addition to 87252 as appropriate)

---

740   ● New Code   ▲ Revised Code   ✳ Starred Procedure   ✛ Add-On Code   ⊘ Modifier -51 Exempt

87260   Infectious agent antigen detection by immunofluorescent technique; adenovirus

87265   Bordetella pertussis/parapertussis

87270   Chlamydia trachomatis

87272   cryptosporidium/giardia

87273   Herpes simplex virus type 2

87274   Herpes simplex virus 1

87275   Influenza B virus

87276   influenza A virus

87277   Legionella micdadei

87278   Legionella pneumophila

87279   Parainfluenza virus, each type

87280   respiratory syncytial virus

87281   Pneumocystis carinii

87283   Rubeola

87285   Treponema pallidum

87290   Varicella zoster virus

87299   not otherwise specified, each organism

87300   Infectious agent antigen detection by immunofluorescent technique, polyvalent for multiple organisms, each polyvalent antiserum

87301   Infectious agent antigen detection by enzyme immunoassay technique, qualitative or semiquantitative, multiple step method; adenovirus enteric types 40/41

87320   Chlamydia trachomatis

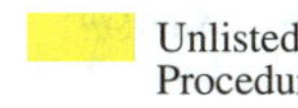

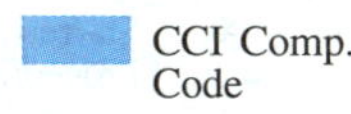

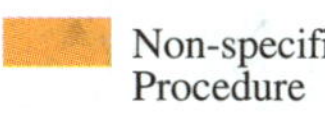

741

87324   Clostridium difficile toxin(s)

87327   Cryptococcus neoformans

(For Cryptococcus latex agglutination, use 86403)

87328   cryptosporidium/giardia

87332   cytomegalovirus

87335   Escherichia coli 0157

(For giardia antigen, use 87328)

87336   Entamoeba histolytica dispar group

87337   Entamoeba histolytica group

87338   Helicobacter pylori, stool

87339   Helicobacter pylori

(For H. pylori, stool, use 87338. For H. pylori, breath and blood by mass spectrometry, see 83013, 83014. For H. pylori, liquid scintillation counter, see 78267, 78268)

87340   hepatitis B surface antigen (HBsAg)

87341   hepatitis B surface antigen (HBsAg) neutralization

87350   hepatitis Be antigen (HBeAg)

87380   hepatitis, delta agent

87385   Histoplasma capsulatum

87390   HIV-1

87391   HIV-2

87400   Influenza, A or B, each

87420   respiratory syncytial virus

87425   rotavirus

● New Code   ▲ Revised Code   ∗ Starred Procedure   ✚ Add-On Code   ⊘ Modifier -51 Exempt

87427 Shiga-like toxin

87430 Streptococcus, group A

87449 Infectious agent antigen detection by enzyme immunoassay technique qualitative or semiquantitative; multiple step method, not otherwise specified, each organism

87450 single step method, not otherwise specified, each organism

87451 multiple step method, polyvalent for multiple organisms, each polyvalent antiserum

87470 Infectious agent detection by nucleic acid (DNA or RNA); Bartonella henselae and Bartonella quintana, direct probe technique

87471 Bartonella henselae and Bartonella quintana, amplified probe technique

87472 Bartonella henselae and Bartonella quintana, quantification

87475 Borrelia burgdorferi, direct probe technique

87476 Borrelia burgdorferi, amplified probe technique

87477 Borrelia burgdorferi, quantification

87480 Candida species, direct probe technique

87481 Candida species, amplified probe technique

87482 Candida species, quantification

87485 Chlamydia pneumoniae, direct probe technique

87486 Chlamydia pneumoniae, amplified probe technique

87487 Chlamydia pneumoniae, quantification

87490 Chlamydia trachomatis, direct probe technique

87491 Chlamydia trachomatis, amplified probe technique

87492 Chlamydia trachomatis, quantification

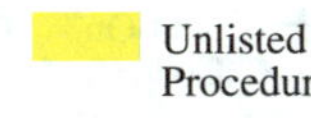

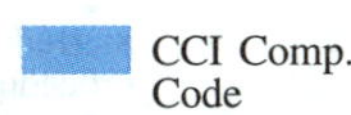

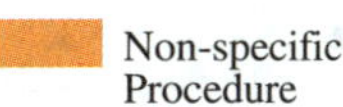

Non-specific
Procedure

87495	cytomegalovirus, direct probe technique
87496	cytomegalovirus, amplified probe technique
87497	cytomegalovirus, quantification
87510	Gardnerella vaginalis, direct probe technique
87511	Gardnerella vaginalis, amplified probe technique
87512	Gardnerella vaginalis, quantification
87515	hepatitis B virus, direct probe technique
87516	hepatitis B virus, amplified probe technique
87517	hepatitis B virus, quantification
87520	hepatitis C, direct probe technique
87521	hepatitis C, amplified probe technique
87522	hepatitis C, quantification
87525	hepatitis G, direct probe technique
87526	hepatitis G, amplified probe technique
87527	hepatitis G, quantification
87528	Herpes simplex virus, direct probe technique
87529	Herpes simplex virus, amplified probe technique
87530	Herpes simplex virus, quantification
87531	Herpes virus-6, direct probe technique
87532	Herpes virus-6, amplified probe technique
87533	Herpes virus-6, quantification
87534	HIV-1, direct probe technique
87535	HIV-1, amplified probe technique

● New Code	▲ Revised Code	✳ Starred Procedure	✛ Add-On Code	⊘ Modifier -51 Exempt

87536	HIV-1, quantification
87537	HIV-2, direct probe technique
87538	HIV-2, amplified probe technique
87539	HIV-2, quantification
87540	Legionella pneumophila, direct probe technique
87541	Legionella pneumophila, amplified probe technique
87542	Legionella pneumophila, quantification
87550	Mycobacteria species, direct probe technique
87551	Mycobacteria species, amplified probe technique
87552	Mycobacteria species, quantification
87555	Mycobacteria tuberculosis, direct probe technique
87556	Mycobacteria tuberculosis, amplified probe technique
87557	Mycobacteria tuberculosis, quantification
87560	Mycobacteria avium-intracellulare, direct probe technique
87561	Mycobacteria avium-intracellulare, amplified probe technique
87562	Mycobacteria avium-intracellulare, quantification
87580	Mycoplasma pneumoniae, direct probe technique
87581	Mycoplasma pneumoniae, amplified probe technique
87582	Mycoplasma pneumoniae, quantification
87590	Neisseria gonorrhoeae, direct probe technique
87591	Neisseria gonorrhoeae, amplified probe technique
87592	Neisseria gonorrhoeae, quantification
87620	papillomavirus,human, direct probe technique

745

87621	papillomavirus,human, amplified probe technique
87622	papillomavirus, human, quantification
87650	Streptococcus, group A, direct probe technique
87651	Streptococcus, group A, amplified probe technique
87652	Streptococcus, group A, quantification
87797	Infectious agent detection by nucleic acid (DNA or RNA), not otherwise specified; direct probe technique, each organism
87798	amplified probe technique, each organism
87799	not otherwise specified, quantification, each organism
87800	Infectious agent detection by nucleic acid (DNA or RNA), multiple organisms; direct probe(s) technique
87801	amplified probe(s) technique
● **87802**	Infectious agent antigen detection by immunoassay with direct optical observation; Streptococcus, group B
● **87803**	Clostridium difficile toxin A
● **87804**	Influenza
87810	Infectious agent detection by immunoassay with direct optical observation; Chlamydia trachomatis
87850	Neisseria gonorrhoeae
87880	Streptococcus, group A
87899	not otherwise specified
87901	Infectious agent genotype analysis by nucleic acid (DNA or RNA) HIV 1, reverse transciptase and protease
	(For infectious agent drug susceptibility phenotype prediction for HIV-1, use Category III code 0023T)
● **87902**	Hepatitis C virus

▲ **87903**   Infectious agent phenotype analysis by nucleic acid (DNA or RNA) with drug resistance tissue culture analysis, HIV 1; first through 10 drugs tested

▲ **+87904**   each additional 1 through 5 drugs tested (List separately in addition to code for primary procedure)

(Use 87904 in conjunction with code 87903)

87999   Unlisted microbiology procedure

ANATOMIC PATHOLOGY

POSTMORTEM EXAMINATION

88000 Necropsy (autopsy), gross examination only; without CNS

88005 with brain

88007 with brain and spinal cord

88012 infant with brain

88014 stillborn or newborn with brain

88016 macerated stillborn

88020 Necropsy (autopsy), gross and microscopic; without CNS

88025 with brain

88027 with brain and spinal cord

88028 infant with brain

88029 stillborn or newborn with brain

88036 Necropsy (autopsy), limited, gross and/or microscopic; regional

88037 single organ

88040 Necropsy (autopsy); forensic examination

88045 coroner's call

88099 Unlisted necropsy (autopsy) procedure

● New Code ▲ Revised Code ✳ Starred Procedure ✚ Add-On Code ⃠ Modifier -51 Exempt

CYTOPATHOLOGY

88104 Cytopathology, fluids, washings or brushings, except cervical or vaginal; smears with interpretation

88106 filter method only with interpretation

88107 smears and filter preparation with interpretation

88108 Cytopathology, concentration technique, smears and interpretation (eg, Saccomanno technique)

(For cervical or vaginal smears, see 88150-88155)

(For gastric intubation with lavage, see 89130-89141, 91055)

(For x-ray localization, use 74340)

88125 Cytopathology, forensic (eg, sperm)

88130 Sex chromatin identification; Barr bodies

88140 peripheral blood smear, polymorphonuclear drumsticks

(For Guard stain, use 88313)

+88141 Cytopathology, cervical or vaginal (any reporting system); requiring interpretation by physician (List separately in addition to code for technical service)

(Use 88141 in conjunction with codes 88142-88154, 88164-88167)

88142 Cytopathology, cervical or vaginal (any reporting system), collected in preservative fluid, automated thin layer preparation; manual screening under physician supervision

88143 with manual screening and rescreening under physician supervision

88144 with manual screening and computer-assisted rescreening under physician supervision

88145 with manual screening and computer-assisted rescreening using cell selection and review under physician supervision

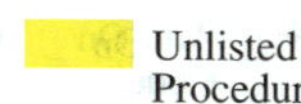

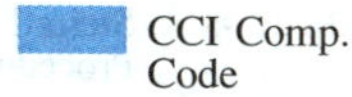

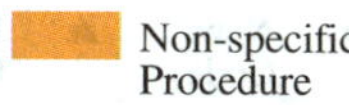

Non-specific
Procedure

88147 Cytopathology smears, cervical or vaginal; screening by automated system under physician supervision

88148 screening by automated system with manual rescreening under physician supervision

88150 Cytopathology, slides, cervical or vaginal; manual screening under physician supervision

88152 with manual screening and computer-assisted rescreening under physician supervision

88153 with manual screening and rescreening under physician supervision

88154 with manual screening and computer-assisted rescreening using cell selection and review under physician supervision

+88155 Cytopathology, slides, cervical or vaginal, definitive hormonal evaluation (eg, maturation index, karyopyknotic index, estrogenic index) (List separately in addition to code(s) for other technical and interpretation services)

(Use 88155 in conjunction with 88142-88154, 88164-88167)

88160 Cytopathology, smears, any other source; screening and interpretation

88161 preparation, screening and interpretation

88162 extended study involving over 5 slides and/or multiple stains

(For obtaining specimen, see percutaneous needle biopsy under individual organ in Surgery)

(For aerosol collection of sputum, use 89350)

(For special stains, see 88312-88314)

88164 Cytopathology, slides, cervical or vaginal (the Bethesda System); manual screening under physician supervision

88165 with manual screening and rescreening under physician supervision

88166 with manual screening and computer-assisted rescreening under physician supervision

---

● New Code   ▲ Revised Code   * Starred Procedure   + Add-On Code   ⊘ Modifier -51 Exempt

88167   with manual screening and computer-assisted rescreening using cell selection and review under physician supervision

(88170   deleted 2002 edition. To report, use 10021)

(88171   deleted 2002 edition. To report, use 10022)

88172   Cytopathology, evaluation of fine needle aspirate; immediate cytohistologic study to determine adequacy of specimen(s)

88173   interpretation and report

88180   Flow cytometry; each cell surface, cytoplasmic or nuclear marker

88182   cell cycle or DNA analysis

(For tumor morphometry and DNA and ploidy analysis by imaging techniques, use 88358)

88199   Unlisted cytopathology procedure

(For electron microscopy, see 88348, 88349)

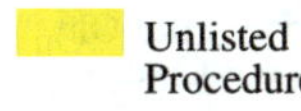 Separate Procedure

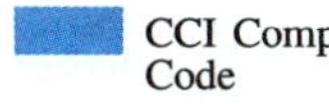 Unlisted Procedure

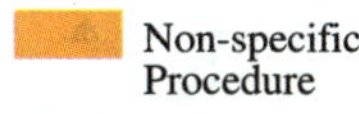 CCI Comp. Code

Non-specific Procedure

CYTOGENETIC STUDIES

(For acetylcholinesterase, use 82013)

(For alpha-fetoprotein, serum or amniotic fluid, see 82105, 82106)

(For laser microdissection of cells from tissue sample, see 88380)

88230 Tissue culture for non-neoplastic disorders; lymphocyte

88233 skin or other solid tissue biopsy

88235 amniotic fluid or chorionic villus cells

88237 Tissue culture for neoplastic disorders; bone marrow, blood cells

88239 solid tumor

88240 Cryopreservation, freezing and storage of cells, each cell line

88241 Thawing and expansion of frozen cells, each aliquot

88245 Chromosome analysis for breakage syndromes; baseline Sister Chromatid Exchange (SCE), 20-25 cells

88248 baseline breakage, score 50-100 cells, count 20 cells, 2 karyotypes (eg, for ataxia telangiectasia, Fanconi anemia, fragile X)

88249 score 100 cells, clastogen stress (eg, diepoxybutane, mitomycin C, ionizing radiation, UV radiation)

88261 Chromosome analysis; count 5 cells, 1 karyotype, with banding

88262 count 15-20 cells, 2 karyotypes, with banding

88263 count 45 cells for mosaicism, 2 karyotypes, with banding

88264 analyze 20-25 cells

88267 Chromosome analysis, amniotic fluid or chorionic villus, count 15 cells, 1 karyotype, with banding

---

752   ● New Code   ▲ Revised Code   * Starred Procedure   + Add-On Code   ⊘ Modifier -51 Exempt

88269   Chromosome analysis, in situ for amniotic fluid cells, count cells from 6-12 colonies, 1 karyotype, with banding

88271   Molecular cytogenetics; DNA probe, each (eg, FISH)

88272   chromosomal in situ hybridization, analyze 3-5 cells (eg, for derivatives and markers)

88273   chromosomal in situ hybridization, analyze 10-30 cells (eg, for microdeletions)

88274   interphase in situ hybridization, analyze 25-99 cells

88275   interphase in situ hybridization, analyze 100-300 cells

88280   Chromosome analysis; additional karyotypes, each study

88283   additional specialized banding technique (eg, NOR, C-banding)

88285   additional cells counted, each study

88289   additional high resolution study

88291   Cytogenetics and molecular cytogenetics, interpretation and report

88299   Unlisted cytogenetic study

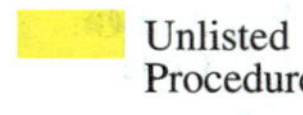
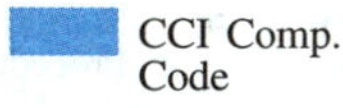

Separate Procedure   Unlisted Procedure   CCI Comp. Code   Non-specific Procedure

SURGICAL PATHOLOGY

88300   Level I - Surgical pathology, gross examination only

88302   Level II - Surgical pathology, gross and microscopic examination

Appendix, Incidental
Fallopian Tube, Sterilization
Fingers/Toes, Amputation, Traumatic
Foreskin, Newborn
Hernia Sac, Any Location
Hydrocele Sac
Nerve
Skin, Plastic Repair
Sympathetic Ganglion
Testis, Castration
Vaginal Mucosa, Incidental
Vas Deferens, Sterilization

▲ **88304**   Level III - Surgical pathology, gross and microscopic examination

Abortion, Induced
Abscess
Aneurysm - Arterial/Ventricular
Anus, Tag
Appendix, Other than Incidental
Artery, Atheromatous Plaque
Bartholin's Gland Cyst
Bone Fragment(s), Other than Pathologic Fracture
Bursa/Synovial Cyst
Carpal Tunnel Tissue
Cartilage, Shavings
Cholesteatoma
Colon, Colostomy Stoma
Conjunctiva - Biopsy/Pterygium
Cornea
Diverticulum - Esophagus/Small Intestine
Dupuytren's Contracture Tissue
Femoral Head, Other than Fracture
Fissue/Fistula
Foreskin, Other than Newborn
Gallbladder
Ganglion Cyst
Hematoma
Hemorrhoids
Hydatid of Morgagni
Intervertebral Disc
Joint, Loose Body

| ● New Code | ▲ Revised Code | * Starred Procedure | + Add-On Code | ⊘ Modifier -51 Exempt |

Meniscus
Mucocele, Salivary
Neuroma - Morton's/Traumatic
Pilonidal Cyst/Sinus
Polyps, Inflammatory - Nasal/Sinusoidal
Skin - Cyst/Tag/Debridement
Soft Tissue, Debridement
Soft Tissue, Lipoma
Spermatocele
Tendon/Tendon Sheath
Testicular Appendage
Thrombus or Embolus
Tonsil and/or Adenoids
Varicocele
Vas Deferens, Other than Sterilizaton
Vein, Varicosity

▲ **88305** Level IV - Surgical pathology, gross and microscopic examination

Abortion - Spontaneous/Missed
Artery, Biopsy
Bone Marrow, Biopsy
Bone Exostosis
Brain/Meninges, Other than for Tumor Resection
Breast Biopsy, Not Requiring Microscopic Evaluation of
  Surgical Margins
Breast, Reduction Mammoplasty
Bronchus, Biopsy
Cell Block, Any Source
Cervix, Biopsy
Colon, Biopsy
Duodenum, Biopsy
Endocervix, Curettings/Biopsy
Endometrium, Currettings/Biopsy
Esophagus, Biopsy
Extremity, Amputation, Traumatic
Fallopian Tube, Biopsy
Fallopian Tube, Ectopic Pregnancy
Femoral Head, Fracture
Fingers/Toes, Amputation, Non-Traumatic
Gingiva/Oral Mucosa, Biopsy
Heart Valve
Joint, Resection
Kidney, Biopsy
Larynx, Biopsy
Leiomyoma(s), Uterine Myomectomy - without Uterus
Lip, Biopsy/Wedge Resection
Lung, Transbronchial Biopsy

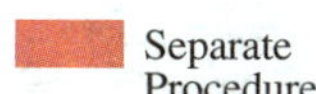

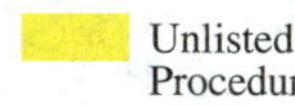

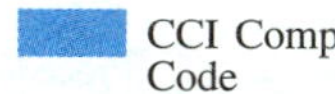

Non-specific
Procedure

Lymph Node, Biopsy
Muscle, Biopsy
Nasal Mucosa, Biopsy
Nasopharynx/Oropharynx, Biopsy
Nerve, Biopsy
Odontogenic/Dental Cyst
Omentum, Biopsy
Ovary with or without Tube, Non-neoplastic
Ovary, Biopsy/Wedge Resection
Parathyroid Gland
Peritoneum, Biopsy
Pituitary Tumor
Placenta, Other than Third Trimester
Pleura/Pericardium - Biopsy/Tissue
Polyp, Cervical/Endometrial
Polyp, Colorectal
Polyp, Stomach/Small Intestine
Prostate, Needle Biopsy
Prostate, TUR
Salivary Gland, Biopsy
Sinus, Paranasal Biopsy
Skin, Other than Cyst/Tag/Debridement/Plastic Repair
Small Intestine, Biopsy
Soft Tissue, Other than Tumor/Mass/Lipoma/Debridement
Spleen
Stomach, Biopsy
Synovium
Testis, Other than Tumor/Biopsy/Castration
Thyroglossal Duct/Brachial Cleft Cyst
Tongue, Biopsy
Tonsil, Biopsy
Trachea, Biopsy
Ureter, Biopsy
Urethra, Biopsy
Urinary Bladder, Biopsy
Uterus, with or without Tubes and Ovaries, for Prolapse
Vagina, Biopsy
Vulva/Labia, Biopsy

88307   Level V - Surgical pathology, gross and microscopic
examination

Adrenal, Resection
Bone - Biopsy/Curettings
Bone Fragment(s), Pathologic Fracture
Brain, Biopsy
Brain/Meninges, Tumor Resection
Breast, Excision of Lesion, Requiring Microscopic Evaluation
   of Surgical Margins

Breast, Mastectomy - Partial/Simple
Cervix, Conization
Colon, Segmental Resection, Other than for Tumor
Extremity, Amputation, Non-traumatic
Eye, Enucleation
Kidney, Partial/Total Nephrectomy
Larynx, Partial/Total Resection
Liver, Biopsy - Needle/Wedge
Lung, Wedge Biopsy
Lymph Nodes, Regional Resection
Mediastinum, Mass
Myocardium, Biopsy
Odontogenic Tumor
Ovary with or without Tube, Neoplastic
Pancreas, Biopsy
Placenta, Third Trimester
Prostate, Except Radical Resection
Salivary Gland
Sentinel Lymph Node
Small Intestine, Resection, Other Than for Tumor
Soft Tissue Mass (except Lipoma) - Biopsy/Simple Excision
Stomach - Subtotal/Total Resection, Other than for Tumor
Testis, Biopsy
Thymus, Biopsy
Thyroid, Total/Lobe
Ureter, Resection
Urinary Bladder, TUR
Uterus, with or without Tubes and Ovaries, Other than
   Neoplastic/Prolapse

88309   Level VI - Surgical pathology, gross and microscopic
examination

Bone Resection
Breast, Mastectomy - with Regional Lymph Nodes
Colon, Segmental Resection for Tumor
Colon, Total Resection
Esophagus, Partial/Total Resection
Extremity, Disarticulation
Fetus, with Dissection
Larynx, Partial/Total Resection - with Regional Lymph Nodes
Lung - Total/Lobe/Segment Resection
Pancreas, Total/Subtotal Resection
Prostate, Radical Resection
Small Intestine, Resection for Tumor
Soft Tissue Tumor, Extensive Resection
Stomach - Subtotal/Total Resection for Tumor
Testis, Tumor
Tongue/Tonsil - Resection for Tumor

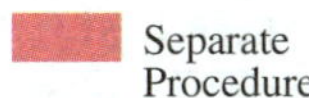

Separate
Procedure

Unlisted
Procedure

CCI Comp.
Code

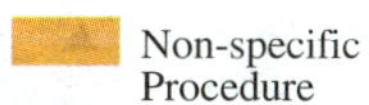

Non-specific
Procedure

757

Urinary Bladder, Partial/Total Resection
Uterus, with or without Tubes and Ovaries, Neoplastic
Vulva, Total/Subtotal Resection

(For fine needle aspiration, see 10021, 10022)

(For evaluation of fine needle aspirate, see 88172-88173)

+88311 Decalcification procedure (List separately in addition to code for surgical pathology examination)

+88312 Special stains (List separately in addition to code for surgical pathology examination); Group I for microorganisms (eg, Gridley, acid fast, methenamine silver), each

+88313 Group II, all other, (eg, iron, trichrome), except immunocytochemistry and immunoperoxidase stains, each

(For immunocytochemistry and immunoperoxidase tissue studies, use 88342)

+88314 histochemical staining with frozen section(s)

88318 Determinative histochemistry to identify chemical components (eg, copper, zinc)

88319 Determinative histochemistry or cytochemistry to identify enzyme constituents, each

88321 Consultation and report on referred slides prepared elsewhere

88323 Consultation and report on referred material requiring preparation of slides

88325 Consultation, comprehensive, with review of records and specimens, with report on referred material

88329 Pathology consultation during surgery;

88331 first tissue block, with frozen section(s), single specimen

88332 each additional tissue block with frozen section(s)

88342 Immunocytochemistry (including tissue immunoperoxidase), each antibody

88346 Immunofluorescent study, each antibody; direct method

● New Code ▲ Revised Code ∗ Starred Procedure + Add-On Code ⃠ Modifier -51 Exempt

88347   indirect method

88348 Electron microscopy; diagnostic

88349   scanning

88355 Morphometric analysis; skeletal muscle

88356   nerve

88358   tumor

(When semi-thin plastic-embedded sections are performed in conjunction with morphometric analysis, only the morphometric analysis should be coded; if performed as an independent procedure, see codes 88300-88309 for surgical pathology)

88362 Nerve teasing preparations

(For physician interpretation of peripheral blood smear, use 85060)

88365 Tissue in situ hybridization, interpretation and report

88371 Protein analysis of tissue by Western Blot, with interpretation and report;

88372   immunological probe for band identification, each

● **88380** Microdissection (eg, mechanical, laser capture)

88399 Unlisted surgical pathology procedure

TRANSCUTANEOUS PROCEDURES

88400 Bilirubin, total transcutaneous

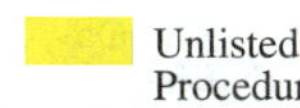

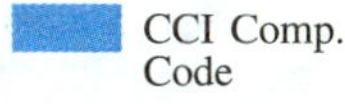

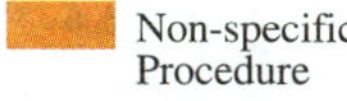

OTHER PROCEDURES

(Basal metabolic rate has been deleted. If necessary to report, use 89399)

▲ **89050** Cell count, miscellaneous body fluids (eg, cerebrospinal fluid, joint fluid), except blood;

89051 with differential count

89060 Crystal identification by light microscopy with or without polarizing lens analysis, any body fluid (except urine)

89100 Duodenal intubation and aspiration; single specimen (eg, simple bile study or afferent loop culture) plus appropriate test procedure

89105 collection of multiple fractional specimens with pancreatic or gallbladder stimulation, single or double lumen tube

(For radiological localization, use 74340)

(For chemical analyses, see Chemistry, this section)

(Electrocardiogram, see 93000-93268)

(Esophagus acid perfusion test (Bernstein), see 91030)

89125 Fat stain, feces, urine, or respiratory secretions

89130 Gastric intubation and aspiration, diagnostic, each specimen, for chemical analyses or cytopathology;

89132 after stimulation

89135 Gastric intubation, aspiration, and fractional collections (eg, gastric secretory study); one hour

89136 two hours

89140 two hours including gastric stimulation (eg, histalog, pentagastrin)

89141 three hours, including gastric stimulation

(For gastric lavage, thereapeutic, use 91105)

(For radiologic localization of gastric tube, use 74340)

760

● New Code   ▲ Revised Code   ✱ Starred Procedure   ✚ Add-On Code   ⊘ Modifier -51 Exempt

(For chemical analyses, see 82926, 82928)

(Joint fluid chemistry, see Chemistry, this section)

89160 Meat fibers, feces

89190 Nasal smear for eosinophils

(Occult blood, feces, use 82270)

(Paternity tests, use 86910)

89250 Culture and fertilization of oocyte(s);

89251   with co-culture of embryos

89252 Assisted oocyte fertilization, microtechnique (any method)

89253 Assisted embryo hatching, microtechniques (any method)

89254 Oocyte identification from follicular fluid

89255 Preparation of embryo for transfer (any method)

89256 Preparation of cryopreserved embryos for transfer (includes thaw)

89257 Sperm identification from aspiration (other than seminal fluid)

(For semen analysis, see 89300-89320)

(For sperm identification from testis tissue, use 89264)

89258 Cryopreservation; embryo

89259   sperm

89260 Sperm isolation; simple prep (eg, sperm wash and swim-up) for insemination or diagnosis with semen analysis

89261   complex prep (eg, Percoll gradient, albumin gradient) for insemination or diagnosis with semen analysis

(For semen analysis without sperm wash or swim-up, use 89320)

89264 Sperm identification from testis tissue, fresh or cryopreserved

	Separate Procedure		Unlisted Procedure		CCI Comp. Code		Non-specific Procedure

(For biopsy of testis, see 54500, 54505)

(For sperm identification from aspiration, use 89257)

(For semen analysis, see 89300-89320)

89300 Semen analysis; presence and/or motility of sperm including Huhner test (post coital)

89310 motility and count

89320 complete (volume, count, motility, and differential)

(Skin tests, see 86485-86585 and 95010-95199)

89321 Semen analysis, presence and/or motility of sperm

89325 Sperm antibodies

(For medicolegal identification of sperm, use 88125)

89329 Sperm evaluation; hamster penetration test

89330 cervical mucus penetration test, with or without spinnbarkeit test

89350 Sputum, obtaining specimen, aerosol induced technique (separate procedure)

89355 Starch granules, feces

89360 Sweat collection by iontophoresis

(For chloride and sodium analysis, use 84295)

89365 Water load test

89399 Unlisted miscellaneous pathology test

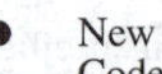 New Code   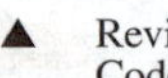 Revised Code   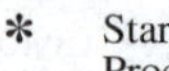 Starred Procedure   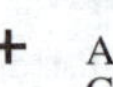 Add-On Code   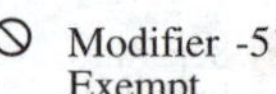 Modifier -51 Exempt

MEDICINE SECTION OVERVIEW

The sixth section of the CPT coding system is the medicine section, which includes codes for immunizations, therapeutic or diagnostic injections, psychiatric services, dialysis, ophthalmology services, specialty specific diagnostic services, chemotherapy administration, physical medicine and rehabilitation services, osteopathic and chiropractic services. Within each subsection, the CPT codes are arranged by the type of service provided.

MEDICINE SUBSECTIONS

The MEDICINE section of CPT is divided into 27 subsections:

Immune Globulins	90280-90399
Immunization Administration for Vaccines/Toxoids	90471-90472
Vaccines, Toxoids	90476-90749
Therapeutic or Diagnostic Infusions (excludes chemotherapy)	90780-90781
Therapeutic, Prophylactic or Diagnostic Injections	90782-90799
Psychiatry	90801-90899
Biofeedback	90900-90915
Dialysis	90935-90989
Gastroenterology	91000-92199
Ophthalmology	92002-92499
Special Otorhinolaryngologic Services	92502-92599
Cardiovascular	92950-93799
Non-Invasive Vascular Diagnostic Studies	93875-93979
Pulmonary	94010-94799
Allergy and Clinical Immunology	95000-95199
Neurology and Neuromuscular Procedures	95805-95999
Central Nervous System Assessments/Tests	96100-96117
Chemotherapy Administration	96400-96549
Photodynamic Therapy	96570-96571
Special Dermatological Procedures	96900-96999
Physical Medicine and Rehabilitation	97010-97799
Osteopathic Manipulative Treatment	98925-98929
Chiropractic Manipulative Treatment	98940-98943
Special Services, Procedures and Reports	99000-99199
Qualifying Circumstances for Anesthesia	99100-99140
Sedation With or Without Analgesia	99141-99142
Other Services and Procedures	99170-99199

MED 90000

Most of the subsections have special needs or instructions unique to that section which should be reviewed carefully before reporting.

 Separate Procedure

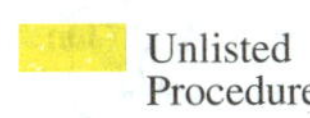 Unlisted Procedure

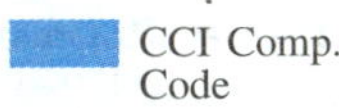 CCI Comp. Code

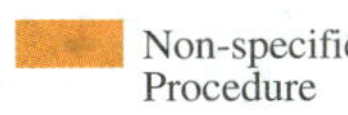 Non-specific Procedure

MEDICINE SERVICES MODIFIERS

MEDICINE services and procedures may be modified under certain circumstances. When applicable, the modifying circumstance is identified by the addition of the appropriate modifier code. The following modifiers are frequently used with MEDICINE services.

-22 Unusual services

-26 Professional component

-51 Multiple procedures

This modifier may be used to report multiple medical procedures performed at the same session, as well as a combination of medical and surgical procedures.

-52 Reduced services

-76 Repeat procedure by same physician

-77 Repeat procedure by another physician

-90 Reference (outside) laboratory

-99 Multiple modifiers

● New Code   ▲ Revised Code   ✴ Starred Procedure   ✛ Add-On Code   ⊘ Modifier -51 Exempt

MEDICINE CODES

IMMUNE GLOBULINS

Immune globulins are administered to provide protection from hepatitis B, diphtheria, rabies, respiratory viruses, tetanus and other diseases. Immune globulin CPT codes 90281-90399 identify the immune globulin product only and must be reported in addition to immunization administration CPT codes.

⊘ **90281**   Immune globulin (Ig), human, for intramuscular use

⊘ **90283**   Immune globulin (IgIV), human, for intravenous use

⊘ **90287**   Botulinum antitoxin, equine, any route

⊘ **90288**   Botulism immune globulin, human, for intravenous use

⊘ **90291**   Cytomegalovirus immune globulin (CMV-IgIV), human, for intravenous use

⊘ **90296**   Diphtheria antitoxin, equine, any route

⊘ **90371**   Hepatitis B immune globulin (HBIg), human, for intramuscular use

⊘ **90375**   Rabies immune globulin (RIg), human, for intramuscular and/or subcutaneous use

⊘ **90376**   Rabies immune globulin, heat-treated (RIg-HT), human, for intramuscular and/or subcutaneous use

⊘ **90378**   Respiratory syncytial virus immune globulin (RSV-IgIM), for intramuscular use, 50 mg, each

⊘ **90379**   Respiratory syncytial virus immune globulin (RSV-IgIV), human, for intravenous use

⊘ **90384**   Rho(D) immune globulin (RhIg), human, full-dose, for intramuscular use

⊘ **90385**   Rho(D) immune globulin (RhIg), human, mini-dose, for intramuscular use

⊘ **90386**   Rho(D) immune globulin (RhIgIV), human, for intravenous use

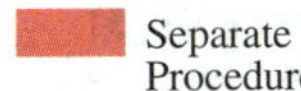 Separate Procedure

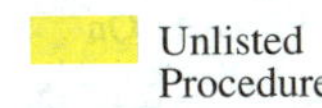 Unlisted Procedure

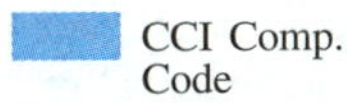 CCI Comp. Code

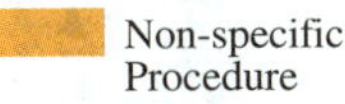 Non-specific Procedure

⊘ **90389**   Tetanus immune globulin (TIg), human, for intramuscular use

⊘ **90393**   Vaccinia immune globulin, human, for intramuscular use

⊘ **90396**   Varicella-zoster immune globulin, human, for intramuscular use

⊘ **90399**   Unlisted immune globulin

IMMUNIZATION ADMINISTRATION FOR VACCINES/TOXOIDS

Immunization is the administration of a vaccine or toxoid to stimulate the immune system to provide protection against disease. Immunizations are usually given in conjunction with an evaluation and management service. When an immunization is the only service performed, a minimal evaluation and management service code may be listed in addition to the injection code.

Coding Rules

1. When an immunization is the only service provided, evaluation and management service code 99221, Minimal service, may be reported in addition to the immunization.

2. Immunization administration CPT codes must be reported in addition to the vaccine and toxoid CPT codes.

3. Supplies or equipment used to inject the vaccine or toxoid are not reported separately.

IMMUNIZATION ADMINISTRATION

(For allergy testing, see 95004 et seq)

(For skin testing of bacterial, viral, fungal extracts, see 86485-86586)

(For therapeutic or diagnostic injections, see 90782-90799)

▲ **90471**   Immunization administration (includes percutaneous, intradermal, subcutaneous, intramuscular and jet injections); one vaccine (single or combination vaccine/toxoid)

+**90472**   each additional vaccine (single or combination vaccine/toxoid) (List separately in addition to code for primary procedure)

(Use 90472 in conjunction with code 90471)

● New Code ▲ Revised Code ＊ Starred Procedure ＋ Add-On Code ⊘ Modifier -51 Exempt

(For administration of immune globulins, use 90780-90784, and see 90281-90399)

(For intravesical administration of BCG vaccine, use 51720, and see 90586)

● **90473** Immunization administration by intranasal or oral route; one vaccine (single or combination vaccine/toxoid)

●+**90474** each additional vaccine (single or combination vaccine/toxoid) (List separately in addition to code for primary procedure)

(Use 90474 in conjunction with code 90473)

VACCINES, TOXOIDS

Vaccines and toxoids are administered to provide protection from hepatitis, influenza, typhoid, measles, mumps, polio, and other diseases. Vaccine and toxoid CPT codes 90476-90749 identify the vaccine or toxoid only and must be reported in addition to immunization administration CPT codes.

(For immune globulins, see codes 90281-90399, and 90780-90784 for administration of immune globulins)

⊘ **90476** Adenovirus vaccine, type 4, live, for oral use

⊘ **90477** Adenovirus vaccine, type 7, live, for oral use

⊘ **90581** Anthrax vaccine, for subcutaneous use

⊘ **90585** Bacillus Calmette-Guerin vaccine (BCG) for tuberculosis, live, for percutaneous use

⊘ **90586** Bacillus Calmette-Guerin vaccine (BCG) for bladder cancer, live, for intravesical use

⊘ **90632** Hepatitis A vaccine, adult dosage, for intramuscular use

⊘ **90633** Hepatitis A vaccine, pediatric/adolescent dosage-2 dose schedule, for intramuscular use

⊘ **90634** Hepatitis A vaccine, pediatric/adolescent dosage-3 dose schedule, for intramuscular use

⊘ **90636** Hepatitis A and hepatitis B vaccine (HepA-HepB), adult dosage, for intramuscular use

767

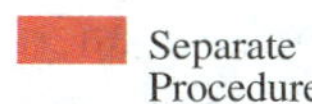

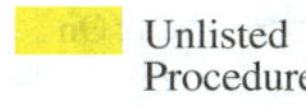

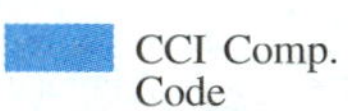

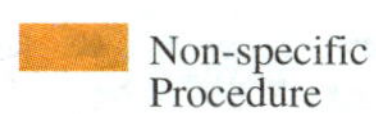

⊘ **90645**   Hemophilus influenza B vaccine (Hib), HbOC conjugate (4 dose schedule), for intramuscular use

⊘ **90646**   Hemophilus influenza B vaccine (Hib), PRP-D conjugate, for booster use only, intramuscular use

⊘ **90647**   Hemophilus influenza B vaccine (Hib), PRP-OMP conjugate (3 dose schedule), for intramuscular use

⊘ **90648**   Hemophilus influenza B vaccine (Hib),PRP-T conjugate (4 dose schedule), for intramuscular use

⊘ **90657**   Influenza virus vaccine, split virus, 6-35 months dosage, for intramuscular or jet injection use

⊘ **90658**   Influenza virus vaccine, split virus, 3 years and above dosage, for intramuscular or jet injection use

⊘ **90659**   Influenza virus vaccine, whole virus, for intramuscular or jet injection use

⊘ **90660**   Influenza virus vaccine, live, for intranasal use

⊘ **90665**   Lyme disease vaccine, adult dosage, for intramuscular use

⊘ **90669**   Pneumococcal conjugate vaccine, polyvalent, for children under five years, for intramuscular use

⊘ **90675**   Rabies vaccine, for intramuscular use

⊘ **90676**   Rabies vaccine, for intradermal use

⊘ **90680**   Rotavirus vaccine, tetravalent, live, for oral use

⊘ **90690**   Typhoid vaccine, live, oral

⊘ **90691**   Typhoid vaccine, Vi capsular polysaccharide (ViCPs), for intramuscular use

⊘ **90692**   Typhoid vaccine, heat- and phenol-inactivated (H-P), for subcutaneous or intradermal use

⊘ **90693**   Typhoid vaccine, acetone-killed, dried (AKD), for subcutaneous or jet injection use (U.S. military)

---

768   ● New Code   ▲ Revised Code   ✳ Starred Procedure   ✚ Add-On Code   ⊘ Modifier -51 Exempt

⊘ **90700** Diphtheria, tetanus toxoids, and acellular pertussis vaccine (DTaP), for intramuscular use

⊘ **90701** Diphtheria, tetanus toxoids, and whole cell pertussis vaccine (DTP), for intramuscular use

⊘ **90702** Diphtheria and tetanus toxoids (DT) adsorbed for use in individuals younger than seven years, for intramuscular use

⊘ **90703** Tetanus toxoid adsorbed, for intramuscular or jet injection use

⊘ **90704** Mumps virus vaccine, live, for subcutaneous or jet injection use

⊘ **90705** Measles virus vaccine, live, for subcutaneous or jet injection use

⊘ **90706** Rubella virus vaccine, live, for subcutaneous or jet injection use

⊘ **90707** Measles, mumps and rubella virus vaccine (MMR), live, for subcutaneous or jet injection use

⊘ **90708** Measles and rubella virus vaccine, live, for subcutaneous or jet injection use

⊘ **90709** Rubella and mumps virus vaccine, live, for subcutaneous use

⊘ **90710** Measles, mumps, rubella, and varicella vaccine (MMRV), live, for subcutaneous use

⊘ **90712** Poliovirus vaccine, (any type(s)) (OPV), live, for oral use

⊘ **90713** Poliovirus vaccine, inactivated, (IPV), for subcutaneous use

⊘ **90716** Varicella virus vaccine, live, for subcutaneous use

⊘ **90717** Yellow fever vaccine, live, for subcutaneous use

⊘ **90718** Tetanus and diphtheria toxoids (Td) adsorbed for use in individuals seven years or older, for intramuscular or jet injection

⊘ **90719** Diphtheria toxoid, for intramuscular use

⊘ **90720** Diphtheria, tetanus toxoids, and whole cell pertussis vaccine and Hemophilus influenza B vaccine (DTP-Hib), for intramuscular use

---

| Separate Procedure | Unlisted Procedure | CCI Comp. Code | Non-specific Procedure |

⊘ **90721**   Diphtheria, tetanus toxoids, and acellular pertussis vaccine and Hemophilus influenza B vaccine (DtaP-Hib), for intramuscular use

⊘ **90723**   Diphtheria, tetanus toxoids, acellular pertussis vaccine, Hepatitis B, and poliovirus vaccine, inactivated (DtaP-HepB-IPV), for intramuscular use

⊘ **90725**   Cholera vaccine for injectable use

(For oral cholera, use 90592)

⊘ **90727**   Plague vaccine, for intramuscular or jet injection use

⊘ ▲ **90732**   Pneumococcal polysaccharide vaccine, 23-valent, adult or immunosuppressed patient dosage, for use in individuals 2 years or older, for subcutaneous or intramuscular use

⊘ **90733**   Meningococcal polysaccharide vaccine (any group(s)), for subcutaneous or jet injection use

⊘ **90735**   Japanese encephalitis virus vaccine, for subcutaneous use

⊘ **90740**   Hepatitis B vaccine, dialysis or immunosuppressed patient dosage (3 dose schedule), for intramuscular use

⊘ **90743**   Hepatitis B vaccine, adolescent (2 dose schedule), for intramuscular use

⊘ **90744**   Hepatitis B vaccine, pediatric/adolescent dosage (3 dose schedule), for intramuscular use

⊘ **90746**   Hepatitis B vaccine, adult dosage, for intramuscular use

⊘ **90747**   Hepatitis B vaccine, dialysis or immunosuppressed patient dosage (4 dose schedule), for intramuscular use

⊘ **90748**   Hepatitis B and Hemophilus influenza B vaccine (HepB-Hib), for intramuscular use

⊘ **90749**   Unlisted vaccine/toxoid

● New Code   ▲ Revised Code   ✻ Starred Procedure   ✚ Add-On Code   ⊘ Modifier -51 Exempt

THERAPEUTIC OR DIAGNOSTIC INFUSIONS (EXCLUDES CHEMOTHERAPY)

Infusion is the therapeutic introduction of a fluid, other than blood, into a vein. An infusion flows in by gravity whereas an injection is forced in by a syringe. Infusion therapy CPT codes are used to report prolonged intravenous injections requiring the presence of a physician during the infusion. These CPT codes are time specific codes covering the first hour, and each additional hour of therapy up to eight (8) hours.

Coding Rules

1.   Presence of the physician during the infusion is required.

2.   Infusion CPT codes may not be used for chemotherapy infusions.

3.   Infusion CPT codes may not be used for intradermal, subcutaneous, intramuscular, or routine intravenous drug injections.

4.   Infusion CPT codes may not be reported in addition to prolonged services CPT codes.

▲ **90780**   Intravenous infusion for therapy/diagnosis, administered by physician or under direct supervision of physician; up to one hour

+90781   each additional hour, up to eight (8) hours (List separately in addition to code for primary procedure)

(Use 90781 in conjunction with code 90780)

THERAPEUTIC, PROPHYLACTIC OR DIAGNOSTIC INJECTIONS

An injection is the process of forcing a liquid, usually via a needle and syringe, into the skin, muscles, arteries or veins. Therapeutic or diagnostic injection CPT codes are used for reporting therapeutic injections of medication, via subcutaneous, intramuscular, intra-arterial or intravenous routes and for reporting intramuscular injection of antibiotics.

Coding Rules

1.   When reporting therapeutic or diagnostic injection CPT codes, the injected material should be specified.

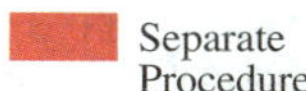

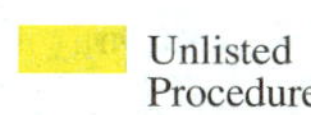

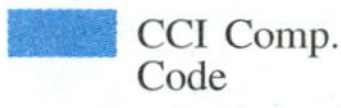

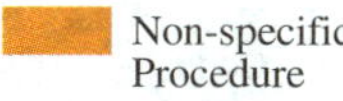

2. Therapeutic or diagnostic injection CPT codes may not be used for allergen immunotherapy.

3. Use CPT therapeutic or diagnostic injection CPT codes when reporting injections to commercial health insurance companies, unless otherwise instructed by specific companies.

4. Use HCPCS Level II codes instead of CPT codes to report therapeutic or diagnostic injections on health insurance claims to Medicare.

90782 Therapeutic, prophylactic or diagnostic injection (specify material injected); subcutaneous or intramuscular

(For administration of vaccines/toxoids, see 90471-90472)

90783 intra-arterial

90784 intravenous

(90782-90784 do not include injections for allergen immunotherapy. For allergen immunotherapy injections, see 95115-95117)

90788 Intramuscular injection of antibiotic (specify)

90799 Unlisted therapeutic, prophylactic or diagnostic injection

(For allergy immunizations, see 95004 et seq)

PSYCHIATRY

(For repetitive transcranial magnetic stimulation for treatment of clinical depression, use Category III code 0018T)

Psychiatry is the study, treatment and prevention of mental disorders. Psychiatric services include diagnostic and therapeutic services in the hospital, office, or other outpatient setting. Psychiatric service CPT codes are used to report general psychiatry, clinical psychiatry, and psychiatric therapeutic services and procedures. Key coding issues include the type of psychotherapy, the place of service, the face-to-face time spent with the patient during psychotherapy, and whether evaluation and management services are furnished on the same date of service as psychotherapy.

| ● New Code | ▲ Revised Code | * Starred Procedure | + Add-On Code | ⊘ Modifier -51 Exempt |

Coding Rules

1. Attending physicians reporting hospital care services in treating a psychiatric inpatient may use the full range of hospital evaluation and management service codes.

2. If the physician is active in the leadership or direction of a treatment team, a code may be selected based upon the services provided that day using Case Management CPT codes from evaluation and management services codes 99361-99362.

3. All procedures performed in addition to hospital care, such as electroconvulsive therapy or medical psychotherapy should be listed in addition to hospital care.

4. Psychiatric care may be reported without time dimensions, using CPT codes 90841 or 90845, or with time dimensions, using CPT codes 90843 or 90844, based upon practices customary in the local area.

5. The modifiers -52, reduced service, or -22, unusual service, may be used to report services that were less or more lengthy that the time-specified CPT codes define.

PSYCHIATRIC CONSULTATIONS

Consultation for psychiatric evaluation of a patient includes examination of a patient and exchange of information with primary physician and others, such as nurses or family members, and preparation of report.

Consultation services provided by psychiatrists are reported with evaluation and management consultation CPT codes. Psychiatric consultation services are limited to initial or follow-up evaluation and do not involve psychiatric treatment.

PSYCHIATRIC DIAGNOSTIC OR EVALUATIVE INTERVIEW PROCEDURES

90801 Psychiatric diagnostic interview examination

90802 Interactive psychiatric diagnostic interview examination using play equipment, physical devices, language interpreter, or other mechanisms of communication

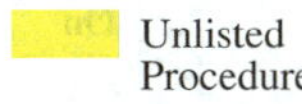

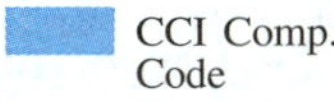

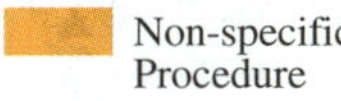

Non-specific
Procedure

PSYCHIATRIC THERAPEUTIC PROCEDURES

OFFICE OR OTHER OUTPATIENT FACILITY

Insight Oriented, Behavior Modifying and/or Supportive Psychotherapy

90804 Individual psychotherapy, insight oriented, behavior modifying and/or supportive, in an office or outpatient facility, approximately 20 to 30 minutes face-to-face with the patient;

90805 with medical evaluation and management services

90806 Individual psychotherapy, insight oriented, behavior modifying and/or supportive, in an office or outpatient facility, approximately 45 to 50 minutes face-to-face with the patient;

90807 with medical evaluation and management services

90808 Individual psychotherapy, insight oriented, behavior modifying and/or supportive, in an office or outpatient facility, approximately 75 to 80 minutes face-to-face with the patient;

90809 with medical evaluation and management services

Interactive Psychotherapy

90810 Individual psychotherapy, interactive, using play equipment, physical devices, language interpreter, or other mechanisms of non-verbal communication, in an office or outpatient facility, approximately 20 to 30 minutes face-to-face with the patient;

90811 with medical evaluation and management services

90812 Individual psychotherapy, interactive, using play equipment, physical devices, language interpreter, or other mechanisms of non-verbal communication, in an office or outpatient facility, approximately 45 to 50 minutes face-to-face with the patient;

90813 with medical evaluation and management services

90814 Individual psychotherapy, interactive, using play equipment, physical devices, language interpreter, or other mechanisms of non-verbal communication, in an office or outpatient facility, approximately 75 to 80 minutes face-to-face with the patient;

90815 with medical evaluation and management services

● New Code   ▲ Revised Code   ✳ Starred Procedure   + Add-On Code   ⊘ Modifier -51 Exempt

INPATIENT HOSPITAL, PARTIAL HOSPITAL OR RESIDENTIAL CARE FACILITY

Insight Oriented, Behavior Modifying and/or Supportive Psychotherapy

90816 Individual psychotherapy, insight oriented, behavior modifying and/or supportive, in an inpatient hospital, partial hospital or residential care setting, approximately 20 to 30 minutes face-to-face with the patient;

90817 with medical evaluation and management services

90818 Individual psychotherapy, insight oriented, behavior modifying and/or supportive, in an inpatient hospital, partial hospital or residential care setting, approximately 45 to 50 minutes face-to-face with the patient;

90819 with medical evaluation and management services

90821 Individual psychotherapy, insight oriented, behavior modifying and/or supportive, in an inpatient hospital, partial hospital or residential care setting, approximately 75 to 80 minutes face-to-face with the patient;

Interactive Psychotherapy

90822 with medical evaluation and management services

90823 Individual psychotherapy, interactive, using play equipment, physical devices, language interpreter, or other mechanisms of non-verbal communication, in an inpatient hospital, partial hospital or residential care setting, approximately 20 to 30 minutes face-to-face with the patient;

90824 with medical evaluation and management services

90826 Individual psychotherapy, interactive, using play equipment, physical devices, language interpreter, or other mechanisms of non-verbal communication, in an inpatient hospital, partial hospital or residential care setting, approximately 45 to 50 minutes face-to-face with the patient;

90827 with medical evaluation and management services

90828 Individual psychotherapy, interactive, using play equipment, physical devices, language interpreter, or other mechanisms of non-verbal communication, in an inpatient hospital, partial

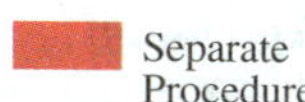

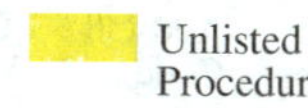

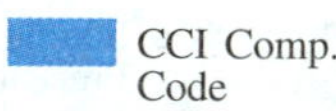

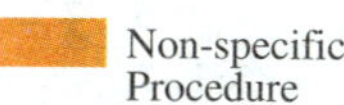

hospital or residential care setting, approximately 75 to 80 minutes face-to-face with the patient;

90829   with medical evaluation and management services

OTHER PSYCHOTHERAPY

90845 Psychoanalysis

90846 Family psychotherapy (without the patient present)

90847 Family psychotherapy (conjoint psychotherapy) (with patient present)

90849 Multiple-family group psychotherapy

90853 Group psychotherapy (other than of a multiple-family group)

90857 Interactive group psychotherapy

OTHER PSYCHIATRIC SERVICES OR PROCEDURES

90862 Pharmacologic management, including prescription, use, and review of medication with no more than minimal medical psychotherapy

90865 Narcosynthesis for psychiatric diagnostic and therapeutic purposes (eg, sodium amobarbital (Amytal) interview)

90870 Electroconvulsive therapy (includes necessary monitoring); single seizure

90871   multiple seizures, per day

90875 Individual psychophysiological therapy incorporating biofeedback training by any modality (face-to-face with the patient), with psychotherapy (eg, insight oriented, behavior modifying or supportive psychotherapy); approximately 20-30 minutes

90876   approximately 45-50 minutes

90880 Hypnotherapy

● New Code   ▲ Revised Code   * Starred Procedure   + Add-On Code   ∅ Modifier -51 Exempt

90882 Environmental intervention for medical management purposes on a psychiatric patients behalf with agencies, employers, or institutions

90885 Psychiatric evaluation of hospital records, other psychiatric reports, psychometric and/or projective tests, and other accumulated data for medical diagnostic purposes

90887 Interpretation or explanation of results of psychiatric, other medical examinations and procedures, or other accumulated data to family or other responsible persons, or advising them how to assist patient

90889 Preparation of report of patients psychiatric status, history, treatment, or progress (other than for legal or consultative purposes) for other physicians, agencies, or insurance carriers

90899 Unlisted psychiatric service or procedure

BIOFEEDBACK

Biofeedback is the process of detecting information about a patient's biological functions, eg. heart rate, breathing rate, skin temperature, and amount of muscle tension, picked up by surface electrodes (sensors) and electronically amplified to provide feedback, usually in the form of an audio-tone and/or visual read-out to the patient. Biofeedback training uses the information that has been monitored from the sensors attached to a muscle on the skin's surface, or to the skin only for thermal or other readings. With the help of a trained clinician, the patient can learn how to make voluntary changes in those biological functions and bring them under control.

(For psychophysiological therapy incorporating biofeedback training, see 90875, 90876)

90901 Biofeedback training by any modality

90911 Biofeedback training, perineal muscles, anorectal or urethral sphincter, including EMG and/or manometry

777

DIALYSIS

Dialysis is the process of passing body fluids through a membrane to remove harmful substances. Dialysis is used in the treatment of kidney failure. Key coding issues include the type of dialysis and the location of the service.

Coding Rules

1. All evaluation and management services related to the patient's end stage renal disease that are rendered on a day when dialysis is performed and all other patient care services that are rendered during the dialysis procedure are included in the dialysis procedure CPT codes.

2. All evaluation and management services unrelated to the dialysis procedure that cannot be rendered during the dialysis session may be reported in addition to the dialysis procedure.

3. Supplies provided to dialysis patients not considered to be included with the dialysis service or procedure are reported using CPT code 99070 or HCPCS codes E1500-E1699 for DME, and A4650-A5149 for supplies for ESRD.

END STAGE RENAL DISEASE SERVICES

90918   End stage renal disease (ESRD) related services per full month; for patients under two years of age to include monitoring for the adequacy of nutrition, assessment of growth and development, and counseling of parents

90919   for patients between two and eleven years of age to include monitoring for the adequacy of nutrition, assessment of growth and development, and counseling of parents

90920   for patients between twelve and nineteen years of age to include monitoring for the adequacy of nutrition, assessment of growth and development, and counseling of parents

90921   for patients twenty years of age and over

90922   End stage renal disease (ESRD) related services (less than full month), per day; for patients under two years of age

90923   for patients between two and eleven years of age

90924   for patients between twelve and nineteen years of age

---

● New Code   ▲ Revised Code   ✳ Starred Procedure   ✚ Add-On Code   ⊘ Modifier -51 Exempt

90925   for patients twenty years of age and over

HEMODIALYSIS

(For home visit hemodialysis services performed by a non-physician health care professional, use 99512)

(For cannula declotting, see 36831, 36833, 36860, 36861)

(For declotting of implanted vascular access device or catheter by thrombolytic agent, use 36550)

(For collection of blood specimen from a partially or completely implantable venous access device, use 36540)

(For prolonged physician attendance, see 99354-99360)

90935 Hemodialysis procedure with single physician evaluation

90937 Hemodialysis procedure requiring repeated evaluation(s) with or without substantial revision of dialysis prescription

● **90939** Hemodialysis access flow study to determine blood flow in grafts and arteriovenous fistulae by an indicator dilution method, hook-up; transcutaneous measurement and disconnection.

90940   measurement and disconnection

(For duplex scan of hemodialysis access, use 93990)

MISCELLANEOUS DIALYSIS PROCEDURES

(For insertion of intraperitoneal cannula or catheter, see 49420, 49421)

(For prolonged physician attendance, see 99354-99360)

90945 Dialysis procedure other than hemodialysis (eg, peritoneal, hemofiltration or other continuous replacement therapies), with single physician evaluation

(For home infusion of peritoneal dialysis, use 99559)

90947 Dialysis procedure other than hemodialysis (eg, peritoneal dialysis, hemofiltration, or other continuous renal replacement therapies) requiring repeated physician evaluations, with or without substantial revision of dialysis prescription

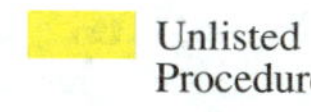

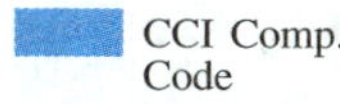

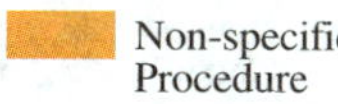

Non-specific
Procedure

779

90989   Dialysis training, patient, including helper where applicable, any mode, completed course

90993   Dialysis training, patient, including helper where applicable, any mode, course not completed, per training session

90997   Hemoperfusion (eg, with activated charcoal or resin)

90999   Unlisted dialysis procedure, inpatient or outpatient

GASTROENTEROLOGY

Gastroenterology is the study and treatment of diseases of the stomach and digestive system. CPT codes listed in this subsection are used to report diagnostic services of the esophagus and/or stomach contents, and therapeutic services such as gastric intubation and lavage. Gastroenterology services are usually performed in conjunction with an evaluation and management service, such as a consultation or visit, and should be reported separately in addition to the evaluation and management service.

(For duodenal intubation and aspiration, see 89100-89105)

(For gastrointestinal radiologic procedures, see 74210-74363)

(For esophagoscopy procedures, see 43200-43228; upper GI endoscopy 43234-43259; endoscopy, small intestine and stomal 44360-44393; proctosigmoidoscopy 45300-45321; sigmoidoscopy 45330-45339; colonscopy 45355-45385; anoscopy 46600-46615)

91000   Esophageal intubation and collection of washings for cytology, including preparation of specimens (separate procedure)

91010   Esophageal motility (manometric study of the esophagus and/or gastroesophageal junction) study;

91011   with mecholyl or similar stimulant

91012   with acid perfusion studies

91020   Gastric motility (manometric) studies

91030   Esophagus, acid perfusion (Bernstein) test for esophagitis

91032   Esophagus, acid reflux test, with intraluminal pH electrode for detection of gastroesophageal reflux;

● New Code   ▲ Revised Code   ＊ Starred Procedure   ✚ Add-On Code   ⊘ Modifier -51 Exempt

91033 prolonged recording

91052 Gastric analysis test with injection of stimulant of gastric secretion (eg, histamine, insulin, pentagastrin, calcium and secretin)

(For gastric biopsy by capsule, peroral, via tube, one or more specimens, use 43600)

(For gastric laboratory procedures, see also 89130-89141)

91055 Gastric intubation, washings, and preparing slides for cytology (separate procedure)

(For gastric lavage, therapeutic, use 91105)

91060 Gastric saline load test

(For biopsy by capsule, small intestine, per oral, via tube (one or more specimens), use 44100)

91065 Breath hydrogen test (eg, for detection of lactase deficiency)

91100 Intestinal bleeding tube, passage, positioning and monitoring

91105 Gastric intubation, and aspiration or lavage for treatment (eg, for ingested poisons)

(For cholangiography, see 47500, 74320)

(For abdominal paracentesis, see 49080, 49081; with instillation of medication, see 96440, 96445)

(For peritoneoscopy, use 49320; with biopsy, use 49321)

(For peritoneoscopy and guided transhepatic cholangiography, use 47560; with biopsy, use 47561)

(For splenoportography, see 38200, 75810)

91122 Anorectal manometry

● **91123** Pulsed irrigation of fecal impaction

GASTRIC PHYSIOLOGY

91132 Electrogastrography, diagnostic, transcutaneous;

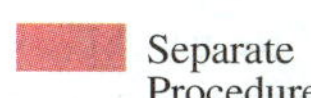 Separate Procedure

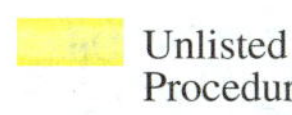 Unlisted Procedure

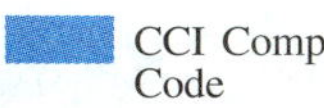 CCI Comp. Code

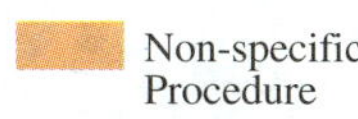 Non-specific Procedure

781

91133   with provocative testing

OTHER PROCEDURES

91299 Unlisted diagnostic gastroenterology procedure

OPHTHALMOLOGY

(For surgical procedures, see Surgery, Eye and Ocular Adnexa, 65091 et seq)

Ophthalmology is the study and treatment of diseases of the eye. Ophthalmological diagnostic and treatment services are reported using CPT Medicine codes 92002-92499.

Coding Rules

1. Minimal, brief and limited office services, and hospital, home, extended care, emergency department and consultations are reported using appropriate evaluation and management service codes.

2. Surgical procedures on the eye(s) are reported using CPT codes from the Eye and Ocular Adnexa subsection of the SURGERY section of CPT.

3. To report **intermediate** ophthalmological services, the following must be performed and documented: a) evaluation of new or existing condition, b) complications of new diagnostic or management problems (not necessarily related to the primary diagnosis), c) history, d) general medical observation e) external ocular and adnexal examination, f) other diagnostic procedures as indicated, and g) may include the use of mydriasis. Intermediate ophthalmological services do not usually include determination of refractive state but may in an established patient under continuing active treatment.

4. To report **comprehensive** ophthalmological services the following must be performed and documented: a) reported as a single service but may be performed at more than one session, b) history, c) general medical observation, d) external and ophthalmoscopic examination, e) gross visual fields, f) basic sensorimotor examination, g. may include, as indicated; biomicroscopy, examination with cycloplegia or mydriasis and tonometry, h) always includes initiation of diagnostic and treatment programs.

● New Code   ▲ Revised Code   ✳ Starred Procedure   ＋ Add-On Code   ⊘ Modifier -51 Exempt

5. For both intermediate and comprehensive ophthalmological services, service components, such as slip lamp examination, keratomy, ophthalmoscopy, retinoscopy, tonometry and motor evaluation are not reported separately.

GENERAL OPHTHALMOLOGICAL SERVICES

NEW PATIENT

92002 Ophthalmological services: medical examination and evaluation with initiation of diagnostic and treatment program; intermediate, new patient

92004 comprehensive, new patient, one or more visits

ESTABLISHED PATIENT

92012 Ophthalmological services: medical examination and evaluation, with initiation or continuation of diagnostic and treatment program; intermediate, established patient

92014 comprehensive, established patient, one or more visits

(For surgical procedures, see Surgery, Eye and Ocular Adnexa, 65091 et seq)

SPECIAL OPHTHALMOLOGICAL SERVICES

Special ophthalmological services are defined as a level of service in which a special evaluation of part of the visual system is made which goes beyond the services usually included under general ophthalmological services, or in which special treatment is given. Fluorescein angioscopy, quantitative visual field examination, or extended color vision examination should be specifically reported as special ophthalmological services.

92015 Determination of refractive state

92018 Ophthalmological examination and evaluation, under general anesthesia, with or without manipulation of globe for passive range of motion or other manipulation to facilitate diagnostic examination; complete

92019 limited

92020 Gonioscopy (separate procedure)

(For gonioscopy under general anesthesia, use 92018)

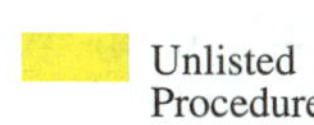

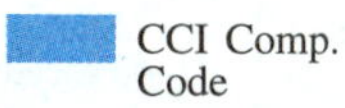

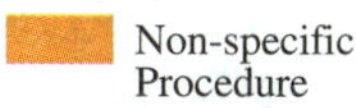

92060 Sensorimotor examination with multiple measurements of ocular deviation (eg, restrictive or paretic muscle with diplopia) with interpretation and report (separate procedure)

92065 Orthoptic and/or pleoptic training, with continuing medical direction and evaluation

92070 Fitting of contact lens for treatment of disease, including supply of lens

92081 Visual field examination, unilateral or bilateral, with interpretation and report; limited examination (eg, tangent screen, Autoplot, arc perimeter, or single stimulus level automated test, such as Octopus 3 or 7 equivalent)

92082 intermediate examination (eg, at least 2 isopters on Goldmann perimeter, or semiquantitative, automated suprathreshold screening program, Humphrey suprathreshold automatic diagnostic test, Octopus program 33)

92083 extended examination (eg, Goldmann visual fields with at least 3 isopters plotted and static determination within the central 30 degrees, or quantitative, automated threshold perimetry, Octopus programs G-1, 32 or 42, Humphrey visual field analyzer full threshold programs 30-2, 24-2, or 30/60-2)

(Gross visual field testing (eg, confrontation testing) is a part of general ophthalmological services and is not reported separately)

92100 Serial tonometry (separate procedure) with multiple measurements of intraocular pressure over an extended time period with interpretation and report, same day (eg, diurnal curve or medical treatment of acute elevation of intraocular pressure)

92120 Tonography with interpretation and report, recording indentation tonometer method or perilimbal suction method

92130 Tonography with water provocation

92135 Scanning computerized ophthalmic diagnostic imaging (eg, scanning laser) with interpretation and report, unilateral

● **92136** Ophthalmic biometry by partial coherence interferometry with intraocular lens power calculation

---

● New Code   ▲ Revised Code   ∗ Starred Procedure   ✚ Add-On Code   ⊘ Modifier -51 Exempt

92140   Provocative tests for glaucoma, with interpretation and report, without tonography

OPHTHALMOSCOPY

92225   Ophthalmoscopy, extended, with retinal drawing (eg, for retinal detachment, melanoma), with interpretation and report; initial

92226   subsequent

92230   Fluorescein angioscopy with interpretation and report

92235   Fluorescein angiography (includes multiframe imaging) with interpretation and report

92240   Indocyanine-green angiography (includes multiframe imaging) with interpretation and report

92250   Fundus photography with interpretation and report

92260   Ophthalmodynamometry

(For opthalmoscopy under general anesthesia, use 92018)

OTHER SPECIALIZED SERVICES

92265   Needle oculoelectromyography, one or more extraocular muscles, one or both eyes, with interpretation and report

92270   Electro-oculography with interpretation and report

92275   Electroretinography with interpretation and report

(For electronystagmography for vestibular function studies, see 92541 et seq)

(For ophthalmic echography (diagnostic ultrasound), see 76511-76529)

92283   Color vision examination, extended, eg, anomaloscope or equivalent

(Color vision testing with pseudoisochromatic plates (such as HRR or Ishihara) is not reported separately. It is included in the appropriate general or ophthalmological service, or 99172)

92284   Dark adaptation examination with interpretation and report

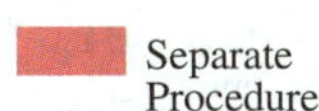

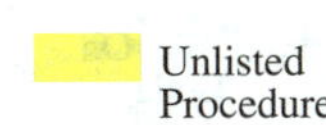

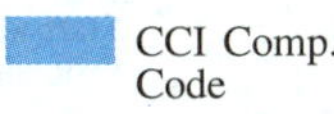

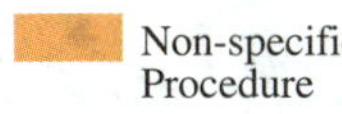

| 92285 | External ocular photography with interpretation and report for documentation of medical progress (eg, close-up photography, slit lamp photography, goniophotography, stereo-photography) |

92286 Special anterior segment photography with interpretation and report; with specular endothelial microscopy and cell count

| 92287 | with fluorescein angiography |

CONTACT LENS SERVICES

(For therapeutic or surgical use of contact lens, see 68340, 92070)

92310 Prescription of optical and physical characteristics of and fitting of contact lens, with medical supervision of adaptation; corneal lens, both eyes, except for aphakia

(For prescription and fitting of one eye, add modifier -52)

| 92311 | corneal lens for aphakia, one eye |

| 92312 | corneal lens for aphakia, both eyes |

| 92313 | corneoscleral lens |

92314 Prescription of optical and physical characteristics of contact lens, with medical supervision of adaptation and direction of fitting by independent technician; corneal lens, both eyes except for aphakia

(For prescription and fitting of one eye, add modifier -52)

| 92315 | corneal lens for aphakia, one eye |

| 92316 | corneal lens for aphakia, both eyes |

| 92317 | corneoscleral lens |

| 92325 | Modification of contact lens (separate procedure), with medical supervision of adaptation |

| 92326 | Replacement of contact lens |

● New Code   ▲ Revised Code   * Starred Procedure   + Add-On Code   ⊘ Modifier -51 Exempt

OCULAR PROSTHETICS, ARTIFICIAL EYE

92330 Prescription, fitting, and supply of ocular prosthesis (artificial eye), with medical supervision of adaptation

(If supply is not included, use modifier -26; to report supply separately, use 92393)

92335 Prescription of ocular prosthesis (artificial eye) and direction of fitting and supply by independent technician, with medical supervision of adaptation

SPECTACLE SERVICES (INCLUDING PROSTHESIS FOR APHAKIA)

92340 Fitting of spectacles, except for aphakia; monofocal

92341   bifocal

92342   multifocal, other than bifocal

92352 Fitting of spectacle prosthesis for aphakia; monofocal

92353   multifocal

92354 Fitting of spectacle mounted low vision aid; single element system

92355   telescopic or other compound lens system

92358 Prosthesis service for aphakia, temporary (disposable or loan, including materials)

92370 Repair and refitting spectacles; except for aphakia

92371   spectacle prosthesis for aphakia

SUPPLY OF MATERIALS

92390 Supply of spectacles, except prosthesis for aphakia and low vision aids

92391 Supply of contact lenses, except prosthesis for aphakia

(For supply of contact lenses reported as part of the service of fitting, see 92310-92313)

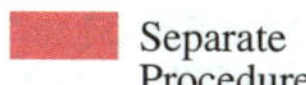 Separate Procedure

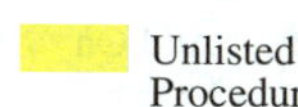 Unlisted Procedure

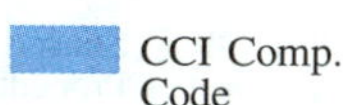 CCI Comp. Code

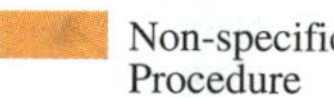 Non-specific Procedure

787

(For replacement of contact lens, use 92326)

92392   Supply of low vision aids (A low vision aid is any lens or device used to aid or improve visual function in a person whose vision cannot be normalized by conventional spectacle correction. Includes reading additions up to 4D.)

92393   Supply of ocular prosthesis (artificial eye)

(For supply reported as part of the service of fitting, use 92330)

92395   Supply of permanent prosthesis for aphakia; spectacles

(For temporary spectacle correction, use 92358)

92396   contact lenses

(For supply reported as part of the service of fitting, see 92311, 92312)

(Use 99070 for the supply of other materials, drugs, trays, etc.)

OTHER PROCEDURES

92499   Unlisted ophthalmological service or procedure

SPECIAL OTORHINOLARYNGOLOGIC SERVICES

Otorhinolaryngology is the study and treatment of diseases of the head and neck, including the ears, nose and throat. Diagnostic or treatment procedures usually included in a comprehensive otorhinolaryngologic evaluation or office visit, are reported as an integrated medical service, using CPT evaluation and management service codes.

Coding Rules

1.   Component procedures, such as otoscopy, rhinoscopy, tuning fork test, which may be provided as part of a comprehensive service are not reported separately.

2.   Special otorhinolaryngologic diagnostic or treatment services not usually included in a comprehensive otorhinolaryngologic evaluation or office visit are reported separately.

● New Code   ▲ Revised Code   ✱ Starred Procedure   + Add-On Code   ⊘ Modifier -51 Exempt

3. All otorhinolaryngologic services include medical diagnostic evaluation. Technical procedures, which may or may not be performed by the physician personally, are often part of the service, but should not be mistaken to constitute the service itself.

(For laryngoscopy with stroboscopy, use 31579)

92502 Otolaryngologic examination under general anesthesia

92504 Binocular microscopy (separate diagnostic procedure)

92506 Evaluation of speech, language, voice, communication, auditory processing, and/or aural rehabilitation status

92507 Treatment of speech, language, voice, communication, and/or auditory processing disorder (includes aural rehabilitation); individual

92508 group, two or more individuals

92510 Aural rehabilitation following cochlear implant (includes evaluation of aural rehabilitation status and hearing, therapeutic services) with or without speech processor programming

92511 Nasopharyngoscopy with endoscope (separate procedure)

92512 Nasal function studies (eg, rhinomanometry)

92516 Facial nerve function studies (eg, electroneuronography)

92520 Laryngeal function studies

92525 Evaluation of swallowing and oral function for feeding

92526 Treatment of swallowing dysfunction and/or oral function for feeding

VESTIBULAR FUNCTION TESTS, WITH OBSERVATION AND EVALUATION BY PHYSICIAN, WITHOUT ELECTRICAL RECORDING

92531 Spontaneous nystagmus, including gaze

▲ **92532** Positional nystagmus test

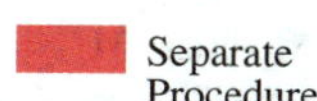

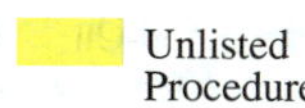

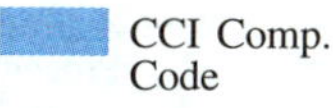

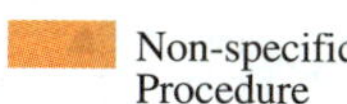

92533 Caloric vestibular test, each irrigation (binaural, bithermal stimulation constitutes four tests)

▲ **92534** Optokinetic nystagmus test

VESTIBULAR FUNCTION TESTS, WITH RECORDING (eg, ENG, PENG), AND MEDICAL DIAGNOSTIC EVALUATION

92541 Spontaneous nystagmus test, including gaze and fixation nystagmus, with recording

92542 Positional nystagmus test, minimum of 4 positions, with recording

92543 Caloric vestibular test, each irrigation (binaural, bithermal stimulation constitutes four tests), with recording

92544 Optokinetic nystagmus test, bidirectional, foveal or peripheral stimulation, with recording

92545 Oscillating tracking test, with recording

92546 Sinusoidal vertical axis rotational testing

+92547 Use of vertical electrodes (List separately in addition to code for primary procedure)

(Use 92547 in conjunction with codes 92541-92546)

(For unlisted vestibular tests, use 92599)

92548 Computerized dynamic posturography

AUDIOLOGIC FUNCTION TESTS WITH MEDICAL DIAGNOSTIC EVALUATION

(For evaluation of speech, language and/or hearing problems through observation and assessment of performance, use 92506)

92551 Screening test, pure tone, air only

92552 Pure tone audiometry (threshold); air only

92553   air and bone

● New Code   ▲ Revised Code   ✻ Starred Procedure   ✚ Add-On Code   ⊘ Modifier -51 Exempt

92555   Speech audiometry threshold;

92556   with speech recognition

92557   Comprehensive audiometry threshold evaluation and speech recognition (92553 and 92556 combined)

(For hearing aid evaluation and selection, see 92590-92595)

92559   Audiometric testing of groups

92560   Bekesy audiometry; screening

92561   diagnostic

92562   Loudness balance test, alternate binaural or monaural

92563   Tone decay test

92564   Short increment sensitivity index (SISI)

92565   Stenger test, pure tone

92567   Tympanometry (impedance testing)

92568   Acoustic reflex testing

92569   Acoustic reflex decay test

92571   Filtered speech test

92572   Staggered spondaic word test

92573   Lombard test

92575   Sensorineural acuity level test

92576   Synthetic sentence identification test

92577   Stenger test, speech

92579   Visual reinforcement audiometry (VRA)

92582   Conditioning play audiometry

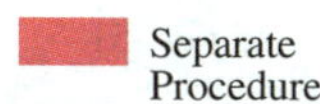

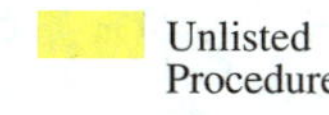

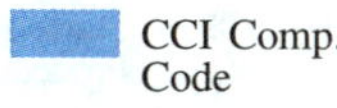

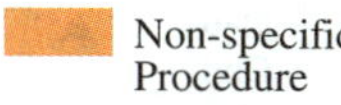

92583   Select picture audiometry

92584   Electrocochleography

92585   Auditory evoked potentials for evoked response audiometry and/or testing of the central nervous system; comprehensive

92586   limited

92587   Evoked otoacoustic emissions; limited (single stimulus level, either transient or distortion products)

92588   comprehensive or diagnostic evaluation (comparison of transient and/or distortion product otoacoustic emissions at multiple levels and frequencies)

92589   Central auditory function test(s) (specify)

92590   Hearing aid examination and selection; monaural

92591   binaural

92592   Hearing aid check; monaural

92593   binaural

92594   Electroacoustic evaluation for hearing aid; monaural

92595   binaural

92596   Ear protector attenuation measurements

92597   Evaluation for use and/or fitting of voice prosthetic or augmentative/alternative communication device to supplement oral speech

92598   Modification of voice prosthetic or augmentative/alternative communication device to supplement oral speech

OTHER PROCEDURES

92599   Unlisted otorhinolaryngological service or procedure

CARDIOVASCULAR

Cardiovascular services refers to the study and treatment of diseases of the heart and vascular (arteries and veins) system. Cardiovascular services CPT codes are used to report therapeutic services such as cardiopulmonary resuscitation (CPR), cardioversion and percutaneous transluminal coronary angioplasty (PTCA) and diagnostic procedures such as electrocardiography, echocardiography and cardiac catheterization.

Coding Rules

1. Cardiovascular services are usually performed in addition to evaluation and management services, such as a consultation or visit, and should be reported in addition to the evaluation and management service.

2. Many cardiovascular services fall under the Medicare Purchased Diagnostic Services guidelines, therefore reporting should be as instructed by your local Medicare carrier.

THERAPEUTIC SERVICES

(For non-surgical septal reduction therapy (eg, alcohol ablation), use Category III code 0024T)

92950 Cardiopulmonary resuscitation (eg, in cardiac arrest)

(See also critical care services, 99291, 99292)

92953 Temporary transcutaneous pacing

(For physician direction of ambulance or rescue personnel outside the hospital, use 99288)

92960 Cardioversion, elective, electrical conversion of arrhythmia; external

92961 internal (separate procedure)

(Do not report 92961 in addition to codes 93662, 93618-93624, 93631, 93640-93642, 93650-93652, 93741-93744)

92970 Cardioassist-method of circulatory assist; internal

92971 external

(For balloon atrial-septostomy, use 92992)

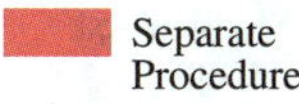

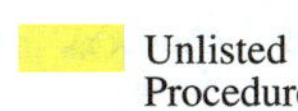

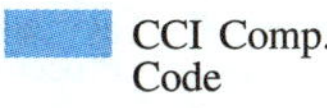

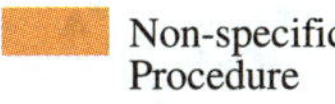

(For placement of catheters for use in circulatory assist devices such as intra-aortic balloon pump, use 33970)

●+**92973**   Percutaneous transluminal coronary thrombectomy (List separately in addition to code for primary procedure)

(Use 92973 in conjunction with codes 92980, 92982)

●+**92974**   Transcatheter placement of radiation delivery device for subsequent coronary intravascular brachytherapy (List separately in addition to code for primary procedure)

(Use 92974 in conjunction with codes 92980, 92982, 93508)

(For intravascular radioelement application, see 77781-77784)

92975   Thrombolysis, coronary; by intracoronary infusion, including selective coronary angiography

92977   by intravenous infusion

(For thrombolysis of vessels other than coronary, see 37201, 75896)

(For cerebral thrombolysis, use 37195)

+**92978**   Intravascular ultrasound (coronary vessel or graft) during diagnostic evaluation and/or therapeutic intervention including imaging supervision, interpretation and report; initial vessel (List separately in addition to code for primary procedure)

+**92979**   each additional vessel (List separately in addition to code for primary procedure)

(Use 92979 in conjunction with code 92978)

(Intravascular ultrasound services include all transducer manipulations and repositioning within the specific vessel being examined, both before and after therapeutic intervention (eg, stent placement)

92980   Transcatheter placement of an intracoronary stent(s), percutaneous, with or without other therapeutic intervention, any method; single vessel

+**92981**   each additional vessel (List separately in addition to code for primary procedure)

(Use 92981 in conjunction with code 92980)

● New Code   ▲ Revised Code   ✳ Starred Procedure   ✛ Add-On Code   ⃠ Modifier -51 Exempt

(To report additional vessels treated by angioplasty or atherectomy only during the same session, see 92984, 92996)

(To report transcatheter placement of radiation delivery device for coronary intravascular brachytherapy, use 92974)

(For intravascular radioelement application, see 77781-77784)

92982 Percutaneous transluminal coronary balloon angioplasty; single vessel

+92984 each additional vessel (List separately in addition to code for primary procedure)

(Use 92984 in conjunction with codes 92980, 92982, 92995)

(For stent placement following completion of angioplasty or atherectomy, see 92980, 92981)

(To report transcatheter placement of radiation delivery device for coronary intravascular brachytherapy, use 92974)

(For intravascular radioelement application, see 77781-77784)

92986 Percutaneous balloon valvuloplasty; aortic valve

92987 mitral valve

92990 pulmonary valve

92992 Atrial septectomy or septostomy; transvenous method, balloon (eg, Rashkind type) (includes cardiac catheterization)

92993 blade method (Park septostomy) (includes cardiac catheterization)

92995 Percutaneous transluminal coronary atherectomy, by mechanical or other method, with or without balloon angioplasty; single vessel

+92996 each additional vessel (List separately in addition to code for primary procedure)

(Use 92996 in conjunction with code(s) 92980, 92982, 92995)

(For stent placement following completion of angioplasty or atherectomy, see 92980, 92981)

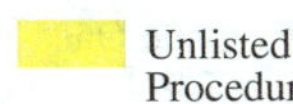

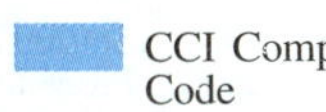

Non-specific
Procedure

795

(To report additional vessels treated by angioplasty only during the same session, use 92984)

92997   Percutaneous transluminal pulmonary artery balloon angioplasty; single vessel

+92998   each additional vessel (List separately in addition to code for primary procedure)

(Use 92998 in conjunction with code 92997)

CARDIOGRAPHY

(For echocardiography, see 93303-93350)

93000   Electrocardiogram, routine ECG with at least 12 leads; with interpretation and report

93005   tracing only, without interpretation and report

93010   interpretation and report only

(For ECG monitoring, see 99354-99360)

93012   Telephonic transmission of post-symptom electrocardiogram rhythm strip(s), per 30 day period of time; tracing only

93014   physician review with interpretation and report only

93015   Cardiovascular stress test using maximal or submaximal treadmill or bicycle exercise, continuous electrocardiographic monitoring, and/or pharmacological stress; with physician supervision, with interpretation and report

93016   physician supervision only, without interpretation and report

93017   tracing only, without interpretation and report

93018   interpretation and report only

93024   Ergonovine provocation test

● **93025**   Microvolt T-wave alternans for assessment of ventricular arrhythmias

93040   Rhythm ECG, one to three leads; with interpretation and report

● New Code   ▲ Revised Code   ✳ Starred Procedure   ＋ Add-On Code   ⊘ Modifier -51 Exempt

93041 tracing only without interpretation and report

93042 interpretation and report only

93224 Electrocardiographic monitoring for 24 hours by continuous original ECG waveform recording and storage, with visual superimposition scanning; includes recording, scanning analysis with report, physician review and interpretation

93225 recording (includes hook-up, recording, and disconnection)

93226 scanning analysis with report

93227 physician review and interpretation

93230 Electrocardiographic monitoring for 24 hours by continuous original ECG waveform recording and storage without superimposition scanning utilizing a device capable of producing a full miniaturized printout; includes recording, microprocessor-based analysis with report, physician review and interpretation

93231 recording (includes hook-up, recording, and disconnection)

93232 microprocessor-based analysis with report

93233 physician review and interpretation

93235 Electrocardiographic monitoring for 24 hours by continuous computerized monitoring and non-continuous recording, and real-time data analysis utilizing a device capable of producing intermittent full-sized waveform tracings, possibly patient activated; includes monitoring and real-time data analysis with report, physician review and interpretation

93236 monitoring and real-time data analysis with report

93237 physician review and interpretation

93268 Patient demand single or multiple event recording with presymptom memory loop, per 30 day period of time; includes transmission, physician review and interpretation

93270 recording (includes hook-up, recording,and disconnection)

93271 monitoring, receipt of transmissions, and analysis

Separate Procedure	Unlisted Procedure	CCI Comp. Code	Non-specific Procedure

93272   physician review and interpretation only

(For postsymptom recording, see 93012, 93014)

(For implanted patient activated cardiac event recording, see 33282, 93727)

93278 Signal-averaged electrocardiography (SAECG), with or without ECG

(For interpretation and report only, use 93278 with modifier -26)

(For unlisted cardiographic procedure, use 93799)

ECHOCARDIOGRAPHY

(For fetal echocardiography, see 76825-76828)

93303 Transthoracic echocardiography for congenital cardiac anomalies; complete

93304   follow-up or limited study

93307 Echocardiography, transthoracic, real-time with image documentation (2D) with or without M-mode recording; complete

93308   follow-up or limited study

93312 Echocardiography, transesophageal, real time with image documentation (2D) (with or without M-mode recording); including probe placement, image acquisition, interpretation and report

93313   placement of transesophageal probe only

93314   image acquisition, interpretation and report only

93315 Transesophageal echocardiography for congenital cardiac anomalies; including probe placement, image acquisition, interpretation and report

93316   placement of transesophageal probe only

93317   image acquisition, interpretation and report only

● New Code   ▲ Revised Code   ✳ Starred Procedure   ✦ Add-On Code   ⊘ Modifier -51 Exempt

93318 Echocardiography, transesophageal (TEE) for monitoring purposes, including probe placement, real time 2-dimensional image acquisition and interpretation leading to ongoing (continuous) assessment of (dynamically changing) cardiac pumping function and to therapeutic measures on an immediate time basis

+93320 Doppler echocardiography, pulsed wave and/or continuous wave with spectral display (List separately in addition to codes for echocardiographic imaging); complete

(Use 93320 in conjunction with codes 93303, 93304, 93307, 93308, 93312, 93314, 93315, 93317, 93350)

+93321 follow-up or limited study (List separately in addition to codes for echocardiographic imaging)

(Use 93321 in conjunction with codes 93303, 93304, 93307, 93308, 93312, 93314, 93315, 93317, 93350)

+93325 Doppler echocardiography color flow velocity mapping (List separately in addition to codes for echocardiography)

(Use 93325 in conjunction with codes 76825, 76826, 76827, 76828, 93303, 93304, 93307, 93308, 93312, 93314, 93315, 93317, 93320, 93321, 93350)

93350 Echocardiography, transthoracic, real-time with image documentation (2D), with or without M-mode recording, during rest and cardiovascular stress test using treadmill, bicycle exercise and/or pharmacologically induced stress, with interpretation and report

(The appropriate stress testing code from the 93015-93018 series should be reported in addition to 93350 to capture the exercise stress portion of the study)

CARDIAC CATHETERIZATION

93501 Right heart catheterization

(For bundle of His recording, use 93600)

93503 Insertion and placement of flow directed catheter (eg, Swan-Ganz) for monitoring purposes

93505 Endomyocardial biopsy

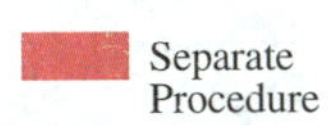 Separate Procedure

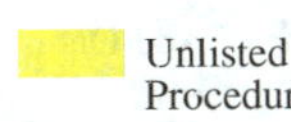 Unlisted Procedure

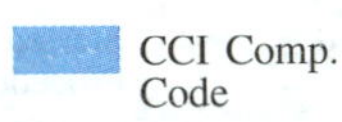 CCI Comp. Code

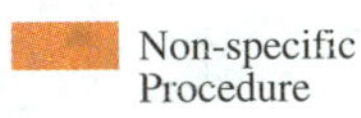 Non-specific Procedure

⊘ 93508 Catheter placement in coronary artery(s), arterial coronary conduit(s), and/or venous coronary bypass graft(s) for coronary angiography without concomitant left heart catheterization

(93508 is to be used only when left heart catheterization 93510, 93511, 93524, 93526 is not performed)

(93508 is to be used only once per procedure)

(To report transcatheter placement of radiation delivery device for coronary intravascular brachytherapy, use 92974)

(For intravascular radioelement application, see 77781-77784)

⊘ 93510 Left heart catheterization, retrograde, from the brachial artery, axillary artery or femoral artery; percutaneous

⊘ 93511 by cutdown

⊘ 93514 Left heart catheterization by left ventricular puncture

⊘ 93524 Combined transseptal and retrograde left heart catheterization

⊘ 93526 Combined right heart catheterization and retrograde left heart catheterization

⊘ 93527 Combined right heart catheterization and transseptal left heart catheterization through intact septum (with or without retrograde left heart catheterization)

⊘ 93528 Combined right heart catheterization with left ventricular puncture (with or without retrograde left heart catheterization)

⊘ 93529 Combined right heart catheterization and left heart catheterization through existing septal opening (with or without retrograde left heart catheterization)

⊘ 93530 Right heart catheterization, for congenital cardiac anomalies

⊘ 93531 Combined right heart catheterization and retrograde left heart catheterization, for congenital cardiac anomalies

⊘ 93532 Combined right heart catheterization and transseptal left heart catheterization through intact septum with or without retrograde left heart catheterization, for congenital cardiac anomalies

---

800

● New Code　　▲ Revised Code　　* Starred Procedure　　+ Add-On Code　　⊘ Modifier -51 Exempt

⊘ **93533** Combined right heart catheterization and transseptal left heart catheterization through existing septal opening, with or without retrograde left heart catheterization, for congenital cardiac anomalies

(93536 deleted 2002 edition. To report, use 33967)

(When injection procedures are performed in conjunction with cardiac catheterization, these services do not include introduction of catheters but do include repositioning of catheters when necessary and use of automatic power injectors. Injection procedures 93539-93545 represent separate identifiable services and may be coded in conjunction with one another when appropriate. The technical details of angiography, supervision of filming and processing, interpretation and report are not included. To report imaging supervision, interpretation and report, use 93555 and/or 93556. Modifier -51 should not be appended to 93539-93556)

⊘ **93539** Injection procedure during cardiac catheterization; for selective opacification of arterial conduits (eg, internal mammary), whether native or used for bypass

⊘ **93540** for selective opacification of aortocoronary venous bypass grafts, one or more coronary arteries

⊘ **93541** for pulmonary angiography

⊘ **93542** for selective right ventricular or right atrial angiography

⊘ **93543** for selective left ventricular or left atrial angiography

⊘ **93544** for aortography

⊘ **93545** for selective coronary angiography (injection of radiopaque material may be by hand)

⊘ **93555** Imaging supervision, interpretation and report for injection procedure(s) during cardiac catheterization; ventricular and/or atrial angiography

⊘ **93556** pulmonary angiography, aortography, and/or selective coronary angiography including venous bypass grafts and arterial conduits (whether native or used in bypass)

(Codes 93561 and 93562 are not to be used with cardiac catheterization codes)

Separate Procedure

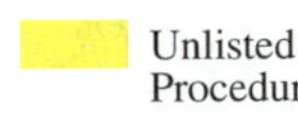
Unlisted Procedure

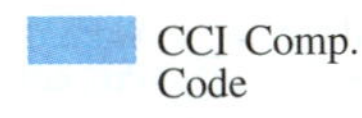
CCI Comp. Code

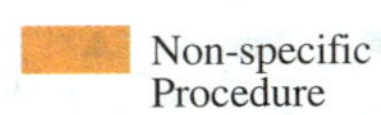
Non-specific Procedure

93561 Indicator dilution studies such as dye or thermal dilution, including arterial and/or venous catheterization; with cardiac output measurement (separate procedure)

93562 subsequent measurement of cardiac output

(For radioisotope method of cardiac output, see 78472, 78473 or 78481)

+93571 Intravascular doppler velocity and/or pressure derived coronary flow reserve measurement (coronary vessel or graft) during coronary angiography including pharmacologically induced stress; initial vessel (List separately in addition to code for primary procedure)

+93572 each additional vessel (List separately in addition to code for primary procedure)

(For unlisted cardiac catheterization procedure, use 93799)

INTRACARDIAC ELECTROPHYSIOLOGICAL PROCEDURES/STUDIES

⊘ **93600** Bundle of His recording

⊘ **93602** Intra-atrial recording

⊘ **93603** Right ventricular recording

(93607 deleted 2002 edition. To report, use 93622)

▲ **+93609** Intraventricular and/or intra-atrial mapping of tachycardia site(s) with catheter manipulation to record from multiple sites to identify origin of tachycardia (List separately in addition to code for primary procedure)

(Use 93609 in conjunction with codes 93620, 93651, 93652)

⊘ **93610** Intra-atrial pacing

⊘ **93612** Intraventricular pacing

(Do not report 93612 in conjunction with codes 93620-93622)

●**+93613** Intracardiac electrophysiologic 3-dimensional mapping (List separately in addition to code for primary procedure)

| ● | New Code | ▲ | Revised Code | * | Starred Procedure | + | Add-On Code | ⊘ | Modifier -51 Exempt |

(Use 93613 in conjunction with codes 93620, 93651, 93652)

⊘ **93615** Esophageal recording of atrial electrogram with or without ventricular electrogram(s);

⊘ **93616** with pacing

⊘ **93618** Induction of arrhythmia by electrical pacing

(For intracardiac phonocardiogram, use 93799)

⊘▲**93619** Comprehensive electrophysiologic evaluation with right atrial pacing and recording, right ventricular pacing and recording, His bundle recording, including insertion and repositioning of multiple electrode catheters without induction or attempted induction of arrhythmia

(Do not report 93619 in conjunction with codes 93600, 93602, 93610, 93612, 93618 or 93620-93622)

⊘▲**93620** Comprehensive electrophysiologic evaluation with right atrial pacing and recording, right ventricular pacing and recording, His bundle recording, including insertion and repositioning of multiple electrode catheters with induction or attempted induction of arrhythmia;

(Do not report 93620 in conjunction with codes 93600, 93602, 93610, 93612, 93618 or 93619)

▲**+93621** with left atrial pacing and recording from coronary sinus or left atrium (List separately in addition to code for primary procedure)

(Use 93621 in conjunction with code 93620)

▲**+93622** with left ventricular pacing and recording (List separately in addition to code for primary procedure)

(Use 93622 in conjunction with code 93620)

+93623 Programmed stimulation and pacing after intravenous drug infusion (List separately in addition to code for primary procedure)

(Use 93623 in conjunction with codes 93619, 93620)

⊘ **93624** Electrophysiologic follow-up study with pacing and recording to test effectiveness of therapy, including induction or attempted induction of arrhythmia

⊘ **93631** Intra-operative epicardial and endocardial pacing and mapping to localize the site of tachycardia or zone of slow conduction for surgical correction

⊘ **93640** Electrophysiologic evaluation of single or dual chamber pacing cardioverter-defibrillator leads including defibrillation threshold evaluation (induction of arrhythmia, evaluation of sensing and pacing for arrhythmia termination) at time of initial implantation or replacement;

⊘ **93641** with testing of single or dual chamber pacing cardioverter-defibrillator pulse generator

⊘ **93642** Electrophysiologic evaluation of single or dual chamber pacing cardioverter-defibrillator (includes defibrillation threshold evaluation, induction of arrhythmia, evaluation of sensing and pacing for arrhythmia termination, and programming or reprogramming of sensing or therapeutic parameters)

(For subsequent or periodic electronic analysis and/or reprogramming of single or dual chamber pacing cardioverter-defibrillators, see 93642, 93741-93744)

⊘ **93650** Intracardiac catheter ablation of atrioventricular node function, atrioventricular conduction for creation of complete heart block, with or without temporary pacemaker placement

⊘ **93651** Intracardiac catheter ablation of arrhythmogenic focus; for treatment of supraventricular tachycardia by ablation of fast or slow atrioventricular pathways, accessory atrioventricular connections or other atrial foci, singly or in combination

⊘ **93652** for treatment of ventricular tachycardia

⊘ **93660** Evaluation of cardiovascular function with tilt table evaluation, with continuous ECG monitoring and intermittent blood pressure monitoring, with or without pharmacological intervention

(For testing of autonomic nervous system function, see 95921-95923)

● New Code ▲ Revised Code ＊ Starred Procedure ＋ Add-On Code ⊘ Modifier -51 Exempt

+93662 Intracardiac echocardiography during therapeutic/diagnostic intervention, including imaging supervision and interpretation (List separately in addition to code for primary procedure)

(Use 93662 in conjunction with codes 93621, 93622, 93651 or 93652, as appropriate)

(Do not report 92961 in addition to 93662)

PERIPHERAL ARTERIAL DISEASE REHABILITATION

93668 Peripheral arterial disease (PAD) rehabilitation, per session

OTHER VASCULAR STUDIES

(For arterial cannulization and recording of direct arterial pressure, use 36620)

(For radiographic injection procedures, see 36000-36299)

(For vascular cannulization for hemodialysis, see 36800-36821)

(For chemotherapy for malignant disease, see 96408-96549)

(For penile plethysmography, use 54240)

● **93701** Bioimpedance, thoracic, electrical

93720 Plethysmography, total body; with interpretation and report

93721 tracing only, without interpretation and report

93722 interpretation and report only

(For regional plethysmography, see 93875-93931)

93724 Electronic analysis of antitachycardia pacemaker system (includes electrocardiographic recording, programming of device, induction and termination of tachycardia via implanted pacemaker, and interpretation of recordings)

93727 Electronic analysis of implantable loop recorder (ILR) system (includes retrieval of recorded and stored ECG data, physician review and interpretation of retrieved ECG data and reprogramming)

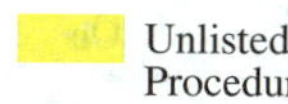
Separate Procedure

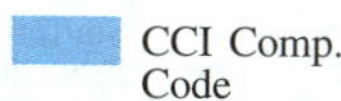
Unlisted Procedure

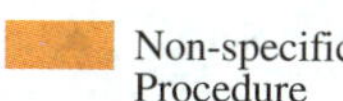
CCI Comp. Code

Non-specific Procedure

93731   Electronic analysis of dual-chamber pacemaker system (includes evaluation of programmable parameters at rest and during activity where applicable, using electrocardiographic recording and interpretation of recordings at rest and during exercise, analysis of event markers and device response); without reprogramming

93732   with reprogramming

93733   Electronic analysis of dual chamber internal pacemaker system (may include rate, pulse amplitude and duration, configuration of wave form, and/or testing of sensory function of pacemaker), telephonic analysis

93734   Electronic analysis of single chamber pacemaker system (includes evaluation of programmable parameters at rest and during activity where applicable, using electrocardiographic recording and interpretation of recordings at rest and during exercise, analysis of event markers and device response); without reprogramming

93735   with reprogramming

93736   Electronic analysis of single chamber internal pacemaker system (may include rate, pulse amplitude and duration, configuration of wave form, and/or testing of sensory function of pacemaker), telephonic analysis

(93737   deleted 2002 edition. To report, use 93741 or 93743)

(93738   deleted 2002 edition. To report, use 93742 or 93744)

93740   Temperature gradient studies

93741   Electronic analysis of pacing cardioverter-defibrillator (includes interrogation, evaluation of pulse generator status, evaluation of programmable parameters at rest and during activity where applicable, using electrocardiographic recording and interpretation of recordings at rest and during exercise, analysis of event markers and device response); single chamber, without reprogramming

93742   single chamber, with reprogramming

93743   dual chamber, without reprogramming

93744   dual chamber, with reprogramming

---

806   ● New Code   ▲ Revised Code   ✻ Starred Procedure   ✛ Add-On Code   ⊘ Modifier -51 Exempt

93760   Thermogram; cephalic

93762   peripheral

93770   Determination of venous pressure

(For central venous cannulization and pressure measurements, see 36488-36491, 36500)

93784   Ambulatory blood pressure monitoring, utilizing a system such as magnetic tape and/or computer disk, for 24 hours or longer; including recording, scanning analysis, interpretation and report

93786   recording only

93788   scanning analysis with report

93790   physician review with interpretation and report

OTHER PROCEDURES

93797   Physician services for outpatient cardiac rehabilitation; without continuous ECG monitoring (per session)

93798   with continuous ECG monitoring (per session)

93799   Unlisted cardiovascular service or procedure

NON-INVASIVE VASCULAR DIAGNOSTIC STUDIES

Vascular studies refers to diagnostic procedures performed to determine blood flow and/or the condition of arteries and/or veins. Vascular studies include patient care required to perform the studies, supervision of the studies and interpretation of the study results with copies for patient records of hard copy output with analysis of all data, including bi-directional vascular flow or imaging when provided.

The use of a simple hand-held or other Doppler device that does not produce hard copy output, or that produces a record that does not permit analysis of bi-directional vascular flow, is considered to be part of the physical examination of the vascular system and is not reported separately. To report unilateral non-invasive diagnostic studies, add modifier -52 to the basic code.

A Duplex Scan is defined as "An ultrasonic scanning procedure with display of both two-dimensional structure and motion with time and Doppler ultrasonic signal documentation with spectral analysis and/or color flow velocity mapping or imaging.

Coding Rules

1. Non-invasive vascular studies are usually performed in addition to evaluation and management service, such as a consultation or visit, and should be reported separately in addition to the evaluation and management service.

2. All of the non-invasive vascular services fall under the Medicare Purchased Diagnostic Services guidelines; therefore, reporting should be as instructed by your local Medicare carrier.

CEREBROVASCULAR ARTERIAL STUDIES

93875   Non-invasive physiologic studies of extracranial arteries, complete bilateral study (eg, periorbital flow direction with arterial compression, ocular pneumoplethysmography, Doppler ultrasound spectral analysis)

93880   Duplex scan of extracranial arteries; complete bilateral study

93882   unilateral or limited study

93886   Transcranial Doppler study of the intracranial arteries; complete study

93888   limited study

EXTREMITY ARTERIAL STUDIES (INCLUDING DIGITS)

93922   Non-invasive physiologic studies of upper or lower extremity arteries, single level, bilateral (eg, ankle/brachial indices, Doppler waveform analysis, volume plethysmography, transcutaneous oxygen tension measurement)

93923   Non-invasive physiologic studies of upper or lower extremity arteries, multiple levels or with provocative functional maneuvers, complete bilateral study (eg, segmental blood pressure measurements, segmental Doppler waveform analysis, segmental volume plethysmography, segmental transcutaneous oxygen tension measurements, measurements with postural provocative tests, measurements with reactive hyperemia)

| ● New Code | ▲ Revised Code | ✳ Starred Procedure | ✛ Add-On Code | ⊘ Modifier -51 Exempt |

93924 Non-invasive physiologic studies of lower extremity arteries, at rest and following treadmill stress testing, complete bilateral study

93925 Duplex scan of lower extremity arteries or arterial bypass grafts; complete bilateral study

93926 unilateral or limited study

93930 Duplex scan of upper extremity arteries or arterial bypass grafts; complete bilateral study

93931 unilateral or limited study

EXTREMITY VENOUS STUDIES (INCLUDING DIGITS)

93965 Non-invasive physiologic studies of extremity veins, complete bilateral study (eg, Doppler waveform analysis with responses to compression and other maneuvers, phleborheography, impedance plethysmography)

93970 Duplex scan of extremity veins including responses to compression and other maneuvers; complete bilateral study

93971 unilateral or limited study

VISCERAL AND PENILE VASCULAR STUDIES

93975 Duplex scan of arterial inflow and venous outflow of abdominal, pelvic, scrotal contents and/or retroperitoneal organs; complete study

93976 limited study

93978 Duplex scan of aorta, inferior vena cava, iliac vasculature, or bypass grafts; complete study

93979 unilateral or limited study

93980 Duplex scan of arterial inflow and venous outflow of penile vessels; complete study

93981 follow-up or limited study

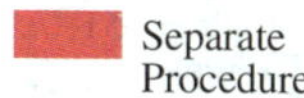 Separate Procedure

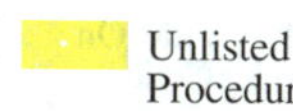 Unlisted Procedure

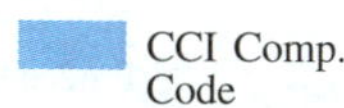 CCI Comp. Code

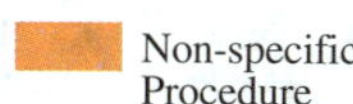 Non-specific Procedure

EXTREMITY ARTERIAL-VENOUS STUDIES

93990 Duplex scan of hemodialysis access (including arterial inflow, body of access and venous outflow)

(For measurement of hemodialysis access flow using indicator dilution methods, use 90940)

PULMONARY

Pulmonary disease is concerned with diseases of the lungs and airways. The Pulmonologist diagnoses and treats pneumonia, cancer, pleurisy, asthma, occupational diseases, bronchitis, sleep disorders, emphysema, and other complex disorders of the lungs. Pulmonologists test lung functions in many ways, endoscope the bronchial airways and prescribe and monitor mechanical assistance to ventilation. Many pulmonary disease physicians are also expert in critical care.

Pulmonary services refer to diagnostic procedures performed to determine air flow, blood gases, and the condition of the lungs and respiratory system. Pulmonary services include the laboratory procedure(s), interpretation, and physician's services (except surgical and anesthesia services) unless otherwise stated. It is common for pulmonologists to provide interpretation services only, under contract to medical facilities.

CODING RULES

1. Pulmonary services are usually performed in addition to evaluation and management service, such as a consultation or visit, and should be coded separately in addition to the evaluation and management service.

2. When reporting physician interpretation only for pulmonary services include the modifier -26 "Professional Component".

3. Most of the pulmonary services fall under the Medicare Purchased Diagnostic Services guidelines; therefore reporting should be as instructed by your local Medicare carrier.

94010 Spirometry, including graphic record, total and timed vital capacity, expiratory flow rate measurement(s), with or without maximal voluntary ventilation

94014 Patient-initiated spirometric recording per 30-day period of time; includes reinforced education, transmission of spirometric tracing, data capture, analysis of transmitted data, periodic recalibration and physician review and interpretation

---

● New Code   ▲ Revised Code   ✳ Starred Procedure   ✛ Add-On Code   ⊘ Modifier -51 Exempt

94015   recording (includes hook-up, reinforced education, data transmission, data capture, trend analysis, and periodic recalibration)

94016   physician review and interpretation only

94060   Bronchospasm evaluation: spirometry as in 94010, before and after bronchodilator (aerosol or parenteral)

(For prolonged exercise test for bronchospasm with pre- and post-spirometry, use 94620)

94070   Prolonged postexposure evaluation of bronchospasm with multiple spirometric determinations after antigen, cold air, methacholine or other chemical agent, with subsequent spirometrics

94150   Vital capacity, total (separate procedure)

94200   Maximum breathing capacity, maximal voluntary ventilation

94240   Functional residual capacity or residual volume: helium method, nitrogen open circuit method, or other method

94250   Expired gas collection, quantitative, single procedure (separate procedure)

94260   Thoracic gas volume

(For plethysmography, see 93720-93722)

94350   Determination of maldistribution of inspired gas: multiple breath nitrogen washout curve including alveolar nitrogen or helium equilibration time

94360   Determination of resistance to airflow, oscillatory or plethysmographic methods

94370   Determination of airway closing volume, single breath tests

94375   Respiratory flow volume loop

94400   Breathing response to CO_2 (CO_2 response curve)

94450   Breathing response to hypoxia (hypoxia response curve)

 Separate Procedure   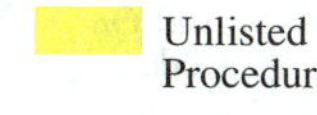 Unlisted Procedure   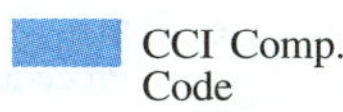 CCI Comp. Code   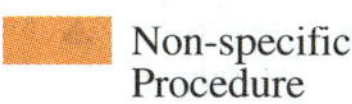 Non-specific Procedure

811

94620   Pulmonary stress testing; simple (eg, prolonged exercise test for bronchospasm with pre- and post-spirometry)

94621   complex (including measurements of CO_2 production, O_2 uptake, and electrocardiographic recordings)

94640   Nonpressurized inhalation treatment for acute airway obstruction

94642   Aerosol inhalation of pentamidine for pneumocystis carinii pneumonia treatment or prophylaxis

94650   Intermittent positive pressure breathing (IPPB) treatment, air or oxygen, with or without nebulized medication; initial demonstration and/or evaluation

94651   subsequent

94652   newborn infants

94656   Ventilation assist and management, initiation of pressure or volume preset ventilators for assisted or controlled breathing; first day

94657   subsequent days

94660   Continuous positive airway pressure ventilation (CPAP), initiation and management

94662   Continuous negative pressure ventilation (CNP), initiation and management

94664   Aerosol or vapor inhalations for sputum mobilization, bronchodilation, or sputum induction for diagnostic purposes; initial demonstration and/or evaluation

94665   subsequent

94667   Manipulation chest wall, such as cupping, percussing, and vibration to facilitate lung function; initial demonstration and/or evaluation

94668   subsequent

94680   Oxygen uptake, expired gas analysis; rest and exercise, direct, simple

---

● New Code   ▲ Revised Code   ✻ Starred Procedure   + Add-On Code   ⊘ Modifier -51 Exempt

94681   including CO_2 output, percentage oxygen extracted

94690   rest, indirect (separate procedure)

(For single arterial puncture, use 36600)

▲ **94720**   Carbon monoxide diffusing capacity (eg, single breath, steady state)

94725   Membrane diffusion capacity

▲ **94750**   Pulmonary compliance study (eg, plethysmography, volume and pressure measurements)

94760   Noninvasive ear or pulse oximetry for oxygen saturation; single determination

(For blood gases, see 82803-82810)

94761   multiple determinations (eg, during exercise)

94762   by continuous overnight monitoring (separate procedure)

94770   Carbon dioxide, expired gas determination by infrared analyzer

(For bronchoscopy, see 31622-31656)

(For placement of flow directed catheter, use 93503)

(For venipuncture, use 36410)

(For central venous catheter placement, see 36488-36491)

(For arterial puncture, use 36600)

(For arterial catheterization, use 36620)

(For thoracentesis, use 32000)

(For phlebotomy, therapeutic, use 99195)

(For lung biopsy, needle, use 32405)

(For intubation, orotracheal or nasotracheal, use 31500)

94772   Circadian respiratory pattern recording (pediatric pneumogram), 12 to 24 hour continuous recording, infant

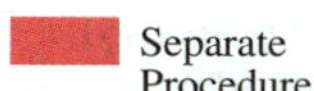

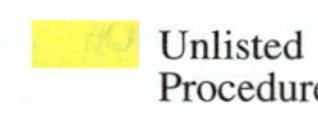

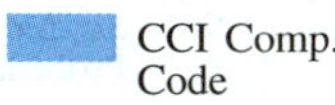

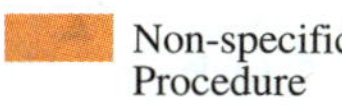

(Separate procedure codes for electromyograms, EEG, ECG, and recordings of respiration are excluded when 94772 is reported)

94799 Unlisted pulmonary service or procedure

ALLERGY AND CLINICAL IMMUNOLOGY

Allergy and Immunology refers to diagnostic services performed to determine a patient's sensitivity to specific substances, the treatment of patients with allergens by the administration or allergenic extracts, and/or medical conference services.

Coding Rules

1. Allergy and immunology services are usually performed in addition to evaluation and management service, such as a consultation or visit, and should be reported separately in addition to the evaluation and management service.

2. Summary or therapeutic conferences following completion of the diagnostic workup, including discussion, avoidance, elimination, symptomatic treatment and immunotherapy should be reported with evaluation and management service codes 99241-99245.

3. Prolonged conferences should be reported with evaluation and management Case Management CPT codes.

ALLERGY TESTING

95004 Percutaneous tests (scratch, puncture, prick) with allergenic extracts, immediate type reaction, specify number of tests

95010 Percutaneous tests (scratch, puncture, prick) sequential and incremental, with drugs, biologicals or venoms, immediate type reaction, specify number of tests

95015 Intracutaneous (intradermal) tests, sequential and incremental, with drugs, biologicals, or venoms, immediate type reaction, specify number of tests

95024 Intracutaneous (intradermal) tests with allergenic extracts, immediate type reaction, specify number of tests

95027 Skin end point titration

● New Code   ▲ Revised Code   * Starred Procedure   + Add-On Code   ⊘ Modifier -51 Exempt

95028 Intracutaneous (intradermal) tests with allergenic extracts, delayed type reaction, including reading, specify number of tests

95044 Patch or application test(s) (specify number of tests)

95052 Photo patch test(s) (specify number of tests)

95056 Photo tests

95060 Ophthalmic mucous membrane tests

95065 Direct nasal mucous membrane test

95070 Inhalation bronchial challenge testing (not including necessary pulmonary function tests); with histamine, methacholine, or similar compounds

95071   with antigens or gases, specify

(For pulmonary function tests, see 94060, 94070)

95075 Ingestion challenge test (sequential and incremental ingestion of test items, eg, food, drug or other substance such as metabisulfite)

95078 Provocative testing (eg, Rinkel test)

(For allergy laboratory tests, see 86000-86999)

(For intravenous therapy, for severe or intractable allergic disease, see 90780, 90781, 90784)

ALLERGEN IMMUNOTHERAPY

Allergen immunotherapy CPT codes include the professional services necessary for allergen immunotherapy. Evaluation and management service codes may be reported in addition to allergen immunotherapy if other identifiable services are provided at the same time.

95115 Professional services for allergen immunotherapy not including provision of allergenic extracts; single injection

95117   two or more injections

95120 Professional services for allergen immunotherapy in prescribing physicians office or institution, including provision of allergenic extract; single injection

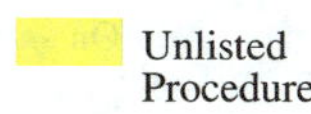
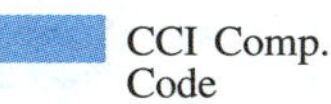
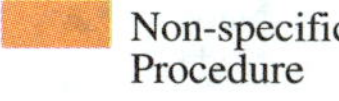

Separate Procedure   Unlisted Procedure   CCI Comp. Code   Non-specific Procedure

95125   two or more injections

95130   single stinging insect venom

95131   two stinging insect venoms

95132   three stinging insect venoms

95133   four stinging insect venoms

95134   five stinging insect venoms

▲ **95144**   Professional services for the supervision of preparation and provision of antigens for allergen immunotherapy; single dose vials(s) (specify number of vials)

(A single dose vial contains a single dose of antigen administered in one injection)

▲ **95145**   Professional services for the supervision of preparation and provision of antigens for allergen immunotherapy (specify number of doses); single stinging insect venom

95146   two single stinging insect venoms

95147   three single stinging insect venoms

95148   four single stinging insect venoms

95149   five single stinging insect venoms

▲ **95165**   Professional services for the supervision of preparation and provision of antigens for allergen immunotherapy; single or multiple antigens (specify number of doses)

95170   whole body extract of biting insect or other arthropod (specify number of doses)

(For allergy immunotherapy reporting, a dose is the amount of antigen(s) administered in a single injection from a multiple dose vial)

▲ **95180**   Rapid desensitization procedure, each hour (eg, insulin, penicillin, equine serum)

95199   Unlisted allergy/clinical immunologic service or procedure

● New Code　　▲ Revised Code　　✳ Starred Procedure　　✚ Add-On Code　　⊘ Modifier -51 Exempt

(For skin testing of bacterial, viral, fungal extracts, see 95028, 86485-86586)

(For special reports on allergy patients, use 99080)

(For testing procedures such as radioallergosorbent testing (RAST), rat mast cell technique (RMCT), mast cell degranulation test (MCDT), lymphocytic transformation test (LTT), leukocyte histamine release (LHR), migration inhibitory factor test (MIF), transfer factor test (TFT), nitroblue tetrazolium dye test (NTD), see Immunology section in Pathology or use 95199)

ENDOCRINOLOGY

● **95250** Glucose monitoring for up to 72 hours by continuous recording and storage of glucose values from interstitial tissue fluid via a subcutaneous sensor (includes hook-up, calibration, patient initiation and training, recording, disconnection, downloading with printout of data)

(Do not report 95250 in conjunction with 99091)

(To report physician review, interpretation and written report associated with code 95250, see Evaluation and Management services codes)

NEUROLOGY AND NEUROMUSCULAR PROCEDURES

Neurology refers to the study and treatment of the nervous system. Neurology services are usually performed in conjunction with a medical consultation. The consultation should be reported separately using the appropriate evaluation and management consultation code.

Coding Rules

1. All EEG services listed include the tracing, interpretation and report.

2. For interpretation of EEG only, add modifier -26 to the basic procedure code.

3. Most of the neurology and neuromuscular procedures fall under the Medicare Purchased Diagnostic Services guidelines; therefore, reporting should be as instructed by your local Medicare carrier.

(For repetitive transcranial magnetic stimulation for treatment of clinical depression, use Category III code 0018T)

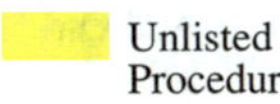

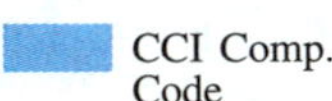

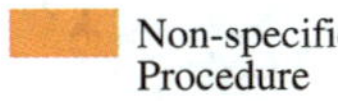

(Do not report codes 95860-95875 in addition to 96000-96004)

SLEEP TESTING

(Report with a -52 modifier if less than 6 hours of recording or in other cases of reduced services as appropriate)

(For unattended sleep study, use 95806)

95805 Multiple sleep latency or maintenance of wakefulness testing, recording, analysis and interpretation of physiological measurements of sleep during multiple trials to assess sleepiness

95806 Sleep study, simultaneous recording of ventilation, respiratory effort, ECG or heart rate, and oxygen saturation, unattended by a technologist

95807 Sleep study, simultaneous recording of ventilation, respiratory effort, ECG or heart rate, and oxygen saturation, attended by a technologist

95808 Polysomnography; sleep staging with 1-3 additional parameters of sleep, attended by a technologist

95810 sleep staging with 4 or more additional parameters of sleep, attended by a technologist

95811 sleep staging with 4 or more additional parameters of sleep, with initiation of continuous positive airway pressure therapy or bilevel ventilation, attended by a technologist

95812 Electroencephalogram (EEG) extended monitoring; up to one hour

95813 greater than one hour

95816 Electroencephalogram (EEG) including recording awake and drowsy (including hyperventilation and/or photic stimulation when appropriate)

(For extended EEG monitoring, see 95812, 95813)

95819 Electroencephalogram (EEG) including recording awake and asleep (including hyperventilation and/or photic stimulation when appropriate)

(For extended EEG monitoring, see 95812, 95813)

● New Code   ▲ Revised Code   * Starred Procedure   + Add-On Code   ⊘ Modifier -51 Exempt

(For digital analysis of EEG, use 95957)

95822 Electroencephalogram (EEG); sleep only

(For extended EEG monitoring, see 95812, 95813)

95824 cerebral death evaluation only

95827 all night sleep only

(For ambulatory 24-hour EEG monitoring, use 95950)

(For EEG during nonintracranial surgery, use 95955)

(For Wada activation test, use 95958)

(For recording of circadian respiratory patterns of infants, use 94772)

95829 Electrocorticogram at surgery (separate procedure)

95830 Insertion by physician of sphenoidal electrodes for electroencephalographic (EEG) recording

95831 Muscle testing, manual (separate procedure) with report; extremity (excluding hand) or trunk

95832 hand, with or without comparison with normal side

95833 total evaluation of body, excluding hands

95834 total evaluation of body, including hands

95851 Range of motion measurements and report (separate procedure); each extremity (excluding hand) or each trunk section (spine)

95852 hand, with or without comparison with normal side

95857 Tensilon test for myasthenia gravis;

95858 with electromyographic recording

95860 Needle electromyography, one extremity with or without related paraspinal areas

95861 Needle electromyography, two extremities with or without related paraspinal areas

---

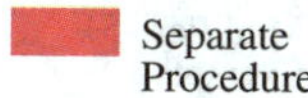

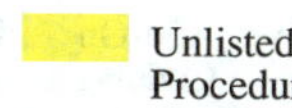

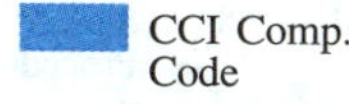

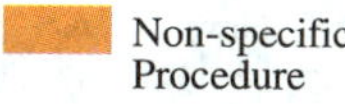

(For dynamic electromyography performed during motion analysis studies, see 96002-96003)

95863   Needle electromyography, three extremities with or without related paraspinal areas

95864   Needle electromyography, four extremities with or without related paraspinal areas

95867   Needle electromyography, cranial nerve supplied muscles, unilateral

95868   Needle electromyography, cranial nerve supplied muscles, bilateral

95869   Needle electromyography; thoracic paraspinal muscles

95870   limited study of muscles in one extremity or non-limb (axial) muscles (unilateral or bilateral), other than thoracic paraspinal, cranial nerve supplied muscles, or sphincters

(To report a complete study of the extremities, see 95860-95864)

(For needle electromyography of cranial supplied muscles, see 95867, 95868)

(For anal or urethral sphincter, detrusor, urethra, perineum musculature, see 51785-51792)

(For eye muscles, use 92265)

95872   Needle electromyography using single fiber electrode, with quantitative measurement of jitter, blocking and/or fiber density, any/all sites of each muscle studied

▲ **95875**   Ischemic limb exercise test with serial specimen(s) acquisition for muscle metabolite(s)

NERVE CONDUCTION STUDIES

⊘ **95900**   Nerve conduction, amplitude and latency/velocity study, each nerve; motor, without F-wave study

⊘ **95903**   motor, with F-wave study

⊘▲**95904**   sensory

● New Code   ▲ Revised Code   * Starred Procedure   + Add-On Code   ⊘ Modifier -51 Exempt

(Report 95900, 95903, and/or 95904 only once when multiple sites on the same nerve are stimulated or recorded)

+95920 Intraoperative neurophysiology testing, per hour (List separately in addition to code for primary procedure)

(Use code 95920 in conjunction with the study performed, 92585, 95822, 95860, 95861, 95867, 95868, 95900, 95904, 95925, 95926, 95927, 95930, 95933, 95934, 95936, 95937)

(Code 95920 describes ongoing electrophysiologic testing and monitoring performed during surgical procedures. Code 95920 is reported per hour of service, and includes only the ongoing electrophysiologic monitoring time distinct from performance of specific type(s) of baseline electrophysiologic study(ies) (95860, 95861, 95867, 95868, 95900, 95904, 95933, 95934, 95936, 95937) or interpretation of specific type(s) of baseline electrophysiologic study(ies) (92585, 95822, 95925, 95926, 95927, 95930). The time spent performing or interpreting the baseline electrophysiologic study(ies) should not be counted as intraoperative monitoring, but represents separately reportable procedures. Code 95920 should be used once per hour even if multiple electrophysiologic studies are performed. The baseline electrophysiologic study(ies) should be used once per operative session.)

95921 Testing of autonomic nervous system function; cardiovagal innervation (parasympathetic function), including two or more of the following: heart rate response to deep breathing with recorded R-R interval, Valsalva ratio, and 30:15 ratio

95922 vasomotor adrenergic innervation (sympathetic adrenergic function), including beat-to-beat blood pressure and R-R interval changes during Valsalva maneuver and at least five minutes of passive tilt

95923 sudomotor, including one or more of the following: quantitative sudomotor axon reflex test (QSART), silastic sweat imprint, thermoregulatory sweat test, and changes in sympathetic skin potential

95925 Short-latency somatosensory evoked potential study, stimulation of any/all peripheral nerves or skin sites, recording from the central nervous system; in upper limbs

95926 in lower limbs

95927 in the trunk or head

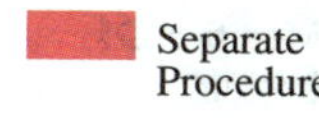

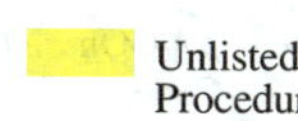

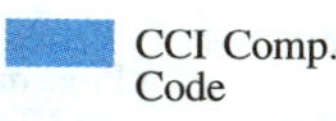

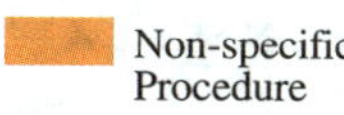

(To report a unilateral study, use modifier -52)

(For visual evoked potentials, use 95930)

(For brainstem evoked response recording, use 92585)

(For auditory evoked potentials, use 92585)

95930   Visual evoked potential (VEP) testing central nervous system, checkerboard or flash

95933   Orbicularis oculi (blink) reflex, by electrodiagnostic testing

95934   H-reflex, amplitude and latency study; record gastrocnemius/soleus muscle

95936   record muscle other than gastrocnemius/soleus muscle

(To report a bilateral study, use modifier -50)

95937   Neuromuscular junction testing (repetitive stimulation, paired stimuli), each nerve, any one method

95950   Monitoring for identification and lateralization of cerebral seizure focus, electroencephalographic (eg, 8 channel EEG) recording and interpretation, each 24 hours

95951   Monitoring for localization of cerebral seizure focus by cable or radio, 16 or more channel telemetry, combined electroencephalographic (EEG) and video recording and interpretation (eg, for presurgical localization), each 24 hours

95953   Monitoring for localization of cerebral seizure focus by computerized portable 16 or more channel EEG, electroencephalographic (EEG) recording and interpretation, each 24 hours

95954   Pharmacological or physical activation requiring physician attendance during EEG recording of activation phase (eg, thiopental activation test)

(For digital analysis of EEG, use 95957)

95955   Electroencephalogram (EEG) during nonintracranial surgery (eg, carotid surgery)

   ● New Code   ▲ Revised Code   * Starred Procedure   + Add-On Code   ⊘ Modifier -51 Exempt

95956 Monitoring for localization of cerebral seizure focus by cable or radio,16 or more channel telemetry, electroencephalographic (EEG) recording and interpretation, each 24 hours

95957 Digital analysis of electroencephalogram (EEG) (eg, for epileptic spike analysis)

95958 Wada activation test for hemispheric function, including electroencephalographic (EEG) monitoring

95961 Functional cortical and subcortical mapping by stimulation and/or recording of electrodes on brain surface, or of depth electrodes, to provoke seizures or identify vital brain structures; initial hour of physician attendance

+95962 each additional hour of physician attendance (List separately in addition to code for primary procedure)

(Use 95962 in conjunction with code 95961)

● **95965** Magnetoencephalography (MEG), recording and analysis; for spontaneous brain magnetic activity (eg, epileptic cerebral cortex localization)

● **95966** for evoked magnetic fields, single modality (eg, sensory, motor, language, or visual cortex localization)

●**+95967** for evoked magnetic fields, each additional modality (eg, sensory, motor, language, or visual cortex localization) (List separately in addition to code for primary procedure)

(Use 95967 in conjunction with code 95966)

(For electroencephalography performed in addition to magnetoencephalography, see 95812-95827)

(For somatosensory evoked potentials, auditory evoked potentials, and visual evoked potentials performed in addition to magnetic evoked field responses, see 92585, 95925, 95926, and/or 95930)

(For computerized tomography performed in addition to magnetoencephalography, see 70450-70470, 70496)

(For magnetic resonance imaging perfomed in addition to magnetoencephalography, see 70551-70553)

NEUROSTIMULATORS, ANALYSIS-PROGRAMMING

(For insertion of neurostimulator pulse generator, see 61885, 63685, 63688, 64590)

(For revision or removal of neurostimulator pulse generator or receiver, see 61888, 63688, 64595)

(For implantation of neurostimulator electrodes, see 61850-61875, 63650-63655, 64553-64580. For revision or removal of neurostimulator electrodes, see 61880, 63660, 64585)

95970   Electronic analysis of implanted neurostimulator pulse generator system (eg, rate, pulse amplitude and duration, configuration of wave form, battery status, electrode selectability, output modulation, cycling, impedance and patient compliance measurements); simple or complex brain, spinal cord, or peripheral (ie, cranial nerve, peripheral nerve, autonomic nerve, neuromuscular) neurostimulator pulse generator/transmitter, without reprogramming

95971   simple brain, spinal cord, or peripheral (ie, peripheral nerve, autonomic nerve, neuromuscular) neurostimulator pulse generator/transmitter, with intraoperative or subsequent programming

95972   complex brain, spinal cord, or peripheral (except cranial nerve) neurostimulator pulse generator/transmitter, with intraoperative or subsequent programming, first hour

+95973   complex brain, spinal cord, or peripheral (except cranial nerve) neurostimulator pulse generator/transmitter, with intraoperative or subsequent programming, each additional 30 minutes after first hour (List separately in addition to code for primary procedure)

(Use 95973 in conjunction with code 95972)

95974   complex cranial nerve neurostimulator pulse generator/transmitter, with intraoperative or subsequent programming, with or without nerve interface testing, first hour

+95975   complex cranial nerve neurostimulator pulse generator/transmitter, with intraoperative or subsequent programming, each additional 30 minutes after first hour (List separately in addition to code for primary procedure)

(Use 95975 in conjuntion with code 95974)

● New Code   ▲ Revised Code   ✳ Starred Procedure   **+** Add-On Code   ⊘ Modifier -51 Exempt

OTHER PROCEDURES

95999 Unlisted neurological or neuromuscular diagnostic procedure

MOTION ANALYSIS

(For performance of needle electromyography procedures, see 95860-95875)

(For gait training, use 97116)

● **96000** Comprehensive computer-based motion analysis by video-taping and 3-D kinematics;

● **96001** with dynamic plantar pressure measurements during walking

● **96002** Dynamic surface electromyography, during walking or other functional activities, 1-12 muscles

● **96003** Dynamic fine wire electromyography, during walking or other functional activities, 1 muscle

(Do not repot codes 95860-95875 in addition to 96002, 96003)

● **96004** Physician review and interpretation of comprehensive computer based motion analysis, dynamic plantar pressure measurements, dynamic surface electromyography during walking or other functional activities, and dynamic fine wire electromyography, with written report

CENTRAL NERVOUS SYSTEM ASSESSMENTS/TESTS

96100 Psychological testing (includes psychodiagnostic assessment of personality, psychopathology, emotionality, intellectual abilities, eg, WAIS-R, Rorschach, MMPI) with interpretation and report, per hour

96105 Assessment of aphasia (includes assessment of expressive and receptive speech and language function, language comprehension, speech production ability, reading, spelling, writing, eg, by Boston Diagnostic Aphasia Examination) with interpretation and report, per hour

 Separate Procedure

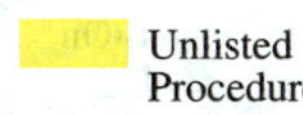 Unlisted Procedure

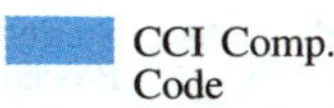 CCI Comp. Code

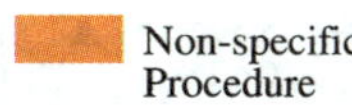 Non-specific Procedure

96110 Developmental testing; limited (eg, Developmental Screening Test II, Early Language Milestone Screen), with interpretation and report

96111 extended (includes assessment of motor, language, social, adaptive and/or cognitive functioning by standardized developmental instruments, eg, Bayley Scales of Infant Development) with interpretation and report, per hour

96115 Neurobehavioral status exam (clinical assessment of thinking, reasoning and judgment, eg, acquired knowledge, attention, memory, visual spatial abilities, language functions, planning) with interpretation and report, per hour

(For mini-mental status examination performed by a physician, see Evaluation and Management services codes)

96117 Neuropsychological testing battery (eg, Halstead-Reitan, Luria, WAIS-R) with interpretation and report, per hour

HEALTH AND BEHAVIOR ASSESSMENT/INTERVENTION

● **96150** Health and behavior assessment (eg, health-focused clinical interview, behavioral observations, psychophysicological monitoring, health-oriented questionnaires), each 15 minutes face-to-face with the patient; intial assessment

● **96151** re-assessment

● **96152** Health and behavior intervention, each 15 minutes, face-to-face; individual

● **96153** group (2 or more patients)

● **96154** family (with the patient present)

● **96155** family (without the patient present),

(For health and behavior assessment and/or intervention performed by a physician, see Evaluation and Management or Preventive Medicine services codes)

● New Code ▲ Revised Code ✱ Starred Procedure ✛ Add-On Code ⊘ Modifier -51 Exempt

CHEMOTHERAPY ADMINISTRATION

Chemotherapy is the process of treating cancer with chemicals formulated to harm or destroy the cancer cells. Chemotherapy agents are administered via intravenous or infusion methods. Chemotherapy administration may be coded when administered by a physician or a qualified assistant under the supervision of a physician, excluding chemotherapy administered by hospital or home health agency personnel.

Coding Rules

1. Chemotherapy administration is independent of the patient's office visit.

2. The injection procedures may occur independently, or on the same day as an office visit.

3. Visit services should be reported using the appropriate evaluation and management service code in addition to the chemotherapy administration code.

4. Regional (isolation) chemotherapy perfusion should be reported using existing CPT codes for arterial infusion.

5. Placement of the intra-arterial catheter should be reported using the appropriate code from the Cardiovascular Surgery section.

CHEMOTHERAPY DRUGS

Chemotherapy administration CPT codes do not include provision of the chemotherapy agent. CPT code 96545 is used to report provision of the chemotherapy agent for non-Medicare patients. For Medicare patients, choose HCPCS codes from the series J9000-J9999 to report chemotherapy drugs.

Preparation of chemotherapy agent(s) is included in the service for administration of the agent. Report separate CPT codes for each parenteral method of administration employed when chemotherapy is administered by different techniques.

CHEMOTHERAPY ADMINISTRATION

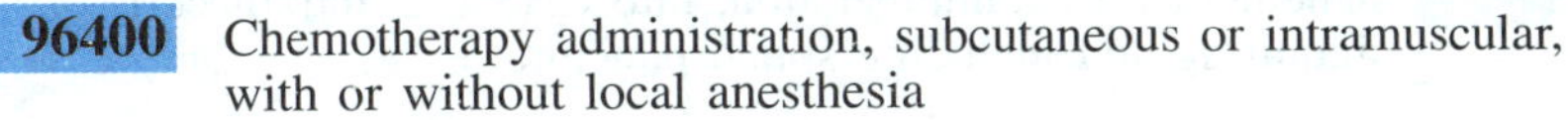 Chemotherapy administration, subcutaneous or intramuscular, with or without local anesthesia

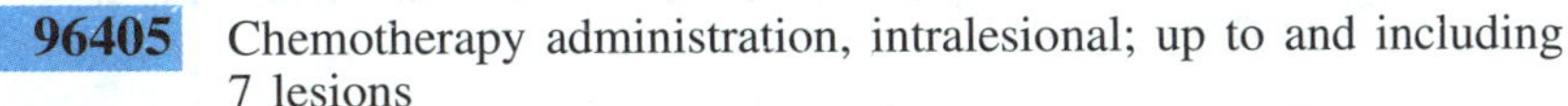 Chemotherapy administration, intralesional; up to and including 7 lesions

96406 more than 7 lesions

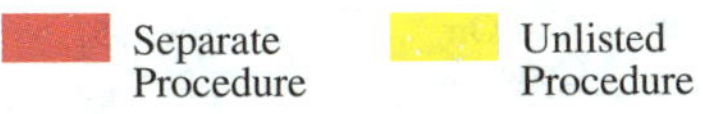 Separate Procedure   Unlisted Procedure   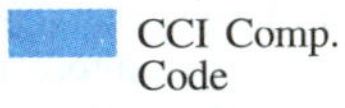 CCI Comp. Code   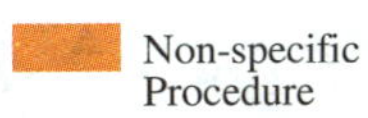 Non-specific Procedure

96408   Chemotherapy administration, intravenous; push technique

96410   infusion technique, up to one hour

+96412   infusion technique, one to 8 hours, each additional hour
(List separately in addition to code for primary procedure)

(Use 96412 in conjunction with code 96410)

96414   infusion technique, initiation of prolonged infusion (more
than 8 hours), requiring the use of a portable or
implantable pump

(For pump or reservoir refilling, see 96520, 96530)

96420   Chemotherapy administration, intra-arterial; push technique

96422   infusion technique, up to one hour

+96423   infusion technique, one to 8 hours, each additional hour
(List separately in addition to code for primary procedure)

(Use 96423 in conjunction with code 96422)

(For regional chemotherapy perfusion via membrane oxygenator
perfusion pump to an extremity, use 36823)

96425   infusion technique, initiation of prolonged infusion (more
than 8 hours), requiring the use of a portable or
implantable pump

(For implanted pump or reservoir refilling, see 96520, 96530)

96440   Chemotherapy administration into pleural cavity, requiring and
including thoracentesis

96445   Chemotherapy administration into peritoneal cavity, requiring
and including peritoneocentesis

▲ **96450**   Chemotherapy administration, into CNS (eg, intrathecal),
requiring and including spinal puncture

(For intravesical (bladder) chemotherapy administration, use
51720)

(For insertion of subarachnoid catheter and reservoir for
infusion of drug, see 62350, 62351, 62360, 62361, 62362; for

insertion of intraventricular catherter and reservoir, see 61210, 61215)

96520 Refilling and maintenance of portable pump

96530 Refilling and maintenance of implantable pump or reservoir

(For collection of blood specimen from a partially or completely implantable venous access device, use 36540)

96542 Chemotherapy injection, subarachnoid or intraventricular via subcutaneous reservoir, single or multiple agents

96545 Provision of chemotherapy agent

(For radioactive isotope therapy, see 79000-79999)

96549 Unlisted chemotherapy procedure

PHOTODYNAMIC THERAPY

Photodynamic therapy (PDT) is a two-part treatment for esophageal cancer, gastric cancer, and lung cancer using a photosensitizing drug activated by red, non-thermal laser light.

● **96567** Photodynamic therapy by external application of light to destroy premalignant and/or malignant lesions of the skin and adjacent mucosa (eg, lip) by activation of photosensitive drug(s), each phototherapy exposure session

(96570, 96571 are to be used in addition to bronchoscopy, endoscopy codes)

(To report ocular photodynamic therapy, use 67221)

+96570 Photodynamic therapy by endoscopic application of light to ablate abnormal tissue via activation of photosensitive drug(s); first 30 minutes (List separately in addition to code for endoscopy or bronchoscopy procedures of lung and esophagus)

+96571 each additional 15 minutes (List separately in addition to code for endoscopy or bronchoscopy procedures of lung and esophagus)

(Ue 96570, 96571 in conjunction with codes 31641, 43228 as appropriate)

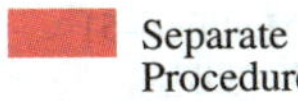 Separate Procedure
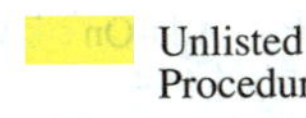 Unlisted Procedure
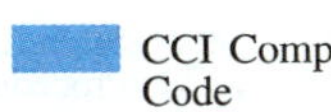 CCI Comp. Code
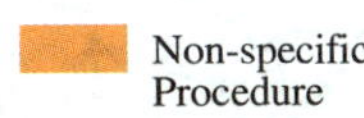 Non-specific Procedure

SPECIAL DERMATOLOGICAL PROCEDURES

(For intralesional injections, see 11900, 11901)

(For Tzanck smear, use 87207)

96900　Actinotherapy (ultraviolet light)

96902　Microscopic examination of hairs plucked or clipped by the examiner (excluding hair collected by the patient) to determine telogen and anagen counts, or structural hair shaft abnormality

96910　Photochemotherapy; tar and ultraviolet B (Goeckerman treatment) or petrolatum and ultraviolet B

96912　　psoralens and ultraviolet A (PUVA)

96913　Photochemotherapy (Goeckerman and/or PUVA) for severe photoresponsive dermatoses requiring at least four to eight hours of care under direct supervision of the physician (includes application of medication and dressings)

96999　Unlisted special dermatological service or procedure

PHYSICAL MEDICINE AND REHABILITATION

Physical medicine is the diagnosis, treatment, and prevention of disease with the aid of physical agents such as light, heat, cold, water, electricity or with mechanical devices. Physical medicine services may be provided by physicians or physical therapists. Physical medicine and rehabilitation CPT codes are divided into three sections: Modalities, Procedures and Tests and Measurements. Other services performed by medical professionals specializing in physical medicine and/or physical therapy include: muscle testing, range of joint motion, electromyography, biofeedback training by EMG, and transcutaneous nerve stimulation (TNS).

Coding Rules

1.　The physician or therapist is required to be in constant attendance when reporting CPT codes for modalities and procedures.

2.　The physical medicine procedure CPT codes specify treatment to one area, initial 30 minutes, and provide CPT codes to report each additional 15 minutes of treatment.

● New Code　▲ Revised Code　✳ Starred Procedure　✚ Add-On Code　⊘ Modifier -51 Exempt

SPECIAL PHYSICAL MEDICINE CODING ISSUES

Many worker's compensation and casualty insurance companies use pre-CPT coding systems, such as CRVS, and do not use any form of diagnostic coding, relying instead on special reports to justify the procedures performed and services provided. As the majority of physical medicine services are performed for accidents and injuries, many work related, the medical professional performing these services must be informed of the specific reporting requirements in the area that they practice.

PHYSICAL MEDICINE AND REHABILITATION SERVICES

(For muscle testing, range of joint motion, electromyography, see 95831 et seq)

(For biofeedback training by EMG, use 90901)

(For transcutaneous nerve stimulation (TNS), use 64550)

97001 Physical therapy evaluation

97002 Physical therapy re-evaluation

97003 Occupational therapy evaluation

97004 Occupational therapy re-evaluation

● **97005** Athletic training evaluation

● **97006** Athletic training re-evaluation

MODALITIES, SUPERVISED

97010 Application of a modality to one or more areas; hot or cold packs

97012 traction, mechanical

97014 electrical stimulation (unattended)

(For acupuncture with electrical stimulation, use 97781)

97016 vasopneumatic devices

97018 paraffin bath

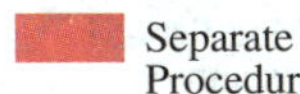 Separate Procedure

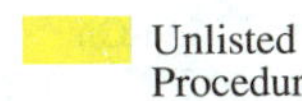 Unlisted Procedure

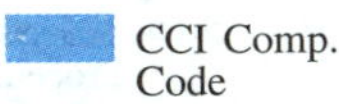 CCI Comp. Code

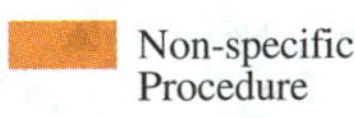 Non-specific Procedure

97020	microwave
97022	whirlpool
97024	diathermy
97026	infrared
97028	ultraviolet

MODALITIES, CONSTANT ATTENDANCE

97032	Application of a modality to one or more areas; electrical stimulation (manual), each 15 minutes
97033	iontophoresis, each 15 minutes
97034	contrast baths, each 15 minutes
97035	ultrasound, each 15 minutes
97036	Hubbard tank, each 15 minutes
97039	Unlisted modality (specify type and time if constant attendance)

THERAPEUTIC PROCEDURES

97110	Therapeutic procedure, one or more areas, each 15 minutes; therapeutic exercises to develop strength and endurance, range of motion and flexibility
▲ 97112	neuromuscular reeducation of movement, balance, coordination, kinesthetic sense, posture, and/or proprioception for sitting and/or standing activities
97113	aquatic therapy with therapeutic exercises
97116	gait training(includes stair climbing)

(Use 96000-96003 to report comprehensive gait and motion analysis procedures)

| 97124 | massage, including effleurage, petrissage and/or tapotement (stroking, compression, percussion) |

(For myofascial release, use 97140)

● New Code ▲ Revised Code ✱ Starred Procedure ✛ Add-On Code ⊘ Modifier -51 Exempt

97139 Unlisted therapeutic procedure (specify)

97140 Manual therapy techniques (eg, mobilization/ manipulation, manual lymphatic drainage, manual traction), one or more regions, each 15 minutes

97150 Therapeutic procedure(s), group (2 or more individuals)

(Report 97150 for each member of group)

(Group therapy procedures involve constant attendance of the physician or therapist, but by definition do not require one-on-one patient contact by the physician or therapist)

(For manipulation under general anesthesia, see appropriate anatomic section in Musculoskeletal System)

(For osteopathic manipulative treatment (OMT), see 98925-98929)

▲ **97504** Orthotic(s) fitting and training, upper extremity(ies), lower extremity(ies), and/or trunk, each 15 minutes

(Code 97504 should not be reported with 97116)

(For casting and strapping of fracture, injury or dislocation, see 29000, 29590)

97520 Prosthetic training, upper and/or lower extremities, each 15 minutes

97530 Therapeutic activities, direct (one-on-one) patient contact by the provider (use of dynamic activities to improve functional performance), each 15 minutes

97532 Development of cognitive skills to improve attention, memory, problem solving, (includes compensatory training), direct (one-on-one) patient contact by the provider, each 15 minutes

97533 Sensory integrative techniques to enhance sensory processing and promote adaptive responses to environmental demands, direct (one-on-one) patient contact by the provider, each 15 minutes

▲ **97535** Self-care/home management training (eg, activities of daily living (ADL) and compensatory training, meal preparation, safety procedures, and instructions in use of assistive technology devices/adaptive equipment) direct one-on-one contact by provider, each 15 minutes

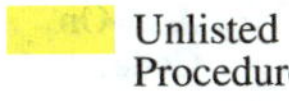

Unlisted
Procedure

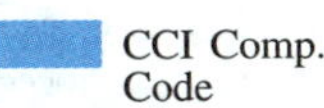

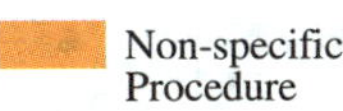

97537 Community/work reintegration training (eg, shopping, transportation, money management, avocational activities and/or work environment/modification analysis, work task analysis), direct one on one contact by provider, each 15 minutes

(For wheelchair management/propulsion training, use 97542)

97542 Wheelchair management/propulsion training, each 15 minutes

97545 Work hardening/conditioning; initial 2 hours

+97546 each additional hour (List separately in addition to code for primary procedure)

(Use 97546 in conjunction with code 97545)

ACTIVE WOUND CARE MANAGEMENT

(Do not report 97601, 97602 in addition to 11040-11044)

▲ **97601** Removal of devitalized tissue from wound(s); selective debridement, without anesthesia (eg, high pressure waterjet, sharp selective debridement with scissors, scalpel and tweezers), including topical application(s), wound assessment, and instruction(s) for ongoing care, per session

97602 non-selective debridement, without anesthesia (eg, wet-to-moist dressing, enzymatic, abrasion), including topical application(w), wound assessment, and instruction(s) for ongoing care, per session

TESTS AND MEASUREMENTS

(For muscle testing, manual or electrical, joint range of motion, electromyography or nerve velocity determination, see 95831-95904)

97703 Checkout for orthotic/prosthetic use, established patient, each 15 minutes

97750 Physical performance test or measurement (eg, musculo-skeletal, functional capacity), with written report, each 15 minutes

● New Code ▲ Revised Code * Starred Procedure + Add-On Code ⊘ Modifier -51 Exempt

OTHER PROCEDURES

(For extracorporeal shock wave musculoskeletal therapy, use Category III code 0019T)

(97770   deleted 2001 edition. To report, see 97532, 97533)

97780   Acupuncture, one or more needles; without electrical stimulation

97781   with electrical stimulation

97799   Unlisted physical medicine/rehabilitation service or procedure

MEDICAL NUTRITION THERAPY

Medical nutrition therapy (MNT) is the assessment of nutritional status followed by nutritional therapy. The nutrition assessment includes review and analysis of 1) medical, nutrition and medication histories, 2) physical examination, 3) anthropometric measurements, and 4) laboratory test values. Nutrition therapy may include 1) diet modification, 2) counseling and education, 3) disease self-management skills training, and 4) administration of specialized therapies such as medical foods, intravenous or tube feedings.

MEDICAL NUTRITION THERAPY CODES

97802   Medical nutrition therapy; initial assessment and intervention, individual, face-to-face with the patient, each 15 minutes

97803   re-assessment and intervention, individual, face-to-face with the patient, each 15 minutes

97804   group (2 or more individual(s)), each 30 minutes

(For medical nutrition therapy assessment and/or intervention performed by a physician, see Evaluation and Management or Preventive Medicine service codes)

OSTEOPATHIC MANIPULATIVE TREATMENT

Osteopathic medicine is a system of therapy based on the theory that the body is capable of making its own remedies against disease and other toxic conditions when it is in normal structural relationship and has favorable environmental conditions and adequate nutrition. Osteopathic manipulative treatment (OMT) is a form of manual treatment applied by a physician to eliminate or alleviate somatic dysfunction and related disorders. This treatment may be accomplished by a variety of techniques.

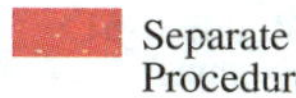
Separate Procedure

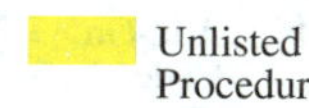
Unlisted Procedure

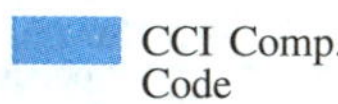
CCI Comp. Code

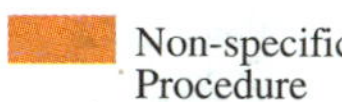
Non-specific Procedure

835

Coding Rules

1. Evaluation and management services may be reported separately, if, and only if the patient's condition requires a significant separately identifiable evaluation and management service, above and beyond the usual pre-service and post service work associated with the osteopathic manipulation.

2. CPT codes in this section are used to report OMT services provided in any location.

OSTEOPATHIC MANIPULATIVE TREATMENT CODES

98925 Osteopathic manipulative treatment (OMT); one to two body regions involved

98926 three to four body regions involved

98927 five to six body regions involved

98928 seven to eight body regions involved

98929 nine to ten body regions involved

CHIROPRACTIC MANIPULATIVE TREATMENT

Chiropractic medicine is a system of diagnosis and treatment based on the theory that irritation of the nervous system by mechanical, chemical or psychic factors is the cause of disease. Chiropractic services may include office visits, diagnostic tests, physical therapy, and/or chiropractic manipulation. Chiropractic manipulation treatment (CMT) is a form of manual treatment applied by a chiropractic physician to eliminate or alleviate somatic dysfunction and related disorders.

Coding Rules

1. Chiropractic manipulation treatment includes a pre-manipulation patient assessment.

2. Evaluation and management services provided in conjunction with CMT may be reported separately with the addition of CPT modifier -25, along with any diagnostic tests or other therapy provided.

---

836   ● New Code   ▲ Revised Code   ✳ Starred Procedure   ✛ Add-On Code   ⊘ Modifier -51 Exempt

REPORTING CHIROPRACTIC MANIPULATION TO MEDICARE

Medicare restricts the number of times the CMT code may be reported, provides a maximum reimbursement amount per year, and requires extensive supporting documentation as described below.

Documentation of Treatment Phase

Proper documentation of the treatment phase is extremely important when submitting claims for chiropractic services to Medicare. The treatment phase consists of the date the course of treatment was initiated and the number of treatments rendered to date. Proper documentation enables Medicare to process your claims quickly and accurately. For payment of chiropractic claims, the following information must be on the HCFA1500 claim form:

1. The service must be manual manipulation of the spine. This service is reported by CPT codes 98940-98943.

2. The primary diagnosis must be subluxation of the spine, either so stated or identified by a term descriptive of the subluxation. The following diagnoses are acceptable because they would always involve a subluxation:

Intervertebral disc disorders	722.0-722.9
Curvatures of the spine	737.0-737.9
Spondylolisthesis	738.4,756.12
Nonallopathic lesions	739.1-739.4
Spondylolysis	756.11

3. The level of subluxation must be stated.

4. The symptoms related to the level of subluxation must be given.

5. The date of the confirming x-ray must be on the claim. Note that the x-ray must have been taken within 12 months prior to or 3 months after the course of treatment was initiated.

6. The date this course of treatment was initiated and the number of treatments rendered since the start of this course must be on the claim.

Special Situations

If a patient returns with a new condition or injury, this represents a new treatment phase. The treatment phase information should reflect when you first saw the patient for this condition. Do not use the date you first saw the patient for an earlier course of treatment. Note on your HCFA1500 claim form that this is a new condition. Remember that a new documenting x-ray may be required.

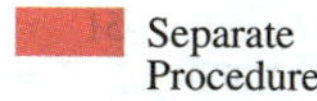 Separate Procedure

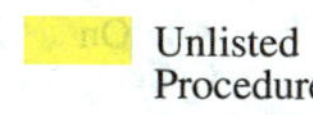 Unlisted Procedure

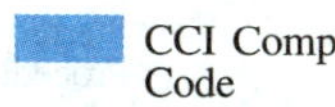 CCI Comp. Code

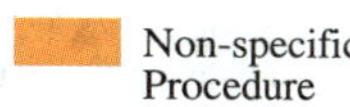 Non-specific Procedure

In the case of chronic conditions, an x-ray older than 12 months may be acceptable. For coverage of chronic conditions such as scoliosis, spondylolysis, and spondylolisthesis, there must be a reasonable expectation that there is a restorative potential. Remember that maintenance care is not covered by Medicare.

CHIROPRACTIC MANIPULATIVE TREATMENT CODES

98940   Chiropractic manipulative treatment (CMT); spinal, one to two regions

98941   spinal, three to four regions

98942   spinal, five regions

98943   extraspinal, one or more regions

SPECIAL SERVICES, PROCEDURES AND REPORTS

The MEDICINE section of CPT includes a subsection Special Services and Reports, with CPT codes 99000-99090 which provides the reporting physician with a means of identifying the completion of special reports and services that are an adjunct to the basic services rendered. The specific special services code reported indicates the special circumstances under which a basic procedure is performed.

The proper use of Special Services CPT codes can result in a significant increase in reimbursement. Most codes in this section are "add on" codes which means that they are used in addition to whatever other CPT codes describe the procedures or services performed.

SPECIMEN HANDLING

99000   Handling and/or conveyance of specimen for transfer from the physician's office to a laboratory

99001   Handling and/or conveyance of specimen for transfer from the patient in other than a physician's office to a laboratory (distance may be indicated)

● New Code ▲ Revised Code ✳ Starred Procedure ✚ Add-On Code ⊘ Modifier -51 Exempt

99002   Handling, conveyance, and/or any other service in connection with the implementation of an order involving devices (eg, designing, fitting, packaging, handling, delivery or mailing) when devices such as orthotics, protectives, prosthetics are fabricated by an outside laboratory or shop but which items have been designed, and are to be fitted and adjusted by the attending physician

(For routine collection of venous blood, use 36415)

SPECIAL VISIT CPT CODES

99024   Postoperative follow-up visit, included in global service

(As a component of a surgical "package," see Surgery guidelines)

99025   Initial (new patient) visit when starred (*) surgical procedure constitutes major service at that visit

SERVICES RENDERED AFTER REGULAR OFFICE HOURS

The office-based physician may provide services after regular office hours, during the evening or night, or on Sundays and/or holidays. The following codes may be reported in addition to the evaluation and management service code used to report the basic service(s).

99050   Services requested after office hours in addition to basic service

99052   Services requested between 10:00 PM and 8:00 AM in addition to basic service

99054   Services requested on Sundays and holidays in addition to basic service

SERVICES RENDERED AT SPECIAL LOCATION

The patient or patient's family may request that services normally provided in the physician's office be provided at another location, eg. hospital emergency room. The following code may be reported in addition to the evaluation and management service code used to report the basic service(s).

99056   Services provided at request of patient in a location other than physician's office which are normally provided in the office

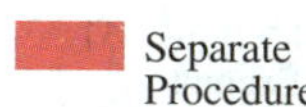 Separate Procedure

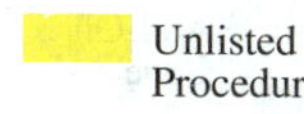 Unlisted Procedure

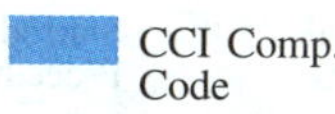 CCI Comp. Code

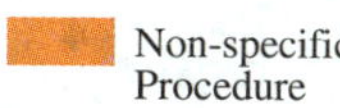 Non-specific Procedure

OFFICE EMERGENCY SERVICES

Occasionally office services may be provided on an emergency basis due either due to patient deterioration during an office visit or the patient presenting at the office for an emergent condition. The following code may be reported in addition to the evaluation and management service code used to report the basic service(s). The ICD-9-CM code(s) listed on the health insurance claim form must clearly justify the nature of the emergency.

99058   Office services provided on an emergency basis

SUPPLIES AND MATERIALS

HCPCS National Level II or Local Level III codes must be used instead of CPT code 99070 when reporting supplies, materials and drugs to Medicare.

99070   Supplies and materials (except spectacles), provided by the physician over and above those usually included with the office visit or other services rendered (list drugs, trays, supplies, or materials provided)

(For spectacles, see 92390-92395)

99071   Educational supplies, such as books, tapes, and pamphlets, provided by the physician for the patient's education at cost to physician

MEDICAL TESTIMONY

This CPT code may be used to report medical testimony provided as part of malpractice, worker's compensation and casualty cases. If the provider appears as an expert witness, appearance and stand-by fees should be negotiated with the attorneys in advance of testimony.

99075   Medical testimony

EDUCATIONAL SERVICES

99078   Physician educational services rendered to patients in a group setting (eg, prenatal, obesity, or diabetic instructions)

● New Code   ▲ Revised Code   * Starred Procedure   **+** Add-On Code   ⊘ Modifier -51 Exempt

SPECIAL REPORTS

This code is used frequently to report review of medical records in worker's compensation and casualty cases.

99080   Special reports such as insurance forms, more than the information conveyed in the usual medical communications or standard reporting form

TRANSPORTATION SERVICES

If the medical professional accompanied the patient on a long hospital transfer by ambulance, air ambulance, or long distance by common carrier, CPT code 99082 is reported in addition to any other services provided.

HCPCS Level II CPT codes A0000-A0999 cover emergency ambulance service using surface, air or water transport, plus non-emergency transportation services. There are also specific Ambulance Service Modifiers and a waiting time table to be used with these CPT codes.

This code may also be used to report travel associated with medical testimony.

99082   Unusual travel (eg, transportation and escort of patient)

DATA ANALYSIS

▲ **99090**   Analysis of clinical data stored in computers (eg, ECGs, blood pressures, hematologic data)

(For physician/health care professional collection and interpretation of physiologic data stored/transmitted by patient/caregiver, see 99091)

(Do not report 99090 if other more specific CPT codes exist, eg, 93014, 93227, 93233, 93272 for cardiographic services; 95250 for continuous glucose monitoring, 97750 for musculoskeletal function testing)

● **99091**   Collection and interpretation of physiologic data (eg, ECG, blood pressure, glucose monitoring) digitally stored and/or transmitted by the patient and/or caregiver to the physician or other qualified health care professional, requiring a minimum of 30 minutes of time

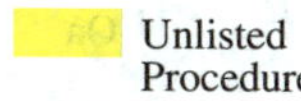 Separate Procedure

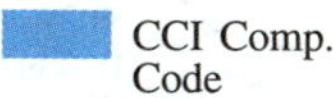 Unlisted Procedure

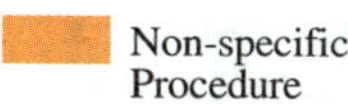 CCI Comp. Code

Non-specific Procedure

841

QUALIFYING CIRCUMSTANCES FOR ANESTHESIA

(For explanation of these services, see Anesthesia guidelines)

+99100 Anesthesia for patient of extreme age, under one year and over seventy (List separately in addition to code for primary anesthesia procedure)

+99116 Anesthesia complicated by utilization of total body hypothermia (List separately in addition to code for primary anesthesia procedure)

+99135 Anesthesia complicated by utilization of controlled hypotension (List separately in addition to code for primary anesthesia procedure)

+99140 Anesthesia complicated by emergency conditions (specify) (List separately in addition to code for primary anesthesia procedure)

SEDATION WITH OR WITHOUT ANALGESIA (CONSCIOUS SEDATION)

(If the sedation with or without analgesia (conscious sedation) is administered in support of a procedure provided by another physician, see Anesthesia section)

⊘ **99141** Sedation with or without analgesia (conscious sedation); intravenous, intramuscular or inhalation

(94760-94762 may not be reported in addition to 99141)

⊘ **99142** oral, rectal and/or intranasal

(94760-94762 may not be reported in addition to 99142)

● New Code   ▲ Revised Code   ✷ Starred Procedure   ✛ Add-On Code   ⊘ Modifier -51 Exempt

OTHER SERVICES AND PROCEDURES

99170	Anogenital examination with colposcopic magnification in childhood for suspected trauma

(For conscious sedation, use 99141, 99142)

99172	Visual function screening, automated or semi-automated bilateral quantitative determination of visual acuity, ocular alignment, color vision by pseudoisochromatic plates, and field of vision (may include all or some screening of the determination(s) for contrast sensitivity, vision under glare)

(This service must employ graduated visual acuity stimuli that allow a quantitative determination of visual acuity (eg, Snellen chart). This service may not be used in addition to a gernal ophthalmological service or an E/M service)

(Do not report 99172 in conjunction with code 99173)

99173	Screening test of visual acuity, quantitative, bilateral

(The screening test used must employ graduated visual acuity stimuli that allow a quantitative estimate of visual acuity (eg, Snellen chart). Other identifiable services unrelated to this screening test provided at the same time may be reported separately (eg, preventive medicine services). When acuity is measured as part of a general ophthalmological service or of an E/M service of the eye, it is a diagnostic examination and not a screening test.)

(Do not report 99173 in conjunction with code 99172)

99175	Ipecac or similar administration for individual emesis and continued observation until stomach adequately emptied of poison

(For diagnostic intubation, see 82926-82928, 89130-89141)

(For gastric lavage for diagnostic purposes, see 91055)

99183	Physician attendance and supervision of hyperbaric oxygen therapy, per session

(Evaluation and Management services and/or procedures (eg, wound debridement) provided in a hyperbaric oxygen treatment facility in conjunction with a hyperbaric oxygen therapy session should be reported separately)

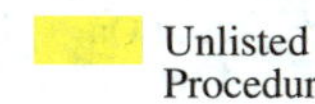
Separate
Procedure

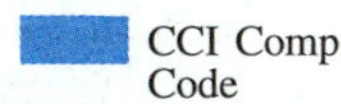
Unlisted
Procedure

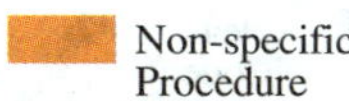
CCI Comp.
Code

Non-specific
Procedure

99185   Hypothermia; regional

99186   total body

99190   Assembly and operation of pump with oxygenator or heat exchanger (with or without ECG and/or pressure monitoring); each hour

99191   3/4 hour

99192   1/2 hour

99195   Phlebotomy, therapeutic (separate procedure)

99199   Unlisted special service, procedure or report

HOME HEALTH PROCEDURES/SERVICES

Home health procedures/services codes are used by non-physician health care professionals to report services provided in the patient's residence.

● **99500**   Home visit for prenatal monitoring and assessment to include fetal heart rate, non-stress test, uterine monitoring, and gestational diabetes monitoring

● **99501**   Home visit for postnatal assessment and follow-up care

● **99502**   Home visit for newborn care and assessment

● **99503**   Home visit for respiratory therapy care (eg, bronchodilator, oxygen therapy, respiratory assessment, apnea evaluation)

● **99504**   Home visit for patients receiving mechanical ventilation

● **99505**   Home visit for stoma care and maintenance including colostomy and cystostomy

● **99506**   Home visit for intramuscular injections

● **99507**   Home visit for care and maintenance of catheter(s) (eg, urinary, drainage, and enteral)

● **99508**   Home visit for polysomnography and sleep studies

---

844

● New Code	▲ Revised Code	* Starred Procedure	+ Add-On Code	⊘ Modifier -51 Exempt

- **99509** Home visit for assistance with activities of daily living and personal care

  (To report self-care/home management training, see 97535)

  (To report home medical nutrition assessment and intervention services, see 97802-97804)

  (To report home speech therapy services, see 92507-92508)

- **99510** Home visit for individual, family, or marriage counseling

- **99511** Home visit for fecal impaction management and enema administration

- **99512** Home visit for hemodialysis, per diem

  (For home infusion of peritoneal dialysis, use 99559)

- **99539** Unlisted home visit service or procedure

HOME INFUSION PROCEDURES

Home infusion procedures codes are used to report per diem home visits for the purpose of administering infusions. With the exception of the infusion drug; all materials, equipments and supplies are included in the basic code. Drugs used for the infusion are coded separately.

- **99551** Home infusion for pain management (intravenous or subcutaneous), per diem

- **99552** Home infusion for pain management (epidural or intrathecal), per diem

- **99553** Home infusion for tocolytic therapy, per diem

- **99554** Home infusion for hematopoietic hormones (eg, erythropoietin, G-CSF, CM-CSF) or platelets, per diem

- **99555** Home infusion for chemotherapy, per diem

- **99556** Home infusion for antibiotics/antifungals/antivirals, per diem

- **99557** Home infusion of continuous anticoagulant therapy (eg, heparin), per diem

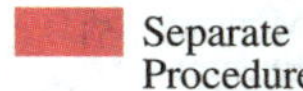 Separate Procedure
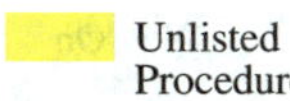 Unlisted Procedure
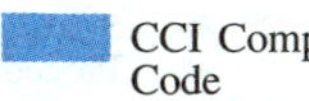 CCI Comp. Code
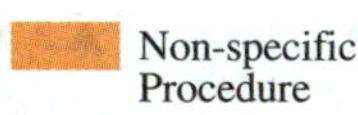 Non-specific Procedure

- **99558** Home infusion of immunotherapy, per diem

- **99559** Home infusion of peritoneal dialysis, per diem

  (For home visit for hemodialysis, use 99512)

- **99560** Home infusion of enteral nutrition, per diem

- **99561** Home infusion of hydration therapy, per diem

- **99562** Home infusion of total parenteral nutrition, per diem

- **99563** Home administration of aerosolized pentamidine, per diem

- **99564** Home infusion for anti-hemophilic agents (eg, Factor VIII), per diem

- **99565** Home infusion of alpha-1-proteinase inhibitor (eg, Prolastin), per diem

- **99566** Home infusion for uninterrupted, long-term intravenous treatment (eg, epoprostenol), per diem

- **99567** Home infusion of sympathomimetic agents (eg, dobutamine), per diem

- **99568** Home infusion of miscellaneous drugs, per diem

- **+99569** Home infusion, each additional therapy given on same day (List separately in addition to code for primary visit)

● New Code　　▲ Revised Code　　＊ Starred Procedure　　+ Add-On Code　　⊘ Modifier -51 Exempt

CATEGORY III CODES

CATEGORY III SECTION OVERVIEW

The seventh section of the CPT coding system is the Category III Emerging Technology section. The primary purpose of this section is to provide classification codes which will allow the collection of data on emerging technology services and procedures.

The assignment of a Category III code to a given service or procedure does not mean that the particular service or procedure is endorsed, approved, safe or has applicability to clinical practice. The Category III code simply provides a mechanism to identify and review emerging services and procedures.

Category III codes consist of four numbers followed by a letter. These is no particular organization to the codes listed in this section.

CATEGORY III CODES

- **0001T**   Endovascular repair of infrarenal abdominal aortic aneurysm or dissection; modular bifurcated prosthesis (two docking limbs)

- **0002T**   aorto-uni-iliac or aorto-unifemoral prosthesis

  (For radiological supervision and interpretation, use 75952 in conjunction with 0001T-0002T)

- **0003T**   Cervicography

- **0005T**   Transcatheter placement of extracranial cerebrovascular artery stent(s), percutaneous; initial vessel

- **+0006T**   each additional vessel (List separately in addition to code for primary procedure)

  (Use 0006T in conjunction with code 0005T)

  (For radiological supervision and interpretation, use 0007T)

- **0007T**   Transcatheter placement of extracranial cerebrovascular artery stent(s), percutaneous, radiological supervision and interpretation, each vessel

  (For procedure, see 0005T, 0006T)

Separate Procedure

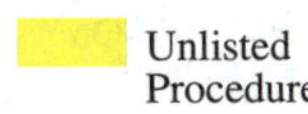
Unlisted Procedure

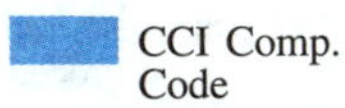
CCI Comp. Code

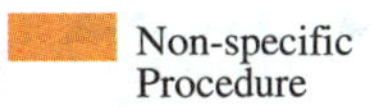
Non-specific Procedure

● **0008T** Upper gastrointestinal endoscopy including esophagus, stomach, and either the duodenum and/or jejunum as appropriate, with suturing of the esophagogastric junction

● **0009T** Endometrial cryoablation with ultrasonic guidance

● **0010T** Tuberculosis test, cell mediated immunity measurement of gamma interferon antigen response

● **0012T** Arthroscopy, knee, surgical, implantation of osteochondral graft(s) for treatment of articular surface defect; autografts

● **0013T**   allografts

● **0014T** Meniscal transplantation, medial or lateral, knee (any method)

● **0016T** Destruction of localized lesion of choroid (eg, choroidal neovascularization), transpupillary thermotherapy

● **0017T** Destruction of macular drusen, photocoagulation

● **0018T** Delivery of high power, focal magnetic pulses for direct stimulation to cortical neurons

● **0019T** Extracorporeal shock wave therapy; involving musculoskeletal system

● **0020T**   involving plantar fascia

● **0021T** Insertion of transcervical or transvaginal fetal oximetry sensor

● **0023T** Infectious agent drug susceptibility phenotype prediction using genotypic comparison to known genotypic/phenotypic database, HIV 1

● **0024T** Non-surgical septal reduction therapy (eg, alcohol ablation), for hypertrophic obstructive cardiomyopathy, with coronary arteriograms, with or without temporary pacemaker

● **0025T** Determination of corneal thickness (eg, pachymetry) with interpretation and report, bilateral

● **0026T** Lipoprotein, direct measurement, intermediate density lipoproteins (IDL) (remnant lipoproteins)

848

●	New Code	▲ Revised Code	✱ Starred Procedure	✚ Add-On Code	⊘ Modifier -51 Exempt

ALPHABETICAL INDEX

The alphabetical index includes listings by procedure, CPT® headings and sub-headings and anatomic site. Procedures and services commonly known by their acronyms, eponyms, homonyms or other designations are also included. The alphabetical index of *CPT® PLUS 2001* is unique in that both indexes to specific page numbers and indexes to CPT code numbers are included.

HOW TO USE THE ALPHABETICAL INDEX

When using the alphabetical index to locate CPT codes, use the following search sequence:

- Look for the CPT HEADING for the general category of surgical procedure(s) or medical service(s) or TOPIC for instructional and/or explanatory information.

- Look for the CPT Sub-heading for the organ system(s) involved or service(s) performed or the TOPIC sub-heading for the instructional or explanatory issue. Scan the index listings to determine if the specific procedure or service or topic is listed.

- For CPT codes, use the thumb-tab indexes to locate the appropriate CPT code section. If the specific procedure or service was listed in the index, locate the procedure or service in the CPT code section and verify the full description of the CPT code before using. If the specific procedure or service was not listed in the index, first locate the organ system and/or medical service sub-heading and then review the CPT code section until you locate the specific procedure and/or service.

- For instructional and/or explanatory topics, turn to the page number specified in the alphabetical index.

- Alternately, look for SYNONYMS, HOMONYMS, EPONYMS or ACRONYMS.

ORGANIZATION OF THE ALPHABETICAL INDEX

When using the alphabetical index, it is important to understand how entries to the index have been made. Index entries fall into one or more of the general categories described on the following page.

MAIN TERMS

1. SURGERY SERVICES CODES 10000-69999
      Auditory system 69000-69979
      Cardiovascular system 33000-37799
      Digestive system 40490-49999
      Endocrine system 60000-60699
      Eye and ocular adnexa 65091-68899.....
Surgical pathology, gross examination only 88300
Surgical preparation or creation recipient site 15000-15001
Surgical treatment
      anal fistula 46270-46285
      ectopic pregnancy 59120-59140

Note that in the above example, the CPT code categories and procedures/services are listed as the heading and a "range" of CPT codes follows. The range of CPT codes directs the coder to the appropriate CPT section where additional information on the procedure(s) or service(s) may be located. All CPT code sections and individual sub-headings are listed in **BOLD UPPER CASE**.

2. PROCEDURE OR SERVICE

Destruction
      benign or premalignant lesions 17000-17004
      celiac plexus by neurolytic agent 64680
      cervical spinal muscles by neurolytic agent 64613
      ciliary body 66700-66740
      cutaneous vascular proliferative lesions 17106-17108
      cyst or lesion, iris or ciliary body 66770
      hemorrhoids 46934-46936
      intercostal nerve by neurolytic agent 64620
      lesion, anus 46900-46924

3. TOPIC

RADIOLOGY SERVICES *557-604*
      Bilateral procedure codes *559*
      Complete procedures *557*
      Modifiers *558*
      Separate or multiple procedures *557*
      Services over-view *557*
      Subject listings *557*
      Subsections *557*
      Supervision and interpretation only *558*

Note that in the above example, the CPT topics and sub-topics are listed as the heading and a page or range of page numbers follows. The page number(s) directs the coder to the specific page(s) where additional information on the topic(s) may be located. All topics referring to CPT code sections or chapter headings are listed in **BOLD UPPER CASE**.

4)   SYNONYMS, EPONYMS AND ACRONYMS

Bankart procedure (capsulorrhaphy, anterior with labral repair) 23455
BCG 90585
Belsey IV procedure (esophagogastric fundoplasty) 43324
Bennett type procedure (quadricepsplasty) 27430
PSA 84153
T3 84480
Torkildsen type operation (ventriculocisternostomy) 62180

A

Aldolase 82085
Aldosterone 82088
Alkaloids, urine, quantitative 82101
Allergen immunotherapy professional services 95115-95134
Allergen immunotherapy supervision and provision antigens 95144-95170
ALLERGY AND CLINICAL IMMUNOLOGY SERVICES 95004-95199
Allergen specific ige 86003-86005
Allograft spine surgery 20930-20931
Alpha-1-antitrypsin 82103-82104
Alpha-fetoprotein 82105-82106
Aluminum 82108
Alveolectomy 41830
Alveoloplasty 41874
Ambulatory blood pressure monitoring 93784-93790
Amines vaginal fluid 82120
Amino acids 82127-82131
Ammonia 82140
Amniocentesis 59000-59001
Amniotic fluid scan 82143
Amphetamine or methamphetamine 82145
Amputation
    ankle 27888
    arm through humerus 24900-24931
    finger/thumb 26951-26952
    foot 28805
    foot (eg, Chopart type procedure) 28800
    forearm 25900-25909
    interpelviabdominal 27290
    leg 27880-27886
    metacarpal, with finger/thumb 26910
    metatarsal, with toe 28810
    penis 54120-54135
    thigh 27590-27596
    toe 28820-28825
Amylase 82150
Analysis information data stored in computers 99090
Anastomosis
    arterial, extracranial-intracranial 61711
    choledochal cyst 47716
    extrahepatic biliary ducts and gastrointestinal tract 47760
    facial-hypoglossal 64868
    facial-phrenic 64870
    facial-spinal accessory 64866
    intrahepatic ducts and gastrointestinal tract 47765
    pancreatic cyst to gastrointestinal tract 48520-48540
    pulmonary artery to aorta (Damus-Kaye-Stansel procedure) 33606
    Roux-en-Y, 47780, 47785

ANATOMIC PATHOLOGY SERVICES 88000-88099
Anatomical illustrations *41-90*
Androstanediol glucuronide 82154
Androstenedione 82157
Androsterone 82160
ANESTHESIA SERVICES *201-222*
    Modifiers *202*
    Qualifying circumstances *203*
    Section overview *201*
ANESTHESIA SERVICES CODES 00100-01999
    Burn excisions/debridement 01951-01953
    Forearm, wrist and hand 01810-01860
    Head 00100-00222
    Intrathoracic 00500-00580
    Knee and popliteal area 01320-01444
    Lower abdomen 00800-00882, 01930
    Lower leg 01462-01522
    Neck 00300-00352
    Obstetric 01960-01969
    Other procedures 01990-01999
    Pelvic (except hip) 01112-01190
    Perineum 00902-00952
    Radiological procedures 01905-01933
    Shoulder and axilla 01610-01682
    Spine and spinal cord 00600-00670
    Thorax (chest wall and shoulder girdle) 00400-00474
    Upper abdomen 00700-00796
    Upper arm and elbow 01710-01782
    Upper leg (except knee) 01320-01444
Anesthesia services for
    access to central venous circulation 00532
    angioplasty 01924-01926
    arteries, forearm, wrist, and hand 01840
    arteries, forearm, wrist, and hand embolectomy 01842
    arteries, knee and popliteal area 01440-01444
    arteries, lower leg 01500-01502
    arteries, shoulder and axilla 01650-01656
    arteries, upper arm and elbow 01770-01772
    arteries, upper leg 01270-01274
    arteriograms, needle, carotid/vertebral 01916
    arteriograms, needle, retrograde, brachial/femoral 01916
    arthroscopic procedures, ankle joint 01464
    arthroscopic procedures, elbow joint 01732
    arthroscopic procedures, hip joint 01202
    arthroscopic procedures, knee joint 01382
    arthroscopic procedures, shoulder joint 01622
    body cast application/revision 01130

Anesthesia services for *(continued)*
    bones, lower leg, ankle, and foot 01480-01486
    bony pelvis 01120
    cardiac catheterization 01920
    cardioverter/defibrillator 00534
    cast applications, removal/repair knee joint 01420
    cervical spine and cord 00600-00604
    chest procedures 00520-00528
    clavicle and scapula 00450-00454
    cleft lip 00102
    complicated by emergency conditions 99140
    complicated controlled hypotension 99135
    complicated total body hypothermia 99116
    ear 00120-00126
    electroconvulsive therapy 00104
    esophagus 00500
    extraperitoneal procedures lower abdomen 00860-00870
    eye 00140-00148
    eyelid 00103
    facial bones 00190-00192
    femur 01220-01234
    forearm, wrist, and hand 01810
    forearm, wrist/hand cast 01860
    head, neck, and posterior trunk 00300
    heart pericardium, and great vessels of chest 00560-00562
    heart transplant or heart/lung transplant 00580
    hernia repairs lower abdomen 00830-00832
    hernia repairs upper abdomen 00750-00756
    hip joint 01200-01214
    humerus and elbow 01730-01760
    injection procedure, diskography, cervical 01905
    injection procedure, diskography, lumbar 01905
    injection procedure, myelography, cervical 01905
    injection procedure, myelography, lumbar 01905
    injection procedure, myelography, posterior fossa 01905
    injection procedure, pneumoencephalography 01905
    integumentary system 00400-00410
    interpelviabdominal amputation 01140
    intracranial procedures 00210-00222
    intraoral procedures 00170-00176
    intraperitoneal procedures, lower abdomen 00840-00851
    intraperitoneal procedures, upper abdomen 00790-00796
    knee joint 01380-01404
    knee popliteal area 01320
    lithotripsy, extracorporeal shock wave 00872-00873
    lower anterior abdominal wall 00800-00802
    lower femur 01340-01360

Angiography
    adrenal 75731-75733
    arteriovenous shunt 75790
    brachial 75658
    carotid 75665-75680
    cervicocerebral 75650
    external carotid 75660-75662
    extremity 75710-75716
    internal mammary 75756
    pelvic 75736
    pulmonary 75741-75746
    renal 75722-75724
    selective 75774
    spinal 75705
    vertebral 75685
    visceral 75726
Angioplasty pulmonary artery 92997-92998
Angioscopy therapeutic intervention 35400
Angiotensin 82163-82164
Animal inoculation 87001-87003
Ankle disarticulation 27889
Anogenital examination 99170
Anoplasty 46700-46705
Anorectal manometry 91122
Anorectal myomectomy 45108
Anoscopy 46600-46615
Antepartum care 59425-59426
Anterior colporrhaphy 57240
Anterior tibial tubercleplasty (eg, Maquet type procedure) 27418
Anterior vesicourethropexy 51841
    Marshall-Marchetti-Krantz, Burch 51840
Anthrax vaccine 90581
Anti-phosphatidylserine antibody 86148
Antibody
    actinomyces 86602
    adenovirus 86603
    aspergillus 86606
    bacterium 86609
    blastomyces 86612
    bordetella 86615
    borrelia 86619
    borrelia burgdorferi (Lyme disease) 86617-86618
    brucella 86622
    campylobacter 86625
    candida 86628
    chlamydia 86631
    chlamydia, igm 86632

Antibody *(continued)*
    protozoa, not elsewhere specified 86753
    respiratory syncytial virus 86756
    rotavirus 86759
    rubella 86762
    rubeola 86765
    salmonella 86768
    screen rbc 86850
    shigella 86771
    tetanus 86774
    toxoplasma 86777
    toxoplasma, IGM 86778
    treponema pallidum (eg, FTA-ABS) 86781
    trichinella 86784
    varicella-zoster 86787
    virus not elsewhere specified 86790
    yersinia 86793
Antihuman globulin test (Coombs test) 86880-86886
Antinuclear antibodies (ANA) 86038-86039
Antistreptolysin 0 screen 86063
Antistreptolysin 0 titer 86060
Aortic suspension 33800
Aortography abdominal 75625-75630
Aortography thoracic 75600-75605
Aortoplasty supravalvular stenosis 33417
Apolipoprotein 82172
Appendectomy 44950-44960
Application
    allograft   skin 15350-15351
    cranial tongs, caliper, stereotactic frame 20660
    halo including removal 20661-20664
    halo type appliance 21100
    interdental fixation device 21110
    intervertebral biomechanical device(s) 22851
    multiplane 20692
    surface neurostimulator 64550
    uniplane 20690
    xenograft skin 15400-15401
Aqueous shunt to extraocular reservoir 66180
Arrest epiphyseal
    combined distal femur, proximal tibia and fibula 27479
    distal femur 27475
    distal fibula 27732
    distal tibia 27730
    distal tibia and fibula 27734
    proximal and distal tibia and fibula 27740-27742
    tibia and fibula 27477

Arthroplasty
    ankle 27700-27703
    elbow 24360-24363
    femoral prosthetic replacement 27130
    glenohumeral joint, hemi 23470
    glenohumeral joint, total shoulder 23472
    intercarpal/carpometacarpal joints 25447
    interphalangeal joint 26535-26536
    knee condyle and plateau 27446-27447
    knee femoral condyles/tibial plateau(s) 27442-27443
    knee hinge prosthesis (eg, Walldius type) 27445
    knee tibial plateau 27440-27441
    metacarpophalangeal joint 26530-26531
    patella 27437-27438
    prosthetic replacement, distal radius 25441-25446
    prosthetic replacement, distal ulna 25442
    prosthetic replacement, lunate 25444
    prosthetic replacement, scaphoid 25443
    prosthetic replacement, trapezium 25445
    radial head 24365-24366
    temporomandibular joint 21240-21243
    wrist 25332
Arthroscopic repair cruciate ligament 29888-29889
Arthroscopic treatment
    fracture, intercondylar spine(s) knee 29850-29851
    fracture, tibia 29855-29856
Arthroscopy
    ankle 29894-29898
    ankle, surgical 29891
    elbow, diagnostic 29830
    elbow, surgical 29834-29838
    hip 29860-29863
    knee 29870-29887
    metacarpophalangeal joint 29900-29902
    shoulder, diagnostic 29805-29807
    shoulder, surgical 29819-29826
    temporomandibular joint 29800-29804
    unlisted, 29999
    wrist, diagnostic 29840
    wrist, surgical 29843-29847
Arthrotomy
    acromioclavicular joint 23101
    acromioclavicular, sternoclavicular joint 23044
    ankle 27610-27626
    biopsy, hip joint 27052
    biopsy, sacroiliac joint 27050
    carpometacarpal joint 26070-26100

Auditory evoked potentials 92585
AUDITORY SYSTEM SURGICAL PROCEDURES 69000-69979
Augmentation mandibular body/angle 21125-21127
Aural rehabilitation following cochlear implant 92510
Autograft spine surgery 20936-20938
Autologous blood/component, collection processing and storage 86890-86891
Autopsy 88000
Avulsion nail plate 11730-11732

B

B-hexosaminidase 83080
Bacillus Calmette-Guerin vaccine (BCG) 90585-90586
Baker's cyst (excision) 27345
Banding pulmonary artery 33690
Bankart procedure (capsulorrhaphy, anterior with labral repair) 23455
Barbiturates 82205
Basic life disability examination 99450
BCG 90585
Behavior assessment and intervention 96150-96155
Bekesy audiometry 92560-92561
Belsey IV procedure (esophagogastric fundoplasty) 43324
Bennett type procedure (quadricepsplasty) 27430
Bile acids 82239-82240
Biliary drainage transhepatic percutaneous 75980
Biliary duct stone extraction 47630
Bilirubin 82247-82252
Binocular microscopy 92504
BIOFEEDBACK 90901-90911
Biopsy
    abdominal or retroperitoneal mass 49180
    anorectal wall 45100
    bone 20220-20245
    bone marrow 38221
    brain stem 61575-61576
    breast 19100-19101
    cervix 57500
    conjunctiva 68100
    cornea 65410
    epididymis 54800
    external auditory canal 69105
    external ear 69100
    extraocular muscle 67350
    eyelid 67810
    floor mouth 41108
    hypopharynx 42802

Biopsy *(continued)*
    intestine 44100
    intranasal 30100
    lacrimal gland 68510
    lacrimal sac 68525
    lip 40490
    liver 47000-47100
    lung/mediastinum 32405
    lymph node(s) 38500-38530
    muscle 20200-20206
    nail unit 11755
    nasopharynx 42804-42806
    nerve 64795
    oropharynx 42800
    ovary 58900
    palate uvula 42100
    pancreas 48100-48102
    penis 54100-54105
    pleura 32400-32402
    prostate 55700-55705
    salivary gland 42400-42405
    skin subcutaneous tissue mucous membrane 11100-11101
    soft tissue, back/flank 21920-21925
    soft tissue, forearm wrist 25065-25066
    soft tissue, leg/ankle area 27613-27614
    soft tissue, neck/thorax 21550
    soft tissue, pelvis and hip area 27040-27041
    soft tissue, shoulder 23065-23066
    soft tissue, thigh/knee area 27323-27324
    soft tissue, upper arm/elbow area 24065-24066
    spinal cord, 62269
    stomach 43600-43605
    testis 54500-54505
    thyroid 60100
    tongue 41100-41105
    urethra 53200
    vaginal mucosa 57100-57105
    vertebral body 20250-20251
    vestibule mouth 40808
    vulva perineum 56605-56606
Biotinidase 82261
Bladder instillation
    anticarcinogenic agent 51720
    irrigation 51700
Blalock-taussig type operation (shunt subclavian to pulmonary artery) 33750
Bleeding time 85002
Blepharoplasty 15820-15823

Blepharotomy drainage abscess eyelid 67700
Blood bank physician services 86077-86079
Blood count
    differential WBC count, buffy coat 85009
    hemoglobin 85018
    hemogram and platelet count, automated 85023-85027
    hemogram automated 85021-85022
    hemogram manual, complete 85031
    manual blood smear examination 85008
    manual differential WBC count 85007
    other than spun hematocrit 85014
    red blood cell (RBC) only 85041
    reticulocyte count 85044-85045
    reticulocytes hemoglobin concentration 85046
    spun microhematocrit 85013
    white blood cell (WBC) 85048
Blood gases 82803
Blood occult 82270-82273
Blood smear peripheral interpretation by physician 85060
Blood typing
    ABO 86900
    antigen screening compatible blood unit 86903-86904
    paternity testing 86910-86911
    RBC antigens, other than ABO/RH (D), each 86905
    RH (D) 86901
    RH phenotyping, complete 86906
Blood-derived peripheral stem cell harvesting 38231
Bone age studies 76020
Bone density study 78350-78351
Bone graft 20900-20902
    femoral head, neck, intertrochanteric/subtrochanteric area 27170
    microvascular anastomosis, fibula 20955
    microvascular anastomosis, iliac crest 20956
    microvascular anastomosis, metatarsal 20957
    microvascular anastomosis, other than fibula 20962
Bone joint imaging 78300-78320
Bone length studies (orthoroentgenogram, scanogram) 76040
Bone marrow
    aspiration 38220
    biopsy 38221
    harvesting 38230
    imaging 78102-78104
    smear interpretation 85097
    transplantation 38240-38241
Botulinum antitoxin 90287
Botulism immune globulin 90288
Bowel imaging 78290

C

Carnitine 82379
Carotene 82380
Carpectomy 25210-25215
Cartilage graft 20910-20912
CASE MANAGEMENT SERVICES 99361-99373
Cast application
   body cast shoulder to hips 29035-29046
   cast elbow to finger 29075
   cast hand and lower forearm 29085
   cast shoulder to hand 29065
   clubfoot cast 29450
   cylinder cast 29365
   finger splint 29130-29131
   halo type body cast 29000
   hip spica cast 29305-29325
   long arm splint 29105
   long leg cast 29345-29358
   long leg splint 29505
   patellar tendon bearing (PTB) cast 29435
   plaster figure-of-eight 29049
   plaster velpeau 29058
   rigid total contact leg cast 29445
   Risser jacket 29010-29015
   short arm splint 29125-29126
   short leg cast 29405-29425
   short leg splint 29515
   shoulder spica 29055
   turnbuckle jacket 29020-29025
Catecholamines 82382-82384
Cathepsin-d 82387
Catheter
   nasotracheal 31720
   tracheobronchial 31725
Catheter introduction
   aorta 36200
   right heart/main pulmonary artery 36013
Catheter placement
   arterial system 36215-36248
   coronary artery(s) 93508
   pulmonary artery 36014-36015
   venous system 36011-36012
Catheterization
   bronchial brush biopsy 31717
   bronchography 31710
   combined endoscopic 74330
   hysterosonography/hysterosalpingography 58340
   transglottic 31700

Catheterization *(continued)*
    umbilical artery 36660
    umbilical vein 36510
    urethra 53670-53675
Cauterization
    ablation, mucosa turbinates 30801-30802
    cervix 57510-57513
Cell count, miscellaneous body fluids 89050-89051
Central auditory function test(s) 92589
CENTRAL NERVOUS SYSTEM ASSESSMENTS/TESTS 96100-96177
Centralization wrist on ulna 25335
Cephalogram, orthodontic 70350
Cerclage
    cervix during pregnancy 59320-59325
    uterine cervix 57700
Cerebral blood flow 78615
Cerebrospinal fluid flow, imaging 78630-78647
Ceruloplasmin 82390
Cervical puncture cisternal/lateral 61050-61055
Cervicoplasty 15819
Cesarean delivery only 59514-59622
Change
    biliary drainage catheter, percutaneous 47525
    cystostomy tube 51705-51710
    nephrostomy/pyelostomy tube 50398
    percutaneous tube/drainage catheter 75984
    ureterostomy tube 50688
Checkout orthotic/prosthetic use 97703
Chelatable iron estimation total body iron 78172
Chemical cauterization granulation tissue 17250
Chemical exfoliation 17360
Chemical peel 15788-15793
Chemical pleurodesis 32005
Chemiluminescent assay 82397
CHEMISTRY 82000-84999
Chemodenervation extraocular muscle 67345
Chemosurgery 17304-17310
Chemosurgery (Mohs micrographic technique) 17305
Chemotaxis assay 86155
CHEMOTHERAPY ADMINISTRATION 96400-96549
Chemotherapy injection 96542
CHIROPRACTIC MANIPULATIVE TREATMENT (CMT) 98940-98943
Chloramphenicol 82415
Chloride 82435-82438
Chlorinated hydrocarbons 82441
Cholangiography 74320
Cholangiography pancreatography 74300-74305

Cholecystectomy 47600-47620
Cholecystoenterostomy 47720-47741
Cholecystography 74290-74291
Cholecystostomy percutaneous 47490
Choledochotomy/choledochostomy 47420-47425, 47480
Cholera vaccine 90725
Cholesterol 82465
Cholinesterase 82480-82482
Chondroitin B sulfate 82485
Chopart type procedure (amputation, foot) 28800
Chorionic villus sampling 59015
Chromatography 82486-82492
Chromium 82495
Chromogenic substrate assay 85130
Chromosome analysis 88280-88289
    amniotic fluid/chorionic villus 88267
    breakage syndromes 88245-88249
    in situ amniotic fluid cells 88269
Chromotubation oviduct 58350
Cineplasty upper extremity 24940
Cineradiography 76120-76125
Circadian respiratory pattern recording 94772
Circumcision 54150-54161
Cisternography, positive contrast 70015
Citrate 82507
Clagett type procedure (closure chest wall) 32810
Claviculectomy 23120-23125
Clayton type procedure (ostectomy all metatarsal heads) 28114
Clinical pathology consultation 80500-80502
Clitoroplasty intersex state 56805
Closure
    anal fistula 46288
    aortico-left ventricular tunnel 33722
    atrioventricular valve 33600
    bladder exstrophy 51940
    chest wall (Clagett type procedure) 32810
    cystostomy 51880
    enteroenteric/enterocolic fistula 44650
    enterostomy 44620-44626
    enterovesical fistula 44660-44661
    esophagostomy/fistula 43420-43425
    gastrocolic fistula 43880
    gastrostomy surgical 43870
    intestinal cutaneous fistula 44640
    laceration vestibule mouth 40830-40831
    lacrimal fistula 68770
    lacrimal punctum 68760-68761

Closure *(continued)*
    nephrocutaneous/pyelocutaneous fistula 50520
    nephrovisceral fistula 50525-50526
    postauricular fistula, mastoid 69700
    rectourethral fistula 45820-45825
    rectovaginal fistula 57300-57308
    rectovesical fistula 45800-45805
    salivary fistula 42600
    semilunar valve 33602
    sternotomy separation 21750
    ureterocutaneous fistula 50920
    ureterovisceral fistula 50930
    urethrocutaneous fistula 53520
    urethrostomy 53520
    urethrovaginal fistula 57310-57311
    ventricular septal defect 33681-33688
    vesicouterine fistula 51920-51925
    vesicovaginal fistula 51900-57330
Clot lysis time 85175
Clot retraction 85170
Clotting factor
    II prothrombin 85210
    IX (PTC or Christmas) 85250
    V 85220
    VII 85230
    VIII (AHG) 85240
    VIII related antigen 85244
    VIII Von Willebrands factor 85247
    VIII vw factor antigen 85246
    VIII vw factor, ristocetin cofactor 85245
    X (Stuart-Prower) 85260
    XI (pta) 85270
    XII (Hageman) 85280
    XIII (fibrin stabilizing) 85290
    XIII (fibrin stabilizing), screen solubility 85291
Clotting high molecular weight kininogen assay (Fitzgerald factor assay) 85293
Clotting inhibitors/anticoagulants
    antithrombin III, activity 85300
    antithrombin III, antigen assay 85301
    protein C, activity 85303
    protein C, antigen 85302
    protein S, free 85306
    protein S, total 85305
Clotting prekallikrein assay (Fletcher factor assay) 85292
CMT 98940
CNP 94662
Coagulation time 85345-85348

Computerized tomography guidance
    cyst aspiration 76365
    needle biopsy 76360
    placement radiation therapy fields 76370
    stereotactic localization 76355
Concentration parasites, ova, or tubercle bacillus (TB, AFB) 87015
Conditioning play audiometry 92582
Condylectomy temporomandibular joint 21050
Conization cervix 57520-57522
Conjunctival flap 68360-68362
Conjunctivoplasty 68320-68328
Conjunctivorhinostomy 68745-68750
Construction
    apical-aortic conduit 33404
    artificial vagina 57291-57292
    intermarginal adhesions 67880-67882
    tracheoesophageal fistula 31611
CONSULTATIONS 99241-99275
CONSULTATIONS CLINICAL PATHOLOGY 80500
Consultations, medical
    confirmatory 99271-99275
    inpatient, initial 99251-99255
    inpatient, follow-up 99261-99263
    office 99241-99245
Consultations, pathology
    comprehensive 88325
    during surgery 88329
Consultations, radiology
    medical physics 77336
    X-ray examination 76140
Contact laser vaporization 52648
Contact lens 92310
Continent diversion 50825
Continent ileostomy (Kock procedure) 44316
Continuous negative pressure ventilation (CNP) 94662
Continuous positive airway pressure ventilation (CPAP) 94660
Contrast injection assessment abscess/cyst 49424
Control nasal hemorrhage
    anterior 30901-30903
    posterior 30905-30906
Control nasopharyngeal hemorrhage 42970-42972
Control oropharyngeal hemorrhage 42960-42962
Coombs test 86880
Copper 82525
Coracoacromial ligament release 23415
Cordocentesis 59012
Corneal relaxing incision 65772

Corneal wedge resection 65775
Coronary angioplasty balloon percutaneous transluminal 92982-92984
Coronary artery bypass
    arterial graft(s) 33533-33536
    vein only 33510-33516
    venous graft(s) and arterial graft(s) 33517-33523
Coronary endarterectomy 33572
Coronoidectomy 21070
Corpora cavernosa corpus spongiosum shunt 54430
Corpora cavernosa glans penis fistulization 54435
Corpora cavernosa saphenous vein shunt 54420
Corpora cavernosography 74445
Correction
    claw finger 26499
    cock-up fifth toe 28286
    everted punctum, cautery 68705
    hallux valgus 28290-28299
    hallux valgus (Keller, Mcbride, Mayo procedure) 28292
    hammertoe 28285
    inverted nipples 19355
    lid retraction 67911
    malrotation 44055
    trichiasis 67820-67835
Corticosterone 82528
Corticotropic releasing hormone (CRH) stimulation panel 80412
Cortisol 82530-82533
Costotransversectomy 21610
Counterimmunoelectrophoresis 86185
CPAP 94660
CPK 82550
CPT CODING
    Additions, changes and deletions 2002 *8-9*
    Coding fundamentals *1-5*
    Coding issues *5-26*
    Definition of new patient and established patient *22*
    Format and conventions *3*
    HCPCS modifiers *34-40*
    Hospital care *23*
    Modifiers *27-34*
    Place of service *23*
    Referral *24*
    Separate or multiple procedures *24*
    Starred procedures *3, 22*
    Structure of *2*
    Supplies and materials supplied by physician *24*
    Supporting documentation *5*
    Unlisted procedures or services *5*

Cranial decompression
    posterior fossa, other 61345
    supratentorial, other 61340
Craniectomy
    bone flap craniotomy tumor 61526-61530
    craniosynostosis 61550-61552
    craniotomy, drainage intracranial abscess 61320-61321
    craniotomy, evacuation hematoma 61312-61315
    craniotomy, excision foreign body from brain 61570
    craniotomy, exploratory 61304-61305
    craniotomy, implantation neurostimulator electrodes 61860
    craniotomy, treatment penetrating wound brain 61571
    excision brain tumor 61518-61521
    excision tumor other bone lesion skull 61500
    implantation neurostimulator electrodes 61870-61875
    infratentorial/posterior fossa excision brain abscess 61522
    infratentorial/posterior fossa excision/fenestration cyst 61524
    osteomyelitis 61501
    suboccipital 61458-61480
    suboccipital with cervical laminectomy 61343
    subtemporal 61450
    trephination, bone flap craniotomy 61510-61516
Craniofacial approach to anterior cranial fossa 61580-61583
Craniofacial separation (Lefort III type)
    closed treatment 21431
    open treatment 21432-21436
Cranioplasty
    autograft 62146-62147
    skull defect 62140-62145
Craniotomy
    craniosynostosis 61556-61557
    elevation bone flap 61533-61545
    hypophysectomy excision pituitary tumor 61546
    lobotomy 61490
    repair dural/CSF leak 62100
    repair encephalocele 62121
    section tentorium cerebelli 61440
Creatine 82540
Creatine kinase (CK), (CPK) 82550-82554
Creatinine 82565-82575
Creation
    arteriovenous fistula 36825-36830
    lesion spinal cord by stereotactic method 63600
    lesion stereotactic method 61720-61791
    pericardial window 33025
    shunt 63740-62223
Cricopharyngeal myotomy 43030

Cystotomy excision
    bladder diverticulum 51525
    bladder tumor 51530
    ureterocele 51535
    vesical neck 51520
Cystourethroplasty 51820
Cystourethroscopy 52000-52340
CYTOGENETIC STUDIES 88230-88299
Cytogenetics and molecular cytogenetics 88291
Cytomegalovirus immune globulin (CMV-IgIV) 90291
CYTOPATHOLOGY 88104-88199
Cytopathology
    cervical or vaginal 88141-88145
    slides cervical or vaginal 88150-88167
    smears cervical or vaginal 88147-88148
    smears other source 88160-88162

D

Dacryocystography nasolacrimal duct 70170
Dacryocystorhinostomy 68720
Daily management epidural or subarachnoid drug administration 01996
Damus-Kaye-Stansel procedure (anastomosis pulmonary artery to aorta) 33606
Dark adaptation examination 92284
Dark field examination 87164-87166
Debridement
    extensive eczematous or infected skin 11000-11001
    mastoidectomy cavity 69220-69222
    nail(s) 11720-11721
    open fracture(s) dislocation(s), skin 11010-11012
    skin 11040-11044
Decalcification procedure 88311
Declotting vascular access device or catheter 36550
Decompression
    facial nerve 69720-69725
    fasciotomy, forearm 24495
    fasciotomy, forearm wrist 25020-25023
    fingers, hand 26035
    internal auditory canal 69960
    lesion, brain stem or upper spinal cord 61575
    orbit 61330
    plantar digital nerve 64726
    spinal cord equina nerve root(s) 63055-63057
    spinal cord nerve root(s) 63064-63066
    unspecified nerve(s) 64722
Decompressive fasciotomy hand 26037

Destruction *(continued)*
    nerve joint, lumbar or sacral by neurolytic agent 64622-64623
    nerve joint, other peripheral nerve or branch by neurolytic agent 64640
    nerve joint, pudendal nerve by neurolytic agent 64630
    rectal tumor 45190
    retinopathy 67227-67228
    trigeminal nerve by neurolytic agent 64600-64610
    vaginal lesion(s) 57061-57065
    warts, molluscum contagiosum, or milia 17110-17111
Determination airway closing volume 94370
Determination central c-v hemodynamics 78414
Determination maldistribution inspired gas 94350
Determination refractive state 92015
Determination resistance to airflow 94360
Determination venous pressure 93770
Determinative histochemistry 88318-88319
Development cognitive skills 97770
Developmental testing 96110-96111
DIAGNOSTIC RADIOLOGY SERVICES 70010-76499
DIAGNOSTIC ULTRASOUND SERVICES 76506-76999
DIALYSIS SERVICES 90918-90999
Dialysis procedure other than hemodialysis 90945-90947
Dialysis training 90989-90993
Diaphragm or cervical cap fitting 57170
Dibucaine number 82638
DIGESTIVE SYSTEM SURGICAL PROCEDURES 40490-49999
Digital analysis electroencephalogram (EEG) 95957
Dihydrocodeinone 82646
Dihydromorphinone 82649
Dihydrotestosterone (DHT) 82651
Dihydroxyvitamin d 82652
Dilatation biliary duct stricture, percutaneous transhepatic 74363
Dilation
    anal sphincter 45905
    catheterization, salivary duct 42660
    cervical canal 57800
    curettage 58120
    curettage, cervical stump 57820
    esophagus 43450-43458
    female urethra 53660-53665
    lacrimal punctum 68801
    nephrostomy, ureters, or urethra 74485
    rectal stricture 45910
    salivary duct 42650
    urethral stricture 53600-53621
    vagina 57400
Dimethadione 82654

Dislocation *(continued)*
    knee, closed treatment 27550-27552
    knee, open treatment 27556-27558
    lunate, closed treatment 25690
    lunate, open treatment 25695
    metacarpophalangeal, closed treatment 26700-26705
    metacarpophalangeal, open treatment 26715
    metacarpophalangeal, percutaneous skeletal fixation 26706
    metatarsophalangeal joint, closed treatment 28630-28635
    metatarsophalangeal joint, open treatment 28645
    metatarsophalangeal joint, percutaneous skeletal fixation 28636
    patellar, closed treatment 27560-27562
    patellar, open treatment 27566
    posterior ring, open treatment 27218
    radiocarpal or intercarpal, closed treatment 25660
    radiocarpal or intercarpal, open treatment 25670
    shoulder, closed treatment 23650-23675
    shoulder, open treatment 23670-23680
    sternoclavicular, closed treatment 23520-23525
    sternoclavicular, open treatment 23530-23532
    talotarsal joint, closed treatment 28570-28575
    talotarsal joint, open treatment 28585
    talotarsal, percutaneous skeletal fixation 28576
    tarsal bone, closed treatment 28540-28545
    tarsal bone, open treatment 28555
    tarsal bone, percutaneous skeletal fixation 28546
    tarsometatarsal joint, closed treatment 28600-28605
    tarsometatarsal joint, open treatment 28615
    tarsometatarsal joint, percutaneous skeletal fixation 28606
    temporomandibular, closed treatment 21480-21485
    temporomandibular, open treatment 21490
    tibiofibular joint, closed treatment 27830-27831
    tibiofibular joint, open treatment 27832
Displacement therapy (Proetz type) 30210
Disruption tibiofibular joint, open treatment 27829
Dissection deep jugular node(s) 38542
Diverticulectomy hypopharynx or esophagus 43130-43135
Division
    aberrant vessel 33802-33803
    plantar fascia and muscle 28250
    scalenus anticus 21700-21705
    sternocleidomastoid torticollis 21720-21725
    stricture rectum 45150

DOCUMENTATION OF EXAMINATIONS *117-153*
    Cardiovascular examination *125*
    Ear, nose and throat examination *128*
    Eye examination *131*
    General multi-system examination *120*
    Genitourinary examination *130*
    Hematologic, lymphatic and/or immunologic examination *137*
    Musculoskeletal examination *139*
    Neurological examination *142*
    Psychiatric examination *145*
    Respiratory examination *148*
    Skin examination *151*
Documentation of medical decision making *154-156*
Documentation of counseling or coordination of care *157*
DOMICILIARY, REST HOME, CUSTODIAL CARE SERVICES
    99321-99333
Donor cardiectomy 33940
Donor cardiectomy-pneumonectomy 33930
Donor hepatectomy 47133-47134
Donor nephrectomy 50300-50320
Donor pancreatectomy 48550
Donor pneumonectomy 32850
Doppler echocardiography 93320-93325
Doppler echocardiography, fetal 76827-76828
Douglas type procedure (suture tongue to lip micrognathia) 41510
Drainage
    abscess, dentoalveolar structures 41800
    abscess, external auditory canal 69020
    abscess, finger 26010-26011
    abscess, hematoma external ear 69000-69005
    abscess, hematoma, nasal 30000
    abscess, hematoma, nasal septum 30020
    abscess, lymph node or lymphadenitis 38300-38305
    abscess, palate, uvula 42000
    abscess, parotid 42300-42305
    abscess, perirenal or renal 50020-50021
    abscess, peritoneal or localized peritonitis 49020-49021
    abscess, periurethral 53040
    abscess, perivesical or prevesical space 51080
    abscess, retroperitoneal 49060-49061
    abscess, scrotal wall 55100
    abscess, subdiaphragmatic or subphrenic 49040-49041
    abscess, submaxillary or sublingual, intraoral 42310
    abscess, submaxillary, external 42320
    abscess, vestibule mouth 40800-40801
    extraperitoneal lymphocele to peritoneal cavity 49062
    ovarian abscess 58820-58822

Drainage *(continued)*
    ovarian cyst(s) 58800-58805
    palmar bursa 26025-26030
    pelvic abscess 58823
    perineal, urinary extravasation 53080-53085
    pseudocyst, pancreas 48510-48511
    skene's gland, abscess or cyst 53060
    tendon sheath, digit palm 26020
Dressing change under anesthesia 15852
Dressings debridement 16010-16030
Drug analysis tissue preparation 80103
Drug assay
    amikacin 80150
    amitriptyline 80152
    benzodiazepines 80154
    carbamazepine 80156
    cyclosporine 80158
    desipramine 80160
    digoxin 80162
    dipropylacetic acid (valproic acid) 80164
    doxepin 80166
    ethosuximide 80168
    gentamicin 80170
    gold 80172
    imipramine 80174
    lidocaine 80176
    lithium 80178
    nortriptyline 80182
    phenobarbital 80184
    phenytoin 80185-80186
    primidone 80188
    procainamide 80190-80192
    quantitation drug, not elsewhere specified 80299
    quinidine 80194
    salicylate 80196
    tacrolimus 80197
    theophylline 80198
    tobramycin 80200
    topiramate 80201
    vancomycin 80202
Drug confirmation 80102
Drug implant(s) 11981-11983
Drug screens 80100-80101
DRUG TESTING 80100-80103
DT 90702
DTaP 90700
DTP 90701

Dual energy x-ray absorptiometry (DEXA), bone density study 76075-76076
Duodenal exclusion with gastrojejunostomy 48547
Duodenal intubation and aspiration 89100-89105
Duodenography, hypotonic 74260
Duodenotomy 44010
Duplex scan
    abdominal pelvic, scrotal contents retroperitoneal organs 93975-93976
    aorta inferior vena cava, iliac vasculature, or bypass grafts 93978-93979
    extracranial arteries 93880-93882
    extremity veins 93970-93971
    hemodialysis access 93990
    lower extremity arteries or arterial bypass grafts 93925-93926
    penile vessels 93980-93981
    upper extremity arteries or arterial bypass grafts 93930-93931
Dural graft spinal 63710
Dwyer type procedure (osteotomy calcaneus) 28300
Dynamic cavernosometry 54231

E

Ear, nose and throat examination, documentation *128*
Ear piercing 69090
Ear protector attenuation measurements 92596
Echocardiography
    fetal 76825-76826
    transesophageal 93312-93314
    transthoracic 93307-93350
Echoencephalography 76506
Echography
    abdominal 76700-76705
    breast(s) 76645
    chest 76604
    extremity 76880
    infant, hips 76885-76886
    intraoperative 76986
    pelvic 76856-76857
    placement radiation therapy fields 76950
    pregnant uterus 76805-76816
    retroperitoneal 76770-76775
    scrotum 76870
    soft tissues head and neck 76536
    spinal canal and contents 76800
    transplanted kidney 76778
    transrectal 76872-76873
    transvaginal 76830
Educational supplies 99071

Egger's type procedure (transfer tendon/muscle, hamstrings to femur) 27400
Electrical stimulation to aid bone healing 20974-20975
Electro-oculography 92270
Electrocardiographic monitoring 93224-93237
Electrocochleography 92584
Electroconvulsive therapy 90870-90871
Electrocorticogram at surgery 95829
Electroejaculation 55870
Electroencephalogram (EEG) 95812-95827
    during nonintracranial surgery 95955
Electrolysis epilation 17380
Electromyography motion analysis 96002, 96003
Electromyography needle 95860-95872
Electromyography studies (EMG) anal or urethral sphincter 51784
Electron microscopy 88348-88349
Electronic analysis
    antitachycardia pacemaker system 93724
    dual chamber internal pacemaker system 93733
    dual-chamber pacemaker system 93731-93732
    implantable loop recorder (ILR) system 93727
    implanted neurostimulator pulse generator system 95970-95975
    pacing cardioverter-defibrillator 93741-93744
    programmable implanted pump 62367-62368
    single chamber internal pacemaker system 93736
    single chamber pacemaker system 93734-93735
Electrophoretic technique 82664
Electrophysiologic evaluation
    comprehensive 93619-93622
    pacing cardioverter-defibrillator 93642
    pacing cardioverter-defibrillator leads 93640-93641
    study with pacing and recording 93624
Electroretinography 92275
Elevation depressed skull fracture 62000-62010
Embolectomy
    axillary, brachial, innominate, subclavian artery 34101
    carotid, subclavian or innominate artery 34001
    femoropopliteal, aortoiliac artery 34201
    innominate, subclavian artery 34051
    popliteal-tibio-peroneal artery 34203
    pulmonary artery 33910
    radial or ulnar artery 34111
    renal, celiac, mesentery, aortoiliac artery 34151
Embryo transfer intrauterine 58974
EMERGENCY DEPARTMENT SERVICES 99281-99288
Emergency department visit 99281-99285

End stage renal disease (ESRD)
   full month 90918-90921
   less than full month 90922-90925
Endocervical curettage 57505
ENDOCRINE SYSTEM SURGICAL PROCEDURES 60000-60699
Endolymphatic sac operation 69805-69806
Endometrial sampling 58100
Endomyocardial biopsy 93505
Endoscopic catheterization 74328-74329
Endoscopic evaluation small intestinal pouch 44385-44386
Endoscopic injection implant material submucosal tissues 51715
Endoscopic plantar fasciotomy 29893
Endoscopic retrograde cholangio-pancreatography (ERCP) 43260-43272
Endoscopy biliary 47550-47556
Endoscopy wrist surgical 29848
Endotoxin bacterial (pyrogens) 87174-87176
Enterectomy resection small intestine 44120-44128
Enteroclysis tube, percutaneous placement 74355
Enterocystoplasty 51960
Enteroenterostomy anastomosis intestine 44130
Enterolysis 44005
Enterostomy or cecostomy, tube 44300
Enterotomy small bowel 44020-44021
Enucleation excision external thrombotic hemorrhoid 46320
Enucleation eye 65101-65105
Environmental intervention medical management purposes 90882
Enzyme activity 82657-82658
Epiandrosterone 82666
Epicardial and endocardial pacing and mapping, intra-operative 93631
Epididymectomy 54860-54861
Epididymovasostomy 54900-54901
Epidurography 72275
Epiglottidectomy 31420
Epikeratoplasty 65767
Epiphyseal arrest distal radius and ulna 25455
Epiphyseal arrest distal radius or ulna 25450
Epiphyseal arrest greater trochanter 27185
Episiotomy or vaginal repair 59300
Ergonovine provocation test 93024
Erythropoietin 82668
Escharotomy 16035
Esophageal intubation and collection washings 91000
Esophageal motility 78258
Esophageal motility study 91010-91012
Esophageal recording atrial electrogram 93615-93616

Esophagectomy
    cervical partial 43116
    distal two-thirds, partial 43117-43121
    thoracoabdominal or abdominal approach, partial 43122-43123
    total 43107-43113
    total or partial 43124
Esophagogastric fundoplasty
    Collis 43326
    Nissen, Belsey IV, Hill procedures 43324
    Thal-Nissen procedure 43325
Esophagogastric tamponade 43460
Esophagogastrostomy (cardioplasty) 43320
Esophagojejunostomy abdominal approach 43340-43341
Esophagomyotomy (Heller type) 43330-43331
Esophagoplasty 43300-43305, 43310-43312, 43313-43314
Esophagoscopy
    ablation tumor(s), polyp(s), or other lesion(s) 43228
    balloon dilation 43220
    band ligation esophageal varices 43205
    biopsy 43202
    control bleeding 43227
    diagnostic 43200
    injection sclerosis esophageal varices 43204
    insertion guide wire 43226
    insertion plastic tube or stent 43219
    removal foreign body 43215
    removal tumor(s), polyp(s), or other lesion(s) 43216-43217
Esophagostomy fistulization esophagus 43350-43352
Esophagotomy with removal foreign body 43020-43045
Esophagus acid perfusion (Bernstein) test 91030
Esophagus acid reflux test 91032-91033
ESRD 90918
Estradiol 82670
Estriol 82677
Estrogens 82671-82672
Estrone 82679
Ethchlorvynol 82690
Ethmoidectomy 31205, 31200-31201
Ethylene glycol 82693
Etiocholanolone 82696
Eustachian tube
    catheterization, transtympanic 69405
    inflation, transnasal 69400-69401
Evacuation subungual hematoma 11740

Excision
  abdominal wall tumor 22900
  ampulla vater 48148
  and repair eyelid 67961-67966
  aural glomus tumor 69550-69554
  aural polyp 69540
  Bartholin's gland or cyst 56740
  benign cyst or tumor, mandible 21040-21041
  benign lesion, arms or legs 11400-11406
  benign lesion, face, ears, eyelids, nose, lips, mucous membrane 11440-11446
  benign lesion, neck, hands, feet, genitalia 11420
  benign lesion, scalp, neck, hands, feet, genitalia 11421-11426
  benign tumor, carpal bones 25130
  benign tumor, clavicle or scapula 23140-23145
  benign tumor, cranial bone 61563-61564
  benign tumor, facial bone 21030
  benign tumor, femur 27355
  benign tumor, humerus 24110
  benign tumor, metacarpal 26200
  benign tumor, phalanx finger 26210
  benign tumor, proximal humerus 23150
  benign tumor, radius or olecranon process 24120
  benign tumor, radius or ulna 25120
  bile duct tumor 47711-47712
  bone clavicle 23180
  bone cyst, carpal bones 25130-25136
  bone cyst, clavicle or scapula 23140-23146
  bone cyst, femur 27355-27358
  bone cyst, humerus 24115-24116
  bone cyst, metacarpal 26200-26205
  bone cyst or benign tumor 27065-27067
  bone cyst or benign tumor, humerus 24110
  bone cyst or benign tumor, phalanges foot 28108
  bone cyst or benign tumor, proximal humerus 23155-23156
  bone cyst or benign tumor, talus or calcaneus 28100-28103
  bone cyst or benign tumor, tarsal or metatarsal bones 28104-28107
  bone cyst or benign tumor, tibia or fibula 27635-27638
  bone cyst, phalanx finger 26210-26215
  bone cyst, proximal humerus 23150
  bone cyst, radius or olecranon process 24120-24126
  bone cyst, radius or ulna 25120-25126
  bone, facial bone(s) 21026
  bone, femur, tibia fibula partial 27360
  bone, fibula 27641
  bone, humerus 24140
  bone, mandible 21025

Excision *(continued)*
    foot lesion tendon, tendon sheath, or capsule 28090
    frenum labial or buccal 40819
    fulguration, carcinoma urethra 53220
    fulguration, skene's glands 53270
    fulguration, urethral caruncle 53265
    fulguration, urethral polyp(s) 53260
    fulguration, urethral prolapse 53275
    ganglion wrist 25111-25112
    hemorrhoid tags 46230
    hydrocele 55040-55041
    hydrocele spermatic cord 55500
    hyperplastic alveolar mucosa 41828
    infected graft, abdomen 35907
    infected graft, extremity 35903
    infected graft, neck 35901
    infected graft, thorax 35905
    interdigital neuroma 28080
    intra-abdominal or retroperitoneal tumors 49200-49201
    intracardiac tumor 33120
    intranasal lesion 30117-30118
    ischial bursa 27060
    ischial pressure ulcer 15940-15946
    lacrimal gland 68500-68505
    lacrimal gland tumor 68540-68550
    lacrimal sac 68520
    lactiferous duct fistula 19112
    lesion, conjunctiva 68110-68130
    lesion, cornea 65400
    lesion, epididymis 54830
    lesion, esophagus 43100-43101
    lesion, eyelid 67840
    lesion, floor mouth 41116
    lesion, meniscus or capsule knee 27347
    lesion, mesentery 44820
    lesion, palate, uvula 42104-42107
    lesion, pancreas 48120
    lesion, pharynx 42808
    lesion, sclera 66130
    lesion, small or large bowel 44110-44111
    lesion, spermatic cord 55520
    lesion, tendon sheath or capsule 26160
    lesion, tendon sheath or capsule leg ankle 27630
    lesion, tendon sheath, forearm wrist 25110
    lesion, testis 54512
    lesion, tongue 41110-41114
    lesion, tumor dentoalveolar structures 41825-41827

Excision *(continued)*
    soft tissue tumor, shoulder 23075-23076
    spermatocele 54840
    sublingual gland 42450
    sublingual salivary cyst 42408
    submandibular (submaxillary) gland 42440
    surgical planing skin nose rhinophyma 30120
    synovial cyst, popliteal space (eg, Baker's cyst) 27345
    tendon, finger 26180
    tendon, palm 26170
    thyroglossal duct cyst or sinus 60280-60281
    toe lesion tendon, tendon sheath, or capsule 28092
    tonsil tags 42860
    torus mandibularis 21031
    tracheal stenosis and anastomosis 31780-31781
    tracheal tumor or carcinoma 31785-31786
    trochanteric bursa or calcification 27062
    trochanteric pressure ulcer 15950-15958
    tumor, foot 28043-28045
    tumor, forearm wrist area 25075-25076
    tumor, hand or finger 26115-26116
    tumor, leg or ankle area 27618-27619
    tumor, pelvis and hip area 27047-27048
    tumor, soft tissue back or flank 21930
    tumor, soft tissue neck or thorax 21555-21556
    tumor, thigh or knee area 27327-27328
    tumor, upper arm or elbow area 24075-24076
    turbinate 30130
    ulcer or benign tumor, stomach 43610
    urachal cyst or sinus 51500
    urethral diverticulum 53230-53235
    vaginal cyst or tumor 57135
    vaginal septum 57130
    varicocele or ligation spermatic veins varicocele 55530-55540
    vertebral body, intrinsic bony lesion 22110-22116
Exclusion small bowel from pelvis 44700
Exenteration orbit 65110-65114
Expired gas collection 94250
Exploration
    carotid artery 35701
    congenital atresia bile ducts 47700
    epididymis 54820
    femoral artery 35721
    forearm or wrist, with removal foreign body 25248
    middle ear 69440
    orbit with biopsy 61332
    orbit with removal foreign body 61334

F

Fasciotomy *(continued)*
   palmar 26040-26045
   thigh, knee decompression 27496-27499
Fat differential, feces 82715
Fat or lipids, feces 82705-82710
Fat stain, feces, urine, or sputum 89125
Fatty acids 82725
Fc receptor 86243
FEMALE GENITAL SYSTEM SURGICAL PROCEDURES 56405-58999
Fenestration semicircular canal 69820
Ferritin 82728
Fetal biophysical profile 76818
Fetal contraction stress test 59020
Fetal fibronectin 82731
Fetal monitoring 59050-59051
Fetal non-stress test 59025
Fetal scalp blood sampling 59030
Fibrin degradation products, d-dimer 85378-85379
Fibrin(ogen) degradation products (fdp)(fsp) 85362-85370
Fibrinogen 85384-85385
Fibrinolysins or coagulopathy screen 85390
Fibrinolytic factors and inhibitors 85400-85421
Filleted finger or toe flap 14350
Filtered speech test 92571
Fimbrioplasty 58760
Fine needle aspiration 10021-10022
Fine needle aspiration orbital contents 67415
Fissurectomy 46200
Fistulization
   sclera glaucoma 66150-66172
   sublingual salivary cyst 42325-42326
Fitting contact lens 92070
Fitting insertion pessary 57160
Fitting low vision aid 92354-92355
Fitting spectacle prosthesis 92352-92353
Fitting spectacles 92340-92342
Fixation contralateral testis 54620
Fixation spinal internal by wiring 22841
Fixation tongue mechanical 41500
Flap island pedicle 15740
Flap neurovascular pedicle 15750
Flexor origin slide forearm wrist 25315-25316
Flexor-plasty elbow 24330-24331
Flow cytometry 88180-88182
Fluorescein angiography 92235
Fluorescein angioscopy 92230
Fluorescent noninfectious agent antibody 86255-86256

Fracture *(continued)*
    carpometacarpal thumb, closed treatment 26645
    carpometacarpal thumb, open treatment 26665
    carpometacarpal thumb, percutaneous skeletal fixation 26650
    clavicular, closed treatment 23500-23505
    clavicular, open treatment 23515
    coccygeal, closed treatment 27200
    coccygeal, open treatment 27202
    complicated frontal sinus, open treatment 21344
    complicated mandible, open treatment 21470
    depressed frontal sinus, open treatment 21343
    depressed malar, open treatment 21360
    depressed zygomatic arch, open treatment 21356
    distal fibular, closed treatment 27786-27788
    distal fibular, open treatment 27792
    distal phalangeal finger or thumb, closed treatment 26750-26755
    distal phalangeal finger or thumb, percutaneous skeletal fixation 26756
    distal radial, closed treatment 25600
    distal radius, closed treatment 25605
    distal radius, open treatment 25620
    distal radius, percutaneous skeletal fixation 25611
    femoral shaft, closed treatment 27500-27508
    femoral shaft, open treatment 27506-27507
    femur, closed treatment 27238-27510
    femur distal end, medial or lateral condyle, open treatment 27514
    femur epiphyseal separation, closed treatment 27516-27517
    femur epiphyseal separation, open treatment 27519
    femur neck, closed treatment 27230-27232
    femur, open treatment 27236-27513
    femur, percutaneous skeletal fixation 27235-27509
    great toe phalanx or phalanges, closed treatment 28490-28495
    great toe phalanx or phalanges, open treatment 28505
    great toe phalanx or phalanges, percutaneous skeletal fixation 28496
    greater humerus tuberosity, closed treatment 23620-23625
    greater humerus tuberosity, open treatment 23630
    greater trochanteric, closed treatment 27246
    greater trochanteric, open treatment 27248
    humerus, closed treatment 23600
    humerus condylar, closed treatment 24576-24577
    humerus condylar, open treatment 24579
    humerus condylar, percutaneous skeletal fixation 24582
    humerus epicondylar, closed treatment 24560-24565
    humerus epicondylar, open treatment 24575
    humerus epicondylar, percutaneous skeletal fixation 24566
    humerus, percutaneous skeletal fixation 24538
    humerus shaft, closed treatment 24500-24505
    humerus shaft, open treatment 24515-24516

Fracture *(continued)*
   pelvic ring, closed treatment 27193-27194
   pelvic ring, percutaneous skeletal fixation 27216
   periarticular elbow, open treatment 24586-24587
   phalangeal finger or thumb, open treatment 26765
   phalangeal shaft, closed treatment 26720-26725
   phalangeal shaft, open treatment 26735
   phalangeal shaft, percutaneous skeletal 26727
   phalanx or phalanges, other than great toe, closed treatment 28510-28515
   phalanx or phalanges, other than great toe, open treatment 28525
   proximal fibula or shaft, closed treatment 27780-27781
   proximal fibula or shaft, open treatment 27784
   proximal humerus, closed treatment 23605
   proximal humerus, open treatment 23615-23616
   radial and ulnar shaft, closed treatment 25560-25565
   radial and ulnar shaft, open treatment 25574-25575
   radial head or neck, closed treatment 24650-24655
   radial head or neck, open treatment 24665-24666
   radial shaft, closed treatment 25500-25520
   radial shaft, open treatment 25515-25526
   rib, closed treatment 21800
   rib, open treatment 21805
   scapular, closed treatment 23570-23575
   scapular, open treatment 23585
   sesamoid, closed treatment 28530
   sesamoid, open treatment 28531
   skull, closed treatment 21300
   sternum, closed treatment 21820
   sternum, open treatment 21825
   talus, closed treatment 28430-28435
   talus, open treatment 28445
   talus, percutaneous skeletal fixation 28436
   tarsal bone, open treatment 28465
   tarsal bone, percutaneous skeletal fixation 28456
   tarsal bone treatment 28450-28455
   tibia, closed treatment 27824-27825
   tibia, open treatment 27826-27828
   tibia proximal, closed treatment 27530-27532
   tibia proximal, open treatment 27535-27536
   tibial shaft, closed treatment 27750-27752
   tibial shaft, open treatment 27758-27759
   tibial shaft, percutaneous skeletal fixation 27756
   treatment rib requiring external fixation 21810
   trimalleolar ankle, closed treatment 27816-27818
   trimalleolar ankle, open treatment 27822-27823
   ulna, closed treatment 24670-24675
   ulna, open treatment 24685

Fracture *(continued)*
    ulnar shaft, closed treatment 25530-25535
    ulnar shaft, open treatment 25545
    ulnar styloid, closed treatment 25650
    vertebra, open treatment 22325-22327
    vertebral body, closed treatment 22310
    vertebral, closed treatment 22315
    vertebral process, closed treatment 22305
Fredet-Ramstedt type operation (pyloromyotomy) 43520
Free fascial flap 15758
Free jejunum transfer with microvascular anastomosis 43496
Free muscle flap 15756
Free omental flap with microvascular anastomosis 49906
Free osteocutaneous flap with microvascular anastomosis
    great toe 20973
    iliac crest 20970
    metatarsal 20972
Free skin flap 15757
Frenoplasty 41520
Fresh frozen plasma 86927
Frost suture (temporary closure eyelids by suture) 67875
Frozen blood preparation 86930-86932
Fructose 82757
Fsh 83001
Functional cortical and subcortical mapping 95961-95962
Functional residual capacity 94240
Fundus photography 92250
Fusion thumb with autogenous graft 26820

G

Galactokinase, RBC 82759
Galactose 82760
Galactose-1-phosphate uridyl transferase 82775-82776
Gamete, zygote, or embryo intrafallopian transfer 58976
Gammaglobulin iga, igd, igg, igm 82784
Gammaglobulin ige 82785
Gammaglobulin immunoglobulin subclasses, (igg1, 2, 3, and 4) 82787
Gases, blood, any combination ph, pco2, po2, co 82803
Gases, blood, ph only 82800
Gastrectomy 43638-43639
Gastrectomy 43620-43622, 43631-43634
Gastric acid 82926-82928
Gastric analysis test 91052
Gastric emptying study 78264

Gastric intubation aspiration
  diagnostic 89130-89132
  fractional collections 89135-89141
  lavage treatment 91105
Gastric intubation washings, and preparing slides cytology 91055
Gastric motility studies 91020
Gastric mucosa imaging 78261
Gastric restrictive procedure 43847
  with gastric bypass 43846
  without gastric bypass 43842-43843
Gastric saline load test 91060
Gastrin 82941
Gastrin after secretin stimulation 82938
Gastrocnemius recession (eg, Strayer procedure) 27687
Gastroduodenostomy 43810
GASTROENTEROLOGY MEDICAL PROCEDURES 91000-91298
Gastroesophageal reflux study 78262
Gastrointestinal endoscopic ultrasound 76975
Gastrointestinal protein loss 78282
Gastrointestinal reconstruction previous esophagectomy 43360-43361
Gastrojejunostomy 43820-43825
Gastrorrhaphy 43840
Gastrostomy 43830-43832
Gastrostomy tube change 43760
Gastrostomy tube, percutaneous placement 43750
Gastrotomy 43500-43510
Gastrotomy tube, percutaneous placement 74350
General multi-system examination, documentation *120*
Generation automated data 78890-78891
Genioplasty 21120-21123
Genitourinary system examination, documentation *133*
Gingivectomy 41820
Gingivoplasty 41872
Glossectomy 41120-41155
Glucagon 82943
Glucagon tolerance panel 80424
Glucagon tolerance test 82946
Glucose 82947-82953
Glucose, blood by glucose monitoring device(s) 82962
Glucose monitoring 95250
Glucose-6-phosphate dehydrogenase (G6PD) 82955-82960
Glucosidase, beta 82963
Glutamate dehydrogenase 82965
Glutamine (glutamic acid amide) 82975
Glutamyltransferase, gamma (GGT) 82977
Glutathione 82978
Glutathione reductase, rbc 82979

Glutethimide 82980
Glycated protein 82985
Goldwaite type procedure (reconstruction dislocating patella) 27422
Gonadotropin follicle stimulating hormone (FSH) 83001
Gonadotropin luteinizing hormone (LH) 83002
Gonadotropin releasing hormone stimulation panel 80426
Gonadotropin, chorionic (HCG) 84702-84703
Gonioscopy 92020
Goniotomy 65820
Graft
    bone mandible 21215
    bone nasal maxillary or malar areas 21210
    composite 15760
    derma-fat-fascia 15770
    ear cartilage 21235
    facial nerve paralysis, free fascia graft   15840
    facial nerve paralysis, free muscle graft 15841-15842
    facial nerve paralysis, regional muscle transfer 15845
    forehead, cheeks, chin, mouth, neck, axillae, genitalia, hands, Feet 15240-
        15241
    nose, ears, eyelids, lips 15260-15261
    rectal incontinence prolapse 46753
    rib cartilage 21230
    scalp, arms, legs 15220-15221
    trunk 15200-15201
Gross type operation (repair omphalocele) 49610
Group psychotherapy 90853
Growth hormone human (HGH) (somatotropin) 83003
Growth hormone human (HGH), antibody 86277
Growth hormone stimulation panel 80428
Growth hormone suppression panel 80430
Guanosine monophosphate (GMP), cyclic 83008

H

H-reflex, amplitude and latency study 95934-95936
Hallux rigidus correction first metatarsophalangeal joint 28289
Handling conveyance specimen 99000-99001
Haptoglobin 83010-83012
Harrington rod technique (posterior non-segmental instrumentation) 22840
Harvest upper extremity vein 35500
Hauser type procedure (reconstruction dislocating patella) 27420
HEALTH AND BEHAVIOR ASSESSMENT/INTERVENTION 96150-96155
Hearing aid
    check 92592-92593
    examination and selection 92590-92591

Heart catheterization, combined
   right and left heart 93529
   right and retrograde left heart 93526-93531
   right and transseptal left heart 93527-93533
   right with left ventricular puncture 93528
   transseptal and retrograde left heart 93524
Heart transplant 33945
Heart-lung transplant 33935
Heavy metal 83015-83018
Heinz bodies 85441-85445
Helicobacter pylori, breath test analysis 83013-83014
Heller type procedure (esophagomyotomy) 43330
Hemagglutination inhibition test (HAI) 86280
Hematologic, lymphatic and/or immunologic system(s) examination,
  documentation *137*
HEMATOLOGY AND COAGULATION 85002-85999
Hemiarthroplasty hip 27125
HEMIC AND LYMPHATIC SYSTEMS SURGICAL PROCEDURES
  38100-38999
Hemiepiphyseal arrest 24470
Hemiphalangectomy or interphalangeal joint excision, toe 28160
Hemodialysis procedure 90935-90937
Hemoglobin 83026-83069
Hemoglobin fractionation and quantitation 83020-83021
Hemoglobin or RBCs, fetal 85460-85461
Hemolysin, acid 85475
Hemolysins and agglutinins 86940-86941
Hemoperfusion 90997
Hemophilus influenza B vaccine (HIB) 90645-90648
Hemorrhage management liver 47350-47362
Hemorrhoidectomy 46221-46262
Hemosiderin 83070-83071
Heparin assay 85520
Heparin neutralization 85525
Heparin-protamine tolerance test 85530
Hepatectomy 47120-47130
Hepatic venography 75889-75891
Hepaticotomy or hepaticostomy 47400
Hepatitis A and hepatitis B vaccine (hepA-hepB) 90636
Hepatitis A antibody (haab) 86708-86709
Hepatitis A vaccine 90632-90634
Hepatitis B and hemophilus influenza B vaccine (hepb-hib) 90748
Hepatitis B core antibody (hbcab) 86704-86705
Hepatitis B immune globulin (hbig) 90371
Hepatitis B surface antibody (hbsab) 86706
Hepatitis B vaccine 90744-90747
Hepatitis Be antibody (hbeab) 86707

Hepatitis C antibody 86803-86804
Hepatobiliary ductal system imaging 78223
Hepatotomy 47010-47011
Heterophile antibodies 86308-86310
Heyman type procedure (capsulotomy, midtarsal) 28264
Hib (hemophilus influenza B vaccine) 90645
Histamine 83088
History and examination normal newborn infant 99431-99435
HLA typing A, B, or C 86812-86813
HLA typing dr/dq 86816-86817
HLA typing lymphocyte culture 86821-86822
HOME HEALTH PROCEDURES 99500-99539
HOME INFUSION PROCEDURES 99551-99569
HOME MEDICAL E/M SERVICES 99341-99350
Home visit
    established patient 99347-99350
    new patient 99341-99345
Homovanillic acid (HVA) 83150
Hospital care
    initial 99221-99223
    subsequent 99231-99233
Hospital discharge day management 99238-99239
HOSPITAL SERVICES 99217-99239
Hydroxycorticosteroids 83491
Hydroxyindolacetic acid 83497
Hydroxyprogesterone 83498-83499
Hydroxyproline 83500-83505
Hymenectomy partial 56700
Hymenotomy 56720
Hyperbaric oxygen therapy 99183
Hyperthermia 77610-77620
Hypnotherapy 90880
Hypophysectomy or excision pituitary tumor 61548
Hypothermia 99185-99186
Hysteroplasty 58540
Hysterorrhaphy 58520
Hysterorrhaphy, ruptured uterus 59350
Hysterosalpingography 74740
Hysteroscopy 58555-58563
Hysterosonography 76831
Hysterotomy, abdominal 59100

I

Ileoscopy through stoma 44380-44382
Ileostomy or jejunostomy, non-tube 44310

Imaging lymphatics and lymph glands 78195
Imbrication diaphragm 39545
Immune complex assay 86332
IMMUNE GLOBULINS 90281-90399
Immune globulin (ig) 90281
Immune globulin (igiv) 90283
IMMUNIZATION ADMINISTRATION VACCINES/TOXOIDS 90471-90474
Immunoassay 83516-83520
Immunoassay
    infectious agent antibody 86317-86318
    tumor antigen 86316
Immunocytochemistry 88342
Immunodiffusion 86329-86331
Immunoelectrophoresis 86320-86327
Immunofixation electrophoresis 86334
Immunofluorescent study 88346-88347
IMMUNOLOGY 86000-86849
Implant, non-biodegradeable drug
    insertion 11981
    removal 11982
    removal and reinsertion 11983
Implant removal
    elbow joint 24160
    radial head 24164
Implantation
    cardiac event recorder 33282
    device intrathecal or epidural drug infusion 62360-62362
    electromagnetic bone conduction hearing device 69710
    intrathecal or epidural catheter 62350-62351
    intravitreal drug delivery system 67027
    mesh or other prosthesis 49568
    nerve end into bone or muscle 64787
    neurostimulator electrode array, percutaneous 63650
    neurostimulator electrodes, autonomic nerve 64560
    neurostimulator electrodes, cranial nerve 64553
    neurostimulator electrodes, neuromuscular 64565
    neurostimulator electrodes, peripheral nerve 64555
    ventricular assist device 33975-33976, 33979
Impression
    auricular prosthesis 21086
    definitive obturator prosthesis 21080
    facial prosthesis 21088
    interim obturator prosthesis 21079
    mandibular resection prosthesis 21081
    nasal prosthesis 21087
    oral surgical splint 21085
    orbital prosthesis 21077

Impression *(continued)*
    palatal augmentation prosthesis 21082
    palatal lift prosthesis 21083
    speech aid prosthesis 21084
    surgical obturator prosthesis 21076
In-situ vein bypass 35582-35587
Incision abscess soft tissue 20000-20005
Incision anal septum 46070
Incision and drainage
    abscess 10060-10061
    abscess, appendiceal 44900-44901
    abscess, intramural, intramuscular, or submucosal 46045
    abscess, ischiorectal or intramural 46060
    abscess, ischiorectal perirectal 46040
    abscess, neck or thorax 21501-21502
    abscess, rectum 45005
    abscess, retropharyngeal or parapharyngeal 42720-42725
    abscess, supralevator, pelvirectal, or retrorectal 45020
    abscess, thigh or knee region 27301
    abscess, vulva or perineum 56405
    Bartholin's gland abscess 56420
    bursa, foot 28001
    epididymis, testis scrotal space 54700
    abscess floor mouth 41015-41018
    foot 28002-28003
    forearm wrist 25028-25031
    hematoma 10140
    leg or ankle 27603-27604
    pelvis or hip joint area 26990-26991
    penis 54015
    perianal abscess 46050
    peritonsillar abscess 42700
    pilonidal cyst 10080-10081
    postoperative wound infection 10180
    shoulder area 23030-23031
    thyroglossal cyst 60000
    abscess tongue/floor mouth 41000-41009
    upper arm or elbow area 23930-23931
Incision and placement
    cranial neurostimulator pulse generator 61885-61886
    peripheral neurostimulator pulse generator 64590
    spinal neurostimulator pulse generator 63685
Incision and reconstruction atria operative 33253
Incision and removal foreign body, subcutaneous tissues 10120-10121
Incision
    bone cortex, femur or knee 27303
    bone cortex, foot 28005

Incision *(continued)*
    bone cortex, forearm OR wrist 25035
    bone cortex, hand or finger 26034
    bone cortex, humerus or elbow 23935
    bone cortex, pelvis hip joint 26992
    bone cortex, shoulder area 23035
    bone cortex, thorax 21510
    conjunctiva, drainage cyst 68020
    drainage, lacrimal gland 68400
    drainage, lacrimal sac 68420
    extensor tendon sheath, wrist 25000
    implantation neurostimulator electrodes, autonomic nerve 64577
    implantation neurostimulator electrodes, cranial nerve 64573
    implantation neurostimulator electrodes, neuromuscular 64580
    implantation neurostimulator electrodes, peripheral nerve 64575
    labial frenum 40806
    leg or ankle 27607
    lingual frenum 41010
    thrombosed hemorrhoid 46083
Indicator dilution studies 93561-93562
Indocyanine-green angiography 92240
Induced abortion 59840-59857
Induction arrhythmia by electrical pacing 93618
Infectious agent antigen detection
    enzyme immunoassay technique 87301-87430
    immunofluorescent technique 87260-87299
Infectious agent detection
    immunoassay direct optical observation 87810-87899
    nucleic acid (DNA or RNA) 87470-87652
Influenza virus vaccine 90657-90660
Infratemporal post-auricular approach to middle cranial fossa 61591
Infratemporal pre-auricular approach to middle cranial fossa 61590
Infusion or instillation radioelement solution 77750
Ingestion challenge test 95075
Inhalation bronchial challenge testing 95070-95071
Injection air or contrast into peritoneal cavity 49400
Injection
    anterior chamber 66020-66030
    contrast medium dacryocystography 68850
    corpora cavernosa 54235
    epidural blood or clot patch 62273
    including catheter placement 62318-62319
    infusion neurolytic substance 62280-62282
    intralesional 11900-11901
    sinus tract 20500-20501
    tendon sheath ligament, trigger points or ganglion cyst 20550
    therapeutic agent into tenon's capsule 67515

Injection *(continued)*
    therapeutic prophylactic or diagnostic 90782-90784
    turbinate(s) 30200
    vitreous substitute 67025
Injection anesthetic agent
    axillary nerve 64417
    brachial plexus 64415
    carotid sinus 64508
    celiac plexus 64530
    cervical plexus 64413
    facial nerve 64402
    greater occipital nerve 64405
    ilioinguinal, iliohypogastric nerves 64425
    intercostal nerve, single 64420
    intercostal nerves, multiple, regional block 64421
    lumbar or thoracic 64520
    paracervical (uterine) nerve 64435
    paravertebral facet joint nerve 64470-64476
    peripheral nerve or branch 64450
    phrenic nerve 64410
    pudendal nerve 64430
    sciatic nerve 64445
    sphenopalatine ganglion 64505
    spinal accessory nerve 64412
    stellate ganglion 64510
    suprascapular nerve 64418
    transforaminal epidural 64479-64484
    trigeminal nerve, any division or branch 64400
    vagus nerve 64408
Injection procedure
    ankle arthrography 27648
    cardiac catheterization 93539-93545
    chemonucleolysis 62292
    cholangiography 47505
    cholangiography, percutaneous transhepatic 47500
    contrast venography 36005
    corpora cavernosography 54230
    cystography or voiding urethrocystography 51600
    diskography 62290-62291
    elbow arthrography 24220
    evaluation previously placed peritoneal-venous shunt 49427
    hip arthrography 27093-27095
    identification sentinel node 38792
    intraoperative pancreatography 48400
    knee arthrography 27370
    lymphangiography 38790
    mammary ductogram or galactogram 19030

Injection procedure *(continued)*
    myelography computerized axial tomography, spinal 62284
    occlusion arteriovenous malformation, spinal 62294
    peyronie disease 54200-54205
    placement chain contrast chain urethrocystography 51605
    pyelography 50394
    retrograde urethrocystography 51610
    sacroiliac joint 27096
    shoulder arthrography 23350
    sialography 42550
    splenoportography 38200
    temporomandibular joint arthrography 21116
    ureterography 50684
    ureteropyelography 50684
    visualization ileal conduit ureteropyelography 50690
    wrist arthrography 25246
Injection sclerosing solution 36470-36471
    hemorrhoids 46500
    spider veins face 36469
    spider veins limb or trunk 36468
Insertion
    arterial and venous cannula 36823
    breast prosthesis 19340-19342
    cannula hemodialysis 36800-36815
    cannula prolonged extracorporeal circulation 36822
    cardioverter-defibrillator electrodes 33245-33246
    cardioverter-defibrillator pulse generator 33240
    cervical dilator 59200
    electrode lead(s) 33249
    flow directed catheter (eg, Swan-Ganz) 93503
    graft aorta or great vessels 33330-33335
    implantable contraceptive capsules 11975
    infusion pump, intra-arterial 36260
    infusion pump, intravenous 36530
    intra-aortic balloon assist device 33970-33973
    intra-aortic balloon catheter, percutaneous 33967
    intraocular lens prosthesis 66985
    intraperitoneal cannula or catheter 49420-49421
    intrauterine device (IUD) 58300
    nasal septal prosthesis 30220
    ocular implant 65130-65140
    pacemaker pulse generator only 33212-33213
    pacemaker, fluoroscopy and radiography 71090
    penile prosthesis 54400-54417
    peritoneal-venous shunt 49425
    permanent pacemaker 33206-33201
    pin-retained palatal prosthesis 42281

Intraventricular intra-atrial mapping tachycardia site(s) 93609
Intraventricular pacing 93612
Intravitreal injection pharmacologic agent 67028
Intrinsic factor 83528
Intrinsic factor antibodies 86340
Introduction
    catheter, superior or inferior vena cava 36010
    guide, renal pelvis ureter 50395
    hemostatic agent or pack, vaginal hemorrhage 57180
    intracatheter or catheter, renal pelvis 50392-74475
    long gastrointestinal tube (eg, Miller-Abbott) 44500-74340
    needle, aortic translumbar 36160
    needle, arteriovenous shunt 36145
    needle, brachial artery 36120
    needle, carotid or vertebral artery 36100
    needle, extremity artery 36140
    needle, vein 36000
    transhepatic catheter, percutaneous 47510
    transhepatic stent, percutaneous 47511
    ureteral catheter 50393-74480
Intubation endotracheal, emergency procedure 31500
Ipecac administration 99175
IPPB treatment 94650
Iridectomy 66600-66635
Iridoplasty by photocoagulation 66762
Iridotomy
    laser surgery 66761
    stab incision 66500-66505
Iron 83540
Iron binding capacity 83550
Iron stain (RBC or bone marrow smears) 85536
Irradiation blood product 86945
Irrigation corpora cavernosa priapism 54220
Irrigation vagina 57150
Ischemic limb exercise 95875
Islet cell antibody 86341
Isocitric dehydrogenase (IDH) 83570
IV infusion therapy/diagnosis 90780-90781

J

Japanese encephalitis virus vaccine 90735
Jatene type operation (repair transposition the great arteries) 33778
Joint survey, single view 76066
Jones type procedure (arthrodesis, great toe, interphalangeal joint) 28760
Joplin type procedure (correction hallux valgus) 28294

K

L

LABORATORY SERVICES CODES 80000-89999
  Anatomic pathology 88000-88099
  Chemistry 82000-84999
  Consultations clinical pathology 80500-80502
  Cytogenetic studies 88230-88299
  Cytopathology 88104-88199
  Drug testing 80100-80103
  Evocative/suppression testing 80400-80440
  Hematology and coagulation 85002-85999
  Immunology 86000-86849
  Microbiology 87001-87999
  Organ or disease oriented panels 80048-80090
  Other pathology and laboratory procedures 89050-89399
  Surgical pathology 88300-88399
  Therapeutic drug assays 80150-80299
  Transfusion medicine 86850-86999
  Urinalysis 81000-81099
Labyrinthectomy 69905-69910
Labyrinthotomy 69801-69802
Lactate (lactic acid) 83605
Lactate dehydrogenase (ld), (ldh) 83615-83625
Lactogen 83632
Lactose 83633-83634
Laminectomy
  biopsy/excision, intraspinal neoplasm 63275-63290
  cordotomy 63194-63199
  drainage, intramedullary cyst/syrinx 63172-63173
  excision intraspinal lesion, intradural 63270-63273
  excision intraspinal lesion neoplasm 63265-63268
  excision arteriovenous malformation spinal cord 63250-63252
  exploration decompression spinal cord 63001-63016
  facetectomy and foraminotomy 63045-63048
  implantation neurostimulator electrodes 63655
  myelotomy 63170
  release tethered spinal cord 63200
  removal abnormal facets pars inter-articularis 63012
  rhizotomy 63185-63190
  section dentate ligaments 63180-63182
  section spinal accessory nerve 63191
Laminotomy decompression nerve root(s) 63020-63042
Laparoscopic treatment ectopic pregnancy 59150-59151
Laparoscopically assisted nephroureterectomy 50548
Laparoscopy
  abdomen, peritoneum, and omentum 49320-49323
  ablation renal cysts 50541
  adrenalectomy 60650
  appendectomy 44970

Laparoscopy *(continued)*
    cholecystectomy 47562
    cholecystectomy with cholangiography 47563
    cholecystectomy with exploration common duct 47564
    cholecystoenterostomy 47570
    donor nephrectomy 50547
    enterolysis 44200
    esophagogastric fundoplasty (eg, Nissen, Toupet procedures) 43280
    fimbrioplasty 58672
    fulguration oviducts 58670
    gastrostomy 43653
    intestinal resection 44202
    jejunostomy 44201
    ligation spermatic veins varicocele 55550
    liver 47370-47379
    lymphatic system 38570-38572
    lysis adhesions 58660
    nephrectomy 50546
    occlusion oviducts by device 58671
    orchiectomy 54690
    orchiopexy 54692
    pyeloplasty 50544
    removal adnexal structures 58661
    removal leiomyomata 58551
    repair inguinal hernia 49491-49507, 49650-49651
    salpingostomy 58673
    sling operation 51992
    splenectomy 38120
    transection vagus nerves 43651-43652
    transhepatic cholangiography 47560-47561
    ureterolithotomy 50945
    urethral suspension 51990
    vaginal hysterectomy 58550
Laparotomy 58960
    hepatic parasitic cyst(s) or abscess(es) 47015
Lapidus type procedure (correction hallux valgus) 28297
Laryngeal function studies 92520
Laryngeal reinnervation 31590
Laryngectomy
    partial 31370-31382
    subtotal 31367-31368
    total 31360-31365
Laryngography contrast 70373
Laryngoplasty 31580-31584
    cricoid split 31587
    not otherwise specified 31588

Laryngoscopy
  direct 31515-31571
  flexible fiberoptic 31575-31578
  flexible or rigid fiberoptic 31579
  indirect 31505-31513
Laryngotomy 31300-31320
Lateral canthopexy 21282
Lateral retinacular release 27425
Lavage by cannulation
  maxillary sinus 31000
  sphenoid sinus 31002
Lavage peritoneal 49080
Layer closure wounds
  face, ears, eyelids, nose, lips mucous membranes 12051-12057
  neck, hands, feet external genitalia 12041-12047
  scalp, axillae, trunk extremities 12031-12037
LDH 83615
Lead 83655
Lecithin-sphingomyelin ratio (l/s ratio) 83661-83662
Left heart catheterization 93510-93514
Left ventricular recording 93622
Lengthening
  hamstring tendon 27393-27395
  palate and pharyngeal flap 42226
  palate with island flap 42227
  shortening flexor or extensor tendon, forearm wrist 25280
  shortening tendon, leg or ankle 27685-27686
  tendon extensor, hand or finger 26476
  tendon flexor, hand or finger 26478
Leucine aminopeptidase (lap) 83670
Leukocyte alkaline phosphatase with count 85540
Leukocyte histamine release test (lhr) 86343
Leukocyte phagocytosis 86344
Leukocyte transfusion 86950
Ligation
  arteries, ethmoidal 30915
  arteries, internal maxillary artery 30920
  banding angioaccess arteriovenous fistula 37607
  biopsy, temporal artery 37609
  common iliac vein 37660
  division and stripping, saphenous veins 37720-37735
  division, long saphenous vein 37700
  division, short saphenous vein 37780
  esophageal varices 43400
  external carotid artery 37600
  femoral vein 37650
  internal hemorrhoids 46945-46946

Ligation *(continued)*
    internal jugular vein 37565
    internal or common carotid artery 37605-37606
    major artery, abdomen 37617
    major artery, chest 37616
    major artery, extremity 37618
    major artery, neck 37615
    perforators, subfascial, radical (Linton type) 37760
    peritoneal-venous shunt 49428
    recurrent or secondary varicose veins 37785
    salivary duct, intraoral 42665
    stapling at gastroesophageal junction 43405
    takedown systemic-to-pulmonary artery shunt 33924
    transection fallopian tube(s) 58600-58611, 58670
    vas deferens 55450
Linton type procedure (ligation perforators) 37760
Lipase 83690
Lipectomy
    head and neck, suction assisted 15876
    lower extremity, suction assisted 15879
    trunk, suction assisted 15877
    upper extremity, suction assisted 15878
Lipoprotein 83715-83721
Lithotripsy extracorporeal shock wave 50590
Liver
    allotransplantation 47135-47136
    function study 78220
    imaging 78201-78202
    imaging (SPECT) 78205-78206
    laparoscopy 47370-47379
    -spleen imaging 78215-78216
    tumor ablation 47380-47382
Lombard test 92573
Loudness balance test 92562
Low intensity ultrasound stimulation 20979
Lung lavage total 32997
Lung transplant 32851-32854
Luteinizing releasing factor (lrh) 83727
Lyme disease vaccine 90665
Lymphadenectomy
    abdominal 38747
    axillary 38740-38745
    cervical 38720-38724
    inguinofemoral 38760-38765
    limited staging 38562-38564
    pelvic 38770
    retroperitoneal transabdominal 38780

Lymphadenectomy *(continued)*
    suprahyoid 38700
    thoracic 38746
Lymphangiography
    extremity 75801-75803
    pelvic/abdominal 75805-75807
Lymphangiotomy lymphatic channels 38308
Lymphocyte transformation 86353
Lymphocytotoxicity assay 86805-86806
Lysis adhesions 58740
Lysis epidural adhesions using solution injection 62263
Lysis intranasal synechia 30560
Lysis labial adhesions 56441

M

Magnesium 83735
Magnetic resonance angiography
    abdomen 74185
    chest 71555
    lower extremity 73725
    pelvis 72198
    spinal canal 72159
    upper extremity 73225
Magnetic resonance imaging (MRI)
    abdomen 74181
    bone marrow blood supply 76400
    brain 70551-70553
    breast 76093-76094
    chest 71550
    lower extremity 73720-73721
    orbit, face, and neck 70540
    pelvis 72196
    spinal canal 72141-72158
    temporomandibular joint 70336
    upper extremity 73220-73221
Magnetic resonance spectroscopy 76390
Magnetoencephalography (MEG) 95965-95967
Magnuson type operation (capsulorrhaphy, anterior) 23450
Major reconstruction chest wall 32820
Malar augmentation, prosthetic material 21270
Malate dehydrogenase 83775
MALE GENITAL SYSTEM SURGICAL PROCEDURES 54000-55899
Mammaplasty augmentation 19324-19325
Mammary ductogram or galactogram 76086-76088
Mammography 76090-76091

Manganese 83785
Manipulation
    ankle, general anesthesia 27860
    chest wall 94667-94668
    elbow 24300
    finger 26340
    hip joint, general anesthesia 27275
    knee joint, general anesthesia 27570
    shoulder joint, anesthesia 23700
    spine, anesthesia 22505
    wrist 25259
Manometric studies 50686
Manometric studies through nephrostomy or pyelostomy tube 50396
Manual therapy techniques 97140
Maquet type procedure (anterior tibial tubercleplasty) 27418
Marshall-Marchetti-Krantz procedure (anterior vesicourethropexy) 51840
Marsupialization
    Bartholin's gland cyst 56440
    cyst or abscess liver 47300
    cyst pancreas 48500
    sublingual salivary cyst 42409
    urethral diverticulum 53240
Mass spectrometry and tandem mass spectrometry (ms, ms/ms) 83788-83789
Mastectomy
    gynecomastia 19140
    modified radical 19240
    partial 19160-19162
    radical 19200-19220
    simple 19180
    subcutaneous 19182
Mastoid obliteration 69670
Mastoidectomy 69502-69511
Mastopexy 19316
Mastotomy 19020
MATERNITY CARE AND DELIVERY PROCEDURES 59000-59899
Maxillary impression palatal prosthesis 42280
Maxillectomy 31225-31230
Maximum breathing capacity 94200
Measles and rubella virus vaccine 90708
Measles mumps and rubella virus vaccine (MMR) 90707
Measles mumps, rubella, and varicella vaccine (MMRV) 90710
Measles virus vaccine 90705
Meat fibers, feces 89160
Meatotomy 53020-53025
Mechanical fragility, RBC 85547
Medial canthopexy 21280
Mediastinoscopy 39400

Mediastinotomy 39000-39010
MEDIASTINUM AND DIAPHRAGM SURGICAL PROCEDURES 39000-39599
Medical conference by physician 99361-99362
MEDICAL NUTRITION THERAPY 97802-97804
Medical testimony 99075
MEDICINE SERVICES *763-846*
   Modifiers *764*
   Overview *763*
   Subsections *763*
MEDICINE SERVICES CODES 90000-99199
   Allergy and clinical immunology 95004-95199
   Biofeedback 90901-90911
   Cardiovascular 92050-93799
   Central nervous system assessments/tests 96100-96177
   Chemotherapy administration 96400-96549
   Chiropractic manipulative treatment 98940-98943
   Dermatological procedures 96900-96999
   Dialysis 90918-90999
   Gastroenterology 91000-91298
   Immune globulins 90281-90399
   Immunization administration for vaccines/toxoids 90471-90474
   Medical nutrition therapy 97802-97804
   Neurology and neuromuscular medical procedures 95805-95999
   Non-invasive vascular diagnostic studies 93875-93990
   Ophthalmology 92002-92499
   Osteopathic manipulative treatment (omt) 98925-98929
   Other services and procedures 99170-99199
   Otorhinolaryngologic services 92502-92599
   Photodynamic therapy 96567-96571
   Physical medicine and rehabilitation 97000-97799
   Psychiatry 90801-90899
   Pulmonary 94010-94799
   Qualifying circumstances for anesthesia 99100-99140
   Sedation with or without analgesia 99141-99142
   Special services, procedures and reports 99000-99090
   Therapeutic or diagnostic infusions 90780-90781
   Therapeutic, prophylactic or diagnostic injections 90782-90799
   Vaccines, toxoids 90476-90749
Membrane diffusion capacity 94725
Meningococcal polysaccharide vaccine 90733
Meniscectomy temporomandibular joint 21060
Meprobamate 83805
Mercury 83825
Metanephrines 83835
Metatarsectomy 28140
Methadone 83840

Myocardial perfusion
  imaging 78460-78465
  study 78478-78480
Myocardial resection 33542
Myoglobin 83874
Myomectomy 58140-58145
Myringoplasty 69620
Myringotomy 69420-69421

N

Narcosynthesis psychiatric diagnostic and therapeutic purposes 90865
Nasal endoscopy 31231
Nasal function studies 92512
Nasal sinus endoscopy 31233-31294
Nasal smear eosinophils 89190
Nasopharyngoscopy 92511
Necropsy (autopsy) 88000-88045
Needle biopsy intrathoracic lesion 71036
Needle electromyography studies (emg) anal or urethral sphincter 51785
Needle oculoelectromyography 92265
Neonatal intensive care
    initial 99295
    subsequent 99296-99298
Nephelometry 83883
Nephrectomy 50220-50240
Nephrolithotomy 50060-50075
Nephrorrhaphy 50500
Nephrostolithotomy, percutaneous 50080-50081
Nephrostomy 50040
Nephrotomy 50045
Nerve conduction study 95900-95904
Nerve graft
    additional nerve 64901-64902
    arm or leg 64892-64897, 64898
    hand or foot 64891-64896
    pedicle transfer 64905-64907
Nerve teasing preparations 88362
NERVOUS SYSTEM SURGICAL PROCEDURES 61000-64999
Neuraxial analgesia/anesthesia labor 01967-01969
Neurectomy
    hamstring muscle 27315
    intrinsic musculature foot 28030
    popliteal 27320
Neurobehavioral status exam 96115
Neurological system examination, documentation *142*

NEUROLOGY AND NEUROMUSCULAR MEDICAL PROCEDURES
95805-95999

O

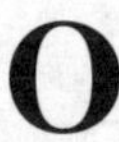

Obliteration
    aortopulmonary septal defect 33813-33814
    arteriovenous malformation 61613
    carotid aneurysm 61613
    carotid-cavernous fistula 61613
Observation care
    discharge day management 99217
    initial 99218-99220
Observation or inpatient hospital care 99234-99236
Occlusion fallopian tube(s) by device 58615
Occupational therapy evaluation 97003
Occupational therapy re-evaluation 97004
Ocular prosthesis 92330
OFFICE SERVICES 99201-99215
Office services provided on an emergency basis 99058
Office visit
    established patient 99211-99215
    new patient 99201-99205
Oligoclonal immunoglobulin 83916
Omental flap 49905
Omentectomy epiploectomy, resection omentum 49255
OMT 98925
Oocyte identification from follicular fluid 89254
Oophorectomy 58940-58943
Open closure major bronchial fistula 32815
Operating microscope 69990
Operculectomy 41821
Ophthalmic biometry 76516-76519
Ophthalmic mucous membrane tests 95060
Ophthalmic ultrasonic foreign body localization 76529
Ophthalmic ultrasound 76511-76513
Ophthalmodynamometry 92260
Ophthalmology examination general anesthesia 92018-92019
OPHTHALMOLOGY MEDICAL SERVICES 92002-92499
Ophthalmoscopy 92225-92226
Opiates 83925
Opponensplasty
    hypothenar muscle transfer 26494
    other methods 26496
    superficialis tendon transfer type 26490
    tendon transfer with graft 26492
Optic nerve decompression 67570
Optokinetic nystagmus 92534
Optokinetic nystagmus test 92544

OPV (oral polio virus) 90712
Orbicularis oculi (blink) reflex 95933
Orbital implant insertion 67550
Orbital implant removal or revision 67560
Orbital repositioning, periorbital osteotomies 21267-21268
Orbitocranial approach to anterior cranial fossa 61584-61585
Orbitocranial zygomatic approach to middle cranial fossa 61592
Orbitotomy
    with bone flap or window 67420-67450
    without bone flap 67400-67414
Orchiectomy 54520-54535
Orchiopexy 54640-54650
ORGAN OR DISEASE ORIENTED PANELS 80048-80090
Organic acids 83918-83919
Orthopantogram 70355
Orthoptic pleoptic training 92065
Orthotics fitting and training 97504
Oscillating tracking test 92545
Osmolality 83930-83935
Osmotic fragility, rbc 85555-85557
Ostectomy
    calcaneus 28118-28119
    metatarsal head 28288
    metatarsal head, complete excision 28111-28113
    metatarsal head, partial excision 28110
    metatarsal heads, complete excision (eg, Clayton type procedure) 28114
    scapula 23190
    sternum 21620
    tarsal coalition excision 28116
Osteocalcin 83937
OSTEOPATHIC MANIPULATIVE TREATMENT (OMT) 98925-98929
Osteoplasty
    facial bones 21208-21209
    femur 27465-27468
    humerus 24420
    metacarpal or phalanx 26568
    radius and ulna, lengthening 25393
    radius and ulna, shortening 25392
    radius or ulna, lengthening 25391
    radius or ulna, shortening 25390
    tibia and fibula, lengthening or shortening 27715
Osteotomies
    humeral shaft, multiple 24410
    radius and ulna, multiple 25370-25375
Osteotomy
    calcaneus (eg, Dwyer or Chambers type procedure) 28300
    clavicle 23480-23485

Osteotomy *(continued)*
    femur neck 27161
    femur shaft or supracondylar 27448-27450
    fibula 27707
    humerus 24400
    iliac acetabular or innominate bone 27146-27156
    intertrochanteric or subtrochanteric 27165
    mandible 21198
    maxilla 21206
    metacarpal 26565
    metatarsal 28306-28308
    metatarsal (eg, Swanson type cavus foot procedure) 28309
    multiple (eg, Sofield type procedure) 27712
    multiple femoral shaft (eg, Sofield type procedure) 27454
    other phalanges 28312
    pelvis bilateral 27158
    phalanx finger 26567
    proximal phalanx 28310
    proximal tibia 27455-27457
    radius 25350-25355
    radius and ulna 25365
    spine anterior 22220-22226
    spine posterior or posterolateral 22210-22216
    talus 28302
    tarsal bones 28304-28305
    tarsal bones, fowler type 28305
    tibia 27705
    tibia and fibula 27709
    transfer greater trochanter 27140
    ulna 25360
Otolaryngologic examination under general anesthesia 92502
Otoplasty protruding ear 69300
OTORHINOLARYNGOLOGIC MEDICAL SERVICES 92502-92599
Outflow tract augmentation 33478
Ova and parasites, smears, concentration and identification 87177
Ovarian cystectomy 58925
Ovulation tests, by visual color comparison methods 84830
Oxalate 83945
Oxygen uptake, expired gas analysis 94680-94690

P

Palatopharyngoplasty 42145
Palatoplasty cleft palate 42200-42225
Pancreatectomy 48140-48160
Pancreaticojejunostomy 48180

Pericardiocentesis 33010-33011
Pericardiotomy 33020
Perineogram 74775
Perineoplasty 56810
Periodontal mucosal grafting 41870
Periorbital osteotomies 21260-21263
Perirectal injection sclerosing solution 45520
Peritoneal-venous shunt patency test 78291
Peritoneocentesis, abdominal paracentesis, or peritoneal lavage 49080-49081
Peritoneogram 74190
Petrous apicectomy 69530
pH body fluid, except blood 83986
Phalangectomy toe 28150
Pharmacologic management 90862
Pharyngectomy 42890
Pharyngoesophageal repair 42953
Pharyngolaryngectomy 31390-31395
Pharyngoplasty 42950
Pharyngostomy 42955
Phencyclidine (PCP) 83992
Phenothiazine 84022
Phenylalanine (PKU), blood 84030
Phenylketones, qualitative 84035
Phlebotomy 99195
Phosphatase 84060-84080
Phosphatidylglycerol 84081
Phosphogluconate, 6-, dehydrogenase, rbc 84085
Phosphohexose isomerase 84087
Phosphorus inorganic 84100-84105
Photo patch test(s) 95052
Photo tests 95056
Photochemotherapy 96910-96912
Photochemotherapy (Goeckerman and/or PUVA) 96913
PHOTODYNAMIC THERAPY 96567-96571
Photopheresis, extracorporeal 36522
PHYSICAL MEDICINE AND REHABILITATION SERVICES 97000-97799
Physical performance test or measurement 97750
Physical therapy evaluation 97001
Physical therapy modality
    contrast baths 97034
    diathermy 97024
    electrical stimulation 97014-97032
    hot or cold packs 97010
    Hubbard tank 97036
    infrared 97026
    iontophoresis 97033
    microwave 97020

Physical therapy modality *(continued)*
    paraffin bath 97018
    traction, mechanical 97012
    ultrasound 97035
    ultraviolet 97028
    vasopneumatic devices 97016
    whirlpool 97022
Physical therapy procedure
    aquatic therapy 97113
    gait training 97116
    massage 97124
    neuromuscular reeducation movement 97112
    therapeutic exercises 97110
Physical therapy re-evaluation 97002
Physician attendance and supervision hyperbaric oxygen therapy 99183
Physician direction emergency medical systems 99288
Physician educational services 99078
Physician services outpatient cardiac rehabilitation 93797-93798
Physician standby service 99360
Physician supervision 99374-99380
Pinch graft 15050
PKU 84030
Placement
    adjustable suture(s) during strabismus surgery 67335
    anal seton 46020
    central venous catheter 36488-36489
    choledochal stent 47801
    drainage catheter, percutaneous 75982
    drains peripancreatic 48000-48001
    IVC filter, percutaneous 75940
    needle intraosseous infusion 36680
Plague vaccine 90727
Plasma radioiron disappearance (turnover) rate 78160
Plasma volume 78110-78111
Plastic repair
    arteriovenous aneurysm 36834
    canaliculi 68700
    cleft lip/nasal deformity 40700-40761
    introitus 56800
    salivary duct, sialodochoplasty 42500-42505
    urethrocele 57230
Platelet 85576-85597
Platelet survival study 78191
Plethysmography total body 93720-93722
Pleural scarification repeat pneumothorax 32215
Pleurectomy parietal 32310
Pneumococcal conjugate vaccine 90669

Pneumococcal polysaccharide vaccine 90732
Pneumonocentesis 32420
Pneumonolysis extraperiosteal 32940
Pneumonostomy 32200-32201
Pneumothorax therapeutic 32960
Poliovirus vaccine (OPV) 90712
Poliovirus vaccine, inactivated, (IPV) 90713
Pollicization digit 26550
Polysomnography 95808-95811
Pooling platelets 86965
Porphobilinogen 84106-84110
Porphyrins 84119-84127
Portoenterostomy (eg, Kasai procedure) 47701
Positional nystagmus 92532
Posterior colporrhaphy 57250
Postoperative biliary duct stone removal 74327
Postoperative follow-up visit 99024
Postpartum care 59430
Potassium 84132-84133
Potts-Smith operation (shunt descending aorta to pulmonary artery) 33762
Prealbumin 84134
Pregnanediol 84135
Pregnanetriol 84138
Pregnenolone 84140
Preoperative placement needle localization wire breast 19290-76096
Preparation cryopreserved embryos transfer 89256
Preparation embryo transfer 89255
Preparation moulage custom breast implant 19396
Preparation report psychiatric status 90889
Prescription contact lens 92310-92317
Prescription ocular prosthesis 92330-92335
Pretreatment RBCs 86970-86972
Pretreatment serum 86975-86978
PREVENTIVE MEDICINE SERVICES 99381-99440
Preventive medicine counseling
   individual 99401-99404
   individuals group setting 99411-99412
Preventive medicine evaluation, new patient, initial 99381-99387
Preventive medicine periodic reevaluation, established patient 99391-99397
Probing lacrimal canaliculi 68840
Probing nasolacrimal duct 68810-68815
Proctectomy 45110-45123
Proctopexy 45540-45541, 45550
Proctoplasty 45500-45505
Proctosigmoidoscopy 45300-45321
Proetz type procedure (displacement therapy) 30210
Progesterone 84144

Programmed stimulation and pacing 93623
Proinsulin 84206
Prolactin 84146
Prolonged extracorporeal circulation 33960-33961
Prolonged physician service
    inpatient 99356-99357
    office 99354-99355
PROLONGED SERVICES 99354-99359
Prophylactic treatment
    clavicle 23490
    femur 27495
    humeral shaft 24498
    proximal humerus 23491
    radius 25490
    radius and ulna 25492
    tibia 27745
    ulna 25491
Prophylaxis retinal detachment 67141-67145
Prostaglandin 84150
Prostate specific antigen (PSA) 84153-84154
Prostatectomy 55801-55845
Prostatotomy 55720-55725
Prosthesis service aphakia 92358
Prosthetic training 97520
Protein 84155-84165
Protein analysis tissue by western blot 88371-88372
Protein western blot 84181-84182
Prothrombin time 85610-85611
Proton beam delivery 77520-77523
Protoporphyrin, rbc 84202-84203
Provision chemotherapy agent 96545
Provision diagnostic radiopharmaceutical(s) 78990
Provision therapeutic radiopharmaceutical(s) 79900
Provocative testing (eg, Rinkel test) 95078
Provocative tests glaucoma 92140
PSA 84153
Psychiatric diagnostic interview examination 90801-90802
Psychiatric examination, documentation *145*
PSYCHIATRY SERVICES 90801-90899
Psychoanalysis 90845
Psychological testing 96100
Psychophysiological therapy incorporating biofeedback training 90875-90876
Psychotherapy
    individual 90804-90829
    multiple-family group 90849
Pterygomaxillary fossa surgery 31040
PTT 85730

Pulmonary artery embolectomy 33910-33915
Pulmonary compliance study 94750
Pulmonary endarterectomy 33916
PULMONARY MEDICAL SERVICES 94010-94799
Pulmonary perfusion imaging 78580-78588
Pulmonary quantitative differential function 78596
Pulmonary stress testing 94620
Pulmonary ventilation imaging 78586-78594
Pump implantable, refilling and maintenance 96530
Pump portable, refilling and maintenance 96520
Punch graft hair transplant 15775-15776
Puncture aspiration
  abscess 10160
  cyst breast 19000-19001
  hydrocele, tunica vaginalis 55000
Puncture shunt tubing or reservoir 61070
Punctures, multiple, anterior cornea 65600
Push transfusion 36440
Putti-platt procedure (capsulorrhaphy, anterior) 23450
Pyeloplasty plastic operation on renal pelvis 50400-50405
Pyelostolithotomy, percutaneous 50080-50081
Pyelotomy 50120-50135
Pyloromyotomy (Fredet-Ramstedt type operation) 43520
Pyloroplasty 43800
Pyridoxal phosphate (vitamin B-6) 84207
Pyruvate 84210
Pyruvate kinase 84220

Q

Quadricepsplasty (eg, Bennett or Thompson type) 27430
QUALIFYING CIRCUMSTANCES FOR ANESTHESIA 99100-99140
Quinine 84228

R

Rabies immune globulin 90375-90376
Rabies vaccine 90675-90676
Radial keratotomy 65771
Radial styloidectomy 25230
Radiation dosimetry calculation 77300
RADIATION ONCOLOGY SERVICES 77261-77799
Radiation therapy management 77431
Radiation treatment delivery 77401-77416

Radiation treatment management 77427
Radical abdominal hysterectomy 58210
Radical excision
    bursa, synovia wrist, or forearm tendon sheaths 25115-25116
    lesion, external auditory canal 69150-69155
Radical resection
    bone tumor, proximal humerus 23220-23222
    capsule, elbow 24149
    metacarpal 26250-26255
    phalanx finger 26260-26262
    sternum 21630-21632
    tonsil 42842-42845
    tumor, acetabulum, pubic rami, or ischium and acetabulum 27076
    tumor, bone 28171-28175
    tumor, bone, femur or knee 27365
    tumor, bone, fibula 27646
    tumor, bone, talus or calcaneus 27647
    tumor, bone, tibia 27645
    tumor, clavicle 23200
    tumor, ilium 27075
    tumor, innominate bone, total 27077
    tumor, ischial tuberosity and greater trochanter femur 27078-27079
    tumor, radial head or neck 24152-24153
    tumor, radius or ulna 25170
    tumor, scapula 23210
    tumor, shaft or distal humerus 24150-24151
    tumor, soft tissue, back or flank 21935
    tumor, soft tissue, face or scalp 21015
    tumor, soft tissue, foot 28046
    tumor, soft tissue, forearm wrist area 25077
    tumor, soft tissue, hand or finger 26117
    tumor, soft tissue, leg or ankle area 27615
    tumor, soft tissue, pelvis and hip area 27049
    tumor, soft tissue, shoulder 23077
    tumor, soft tissue, upper arm or elbow 24077
    tumor, thigh or knee area 27329
    tumor, tissue neck or thorax 21557
Radical trachelectomy 57531
Radioelement supervision, handling, loading 77790
Radiographic absorptiometry (photodensitometry) 76078
Radioiron oral absorption 78162
Radioiron red cell utilization 78170
RADIOLOGY SERVICES *613-660*
    Bilateral procedure codes *614*
    Complete procedures *613*
    Medicare considerations *615*
    Modifiers *614*

Removal *(continued)*
    complete CSF shunt system 62256-62258
    corneal epithelium 65435-65436
    drug implant 11982
    embedded foreign body, eyelid 67938
    entire lumbosubarachnoid shunt system 63746
    epithelial downgrowth, anterior chamber eye 65900
    external fixation system 20694
    fecal impaction or foreign body 45915
    foreign body, deep penile tissue 54115
    foreign body, dentoalveolar structures 41805-41806
    foreign body, esophageal 74235
    foreign body, external auditory canal 69200-69205
    foreign body, external eye 65205-65222
    foreign body, foot 28190-28193
    foreign body, intranasal 30300-30320
    foreign body, intraocular 65235-65265
    foreign body, lacrimal passages 68530
    foreign body, muscle or tendon sheath 20520-20525
    foreign body, orbit 61334
    foreign body, pelvis or hip 27086-27087
    foreign body, pharynx 42809
    foreign body, scrotum 55120
    foreign body, shoulder 23330-23332
    foreign body, thigh region or knee area 27372
    foreign body, upper arm or elbow area 24200-24201
    foreign body, vestibule mouth 40804-40805
    full cast arm or leg 29705
    gauntlet, boot or body cast 29700
    hip prosthesis 27090-27091
    impacted cerumen 69210
    impacted vaginal foreign body 57415
    implant, deep 20680
    implant, non-biodegradeable drug 11982
    implant, finger or hand 26320
    implant, superficial 20670
    implantable contraceptive capsules 11976-11977
    implanted material, anterior segment 65920
    implanted material, posterior segment 67120-67121
    inflatable penile prosthesis 54406, 54410, 54411
    inflatable sphincter 53447
    infusion pump, intra-arterial 36262
    infusion pump, intravenous 36532
    intact mammary implant 19328
    intra-aortic balloon assist device 33968-33974
    intrathecal or epidural catheter 62355
    intrauterine device (IUD) 58301

Removal *(continued)*
    lens material 66840-66940
    lung other than total pneumonectomy 32480-32500
    lung total pneumonectomy 32440-32445
    mammary implant material 19330
    ocular implant 65175
    pacemaker and electrodes 33236-33237
    pacemaker electrode(s) 33234-33235
    pacemaker pulse generator 33233
    pancreatic calculus 48020
    penile prosthesis 54406, 54410, 54411-54417
    perineal prosthesis 53442
    peritoneal foreign body from peritoneal cavity 49085
    peritoneal-venous shunt 49429
    permanent intraperitoneal cannula or catheter 49422
    posterior nonsegmental instrumentation 22850
    posterior segmental instrumentation 22852
    prosthesis knee 27488
    prosthetic rod, hand or finger 26392-26416
    repair electromagnetic bone conduction hearing device 69711
    secondary membranous cataract 66830
    shoulder or hip spica, minerva, or risser jacket, etc. 29710
    skin tags 11201
    subcutaneous reservoir or pump 62365
    subdeltoid calcareous deposits 23000
    sutures under anesthesia 15850-15851
    Thiersch wire or suture, anal canal 46754
    tissue expander(s) 11971
    tongs or halo applied by another physician 20665
    transplanted pancreatic allograft 48556
    transplanted renal allograft 50370
    transvenous electrode(s) 33238
    tumor, temporal bone 69970
    turnbuckle jacket 29715
    venous access device 36535
    ventricular assist device 33977-33978, 33980
    vitreous anterior approach 67005-67010
    wrist prosthesis 25250-25251
Renal allotransplantation
    implantation graft 50360-50365
    reimplantation kidney 50380
Renal biopsy 50200-50205
Renal endoscopy 50551-50580
Renal exploration 50010
Renin 84244
Reopening recent laparotomy 49002

Reoperation
    carotid thromboendarterectomy 35390
    coronary artery bypass procedure or valve procedure 33530
Repair
    achilles tendon 27650-27654
    aneurysm 35001-35162
    ankle disrupted ligament 27695-27698
    anomalous coronary artery 33502-33506
    anomalous venous return 33730
    anterior palate, including vomer flap 42235
    aortic arch 33852-33853
    arteriovenous fistula, extremities 35184-35190
    arteriovenous fistula, head and neck 35180-35188
    arteriovenous fistula, thorax and abdomen 35182-35189
    atrial septal defect 33641
    atrial septal defect and ventricular septal defect 33647
    atrioventricular canal 33660-33670
    bifid digit 26587
    blepharoptosis 67901-67908
    blood vessel, hand, finger 35207
    blood vessel, intra-abdominal 35221-35281
    blood vessel, intrathoracic 35211-35276
    blood vessel, lower extremity 35226-35286
    blood vessel, neck 35201-35261
    blood vessel, upper extremity 35206-35266
    brow ptosis 67900
    cardiac wound 33300-33305
    choanal atresia 30540-30545
    cleft hand 26580
    cloacal anomaly 46744-46748
    collateral ligament, metacarpophalangeal or interphalangeal joint 26540
    complex cardiac anomalies 33610-33617
    complex cardiac anomaly 33608
    complex, eyelids, nose, ears, lips 13150-13153
    complex, forehead, cheeks, chin, mouth, neck, axillae, genitalia, hands, feet
        13131-13133
    complex, scalp, arms,, legs 13120-13122
    complex, truck 13101
    complex, trunk 13100-13102
    cor triatriatum or supravalvular mitral ring 33732
    coronary arteriovenous or arteriocardiac chamber fistula 33500-33501
    defect with autograft radius and/or ulna 25425-25426
    diaphragmatic hernia 39520-39541
    dislocating peroneal tendons 27675-27676
    double outlet right ventricle 33611-33612
    dupuytren's contracture 26040
    dural/CSF leak 63707, 63709

Repair *(continued)*
   ectropion 67914-67917
   elbow ligament 24343-24346
   encephalocele, skull vault 62120
   enterocele 57268-57270
   entropion 67921-67924
   epigastric hernia 49570-49572
   extensor tendon, central slip 26426-26428
   extensor tendon, distal insertion 26433-26434
   extensor tendon, finger 26418-26420
   extensor tendon, hand 26410-26412
   extensor tendon, insertion, closed treatment 26432
   extensor tendon, leg 27664-27665
   fascial defect leg 27656
   femur nonunion or malunion distal to head and neck 27470-27472
   finger, volar plate, interphalangeal joint 26548
   fistula, oromaxillary 30580
   fistula, oronasal 30600
   flexor tendon 26350-26358
   flexor tendon, leg 27658-27659
   graft-enteric fistula 35870
   high imperforate anus 46730-46742
   hypospadias, complications 54340-54348
   hypospadias, cripple 54352
   hypospadias, one stage, distal 54322-54328
   hypospadias, one stage, perineal 54336
   hypospadias, one stage, proximal penile or penoscrotal 54332
   inguinal hernia sliding 49525
   initial femoral hernia 49550-49553
   initial incisional or ventral hernia 49560-49561
   initial inguinal hernia 49491-49507
   intrinsic muscles hand 26591
   iris ciliary body 66680
   laceration, conjunctiva 65270-65273
   laceration, cornea 65275
   laceration, cornea sclera 65280-65286
   laceration, diaphragm 39501
   laceration, floor mouth tongue 41250
   laceration, palate 42182
   laceration, tongue 41251
   laceration, tongue floor mouth 41252
   large omphalocele or gastroschisis 49605-49606
   left ventricular outflow tract obstruction 33414
   lip 40650-40654
   low imperforate anus 46715-46716
   lumbar hernia 49540
   lung hernia through chest wall 32800

Repair *(continued)*
  macrodactylia 26590
  meningocele 63700-63702
  metatarsal nonunion or malunion 28322
  myelomeningocele 63704-63706
  nail bed 11760
  nasal septal perforations 30630
  nasolabial fistula 42260
  neonatal diaphragmatic hernia 39503
  non-union, metacarpal or phalanx 26546
  nonunion or malunion, humerus 24430-24435
  nonunion or malunion, radius and ulna 25415-25420
  nonunion or malunion, radius or ulna 25400-25405
  nonunion, scaphoid bone 25440
  omphalocele (Gross type operation) 49610-49611
  oval window fistula 69666
  paraesophageal hiatus hernia 39502
  patent ductus arteriosus 33820-33824
  postinfarction ventricular septal defect 33545
  profundus tendon 26370-26373
  prosthetic valve dysfunction 33496
  pulmonary artery stenosis 33917
  pulmonary atresia 33918-33920
  rectocele 45560
  recurrent femoral hernia 49555-49557
  recurrent incisional or ventral hernia 49565-49566
  recurrent inguinal hernia 49520-49521
  retinal detachment 67101-67112
  round window fistula 69667
  ruptured musculotendinous cuff 23410-23412
  ruptured spleen 38115
  scleral staphyloma 66220-66225
  single transvenous electrode 33218
  single ventricle 33619
  sinus valsalva aneurysm 33720
  sinus valsalva fistula 33702-33710
  small omphalocele 49600
  spectacles 92370-92371
  spica body cast or jacket 29720
  spigelian hernia 49590
  superficial wounds face, ears, eyelids, nose, lips mucous membranes
      12011-12018
  superficial wounds scalp, neck, axillae, external genitalia, trunk, extremities
      12001-12007
  symblepharon 68330-68340
  syndactyly 26560-26562
  tarsal bones, nonunion or malunion 28320

Resection *(continued)*
    lateral pharyngeal wall or pyriform sinus 42892
    lesion, base anterior cranial fossa 61600-61601
    lesion, infratemporal fossa, parapharyngeal space, petrous apex
        61605-61606
    lesion, parasellar area, cavernous sinus, clivus or midline skull base
        61607-61608
    lip 40530
    lung 32520-32525
    ovarian malignancy 58950-58952
    palate 42120
    pancreas and peripancreatic tissue 48005
    phalangeal base 28126
    pharyngeal wall 42894
    ribs extrapleural 32900
    scrotum 55150
    temporal bone 69535
    transplantation long tendon biceps 23440
Respiratory flow volume loop 94375
Respiratory syncytial virus immune globulin (RSV-igim) 90378
Respiratory syncytial virus immune globulin (RSV-igiv) 90379
Respiratory system examination, documentation *148*
RESPIRATORY SYSTEM SURGICAL PROCEDURES 30000-32999
Rest home visit
    established patient 99331-99333
    new patient 99321-99323
Retrobulbar injection alcohol 67505
Retrobulbar injection medication 67500
Revision
    aqueous shunt to extraocular reservoir 66185
    arteriovenous fistula 36832-36833
    arthroplasty wrist joint 25449
    colostomy 44340-44346
    fenestration operation 69840
    gastric restrictive procedure 43848
    gastroduodenal anastomosis 43850-43855
    gastrojejunal anastomosis 43860-43865
    ileostomy 44312-44314
    infusion pump, intra-arterial 36261
    infusion pump, intravenous 36531
    lower extremity arterial bypass 35879-35881
    mastoidectomy 69601-69605
    operative wound, anterior segment 66250
    orbitocraniofacial reconstruction 21275
    peritoneal-venous shunt 49426
    reconstructed breast 19380
    reinsertion transhepatic tube 47530

Revision *(continued)*
    removal, cranial neurostimulator pulse generator or receiver 61888
    removal, implanted spinal neurostimulator pulse generator 63688
    removal, intracranial neurostimulator electrodes 61880
    removal, peripheral neurostimulator electrodes 64585
    removal, peripheral neurostimulator pulse generator 64595
    removal, spinal neurostimulator electrode 63660
    skin pocket 33223
    skin pocket pacemaker 33222
    stapedectomy or stapedotomy 69662
    total hip arthroplasty 27134-27138
    total knee arthroplasty 27486-27487
    tracheostomy scar 31830
    urinary-cutaneous anastomosis 50727-50728
    venous access device 36534
Rheumatoid factor 86430-86431
Rhinectomy 30150-30160
Rhinoplasty
    nasal deformity 30460-30462
    primary 30400-30420
    secondary 30430-30450
Rho(d) immune globulin (rhig) 90384-90385
Rho(d) immune globulin (rhigiv) 90386
Rhythm ECG, one to three leads 93040-93042
Rhytidectomy
    cheek, chin, and neck 15828
    forehead 15824
    glabellar frown lines 15826
    neck 15825
    superficial musculoaponeurotic system (SMAS) flap 15829
Riboflavin (vitamin B-2) 84252
Right heart catheterization 93501
Right heart catheterization, congenital cardiac anomalies 93530
Right ventricular recording 93603
Right ventricular resection 33476
Rinkel test (provocative testing) 95078
Rotavirus vaccine 90680
Routine obstetric care 59400-59618
Routine venipuncture 36415
Rubella and mumps virus vaccine 90709
Rubella virus vaccine 90706
Ruiz-mora type procedure (correction cock-up toe(s)) 28286
Russell viper venom time 85612-85613

S

Sacrospinous ligament fixation 57282
Salabrasion 15810-15811
Salivary gland function study 78232
Salivary gland imaging 78230-78231
Salpingectomy 58700
Salpingo-oophorectomy 58720, 58953-58954
Salpingostomy 58770
Saphenopopliteal vein anastomosis 34530
Scanning computerized ophthalmic diagnostic imaging 92135
Scapulopexy 23400
Schilling test (vitamin B absorption study) 78270
Schlicter test (serum bactericidal titer) 87197
Scleral reinforcement 67250-67255
Scraping cornea, diagnostic 65430
Screening mammography 76092
Screening test, pure tone, air only 92551
Screening test, visual acuity 99173
Scrotal exploration 55110
Scrotoplasty 55175-55180
Secondary closure surgical wound or dehiscence 13160
Secondary repair dura CSF leak 61618-61619
Section recurrent laryngeal nerve 31595
SEDATION WITH OR WITHOUT ANALGESIA 99141-99142
Seddon-Brookes type procedure (tenoplasty, with muscle transfer) 24320
Sedimentation rate 85651-85652
Select picture audiometry 92583
Selenium 84255
Self care/home management training 97535
Selverstone-Crutchfield type procedure (surgery intracranial aneurysm) 61703
Semen analysis 89300-89320
Senning type operation (repair transposition great arteries) 33774
Sensitivity studies, antibiotic 87181-87192
Sensorimotor examination 92060
Sensorineural acuity level test 92575
Septal or other intranasal dermatoplasty 30620
Septoplasty or submucous resection 30520
Sequestrectomy
    clavicle 23170
    forearm, wrist 25145
    humeral head to surgical neck 23174
    olecranon process 24138
    radial head or neck 24136
    scapula 23172
    shaft or distal humerus 24134

Serial tonometry 92100
Serotonin 84260
Serum bactericidal titer (Schlicter test) 87197
Serum screening cytotoxic percent reactive antibody (PRA) 86807-86808
Services provided in location other than physician's office 99056
Services requested after office hours 99050
Services requested between 10:00 pm and 8:00 am 99052
Services requested on sundays and holidays 99054
Sesamoidectomy 28315
Sesamoidectomy thumb or finger 26185
Sever type procedure (capsular contracture release) 23020
Severing adhesions anterior segment eye 65860-65880
Severing tarsorrhaphy 67710
Sex chromatin identification
    Barr bodies 88130
    peripheral blood smear 88140
Sex hormone binding globulin (SHBG) 84270
SGOT 84450
SGPT 84460
Shaving lesion
    face, ears, eyelids, nose, lips, mucous membrane 11310-11313
    scalp, neck, hands, feet, genitalia 11305-11308
    trunk, arms or legs 11302-11303
Short increment sensitivity index (SISI) 92564
Shortening tendon
    extensor, hand or finger 26477
    flexor, hand or finger 26479
Shunt
    ascending aorta to pulmonary artery (Waterston type operation) 33755
    central 33764
    descending aorta to pulmonary artery (Potts-Smith type operation) 33762
    subclavian to pulmonary artery (Blalock-Taussig type operation) 33750
    superior vena cava to pulmonary artery 33766-33767
Shuntogram 75809
Sialic acid 84275
Sialodochoplasty 42500
Sialography 70390
Sialolithotomy 42330-42340
Sickling RBC, reduction 85660
Sigmoidoscopy 45330-45339
Signal-averaged electrocardiography (SAECG) 93278
Silica 84285
Silver type procedure hallux valgus 28290
Simple cystometrogram (CMG) 51725
Simple uroflowmetry (UFR) 51736
Single event recording patient demand 93268
Sinusoidal vertical axis rotational testing 92546

Sinusotomy
   frontal 31070-31087
   maxillary 31020-31032
   sphenoid 31050-31051
   unilateral 31090
Skin end point titration 95027
Skin examination, documentation *151*
Skin test
   candida 86485
   coccidioidomycosis 86490
   histoplasmosis 86510
   tuberculosis 86580-86585
   unlisted antigen 86586
Sleep latency or maintenance wakefulness testing 95805
Sleep study 95806-95807
Sling operation 57288
Slipped femur epiphysis, open treatment 27177-27181
Slipped femur epiphysis treatment 27175-27176
Slitting prepuce 54000-54001
Small intestinal endoscopy, enteroscopy 44360-44378
Smear primary source, with interpretation 87205-87211
Snip incision lacrimal punctum 68440
Sodium serum 84295
Sodium urine 84300
Sofield type procedure
   osteotomy femoral shaft 27454
   osteotomy multiple 27712
Somatomedin 84305
Somatosensory evoked potential study 95925-95927
Somatostatin 84307
Special anterior segment photography 92286-92287
Special dosimetry 77331
Special medical radiation physics consultation 77370
Special reports 99080
SPECIAL SERVICES, PROCEDURES AND REPORTS 99000-99090
Special stains 88312-88314
Special treatment procedure 77470
Specific gravity 84315
Spectacles 92340
Spectrophotometry 84311
Speech evaluation 70371-92506
Speech treatment 92507
Sperm antibodies 89325
Sperm evaluation 89329-89330
Sperm identification 89264
Sperm identification from aspiration 89257
Sperm isolation 89260-89261

Streptokinase, antibody 86590
Stump elongation, upper extremity 24935
Subconjunctival injection 68200
Subcutaneous hormone pellet implantation 11980
Subcutaneous injection filling material 11950-11954
Subdural implantation strip electrodes 61531
Subdural tap 61000-61001
Subluxation radial head in child, closed treatment 24640
Submucous resection turbinate 30140
Subsequent hospital care normal newborn 99433
Subtotal or total hysterectomy after cesarean delivery 59525
Subtraction in conjunction with contrast studies 76350
Sugars 84376-84379
Sugars chromatographic 84375
Sulfate, urine 84392
Supplies and materials provided by physician 99070
Supply contact lenses 92391
Supply low vision aids 92392
Supply ocular prosthesis 92393
Supply permanent prosthesis 92395-92396
Supply spectacles 92390
Supracervical abdominal hysterectomy 58180
Surface application radioelement 77789
SURGERY SERVICES *223-612*
   Add-on codes *228*
   Global surgical package *223*
   Modifiers *226*
   Multiple surgical procedures *224*
   Separate procedure *226*
   Special report *224*
   Starred procedures *228*
   Subsections *226*
   Surgical supplies *229*
SURGERY SERVICES CODES 10000-69999
   Auditory system 69000-69979
   Cardiovascular system 33000-37799
   Digestive system 40490-49999
   Endocrine system 60000-60699
   Eye and ocular adnexa 65091-68899
   Female genital system 56405-58999
   Hemic and lymphatic systems 38100-38999
   Integumentary system 10000-19999
   Intersex surgery 55970-55980
   Male genital system 54000-55899
   Maternity care and delivery 59000-59899
   Mediastinum and diaphragm 39000-39599
   Musculoskeletal system 20000-29999

SURGERY SERVICES CODES *(continued)*
    Nervous system 61000-64999
    Respiratory system 30000-32999
    Urinary system 50010-53899
Surgical closure tracheostomy or fistula 31820-31825
Surgical correction hydraulic abnormality
    inflatable prosthesis 54408
    inflatable sphincter device 53449
SURGICAL PATHOLOGY 88300-88399
Surgical pathology, gross and microscopic examination 88302-88309
Surgical pathology, gross examination only 88300
Surgical preparation or creation recipient site 15000-15001
Surgical treatment
    anal fistula 46270-46285
    ectopic pregnancy 59120-59140
Suture
    abdominal wall evisceration or dehiscence 49900
    additional major peripheral nerve 64859
    additional nerve, hand or foot 64837
    brachial plexus 64861
    digital nerve, hand or foot 64831-64832
    esophageal wound or injury 43410-43415
    extrahepatic biliary duct 47900
    facial nerve 69740-69745
    facial nerve, extracranial 64864
    facial nerve, infratemporal 64865
    infrapatellar tendon 27380-27381
    iris ciliary body 66682
    large intestine 44604-44605
    ligation thoracic duct 38380-38382
    lumbar plexus 64862
    major peripheral nerve, arm or leg 64856-64857
    mesentery 44850
    nerve 64872-64876
    nerve hand or foot 64834-64836
    pharynx wound or injury 42900
    posterior tibial nerve 64840
    quadriceps or hamstring muscle rupture 27385-27386
    recent wound, eyelid 67930-67935
    removal under anesthesia 15850
    repair aorta or great vessels 33320-33322
    sciatic nerve 64858
    small intestine 44602-44603
    testicular injury 54670
    tongue to lip micrognathia (Douglas type procedure) 41510
    tracheal wound or injury 31800-31805
Swallowing function, pharynx, esophagus 74230

Swan-ganz catheter insertion and placement 93503
Swanson type cavus foot procedure (osteotomy, metatarsal) 28309
Sweat collection 89360
Sympathectomy
   cervical 64802
   cervicothoracic 64804
   digital arteries 64820
   lumbar 64818
   radial artery 64821
   superficial palmar arch 64823
   thoracolumbar 64809
   ulnar artery 64822
Symphysiotomy horseshoe kidney 50540
Syndactylization, toes 28280
Synovectomy
   carpometacarpal joint 26130
   interphalangeal joint 26140
   metacarpophalangeal joint 26135
   tendon sheath foot 28086-28088
   tendon sheath radical flexor tendon 26145
   tendon sheath wrist 25118-25119
Synthetic sentence identification test 92576
Syphilis test 86592-86593

T

T3 84480
Talectomy (astragalectomy) 28130
Tattooing 11920-11922
Telephone call by physician 99371-99373
Telephonic transmission electrocardiogram rhythm strip(s) 93012-93014
Teletherapy isodose plan 77305-77315
Temperature gradient studies 93740
Temporary closure eyelids by suture (eg, Frost suture) 67875
Temporary transcutaneous pacing 92953
Temporomandibular joint arthrography 70332
Tendon graft 20924
Tendon lengthening, upper arm or elbow 24305
Tendon sheath incision 26055
Tendon transplantation forearm, wrist 25310-25312
Tenodesis
   biceps tendon 24340
   distal joint 26474
   long tendon biceps 23430
   proximal interphalangeal joint 26471
   wrist 25300-25301

Tenolysis
    complex extensor tendon, finger 26449
    extensor tendon, foot 28225-28226
    extensor tendon, hand or finger 26445
    flexor or extensor tendon, forearm, wrist 25295
    flexor or extensor tendon, leg, ankle 27680-27681
    flexor tendon, foot 28220-28222
    flexor tendon, palm and finger 26442
    flexor tendon, palm or finger 26440
    triceps, 24332
Tenoplasty with muscle transfer 24320
Tenotomy
    abductor hallucis muscle 28240
    abductors, extensor(s) hip, open 27006
    achilles tendon, percutaneous 27605-27606
    adductor hip 27000-27001
    adductor or hamstring, percutaneous 27306-27307
    adductor subcutaneous 27003
    elbow to shoulder, open 24310
    extensor hand or finger, open 26460
    flexor finger, open 26455
    flexor palm, open 26450
    hip flexor(s), open 27005
    open, extensor, foot or toe 28234
    open, flexor or extensor tendon, forearm, wrist 25290
    open, hamstring, knee to hip 27390-27392
    open, tendon flexor, foot 28230
    open, tendon flexor, toe 28232
    percutaneous 26060
    percutaneous, toe 28010-28011
    shoulder area 23405-23406
Tensilon test myasthenia gravis 95857-95858
Testicular imaging 78760-78761
Testing autonomic nervous system function 95921-95923
Testosterone 84402-84403
Tetanus and diphtheria toxoids (TD) 90718
Tetanus immune globulin (TIG) 90389
Tetanus toxoid adsorbed 90703
Thal-nissen procedure (esophagogastric fundoplasty) 43325
Thawing and expansion frozen cells 88241
Therapeutic activities 97530
Therapeutic apheresis 36520-36521
Therapeutic enema 74283
THERAPEUTIC DRUG ASSAYS 80150-80299
THERAPEUTIC OR DIAGNOSTIC INFUSIONS 90780-90781
THERAPEUTIC, PROPHYLACTIC OR DIAGNOSTIC INJECTIONS
    90782-90799

Therapeutic radiology port film(s) 77417
Therapeutic radiology simulation-aided field setting 77280-77295
Therapeutic radiology treatment planning 77261-77263
Thermogram cephalic 93760
Thermogram peripheral 93762
Thiamine (vitamin B-1) 84425
Thiocyanate 84430
Thompson type procedure (quadricepsplasty) 27430
Thoracentesis
    puncture pleural cavity aspiration 32000
    with insertion tube 32002
Thoracic gas volume 94260
Thoracoplasty Schede type or extrapleural 32905-32906
Thoracoscopy
    diagnostic 32601-32606
    surgical 32650-32665
    with open flap drainage 32036
    with rib resection 32035
Thoracotomy
    biopsy lung or pleura 32095
    cardiac massage 32160
    control traumatic hemorrhage, repair lung tear 32110
    cyst(s) removal 32140
    excision-plication bullae 32141
    exploration and biopsy 32100
    open intrapleural pneumonolysis 32124
    postoperative complications 32120
    removal intrapleural foreign body or fibrin deposit 32150
    removal intrapulmonary foreign body 32151
Thrombectomy
    arterial or venous graft 35875-35876
    arteriovenous fistula 36831
    axillary and subclavian vein 34490
    axillary brachial, innominate, subclavian artery 34101
    carotid subclavian or innominate artery 34001
    femoropopliteal, aortoiliac artery 34201
    innominate subclavian artery 34051
    popliteal-tibio-peroneal artery 34203
    radial or ulnar artery 34111
    renal celiac, mesentery, aortoiliac artery 34151
    subclavian vein 34471
    vena cava 34401-34451
Thrombin time plasma 85670
Thrombin time titer 85675
Thromboendarterectomy 35301-35381
Thrombolysis cerebral 37195
Thrombolysis coronary 92975-92977

Thrombomodulin 85337
Thromboplastin inhibition 85705
Thromboplastin time, partial (PTT) 85730-85732
Thymectomy 60520-60522
Thyroglobulin 84432
Thyroglobulin antibody 86800
Thyroid carcinoma metastases imaging 78015-78018
Thyroid carcinoma metastases uptake 78020
Thyroid hormone (T3 or T4) 84479
Thyroid imaging 78006-78011
Thyroid lobectomy
    partial 60210-60212
    total 60220-60225
Thyroid stimulating hormone (TSH) 84443
Thyroid stimulating immunoglobulins (TSI) 84445
Thyroid uptake 78000-78003
Thyroidectomy 60240-60271
Thyrotropin releasing hormone (TRH) stimulation panel 80438
Thyroxine 84436-84439
Thyroxine binding globulin (TBG) 84442
Tissue ablation
    CAT guidance for 76362
    magnetic resonance guidance for 76394
    ultrasonic guidance for 76490
Tissue culture
    neoplastic disorders 88237-88239
    non-neoplastic disorders 88230-88235
Tissue examination fungi (eg, KOH slide) 87220
Tissue grafts 20926
Tissue in situ hybridization 88365
Tissue transfer
    eyelids, nose, ears, lips 14060-14061
    forehead, cheeks, chin, mouth, neck, axillae, genitalia, hands, feet
        14040-14041
    scalp, arms, legs 14020-14021
    trunk 14000-14001
Tocopherol alpha (vitamin E) 84446
Tone decay test 92563
Tonography 92120-92130
Tonsillectomy 42821-42826
Torkildsen type operation (ventriculocisternostomy) 62180
Toupet procedure (laparoscopy esophagogastric fundoplasty) 43280
Toxin or antitoxin assay, tissue culture 87230
Trabeculoplasty by laser surgery 65855
Trabeculotomy ab externo 65850
Tracheal puncture 31612
Trachelectomy 57530

Trachelorrhaphy 57720
Tracheobronchoscopy 31615
Tracheoplasty
    cervical 31750
    intrathoracic 31760
    tracheopharyngeal fistulization 31755
Tracheostoma revision 31613-31614
Tracheostomy
    emergency procedure 31603-31605
    fenestration procedure 31610
    planned 31600-31601
Tracheotomy tube change 31502
Transcatheter biopsy 37200-75970
Transcatheter introduction intravascular stent(s) 75960
Transcatheter occlusion or embolization 37204
    central nervous system 61624
    non-central nervous system 61626
Transcatheter placement
    intracoronary stent(s) 92980-92981
    intravascular stent(s) 37205-37208
    intravascular foreign body 37203
    intravascular foreign body, percutaneous 75961
Transcatheter therapy 37201-75896
Transcervical catheterization fallopian tube 74742
Transcervical introduction fallopian tube catheter 58345
Transcochlear approach to posterior cranial fossa 61596
Transcondylar lateral) approach to posterior cranial fossa 61597
Transcortin (cortisol binding globulin) 84449
Transcranial doppler study the intracranial arteries 93886-93888
Transduodenal sphincterotomy or sphincteroplasty 47460
Transection
    carotid artery in cavernous sinus 61609-61610
    carotid artery in petrous canal 61611-61612
    esophagus with repair 43401
    facial nerve 64742
    greater occipital nerve 64744
    inferior alveolar nerve 64738
    infraorbital nerve 64734
    lingual nerve 64740
    mental nerve 64736
    obturator nerve 64763-64766
    other cranial nerve 64771
    other spinal nerve 64772
    phrenic nerve 64746
    pudendal nerve 64761
    pulmonary artery 33922
    repositioning aberrant renal vessels 50100

Transection *(continued)*
    supraorbital nerve 64732
    vagi 64755
    vagus nerve abdominal 64760
    vagus nerve transthoracic 64752
Transesophageal echocardiography 93315-93317
Transfer
    adductor to ischium 27098
    external oblique muscle to greater trochanter 27100
    finger to another position 26555
    free toe joint 26556
    iliopsoas to femoral neck 27111
    iliopsoas to greater trochanter 27110
    paraspinal muscle to hip 27105
    pedicle flap 15650
    tendon, hand 26480-26483
    tendon, muscle, hamstrings to femur (eg, Egger's type procedure) 27400
    tendon, palmar 26485-26489
    tendon, to restore intrinsic function 26497-26498
    toe-to-hand 26551-26554
    transplant tendon 27690-27692
Transferase alanine amino (ALT) (SGPT) 84460
Transferase aspartate amino (AST) (SGOT) 84450
Transferrin 84466
Transfusion blood or blood components 36430
Transfusion intrauterine, fetal 36460
TRANSFUSION MEDICINE 86850-86999
Transhepatic portography, percutaneous 75885-75887
Transluminal atherectomy 75992-75995
Transluminal balloon angioplasty 35450-75978
Transluminal peripheral atherectomy 35480-35495
Transmastoid antrotomy 69501
Transmetacarpal amputation 25927-25931
Transmyocardial laser revascularization 33140
Transperineal placement needles or catheters into prostate 55859
Transpetrosal approach to posterior cranial fossa 61598
Transplant hamstring tendon to patella 27396-27397
Transplantation
    pancreatic allograft 48554
    testis(es) to thigh 54680
Transport, patient 99289-99290
Transposition
    ovary(s) 58825
    procedure 67320

Transposition, reimplantation
    carotid to subclavian artery 35695
    subclavian to carotid artery 35694
    vertebral to carotid artery 35691
    vertebral to subclavian artery 35693
Transrectal drainage pelvic abscess 45000
Transtemporal approach to posterior cranial fossa 61595
Transthoracic echocardiography 93303-93304
Transtracheal injection bronchography 31715
Transtracheal introduction needle wire dilator/stent 31730
Transureteroureterostomy 50770
Transurethral balloon dilation prostatic urethra 52510
Transurethral destruction prostate tissue 53850-53852
Transurethral drainage prostatic abscess 52700
Transurethral electrosurgical resection prostate 52601
Transurethral fulguration postoperative bleeding 52606
Transurethral incision prostate 52450
Transurethral resection
    bladder neck 52500
    postoperative bladder neck contracture 52640
    prostate 52612-52614
    regrowth obstructive tissue 52630
    residual obstructive tissue 52620
Transverse arch graft 33870
Transvesical ureterolithotomy 51060
Treatment devices design and construction 77332-77334
Treatment
    first degree burn 16000
    incomplete abortion 59812
    missed abortion 59820-59821
    septic abortion 59830
    speech 92507-92508
    superficial wound dehiscence 12020-12021
    swallowing dysfunction 92526
Tricuspid valve repositioning 33468
Triglycerides 84478
Triiodothyronine t3 84480-84482
Trimming nondystrophic nails 11719
Troponin 84484-84512
Trypsin 84485-84490
TSH 84443
Tube or needle catheter jejunostomy 44015
Tube pericardiostomy 33015
Tube thoracostomy 32020
Tubotubal anastomosis 58750
Tubouterine implantation 58752
Tumor imaging, positron emission tomography (PET) 78810

Tympanic membrane repair 69610
Tympanic neurectomy 69676
Tympanolysis, transcanal 69450
Tympanometry (impedance testing) 92567
Tympanoplasty
    antrotomy or mastoidotomy 69635-69637
    mastoidectomy 69641-69633
Tympanostomy 69433-69436
Typhoid vaccine 90690-90693
Tyrosine 84510

U

U-tube hepaticoenterostomy 47802
Ultrasonic guidance
    amniocentesis 76946
    aspiration ova 76948
    chorionic villus sampling 76945
    compression repair arterial pseudo-aneurysm/arteriovenous fistulae 76936
    cyst or renal pelvis aspiration 76938
    endomyocardial biopsy 76932
    interstitial radioelement application 76965
    intrauterine fetal transfusion or cordocentesis 76941
    needle biopsy 76942
    pericardiocentesis 76930
    placement radiation therapy fields 76960
    thoracentesis or abdominal paracentesis 76934
    tissue ablation 76490
Ultrasound bone density measurement and interpretation 76977
Ultrasound intravascular 92978
Ultrasound ophthalmic 76511
Ultrasound study follow-up 76970
Umbilectomy omphalectomy, excision umbilicus 49250
Unlisted cytogenetic study 88299
Unlisted hysteroscopy procedure, uterus 58579
Unlisted immune globulin 90399
Unlisted laparoscopy procedure
    abdomen, peritoneum and omentum 49329
    appendix 44979
    endocrine system 60659
    hernioplasty, herniorrhaphy, herniotomy 49659
    maternity care and delivery 59898
    oviduct, ovary 58679
    renal 50549
    spermatic cord 55559

Unlisted laparoscopy procedure *(continued)*
    testis 54699
    uterus 58578
Unlisted miscellaneous pathology test 89399
Unlisted procedure
    abdomen, musculoskeletal system 22999
    abdomen, peritoneum and omentum 49999
    accessory sinuses 31299
    allergy/clinical immunologic service 95199
    anesthesia 01999
    anterior segment eye 66999
    anus 46999
    arthroscopy 29999
    biliary tract 47999
    breast 19499
    cardiac surgery 33999
    casting or strapping 29799
    chemistry 84999
    chemotherapy 96549
    clinical brachytherapy 77799
    conjunctiva 68399
    craniofacial and maxillofacial 21299
    cytopathology 88199
    dentoalveolar structures 41899
    diagnostic gastroenterology 91299
    diagnostic nuclear medicine, cardiovascular 78499
    diagnostic nuclear medicine, endocrine 78099
    diagnostic nuclear medicine, gastrointestinal 78299
    diagnostic nuclear medicine, genitourinary 78799
    diagnostic nuclear medicine, miscellaneous 78999
    diagnostic nuclear medicine, musculoskeletal 78399
    diagnostic nuclear medicine, nervous system 78699
    diagnostic nuclear medicine, respiratory 78599
    diagnostic x-ray 76499
    dialysis 90999
    diaphragm 39599
    endocrine system 60699
    esophagus 43499
    external ear 69399
    eyelids 67999
    female genital system 58999
    femur or knee 27599
    foot or toes 28899
    forearm or wrist 25999
    hands or fingers 26989
    hematology and coagulation 85999
    hemic or lymphatic system 38999

Unlisted procedure *(continued)*
    humerus or elbow 24999
    immunology 86849
    inner ear 69949
    intestine 44799
    lacrimal system 68899
    laparoscopy, biliary tract 47579
    laparoscopy, esophagus 43289
    laparoscopy, intestine (except rectum) 44209
    laparoscopy, lymphatic system 38589
    laparoscopy, spleen 38129
    laparoscopy, stomach 43659
    larynx 31599
    leg or ankle 27899
    lips 40799
    liver 47399
    lungs and pleura 32999
    male genital system 55899
    maternity care and delivery 59899
    maxillofacial prosthetics 21089
    Meckel's diverticulum and the mesentery 44899
    mediastinum 39499
    medical radiation physics 77399
    microbiology 87999
    middle ear 69799
    musculoskeletal system, head 21499
    musculoskeletal system, general 20999
    neck or thorax 21899
    necropsy (autopsy) 88099
    nervous system 64999
    neurological or neuromuscular diagnostic 95999
    nose 30999
    ocular muscle 67399
    orbit 67599
    otorhinolaryngology 92599
    palate, uvula 42299
    pancreas 48999
    pelvis or hip joint 27299
    pharynx, adenoids, or tonsils 42999
    physical therapy 97139
    physical therapy modality 97039
    posterior segment 67299
    pressure ulcer 15999
    radiopharmaceutical therapeutic 79999
    rectum 45999
    salivary glands or ducts 42699
    shoulder 23929

Unlisted procedure *(continued)*
    skin, mucous membrane and subcutaneous tissue 17999
    spine 22899
    stomach 43999
    surgical pathology 88399
    temporal bone, middle fossa approach 69979
    therapeutic radiology, clinical treatment planning 77299
    therapeutic radiology, treatment management 77499
    tongue, floor mouth 41599
    trachea bronchi 31899
    transfusion medicine 86999
    ultrasound 76999
    urinalysis 81099
    urinary system 53899
    vascular injection 36299
    vascular surgery 37799
    vestibule mouth 40899
Unlisted service
    cardiovascular 93799
    dermatology 96999
    evaluation and management 99499
    ophthalmology 92499
    physical medicine/rehabilitation 97799
    preventive medicine 99429
    psychiatric 90899
    pulmonary 94799
Unlisted special service procedure or report 99199
Unlisted therapeutic prophylactic or diagnostic injection 90799
Unlisted vaccine/toxoid 90749
Unusual travel 99082
Upgrade pacemaker system 33214
Upper gastrointestinal endoscopy 43234-43259
Urea breath test 78267-78268
Urea nitrogen 84520-84545
Ureteral endoscopy 50951-50980
Ureteral reflux study 78740
Ureterectomy 50650-50660
Ureterocalycostomy 50750
Ureterocolon conduit 50815
Ureteroenterostomy 50800
Ureteroileal conduit 50820
Ureterolithotomy 50610-50630
Ureterolysis 50715-50725
Ureteroneocystostomy 50780-50785
Ureteroplasty 50700
Ureteropyelostomy 50740
Ureterorrhaphy 50900

Ureterosigmoidostomy 50810
Ureterostomy 50860
Ureterotomy 50600-50605
Ureteroureterostomy 50760
Urethral pressure profile studies (UPP) 51772
Urethrectomy 53210-53215
Urethrocystography 74450-74455
Urethromeatoplasty 53450-53460
Urethroplasty 53400-54318
Urethrorrhaphy 53502-53515
Urethrotomy or urethrostomy 53000-53010
Uric acid 84550-84560
URINALYSIS 81000-81020
Urinary bladder residual study 78730
URINARY SYSTEM SURGICAL PROCEDURES 50010-53899
Urinary undiversion 50830
Urine pregnancy test 81025
Urobilinogen 84577-84583
Uroflowmetry complex 51741
Urography 74400-74425
Use vertical electrodes 92547
Uterine evacuation and curettage hydatidiform mole 59870
Uterine suspension 58400-58410
Uvulectomy 42140

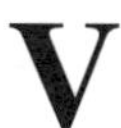

Vaccinia immune globulin 90393
VACCINES, TOXOIDS 90476-90749
Vaginal delivery only 59409-59614
Vaginal hysterectomy 58260-58285
Vaginectomy 57106-57112
Vaginoplasty intersex state 57335
Vagotomy
    partial, distal gastrectomy 43635
    pyloroplasty 43640-43641
Valvectomy tricuspid valve 33460
Valvotomy
    mitral valve 33420-33422
    pulmonary valve 33470-33474
Valvuloplasty
    aortic valve 33400-33403
    balloon, percutaneous 92986-92990
    femoral vein 34501
    mitral valve 33425-33427
    tricuspid valve 33463-33464

Vanillylmandelic acid (VMA), urine 84585
Varicella virus vaccine 90716
Varicella-zoster immune globulin 90396
Vasectomy 55250
    anesthesia for, 00851
Vasoactive intestinal peptide (VIP) 84586
Vasography vesiculography, or epididymography 74440
Vasopressin (ADH) 84588
Vasotomy 55200-55300
Vasovasostomy vasovasorrhaphy 55400
Vein graft cross-over to venous system 34520
Venipuncture 36400-36410
Venipuncture cutdown 36420-36425
Venography
    adrenal 75840-75842
    caval 75825-75827
    epidural 75872
    extremity 75820-75822
    orbital 75880
    renal 75831-75833
    sinus or jugular 75860
    superior sagittal sinus 75870
Venous anastomosis
    caval-mesenteric 37160
    portocaval 37140
    renoportal 37145
    splenorenal distal 37181
    splenorenal proximal 37180
Venous catheterization selective organ blood sampling 36500
Venous sampling through catheter 75893
Venous thrombosis imaging 78457-78458
Venous thrombosis study 78455
Venous valve transposition 34510
Ventilating tube removal 69424
Ventilation assist and management 94656-94657
Ventricular assist device 33975-33980
Ventricular puncture 61020-61026
Ventriculocisternostomy 62180, 62200-62201
Ventriculomyotomy 33416
Vermilionectomy (lip shave) 40500
Vertebral corpectomy 63081-63308
Very long chain fatty acids 82726
Vesiculectomy 55650
Vesiculotomy 55600-55605
Vestibular nerve section 69915-69950
Vestibuloplasty 40840-40845
Virus identification 87250-87253

Viscosity 85810
Visual evoked potential (VEP) testing 95930
Visual field examination 92081-92083
Visual reinforcement audiometry (VRA) 92579
Vital capacity 94150
Vitamin absorption studies combined 78272
Vitamin absorption study (eg, Schilling test) 78270-78271
Vitamin A 84590
Vitamin C 82180
Vitamin K 84597
Vitrectomy 67036-67040
Voiding pressure studies (VP) 51795-51797
Volatiles 84600
Volkmann contracture 25316
Volume measurement timed collection 81050
Vulvectomy 56620-56640

W

Wada activation test hemispheric function 95958
Walldius type procedure (arthroplasty, knee) 27445
Water load test 89365
Waterston type operation (shunt ascending aorta to pulmonary artery) 33755
WBC 85048
Wedge excision skin nail fold 11765
Wedge resection or bisection ovary 58920
Wedging cast 29740
Wedging clubfoot cast 29750
Wheelchair management/propulsion training 97542
Whole blood volume determination 78122
Wilke type procedure (parotid duct diversion) 42509
Windowing cast 29730
Work hardening/conditioning 97545-97546
Work related or medical disability examination 99455-99456

XYZ

X-ray examination
    abdomen 74000-74022
    abscess, fistula or sinus tract study 76080
    acromioclavicular joints 73050
    ankle 73600-73615
    calcaneus 73650
    chest 71010-71035